Basic Physical Pharmacy

Joseph K. H. Ma, PhD
Professor Emeritus
School of Pharmacy, West Virginia University
Morgantown, West Virginia

Boka W. Hadzija, PhD
Professor Emeritus
Eshelman School of Pharmacy
University of North Carolina-Chapel Hill
Chapel Hill, North Carolina

JONES & BARTLETT
LEARNING

World Headquarters
Jones & Bartlett Learning
5 Wall Street
Burlington, MA 01803
978-443-5000
info@jblearning.com
www.jblearning.com

Jones & Bartlett Learning books and products are available through most bookstores and online booksellers. To contact Jones & Bartlett Learning directly, call 800-832-0034, fax 978-443-8000, or visit our website, www.jblearning.com.

Substantial discounts on bulk quantities of Jones & Bartlett Learning publications are available to corporations, professional associations, and other qualified organizations. For details and specific discount information, contact the special sales department at Jones & Bartlett Learning via the above contact information or send an email to specialsales@jblearning.com.

Production Credits
Publisher: William Brottmiller
Acquisitions Editor: Katey Birtcher
Associate Editor: Teresa Reilly
Associate Production Editor: Jill Morton
Marketing Manager: Grace Richards
Composition: Laserwords Private Limited, Chennai, India
Cover Design: Scott Moden
Rights & Photo Research Associate: Amy Rathburn
Cover Image: Upper right, © 18percentgrey/ShutterStock, Inc.; Lower right, © Chris Hellyar/Fotolia.com; Lower left, © Golden Pixels LLC/ShutterStock, Inc.; Upper left, © Ablestock; Top, © Alfred Bondarenko/Shutterstock, Inc.
Printing and Binding: Edwards Brothers Malloy
Cover Printing: Edwards Brothers Malloy

To order this product, use ISBN: 978-1-4496-5334-7

Library of Congress Cataloging-in-Publication Data
Ma, Joseph K. H.
Basic physical pharmacy / by Joseph K. H. Ma and Boka W. Hadzija.
p. ; cm.
Includes bibliographical references and index.
ISBN 978-0-7637-5734-2 — ISBN 0-7637-5734-9
I. Hadzija, Boka. II. Title.
[DNLM: 1. Chemistry, Pharmaceutical. 2. Physicochemical Phenomena. 3. Technology, Pharmaceutical. QV 744]

615.1'9—dc23

2012010775

6048

Printed in the United States of America
16 15 14 13 12 10 9 8 7 6 5 4 3 2 1

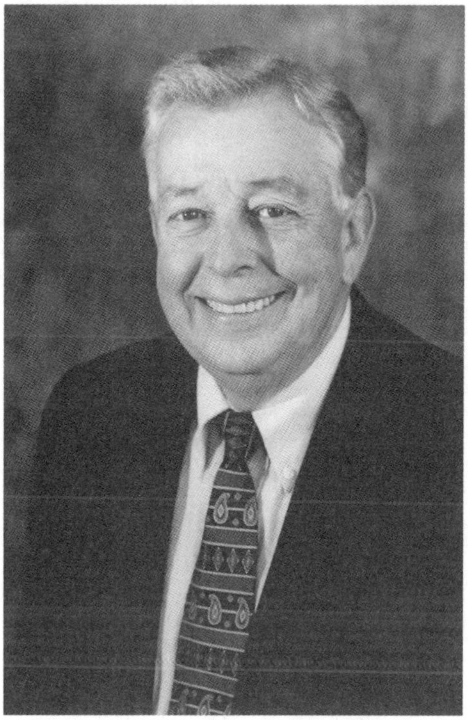

To my friend and mentor
with fond memories.

Louis A. Luzzi (1932–2007)

JKHM

This book is dedicated to my deceased husband,

Professor Arnold Beckett,

who always provided guidance
and useful advice to me.

BWH

CONTENTS

FOREWORD

Physical pharmacy is not only the science upon which the design, manufacturing, and distribution of drug products are based; it also provides the foundation that ensures the stability and proper usage of those products. As such, it is a critical part of all pharmacy curricula.

Basic Physical Pharmacy, by Joseph K. H. Ma, PhD, and Boka W. Hadzija, PhD, provides a comprehensive yet understandable discussion of physical pharmacy and its application in drug formulation and practice. It describes the physicochemical properties of a drug or an excipient, and predicts the bioavailability and its influence on the therapeutic effect of the drug in the body. It also encompasses traditional dosage forms to novel dosage design using nanotechnology. Although current research in targeted drug delivery and product development are very much nanotechnology driven, the fact remains that the traditional drug products are the main revenue generators for the pharmaceutical industry, and ultimately the arena of clinical practice. All relevant subjects are thoroughly discussed and elucidated but in an accessible format that makes it easy for students to comprehend and apply based on their prior knowledge of chemistry.

Until the publication of this book, the availability of comprehensive, understandable physical pharmacy textbooks at the PharmD level was significantly lacking. Most dosage form books deal with pharmaceutical formulation and compounding but do not include in-depth material on physical pharmacy principles.

Joseph K. H. Ma, PhD, has been a faculty member, teacher, and researcher in the West Virginia University School of Pharmacy for 38 years. Dr. Ma is uniquely qualified to shepherd this project, not only because of his academic qualifications—which include a background in physical chemistry and many years of teaching and research—but also thanks to his superior and precise attention to detail and his high level of commitment to the education of tomorrow's pharmacists.

Dr. Ma is nationally recognized, has published extensively, and has mentored countless students over the years. He began his academic career by earning a PhD in physical chemistry from Duquesne University and completed his postdoctoral training in biopharmaceutics at the University of Georgia. He has conducted extensive research in drug formulation and delivery, pulmonary disease, and nanoparticle toxicity, garnering significant federal funding for his research. Having attained emeritus status, he continues to contribute to the future of pharmaceutical sciences through this very important work.

The respect with which Dr. Ma is held in the profession is evident in the distinguished contributors he recruited to provide knowledgeable and helpful contributions to the text, ensuring that all aspects of the subject are well covered. Contributors include another highly respected member of the WVU pharmacy faculty, Yon Rojanasakul, PhD, who authored the chapter on transdermal drug delivery with researcher Sudjit Luanpitpong. Dr. Hing Char and WVU pharmacy graduates and researchers Hae-Young Ahn, PhD; Neelam Azad, PhD; Anand Iyer, PhD; Aniruddha Railkar, PhD; and Jun (Joseph) Shao, PhD also contributed to writing this book. Taken together, the authors of and contributors to this textbook represent an impressive collection of fine pharmaceutical scientists and educators.

As dean of the WVU School of Pharmacy, the publication of this book makes me particularly proud, as it represents the accomplishment of so many colleagues who are or have been affiliated with WVU. It is a point of pride for our school, and I have no doubt that it will make a lasting contribution to our profession for many years to come.

Patricia A. Chase, PhD
Dean, School of Pharmacy
West Virginia University

PREFACE

This book is about learning basic physical pharmacy, the science upon which successful drug formulations are based. A drug cannot be administered to a patient until it is put into a dosage form that ensures the stability of the drug product, minimizes the potential drug toxicity, and is therapeutically effective. Such a dosage form design, however, cannot be achieved without a sound scientific base through which the drug product can be manufactured and evaluated. As the pharmaceutical manufacturers bear the burden in providing safe and efficacious products, it is incumbent upon the pharmacist, who is given the responsibility to care for patients and dispense these products, to understand the scientific basis for which the products are made and ensure that the intended use of a product is achieved. This emphasis on scientific understanding requires that the principles used in product development be thoroughly examined. The term *basic* in the book title indicates a comprehensive approach for the presentation of theories and principles to eliminate potential misuse or misunderstanding of the subject matter. It also indicates a simplified approach so that the subject matter can be easily understood.

Basic Physical Pharmacy consists of four major sections: physical pharmacy in solutions, solid dosage forms, polyphasic systems, and drug delivery and novel drug delivery systems. Appropriate physicochemical principles and their use in dosage form development are described in successive chapters in each major section, which allows the topic of each section to be taught as a learning module. Modern pharmaceutics is built on the foundation of chemistry. Students who have already learned general and organic chemistry before entering pharmacy education will begin to discover how chemical theories are put to use in the development of pharmaceutical dosage forms. Being a subject that is closely related to the student's chemistry background, physical pharmacy in solutions is presented as Part I of this book. This also allows the student to gain a comprehensive view on how drug dosage forms are transformed *in vivo* into therapeutic agents as they study the various dosage forms presented in Parts II and III. Drug delivery, based on route of administration and appropriate dosage form designs, is a subject that requires an integrated knowledge from multiple scientific disciplines. This subject is no more complicated than any other subjects in the book, but it demonstrated the ingenuity of scientists who apply multidisciplinary knowledge to solve a drug delivery problem, which is the hallmark of current pharmaceutical research. This subject is presented as the last module to discuss the trend of current pharmaceutical development as well as to promote the student's appreciation and interest in pursuing creative research.

It is perhaps worthy to note that equations, when properly described, are very effective in representing physicochemical theories, as they always produce a definitive answer. This book provides homework problems for this exercise, which are not designed to be difficult but to reinforce the understanding of the described physical pharmacy phenomena. Despite the emphasis on physicochemical principles, this book is written based on their application to pharmaceutical preparations.

I would like to acknowledge Dr. Boka Hadzija for initiating this project and her contributions to the chapter content. Most gratefully, I thank Drs. Hae-Young Ahn, Ani Railkar, Jun Shao, Hing Char, Sudjit Luanpitpong, Anand Iyer, Neelam Azad, and my colleague and friend Yon Rojanasakul for contributing in writing seven chapters of this book. They provided expertise gained not only from their industrial training, work experience, or research but also from their teaching experiences in the subject matter. My special thanks go to the School of Pharmacy, West Virginia University, where I have worked as a faculty member for 38 years. For a glimpse of this fine institution, I present to the readers a photograph of the school's Cook-Hayman Pharmacy Museum, where on display is a changing view of pharmacy practice from extemporaneous preparations to novel dosage forms with the passage of time.

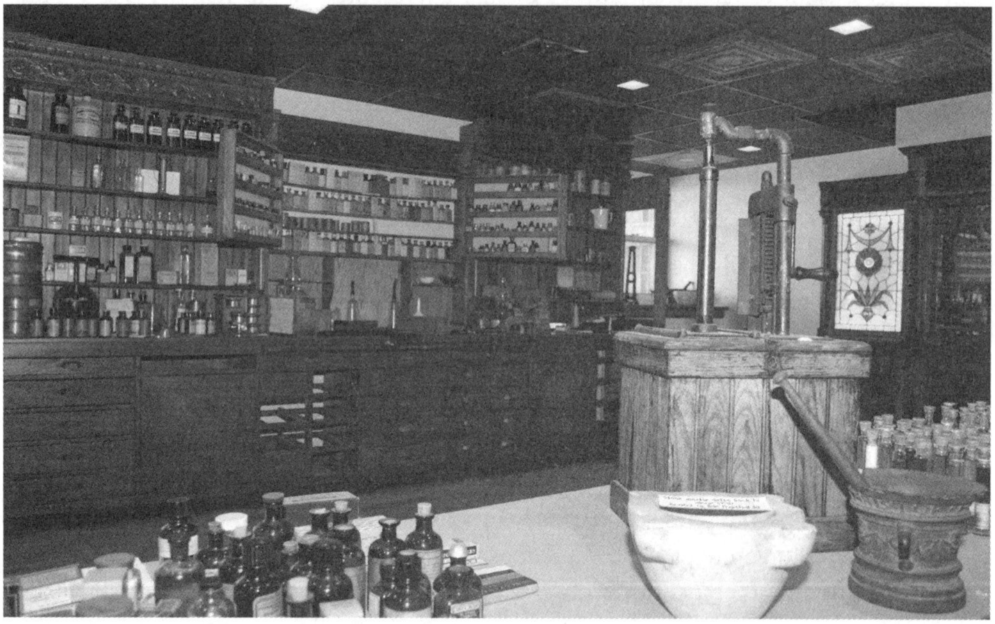

Source: Photo courtesy of the Cook-Hayman Pharmacy Museum of West Virginia University.

I would like to pay a special tribute to my mentor Dr. Louis A. Luzzi, from whom I learned the diverse fields of pharmaceutical sciences. Dr. Luzzi was a formulation scientist and a pioneer in the studies of drug–protein binding and microencapsulation. With even greater achievement, he was a remarkable leader in pharmacy education and served as the Dean of West Virginia University School of Pharmacy and Dean of the College of Pharmacy, University of Rhode Island. With great admiration and fond memories, I dedicate this book to him for his contributions to pharmacy and for being a dear friend to me and my family.

I owe my deepest gratitude to Dr. Carl J. Malanga, a long-time colleague and friend at West Virginia University who taught me how to teach. Dr. Malanga had a long illustrious career as a caring teacher and pharmacy educator. He gave me many thoughtful suggestions on how to write this book, even during the final days of his glorious life.

I thank Dr. Frank D. O'Connell for reading and discussing the content of the book and his critiques on many of the book chapters. Dr. O'Connell's knowledge on the traditional pharmaceutical preparations has helped me in shaping the book content and format.

It is with great gratitude that I thank my wife, Jane, for her understanding and support of me when I was writing this book. As a physical chemist, she constantly reminded me to ensure that the equations used in this book are accurately presented and verified. Indeed, one cannot use an equation with confidence without knowing its accuracy and scientific base. Although I tried to minimize the use of equations and complex mathematical models, this book strives to provide a comprehensive view of the theories so that the equations used are accurately presented and easily understood. Last, but not least, I am pleased to mention my children, Kathy and Kevin, who have given me much support and encouragement. They often came into my thoughts when I worked, as if they were the pharmacy students. I asked as I was formulating a thought: would they be able to learn from this book? In many ways, I wrote this book for them and for students who are excited to enter the pharmacy field.

CONTRIBUTORS

Hae-Young Ahn, PhD
Deputy Director
FDA Office of Clinical Pharmacology
Division of Clinical Pharmacology III
Silver Spring, MD

Hae-Young Ahn is a division deputy director in the Office of Clinical Pharmacology, Center for Drug Evaluation and Research (CDER), Food and Drug Administration (FDA). She has been with the FDA over 20 years and is an expert on clinical pharmacology and biopharmaceutics. She has participated in many coordinating committees and working groups in CDER, FDA, and was involved in establishing the agency's policies and publishing the "guidance for industry" documents. Dr. Ahn is active in professional societies and has organized and chaired several international conferences, symposiums, and workshops. She received her BS in pharmacy from Ewha Women's University, an MS in pharmaceutics from Seoul National University, a PhD in pharmaceutics from West Virginia University, and a postdoctoral fellowship in pharmaceutics at the University of Michigan.

Neelam Azad, PhD
Assistant Professor
Department of Pharmaceutical Sciences
Hampton University
Hampton, VA

Dr. Azad holds a BS in pharmacy from the University of Mumbai and a PhD in pharmaceutical and pharmacological sciences from West Virginia University. She is an established researcher in the area of pulmonary diseases, with focuses on lung fibrosis and lung cancer. Dr. Azad is well published in the area of molecular mechanisms involved in pulmonary fibrosis with NIH funded research.

Hing Char, PhD
HC Consulting, LLC
Nutley, NJ

Hing Char is a registered pharmacist and a pharmaceutical scientist with over 20 years of experience in sterile dosage form development of small molecules and proteins. Currently he is a principal consultant at HC Consulting, LLC, providing consulting services in the area of sterile dosage form development. Previously he worked for Hoffmann-La Roche Inc. as a research leader in the sterile formulation development group. Hing graduated with a BS in pharmacy from Arnold & Marie Schwartz College of Pharmacy and an MS and PhD in pharmaceutical sciences from St. John's University.

Anand Iyer, PhD
Assistant Professor
Department of Pharmaceutical Sciences
Hampton University
Hampton, VA

Dr. Iyer holds a BS in biomedical engineering from the University of Mumbai, an MS in biomedical informatics, and a PhD in cellular and molecular pathology from the University of Pittsburgh. Dr. Iyer, through an NIH funded project, conducts research in the area of a combinatorial approach involving both molecular biology and structural bioinformatics techniques. His work is published in several prominent scientific journals.

Sudjit Luanpitpong, PhD
Research Assistant Professor
School of Pharmacy
West Virginia University
Morgantown, WV

Dr. Sudjit Luanpitpong is a research assistant professor at the West Virginia University School of Pharmacy, with expertise in basic and applied pharmaceutics and biotechnology. Her current research interest is in the area of cellular and molecular mechanisms of gene regulation and targeted drug therapy. She has combined expertise in molecular biotechnology and drug development. Dr. Luanpitpong received her BS in pharmacy and a PhD in pharmaceutical technology from Chulalongkorn University in Thailand.

Aniruddha Railkar, PhD
Assistant Director, Development
Synerx Pharma, LLC
Canonsburg, PA

Aniruddha Railkar is the assistant director of development at Synerx Pharma, LLC. Prior to Synerx, he was a principal scientist and technical team leader in drug product development in J&J PRD. He has over 16 years of experience in pharmaceutical research and development predominantly in oral solid dosage forms. Aniruddha has a BSc in chemistry from Bombay University, an MS in pharmaceutical sciences from West Virginia University, and a PhD from the University of the Sciences in Philadelphia.

Yon Rojanasakul, PhD
Professor
School of Pharmacy
West Virginia University
Morgantown, WV

Dr. Yon Rojanasakul is a professor at West Virginia University School of Pharmacy where he has taught pharmaceutics and pharmaceutical biotechnology for over 20 years. Dr. Rojanasakul received his BS in pharmacy from Mahidol University, an MS in industrial pharmacy from Massachusetts College of Pharmacy, and a PhD in pharmaceutics from the University of Wisconsin. In addition to teaching, he is active in research studying nanobiotechnology and cancer therapeutics. Rojanasakul is a fellow of the American Association of Pharmaceutical Scientists and the Robert C. Byrd Professor and Benedum Distinguished Scholar at West Virginia University.

Jun (Joseph) Shao, PhD
Associate Professor
College of Pharmacy & Allied Health Professions
St. John's University
Queens, NY

Dr. Shao received his PhD in pharmaceutical sciences from West Virginia University. He also holds a BS degree in pharmacy from Zhejian University and an MS degree in biopharmaceutics from China Pharmaceutical University. Dr. Shao completed his postdoctoral training in clinical pharmacokinetics at Janssen Research Foundation, Johnson & Johnson. He is currently an associate professor in the department of pharmaceutical sciences at St. John's University and a three-time recipient, from the college, of the Faculty Recognition Award in teaching and research.

REVIEWERS

Mark A. Best, MD, MBA, MPH
Associate Professor
Lake Erie College of Osteopathic Medicine–Bradenton
Erie, PA

Parag Budukh
Wegmans School of Pharmacy
St. John Fisher College
Rochester, NY

M. Teresa Carvajal, PhD
Faculty Professor
Industrial & Physical Pharmacy
College of Pharmacy & Pharmaceutical Sciences
Purdue University
West Lafayette, IN

S. Craig Dyar, PhD, RPh
Assistant Professor
South University School of Pharmacy
Savannah, GA

Rutesh H. Dave
Long Island University
Brooklyn, NY

Shelley Chambers Fox
Washington State University
Pullman, WA

Werner Geldenhuys, BPharm, PhD
Assistant Professor
Pharmaceutical Sciences
Colleges of Medicine and Pharmacy
Northeastern Ohio Universities
Rootstown, OH

Naushad Khan Ghilzai, PhD
Lake Erie College of Osteopathic Medicine–Bradenton
Erie, PA

Theodore Jochsberger, PhD
Professor Emeritus
Long Island University
Brooklyn, NY

Abby Kahaleh, BPharm, MS, MPH, PhD
LECOM School of Pharmacy
Erie, PA

Arthur H. Kibbe, PhD
Chair and Professor of Pharmaceutical Sciences
Wilkes University
Wilkes-Barre, PA

Maria C. Mancini, MHP, RAC
Senior Faculty
Northeastern University
Boston, MA

Quamrun Masuda, PhD
Assistant Professor (Pharmaceutics)
Appalachian College of Pharmacy
Oakwood, VA

Nina Pavuluri
Assistant Professor
Lake Erie College of Osteopathic Medicine–Bradenton
Erie, PA

Rahmat M. Talukder, PhD
Assistant Professor
College of Pharmacy
Southwestern Oklahoma State University
Weatherford, OK

Xudong Yuan, PhD
Assistant Professor
Department of Pharmaceutical Sciences
College of Pharmacy
Long Island University
Brooklyn, NY

PART I

PHYSICAL PHARMACY IN SOLUTIONS

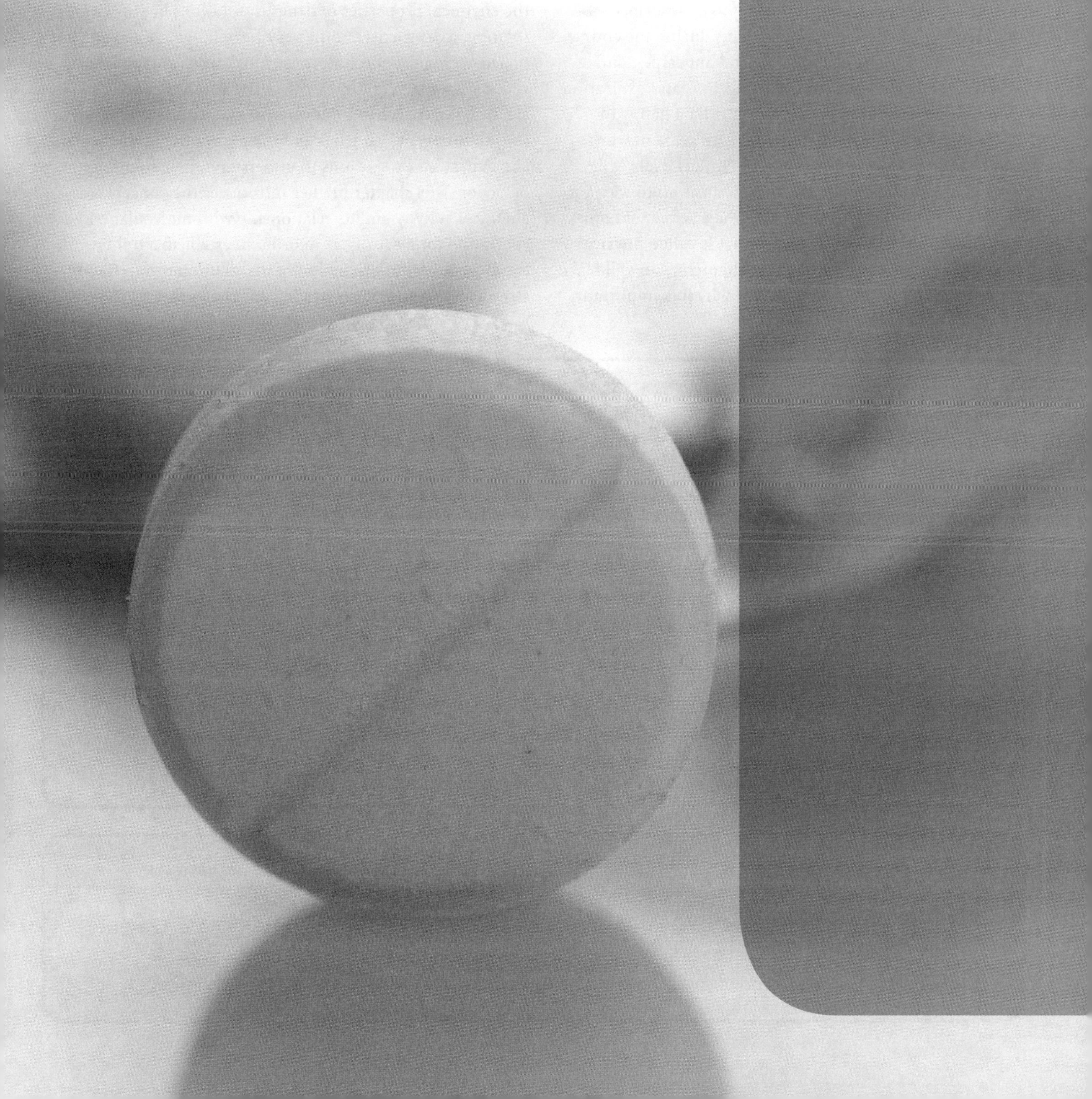

CHAPTER 1

Molecular Expressions and Electrolyte Properties of Drug Molecules

When you visit a pharmacy to have your prescription filled, you will likely receive a well-designed drug product that is (1) uniformly made with precise dose in each dosage form; (2) working according to a prescribed regimen to provide therapeutic effects during the course of treatment; (3) physically stable and appealing; and (4) clearly labeled with storage conditions and expiration date for safe use of the product. You will be happy to know that for a new drug, more than 10 years of work and testing, both in animals and in clinical trials, will have gone into the making of this medication to warrant its safe use and therapeutic effect. The science that must be followed in making such a product is called physical pharmacy. In this and subsequent chapters, you will learn what physical pharmacy entails and why it is important both in preserving the drug action and in making a pharmaceutical product.

Basic physical pharmacy begins with the recognition of the chemical properties of drugs in solutions because in *solution*, a drug exists in the very form in which it exerts its pharmacological effect. Because most drugs and pharmaceutical agents fall into the categories of strong and weak electrolytes, this chapter devotes its discussion to the ionization properties of drugs and the proper use of molecular concentration expressions to understand their solution behavior. This chapter further introduces the concept of chemical activity and its relationship with molecular concentration for electrolytes in order to establish a framework for more in-depth discussion of the solution properties of strong and weak electrolytes in later chapters.

CHAPTER OUTLINE

OBJECTIVES

1. Recognize the ionization property of drugs (as electrolytes, nonelectrolytes, or weak electrolytes) in an aqueous solution.
2. Calculate and/or determine the concentrations of solutes at the molecular, osmolecular, and ionic levels best to describe their solution behavior and pharmacological effects.
3. Understand the concepts of concentration, activity, and activity coefficient in electrolyte solutions.

I. Introduction

The term pharma in all pharmaceutical sciences terminologies derives from the Greek word pharmakon, meaning "drug." The word *drug* refers to any chemical agent that is capable of interacting with the living system (subcellular organelles, cells, tissues, or organs) to produce a biological effect. Thus, in a broad sense, drug molecules include not only those that produce a specific pharmacological effect in a disease state but also chemicals that are necessary for the maintenance of physiological conditions. *Medicine*, in contrast, refers to a formulated drug product to be given by a specific method of drug delivery to produce a therapeutic effect. Hence, the formulation of a drug product bears the responsibility to elicit the drug's therapeutic effect, minimize the drug's potential toxicity, and provide uniform doses so that these effects can be effectively monitored. Drug products may appear in liquid, solid, polyphasic, and aerosolized dosage forms, and it has been well documented that the design of a dosage form for a specific drug is crucial for the drug's therapeutic activity. The science that deals with the development of a drug product is called *pharmaceutics*. The principles that guide the pharmaceutical development compose physical pharmacy, which, in addition to its application in drug product development, provides a sound base of understanding of drug absorption, distribution, metabolism, and elimination during the course of drug treatment.

II. Ionization Properties of Drug Molecules

Drug molecules are diverse but can be classified as nonelectrolytes, strong electrolytes, and weak electrolytes according to their ionization properties when dispersed at the molecular level in an aqueous solution. This section provides a broad discussion of the chemical nature of compounds, both inorganic and organic, that exhibit strong or weak electrolyte properties. Although the main objective of this discussion is to demonstrate the role of electrolyte properties in pharmaceutical development, readers are also encouraged, through this discussion, to actively seek knowledge on the chemical nature of drug molecules. It is worth noting that one of the common mistakes in dosage calculations arises from using incorrect chemical formulas for the drugs in question. Many of these mistakes can be avoided if attention is paid to the composition of the drug based on its electrolyte properties. For example, the compound ephedrine sulfate, $(EphH)_2SO_4$, consists of two protonated ephedrine cations and one sulfate anion, whereas ephedrine hydrochloride, EphHCl, consists of one protonated ephedrine cation and one chloride ion. Although both compounds provide the same drug, they have very different molecular weights and thus dose requirement.

Nonelectrolytes

By nature, nonelectrolytes do not possess dissociable ions. Owing to their significance in pharmaceutical preparations, however, it is worth noting that small alcohols, such as ethanol, propylene glycol, and glycerin, are important pharmaceutical solvents for the preparation of oral liquids. These compounds are freely soluble in water, as are many polyalcohols including the mono- and disaccharides.

Inorganic Acids, Bases, and Salts

The electrolyte properties of compounds composed of metal ions and electronegative elements can be explained in terms of the position of the elements in the periodic table, in which the elements are arranged according to their electron configurations and trends of ionization potential or electron affinity. Removing an electron from an atom to form a cation requires an input of energy known as the *ionization energy* (or potential). *Electron affinity*, in contrast, is the energy change that occurs when an electron is added to a gaseous atom, which represents the ease with which an atom can accept an electron. The term *electronegativity* refers to a measure of the attraction of electrons by an atom in a chemical bond in that the greater the electronegativity of an atom, the greater is its attraction for bonding electrons. The periodic table offers a good guideline on the compounds that can be formed from the elements of varying ionization energy or electron affinity. In general, the ionization energy increases from left to right across a period as the atomic radius decreases; and for a given group, the ionization energy decreases while moving down the periodic table as the atomic radius increases. This indicates that group I elements (alkali metals) have the lowest whereas group VIIA elements (halogens) have the highest electron affinity and electronegativity. Group VIII elements (noble gases) have electron affinities of the order zero because they already possess a stable octet that cannot accept an additional electron.

The alkali metals (Li, Na, K, etc.) have only one loosely bound electron in their outermost shell. With low ionization energies, these metals easily lose their valence electron to form univalent cations. They react readily with nonmetals, especially with halogens, to form neutral salts (such as NaCl) and with water to yield the hydroxide strong bases (LiOH, NaOH, KOH, etc.). The alkaline earths are the elements of group IIA (Be, Mg, Ca, etc.). They have two electrons in their outer shell, which can be removed to form divalent cations when reacting with halogens (such as $CaCl_2$) or hydroxide (such as $Ca(OH)_2$). Boron (B) and aluminum (Al) are both group IIIA elements but exhibit quite different chemical activity. The aluminum metal forms trivalent cations with halides and other anions; boron, however, exhibits both metal and nonmetal characteristics and is known as a metalloid, as this element also forms boron halides similar to those of aluminum but behaves as a nonmetal when reacting with sodium. Boron forms oxide, B_2O_3, with oxygen, which reacts with water to yield the compound $B(OH)_3$. Interestingly, unlike in $Al(OH)_3$, which is a salt, the –OH groups in the boron compound are not ionic. Instead, boric acid, as this compound is known, is a Lewis acid and an important pharmaceutical agent in the preparation of ophthalmic isotonic solutions.

The transition elements, groups IB to VIIIB, are all considered metals. Chemically, transition metals have low ionization energy and may exist in a variety of positively charged forms or oxidation states. This is so because they are capable of losing various numbers of electrons from the *s* and *d* orbitals of their valence shell. For example, in group VIIB, manganese (Mn) may theoretically have seven different oxidation states from +1 to +7. But in reality, manganese only exhibits the +2, +3, +4, +6, or +7 state. Because of this ability to attain positive oxidation states, transition metals form many ionic and partially ionic compounds. Iron (Fe), an important biological element, forms compounds with +2 and +3 oxidation states.

Group VA (N, P) and VIA (O, S) elements occur in the formation of both inorganic and organic compounds. They are the key elements for the formation of various functional groups in organic and biological chemistry. Nitrogen exhibits every integral oxidation number between –3 (as in ammonia, NH_3) and +5 (as in nitric acid, HNO_3). An important phenomenon is that, except in nitric oxide and nitrogen dioxide, nitrogen has either three bonds and one unshared electron pair or four bonds with no unshared electron pair. Hence, compounds such as ammonia and its derivatives (organic amino compounds) can readily accept a proton to form a cationic moiety and exhibit weak base properties. Nitric acid is an inorganic strong acid. For phosphorus, the congener to nitrogen, the –3 state is far less important, but this element forms phosphoric acid (H_3PO_4 with +5 oxidation state), an important weak acid with three dissociable protons that plays a variety of roles in the biological system. In biological fluid, the most frequently encountered phosphate ions are $H_2PO_4^-$ and HPO_4^{2-}.

The abundance of oxygen, which forms oxides with nearly all other elements except the rare gases and some noble metals, makes our world an oxygenated one. Water (H_2O) is arguably the most important compound on Earth, without which life as we know it cannot exist. The chemists have subdivided all oxides into three classes: ionic oxides (as in Li_2O and BaO), covalent oxides (as in

SO_2 and CO_2), and intermediate oxides (as in Fe_2O_3 and ZnO). One can readily see that in reacting with water, the ionic oxides (formed by the alkali and alkaline earth metals) will lose the oxygen, forming a hydroxide (OH^-) ion. These hydroxides are strong bases. The covalent oxides are formed by elements closer to oxygen in the periodic table. In CO_2, for example, oxygen is covalently bound to carbon, and the reaction of CO_2 with water yields not a hydroxide ion but a hydroxide that has a dissociable proton. Many of the intermediate oxides do not react appreciably with water and often exhibit characteristics of both acid and base, known as the amphoteric hydroxides. Oxygen is a key element for the formation of many strong and weak acids, such as the ones noted below.

Strong acids:	Nitric acid, HNO_3; sulfuric acid, H_2SO_4; perchloric acid, $HClO_4$
Weak acids:	Boric acid, $B(OH)_3$; carbonic acid, H_2CO_3 carboxylic acid, compounds with –COOH group; phosphoric acid, H_3PO_4; sulfurous acid, H_2SO_3

Salt is the neutralization product of an acid–base reaction. In an aqueous solution, strong acids and bases are completely ionized in dilute concentrations. Weak acids and bases undergo only partial ionization. However, the salt formed from the reaction of a strong base with a weak acid, such as sodium carbonate, or from the reaction of a strong acid with a weak base, such as the aforementioned ephedrine sulfate, is completely ionized in aqueous solutions. As a summary, strong electrolytes, which are completely ionized in dilute solutions, include strong acids, strong bases, and all salts.

Organic Acids and Bases

The majority of the pharmaceutical and medicinal agents are organic compounds, and many of these agents are classified as weak acids and weak bases, collectively known as the weak electrolytes. According to the Brønsted–Lowry theory, by definition a weak acid is a compound that undergoes partial ionization in an aqueous solution to yield a proton and an anion of the drug, whereas a weak base has the capacity to accept a proton to form a cation (or neutral compound if the weak base is an anion). Even though one cannot always tell whether a drug is a weak acid or weak base based on the name of the chemical, nor can any student know the diverse chemical structures of all drugs, nonetheless students should pay attention to the acid–base behavior of drugs, as the first step in dosage calculations requires the determination of a drug's composition. There are, however, guidelines one can follow to identify the acid or base characteristics of a drug. Aside from dosage determinations, the acid–base phenomenon has a broad effect on the drug's solubility and chemical stability, which are important factors in the development of a suitable drug delivery system for the drug and in the understanding of the drug's pharmacological effects and usage. A few examples that illustrate the roles of acid–base behavior on drug formulation and usage are given in **Table 1-1**.

pK_a and Drug Effects

The acid–base behavior is best described using the concepts of pH and pK_a, which are defined as the negative logarithm of the hydronium ion concentration $[H_3O^+]$ and the negative logarithm of the acidity constant K_a of a weak acid, respectively; that is, $pH = -\log[H_3O^+]$ and $pK_a = -\log K_a$. Applying chemical reaction principles, the ionization of a weak acid (HA) can be written as

$$HA + H_2O \overset{K}{\rightleftarrows} H_3O^+ + A^-$$

$$K = [H_3O^+]\,[A^-]/[HA][H_2O]$$

or

$$K_a = [H_3O^+]\,[A^-]/[HA] \qquad K_a = K[H_2O] \tag{1-1}$$

Table 1-1 Role of Acid–Base Properties in Pharmaceutical Preparations and Therapeutic Application of Drugs

Drug	Structure	pK_a	Preparation	Application
Sulfadiazine	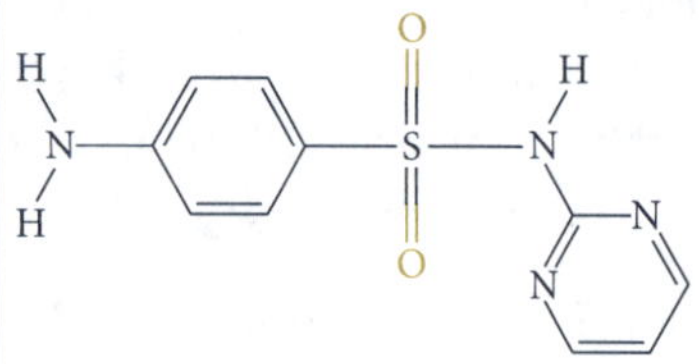	6.3	Sulfadiazine USP tablets Sulfadiazine sodium injection	Systemic infections , e.g., pneumococcal, meningococcal, etc.
Sulfisoxazole	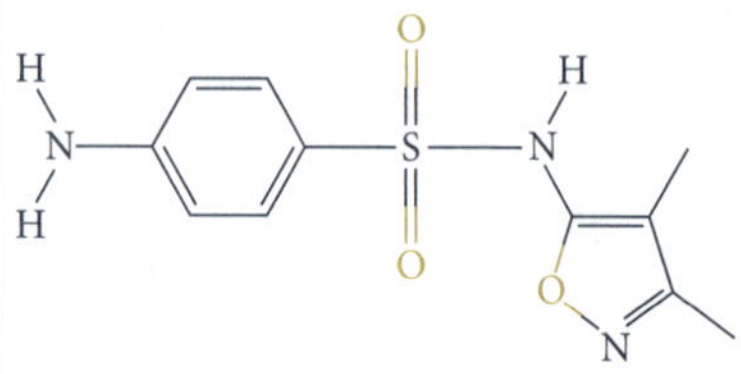	5.0	Sulfisoxazole USP tablets Sulfisoxazole oral suspension	Urinary tract infections
Cefoxitin	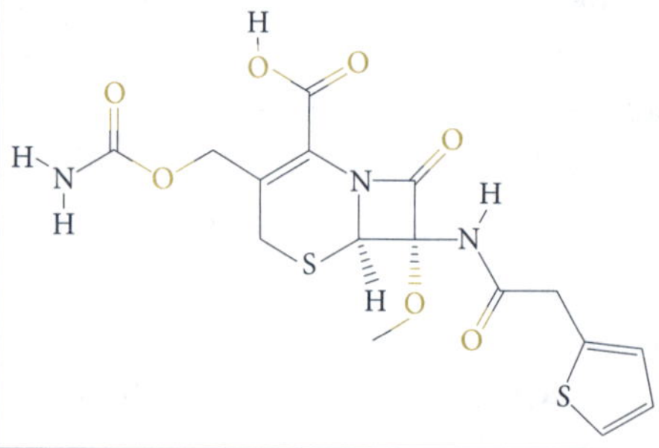	2.2	Sterile cefoxitin sodium for IV, IM injection	Systemic infections
Cephalexin	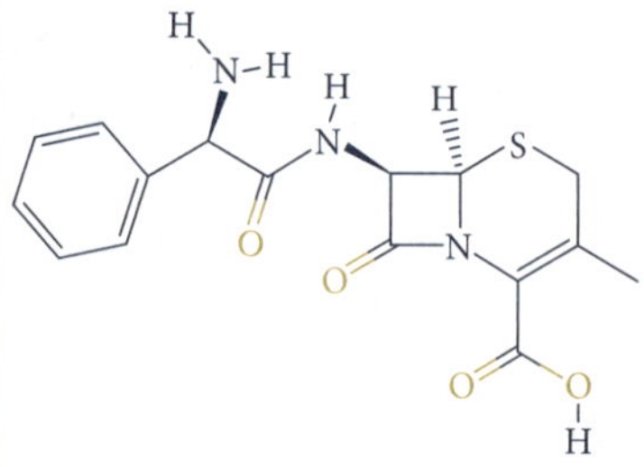	5.2, 7.3†	Cephalexin tablets Cephalexin oral suspension	Urinary tract infections
Atropine	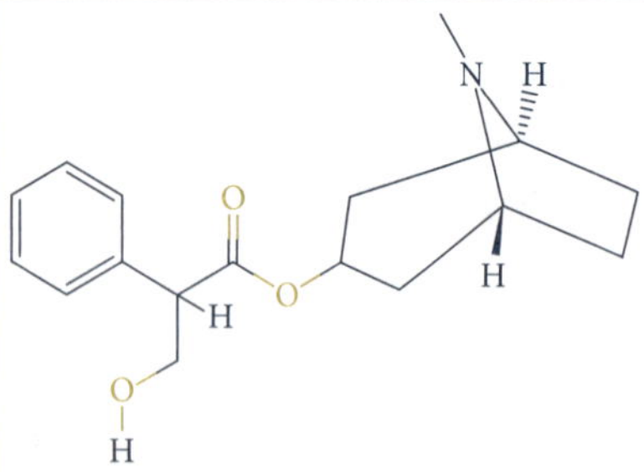	9.7†	Atropine sulfate injection Atropine sulfate ophthalmic solution Atropine sulfate USP tablets	Anticholinergic Topically to the conjunctiva Anticholinergic

†pK_a is given for protonated amine.

where K_a is known as the *acidity constant*. For convenience, the term pK_a is often used, which can be expressed as

$$pK_a = pH - \log([A^-]/[HA]) \tag{1-2}$$

As can be seen, for a weak acid, 50% of the drug will be ionized if the pH of the solution is equal to the drug's pK_a. If the pH is higher than the pK_a, more than 50% of the drug will be in the ionized form.

Sulfadiazine, an anti-infective agent for systemic infections, is a weak acid because of its capacity to release a proton from the substituted sulfonamide ($-SO_2NH-$) group. The pK_a for this drug is 6.3.

In the normal physiological pH range of 7–8, this drug is well ionized (~90% at pH 7.4) to the soluble form. Thus, it is relatively easy to maintain high blood levels. At pH 6 or below, however, less than 50% of the drug will be in the ionized form. This decreases the solubility of the drug as the free (neutral) drug is only poorly soluble. The common side effect of the sulfa drugs with low acidity is the crystallization of the free drug and its *N*-acetyl metabolite in the renal tubules, thereby causing kidney damage. Alkalinization of the urine by giving sodium bicarbonate has been commonly used to reduce the crystallization effect. However, careful selection of drugs based on their pK_a values can also be used to overcome the crystallization problem. For example, sulfisoxazole has a pK_a of 5.0. At pH 6, this drug is well ionized (~90%), and the solubility is sufficiently high in body fluids that the drug is not deposited in the kidneys. For this reason, sulfisoxazole is used for treating urinary tract infections.

The acidic property of the cephalosporins derives from the carboxylic group attached to the bicyclic ring known as cephem. The β-lactam moiety of the bicyclic ring is susceptible to acid-catalyzed hydrolysis that renders the antibiotic inactive. Cefoxitin is poorly absorbed from the gastrointestinal tract and must be administered parenterally or intramuscularly for the treatment of systemic infections. Its poor oral absorption is, in part, attributed to the instability of the β-lactam ring to acid hydrolysis. In comparison, cephalexin is purposely designed to contain an α-amino group at the cephalosporin side chain. This base group, which along with the carboxylic group forms a zwitterion (pI = 4.75), blocks the acid catalysis of the β-lactam ring. Cephalexin is freely soluble in water, resistant to acid, well absorbed orally, and recommended for the treatment of urinary tract infections.

Atropine, a tropine ester of racemic tropic acid, occurs naturally in various Solanaceae. The drug is a weak base owing to its tertiary amine group of the tropane moiety. Atropine is an anticholinergic agent that produces a mydriatic effect by paralyzing the iris and the ciliary muscles; for this reason it is used in treating iritis and corneal inflammations and lesions. It is also a specific antidote to cholinesterase inhibitor–mediated (such as by the organic phosphates) muscarinic effects (due to acetylcholine accumulation) that include vomiting, abdominal cramps, diarrhea, sweating, bronchoconstriction, and excessive bronchial secretion. The free drug, however, is not soluble in water, and hence it has little use as a pharmaceutical agent. But the free base can be made into a salt with sulfuric acid, which is freely soluble in water, without changing the drug's pharmacological effect.

The above examples show that simple acid–base phenomena in fact play a very important role in determining a drug's pharmacological activity. Compounds that possess the carboxylic and substituted amide and sulfonamide groups exhibit weak acid properties. These compounds can react with a strong base such as sodium hydroxide to form soluble salts. Compounds that contain amino and substituted amino groups are weak bases, which can be made into salts with strong acids such as hydrochloric acid or sulfuric acid. An aromatic alcohol, such as phenol, may also exhibit the weak acid property, because the anion formed after losing the proton can be stabilized through delocalization of the negative charge into the aromatic ring. In contrast, the basicity of an amino group attached to an aromatic ring will be much weakened, as the positive charge formed after accepting a proton cannot be delocalized in the aromatic ring, i.e., stabilized through the resonance effect.

III. Molecular Expressions—Quantities and Concentrations

Solution

The term *solution* is used to indicate a multicomponent system in which one (or more) solute(s) is dissolved in a solvent that can be in the gaseous, liquid, or solid state. Studies of drug properties in solution are important because a drug in solution is dispersed at the molecular level, which is essential for the drug to exert its chemical, biochemical, and pharmacological effects. In pharmaceutics, solution is also a necessary and common dosage form for oral, nasal, ophthalmic, and parenteral drug delivery. In comparison to solid dosage forms, a solution has the advantage of producing quick-onset drug action and having an appealing formulation for easy administration and tolerance. However, formulation of a solution dosage form can be difficult because the drug may not have sufficient solubility or may undergo degradation through unwanted chemical reactions. Commonly used pharmaceutical solvents include water and alcohols such as ethanol, propylene glycol, and glycerin.

The Solute

The quantity of a drug that indicates the strength of its chemical and pharmacological activities is not the weight of the drug, but rather the number of molecules or ions available for the drug action. Hence, the *molecular expression* of quantity or concentration (a quantity relative to another quantity in a mixed system) must be used to describe the drug's pharmacological action. For non-electrolytes in ideal solutions, the basic particle (the smallest unit) that indicates the drug's physical and chemical activity is the molecule.

Moles

From a historical point of view, it is worth recalling that the recognition of the molecular nature of matter led to the hypothesis, first proposed by Avogadro in 1811, that equal volumes of different gases at the same temperature and pressure contain the same number of molecules. Because the pressure and volume changes at constant temperature depend on only the number of molecules but not on the chemical nature of the gases, the concept of a mole arises in that 1 mole (mol) of any compound contains the same number of molecules, and this number, known as the *Avogadro number*, has the value of 6.0225×10^{23}. The unit, mole, is a convenient way to express the quantity of a compound that directly relates to the compound's chemical action. The number of moles of a drug with a given weight (wt) in grams can be easily calculated based on the molecular weight (mol wt) of the drug because the molecular weight is defined as weight in grams per mole of molecule. Hence,

$$\text{moles of drug} = \text{wt of drug} / \text{mol wt} \qquad \text{millimoles of drug} = \text{wt of drug} \times 1000/\text{mol wt}$$

It is often desirable to express the number of molecules of a drug in millimoles (mmol), which is equal to moles × 1000.

Osmoles

The mole or millimole is traditionally reserved for the expression of the number of molecules. It would seem to be inadequate, however, to use this term to express the property of an electrolyte that undergoes extensive ionization in a solution. For example, if one hypothetically put 5 molecules of calcium chloride ($CaCl_2$), a strong electrolyte, into a beaker containing water, the theory of ionization would indicate the formation of 5 Ca^{2+} and 10 Cl^- ions. In the resulting solution, the total number of particles (ions) will be 15; the total number of positive (or negative) charges will be 10; and even though 5 molecules were added to the solution, the total number of molecules in solution will be zero. Because one Ca^{2+} ion contributes the same as one Cl^- ion to the physical properties of the drug, such as the osmotic pressure, the physicochemical effect of $CaCl_2$ is in fact 3 times that of a nonelectrolyte. This is known as the van't Hoff modification. For this reason, the term osmole (osmol) or milliosmole (mosmol) has been introduced to indicate the total number of particles in a solution, where the osmole of a drug is equal to the moles of the drug multiplied by the van't Hoff i factor, which indicates the number of ions generated per molecule. Thus,

Osmoles = moles × i milliosmoles = millimoles × i

Charges

The electrolyte property depends on not only the number of ions generated but also the charge characteristics of the dissociated ions. There are equal numbers of total positive and negative charges in an electrolyte solution to maintain electroneutrality. The quantity that has been used to express the charge equivalency is the gram-equivalent weight, defined as the weight of the drug in grams (wt) divided by the equivalent weight. If one defines the number of positive (or negative) charges of a drug as q, then the equivalent weight (eq wt) of a compound is the molecular weight divided by q (eq wt = mol wt / q). Hence,

Gram-equivalent weight = wt / eq wt = wt of drug × q / mol wt = moles × q

The term *milligram-equivalent weight* has been used to express the quantity of all electrolytes and is equal to gram-equivalent weight × 1000. The milligram-equivalent weight is also known as *milliequivalent*, which is abbreviated as mEq. Thus,

mEq = wt of drug × 1000 × q / mol wt = mmol × q

In summary, it is clear from the above discussion that the molecular expressions are designed so that (1) the term mole or millimole indicates the number of molecules, (2) the term osmole or *milliosmole* indicates the total number of particles (including molecules and ions), and (3) milliequivalent indicates the total number of positive or negative charges in solution. Students should study the examples given below for accurate determination of the molecular expressions.

Example 1-1: Calculate the millimoles, milliosmoles, and milliequivalents contained in 5.55 g of $CaCl_2$ (mol wt = 111).

Solution: In water, $CaCl_2 \rightarrow Ca^{2+} + 2\ Cl$

Complete dissociation of calcium chloride yields 3 ions (i = 3); the calcium ion has two positive charges that are balanced by two chloride ions, each with one negative charge. Hence, q = 2. Thus,

Number of molecules (mmol) = 5.55 g × 1000 / 111 g/mol

= 50 mmol

Total number of particles (mosmol) = 50 × 3 = 150 mosmol

Total number of + or − charges (mEq) = 50 × 2 = 100 mEq

Example 1-2: What are the units of mole, osmole, milliequivalent, i, and q?

Answer: Mole is a number but is specifically designated to indicate molecules. Osmole and milliequivalent are numerically equal to mole (that is, 1 mol is 6.0225×10^{23} molecules; 1 milliequivalent is 6.0225×10^{23} charges) but are designated to indicate the number of ions and the total number of charges carried by the ions, respectively. Hence, i bears the unit of mosmol/mmol, whereas q has a unit of mEq/mmol.

Example 1-3: What are the i and q values for NaH_2PO_4, Na_2HPO_4, and NaK_2PO_4?

Answer: For NaH_2PO_4, this compound dissociates in water into 1 Na^+ ion and 1 $H_2PO_4^-$ ion; $i = 2$; $q = 1$; further dissociation of proton from the $H_2PO_4^-$ ion is negligible.

For Na_2HPO_4, this compound dissociates in water into 2 Na^+ ions and 1 HPO_4^{2-} ion; $i = 3$; $q = 2$; further dissociation of proton from the HPO_4^{2-} ion is negligible.

For NaK_2PO_4, this compound dissociates in water into 1 Na^+ ion, 2 K^+ ions, and 1 PO_4^{3-} ion; $i = 4$; $q = 3$. (The q value is for the determination of the total positive or negative charges of this compound.)

Example 1-4: How many milliequivalents of Na^+ and K^+ are in 1.96 g of NaK_2PO_4 (mol wt = 196)?

Solution: Example 1-3 shows that $q = 3$ for the compound. However, one-third of the positive charges come from Na^+, and two-thirds of the positive charges come from K^+, but all negative charges come from PO_4^{3-}; thus, $q_{Na^+} = 1$, $q_{K^+} = 2$, and $q_{PO_4^{3-}} = 3$.

mEq of $Na^+ = 1.96 \times 1000 \times 1 / 196 = 10$ mEq

mEq of $K^+ = 1.96 \times 1000 \times 2 / 196 = 20$ mEq

mEq of $PO_4^{3-} = 1.96 \times 1000 \times 3 / 196 = 30$ mEq

The van't Hoff *i* Value for Weak Electrolytes

A weak electrolyte is only partially dissociated into ions in a solution. As a result, the total number of ions generated is significantly less than the theoretical number of ions that can be expected through complete ionization. The i value can be estimated if the degree of dissociation (usually expressed as percentage of ionization) of the weak electrolyte is known based on the following equation:

$$i = 1 + \alpha (v - 1)$$

where α is the degree of dissociation and v is the theoretical number of ions that can be generated per molecule. For example, the i value for acetic acid (CH_3COOH) in a solution where the weak acid exhibits a 2% dissociation is 1.02 according to the above equation. It is worth pointing out, however, that the sodium salt of acetic acid (CH_3COONa) is a strong electrolyte and has an i value of 2.

Concentrations

A variety of methods of describing concentration in solution exist, some of them rational but rather inconvenient, others convenient but not very rational. The common percent descriptions include grams of solute per 100 mL of solution for solid in liquid solutions (wt/v%) and milliliters of solute in 100 mL of solution (v/v%) for liquid in liquid solutions. For solutions with concentrated solute, such as sulfuric acid, the percentage expression may be expressed as grams of solute per 100 g of solution (wt/wt%). As generally given in the literature, descriptions of concentrations of liquid in liquid solutions are frequently very empiric. The weight percent description at least has the merit that it is readily converted to thermodynamic terms; but the volume percent description provides only the relative volumes of the liquid constituents before mixing but no information about the solution. It is therefore less useful than the weight percent descriptions. Its sole merit is one of experimental convenience.

Table 1-2 Molecular Concentrations of Solutions

Name (Units)	Symbol	Definition	Formula
Molarity (mmol/mL)	M	Moles / liter of solution	$M = \text{wt} \times 1000 / \text{mol wt} \times V^{\dagger}$
Molality (mmol/g)	m	Moles / 1000 grams of solvent	$m = \text{wt}_2 \times 1000 / \text{mol wt} \times \text{wt}_1$ (subscripts 1 and 2 denote solvent and solute, respectively)
Osmolarity (mosmol/mL)	OsM	Osmoles / liter of solution	$\text{OsM} = M \times i$ For nonelectrolyte, $i = 1$; for electrolytes, i = number of ions per molecule
Normality (mEq/mL)	N	Gram-equivalent weight / liter of solution	$N = M \times q$ q is the total number of positive or negative charges
Mole fraction	X	Moles of one component divided by total moles in solution	$X_1 = n_1 / (n_1 + n_2)^{\ddagger}$ $X_2 = n_2 / (n_1 + n_2)$ $X_1 + X_2 = 1$

†V is the volume of the solution in milliliters.

‡Equations are given for a two-component system containing a nonelectrolyte solute; n is the number of moles of the component; subscripts 1 and 2 denote solvent and solute, respectively.

The three most commonly used molecular concentration units are molarity, molality, and mole fraction, which, along with other related concentration descriptions, are listed and defined in **Table 1-2**. In its common but rather imprecise usage, molarity is defined as the number of moles of solute per liter of solution. It is imprecise because the behavior of solutes in solution is not always predictable. For example, when acetic acid is dissolved in benzene, it is largely dimerized. Thus it is correct and precise to describe such a solution prepared by dissolving 60.05 g of acetic acid (mol wt = 60.05) in a sufficient amount of benzene to make a 1 L solution as being 1.0 molar in the component of acetic acid, but it is more useful and informative to describe this solution as being 0.5 molar in a dimer constituent. Furthermore, it will be recalled that for a given solution of NaCl, a strong electrolyte, in water, we already know that the osmotic effect of this agent is not indicated by the molarity of the solution but is increased by a factor of 2 via the van't Hoff modification. The latter gives rise to the need to express the concentration of electrolytes in osmolarity, defined as the number of osmoles of solute per liter of solution. A common description employed by analytical chemists in their acid–base and redox reaction determinations, but much less frequently in physical pharmacy, is the normality. This concentration expression, however, has a unit of gram-equivalent weight per liter or mEq/mL, which is useful in the expression of electrolyte solutions.

Molarity and Molality

In chemical and pharmaceutical studies, few solutions are made in liter or kilogram quantities. Instead, the common units for weight and volume expressions are gram (g) and milliliter (mL), respectively. Thus, for the determination of molarity and molality in gram or milliliter quantities, one can use the following equations for calculation.

$$\begin{aligned} M &= \text{wt of drug} / \text{mol wt} \times \text{liters of solution} \\ &= \text{wt of drug} \times 1000\ (\text{mL/L}) / \text{mol wt} \times V\ (\text{mL}) \end{aligned} \tag{1-3}$$

In Equation (1-3), V is the volume of the solution in milliliters; the unit of molarity is moles per liter (mol/L) or mmoles per milliliter (mmol/mL) of solution. Likewise, one can determine the molality by using the following equation:

$$m = \text{wt of drug} \times 1000\ (\text{g/kg}) / \text{mol wt} \times \text{wt of solvent (g)} \tag{1-4}$$

The unit for molality is moles per kilogram (mol/kg) or millimoles per gram (mmol/g) of solvent.

Example 1-5: What are the molality and molarity of glucose (mol wt = 180) in a solution containing 5.0 g of glucose and 100 g of water? The final solution has a density of 1.015 g/mL.

Solution: The total weight of the solution is 105 g. With the density being 1.015 g/mL, the volume V of this solution is 105/1.015 = 103.4 mL. Thus,

Molarity = 5.0 × 1000 / 180 × 103.4 = 0.2686 M (mmol/mL of solution)

Molality = 5.0 × 1000 / 180 × 100 = 0.2778 m (mmol/g of solvent)

Molality, which avoids the use of volume in its expression and is designed for thermodynamic studies, is significantly different from molarity in concentrated solutions. But in dilute aqueous solutions where the volume of the solution approaches the volume of the solvent alone, these two concentration expressions are interchangeable.

Mole Fraction and Molality

Both concentration expressions are based on the weights of the components. The mole fraction of a solution component is defined as the moles of the component divided by the total moles of all components present in the solution. For a two-component system, the mole fraction of the solute can be easily converted to molality, which is defined as the number of moles of solute per 1000 g of solvent. As can be seen from Table 1-2, for a nonelectrolyte solute in an aqueous solution containing wt_2 of solute and wt_1 of water,

$$X_2 = n_2 / (n_1 + n_2) = \text{moles of solute} / (\text{moles of solute} + \text{moles of water})$$

If one multiplies the numerator and denominator of the right side of the equation by $1000/wt_2$, the above equation becomes

$$X_2 = \frac{\text{moles of solute} \times 1000 / wt_1}{(\text{moles of solute} \times 1000 / wt_1) + (\text{moles of water} \times 1000 / wt_1)}$$

or

$$X_2 = \frac{m}{m + 1000 / \text{mol wt of water}}$$

Because water has a molecular weight of 18.02, the above equation can be written as

$$X_2 = m / (m + 55.5) \qquad (1\text{-}5)$$

In fact, for very dilute solutions when $m \ll 55.5$, then X_2, the mole fraction of the solute, can be approximated as $m/55.5$. For an electrolyte that dissociates into i ions, Equation (1-5) becomes

$$X_2 = mi / (mi + 55.5) \qquad (1\text{-}6)$$

Osmolality (or Osmolarity)

This concentration expression is important for the preparation of pharmaceutical isotonic solutions. Unlike other concentration terms, osmolality is a solution property, and all solute components contribute to the osmolality of a solution. For example, in a solution that contains 0.4 g of sodium chloride (mol wt = 58.5), 2.5 g of dextrose (mol wt = 180), and 0.05 g of calcium chloride (mol wt = 111) per 100 g of the solvent, the osmolality of the solution can be calculated (see formula and definition in Table 1-2) by combining the individual osmolalities of all solute components.

$$\text{Osmolality} = (0.4 \times 1000 \times 2 / 58.5 \times 100) + (2.5 \times 1000 \times 1 / 180 \times 100) + (0.05 \times 1000 \times 3 / 111 \times 100)$$
$$= 0.2801 \text{ OsM (osmol/kg solvent)}$$
($i = 2$, 1, and 3 for NaCl, dextrose, and $CaCl_2$, respectively)

This solution should exhibit the same physical properties as other solutions having the same osmolality, even if they contain different solutes. In the calculation of osmolality or osmolarity, which are not significantly different from each other in dilute solutions, the *i* value for nonelectrolytes such as dextrose is taken to be 1.

IV. Effect of Ionic Interactions on Concentration—The Debye–Hückel Theory

Solutions as a drug delivery system, except those formulated for oral use, must exhibit the same physical and chemical properties as those of the biological fluids. The physiological fluids are inherently ionic, owing to the presence of many electrolytes including, among others, sodium, potassium, calcium, chloride, bicarbonate, and phosphate ions, with a total osmolarity in the range of 0.28 to 0.31 mosmol/mL. Thus, knowing the properties of electrolytes is essential for the development of pharmaceutical products. One of the key effects of electrolytes on solution properties is their ability to alter the effective drug concentrations via ionic interactions. The terms *activity a* and *activity coefficient* γ have been used to describe the ideality of a solution for electrolyte as well as nonelectrolyte solutes.[1] The significance is such that in a nonideal solution, the activity, or the effective concentration of the solute, shows a concentration-dependent deviation from the actual concentration (*C*) prepared, following the relationship that $a = \gamma C$. For nonelectrolytes, the nonideality of a solution can be described in thermodynamic terms involving changes in the heat of mixing and/or the final volume of the solution. In comparison, the nonideality of an ionic solution cannot be readily explained by thermodynamics, but rather there is a somewhat special theory, due to Debye and Hückel, that provides, through the consideration of the electrostatic interactions of ionic species, an interpretation of the activity coefficient of ionic solutes.[2]

Ionic Activity

Consider the ionization of a simple electrolyte (AB) that dissociates into A^+ and B^-; the corresponding activity and activity coefficients are a_+, γ_+ and a_-, γ_-, respectively. The chemical equilibrium for such a compound under the concept of activity is

$$K = a_+a_- \qquad \text{or} \qquad K = \gamma_+\gamma_-[A^+][B^-]$$

where *K* is the equilibrium constant. Thus,

$$a_+a_- = \gamma_+\gamma_-[A^+][B^-]$$

There are no thermodynamic considerations that would lead to methods that can be used to determine the individual ionic activities or activity coefficients. But the concept of a geometric mean for the activity or activity coefficient of the ions, which is a thermodynamic quantity, can be and has been introduced: This has proved to be a very significant development in electrolyte chemistry. The mean ionic activity and *activity coefficient* are defined as follows:

$$a_\pm = (a_+a_-)^{1/2} \qquad \text{and} \qquad \gamma_\pm = (\gamma_+\gamma_-)^{1/2}$$

These relationships show that

$$a_{\pm} = \gamma_{\pm}\,[\mathrm{A}^{+}][\mathrm{B}^{-}] \qquad (1\text{-}7)$$

For an electrolyte that produces x A^{+} and y B^{-} ions per molecule, the mean ionic activity and activity coefficient are

$$a_{\pm} = [(a_{+})^{x}(a_{-})^{y}]^{1/(x+y)} \quad \text{and} \quad \gamma_{\pm} = [(\gamma_{+})^{x}(\gamma_{-})^{y}]^{1/(x+y)} \qquad (1\text{-}8)$$

As will become apparent later, the use of the mean ionic activity contributes to the development of theories for the determination of the activity coefficients of ions in solution.

Ionic Strength

Through the evaluation of the activity coefficient for many systems, Lewis and Randall[3] recognized that the mean ionic activity coefficient could be related to a function of the concentration of charged particles in the solution, and they introduced this function as the *ionic strength* μ. That such a relationship exists reflects the fact that the ionic interactions are primarily responsible for the nonideality of ionic solutes. The ionic strength is a solution property and is defined as

$$\mu = (\Sigma C_i Z_i^2)/2 \qquad (1\text{-}9)$$

where C_i is the concentration, Z_i is the number of charges per ion for each ion, and the summation extends over all the ions in solution. Example 1-6 illustrates the use of Equation (1-9) for the determination of the ionic strength of a solution.

Example 1-6: What is the ionic strength of a solution containing 0.03 *M* K_2HPO_4 and 0.01 *M* KH_2PO_4?

Solution: $\mu = [0.03 \times 2 \times 1^2 + 0.03 \times (-2)^2 + 0.01 \times 1^2 + 0.01 \times (-1)^2] / 2 = 0.10$

Ionic strength is a measure of the nonideality that the solution imposes on any dissociated electrolyte in the solution. One of the key findings by Lewis and Randall was that *in dilute aqueous solutions, the activity coefficient of a given strong electrolyte is the same in all solutions of the same ionic strength*. It is important to keep in mind that the ionic strength is a property of the solution but not a property of any particular ion in the solution. Also, the effect of ionic strength is on ionic species but not on neutral molecules.

The Debye–Hückel Theory on Activity Coefficient

Known as the limiting law, i.e., for dilute solutions, Debye and Hückel showed in 1923 how the activity coefficient of an ion of charge Z can be calculated. Their theory assumed that a strong electrolyte is completely dissociated and each ion is surrounded by ions of opposite charges. Using a number of physical and thermodynamic concepts, the Debye–Hückel theory showed that the difference in chemical potential (or free energy) between nonideal and ideal solutions, which corresponds to $RT\ln\gamma$, is equal to the potential energy change of an ion in an ionic solution. This change in energy is produced by other ions in the solution, and it is directly proportional to the square root of the ionic strength. Thus, a rather simple equation was developed (see Equation (1-10) below) after a series of complicated derivations of the physical and thermodynamic theories involved in ionic interactions, which was in itself a great achievement (the mathematical derivation of the Debye–Hückel theory can be found in Ref. 2).

$$\log \gamma_{+} = -AZ_{+}^{2}\,\mu^{1/2} \qquad \log \gamma_{-} = -AZ_{-}^{2}\,\mu^{1/2} \qquad (1\text{-}10)$$

In Equation (1-10), Z is the charge of either the cation (Z_+) or the anion (Z_-), and the constant A, which is related to the dielectric constant of the solvent and solution temperature, has a numeric value of 0.5091 for the special case of aqueous solutions at 25°C. The thermodynamic expression of the activity coefficient is $\gamma_\pm$. Using Equations (1-8) and (1-9), one obtains

$$\log \gamma_\pm = -0.5091(Z_+Z_-)\,\mu^{1/2} \qquad (1\text{-}11)$$

for the special case of aqueous solutions at 25°C.

A number of experimental methods are available for the determination of activity coefficients of electrolytes in solution. These methods depend on situations in which the nonideality of the ionic solution affects some measurable quantity such as the acidity constants of weak acids, solubility, freezing point depressions, etc. The Debye–Hückel limiting law, although only applicable to dilute solutions of 0.01 M or less, has been shown to be very accurate in predicting the mean ionic activity coefficient when compared to experimental values. In addition, the theory provides a method to determine the activity coefficient and the effective concentrations of ions in an ionic solution that cannot be easily determined using thermodynamic methods.

Activity Coefficients in More-Concentrated Solutions

For solutions with ionic strength greater than 0.01, modified equations of the Debye–Hückel theory have been proposed based on considerations of ion radius and solvent effects. Equations (1-12) and (1-13) have been shown to be applicable for solutions with ionic strength up to 0.1, and they are recommended for use in pharmaceutical considerations. The physiological fluid has an ionic strength of about 0.16. The calculation of the activity and activity coefficient using these equations is given in Example 1-7. For still higher concentrations (0.5 M and higher), the electrolyte solutions exhibit strikingly different ionic behavior from that of dilute solutions. Electrolytes of the same charge type, which should exhibit identical activity coefficients according to the Debye–Huckel theory in dilute solutions, have now very different activity coefficient curves; and for solutes such as calcium chloride and hydrochloric acid, the activity coefficient increases with increasing concentration even to values greater than unity.[4–6] Although some theories, such as the effect of solvation on the concentration of ions, have been suggested for the observed nonideality, the chemistry of ionic interactions at high concentration remains unclear.

$$\log \gamma_i = -0.5091 Z_i^2 \mu^{1/2} / (1 + \mu^{1/2}) \qquad (1\text{-}12)$$

$$\log \gamma_\pm = -0.5091(Z_+Z_-)\mu^{1/2} / (1 + \mu^{1/2}) \qquad (1\text{-}13)$$

Example 1-7: In a solution containing 0.01 M $FeCl_3$, what are (*a*) the mean ionic activity coefficient of $FeCl_3$, (*b*) the ionic activity coefficients of Fe^{3+} and Cl^-, and (*c*) the mean ionic activity of $FeCl_3$?

Solution: The ionic strength of this solution is

$$\mu = [0.01 \times 3^2 + 0.03 \times (-1)^2] / 2 = 0.06$$

(*a*) $\log \gamma_\pm = -0.5091(3 \times 1)(0.06)^{1/2} / [1 + (0.06)^{1/2}] = -0.3005;\ \gamma_\pm = 0.50$

(*b*) $\log \gamma_{Fe} = -0.5091(3 \times 3)(0.06)^{1/2} / [1 + (0.06)^{1/2}] = -0.9014;\ \gamma_{Fe} = 0.125$

$\log \gamma_{Cl} = -0.509(1 \times 1)(0.06)^{1/2} / [1 + (0.06)^{1/2}] = -0.10015;\ \gamma_{Cl} = 0.794$

(*c*) $a_\pm = \gamma_\pm (C_+C_-^{\,3})^{1/4} = \gamma_\pm [(0.01)(3 \times 0.01)^3]^{1/4} = 0.0115\ M$

V. Chapter Summary

This introductory chapter is written to assist students in getting familiar with the various pharmaceutical agents and drugs and their compositions based on their electrolyte properties. The information provided should allow students to apply knowledge they have already learned in chemistry classes. The composition of drugs and their nonionic and ionic characteristics are of particular importance for performing accurate dosage calculations and concentration determinations using the mole, osmole, and milliequivalent expressions. The physiological fluids are ionic in nature. As a result, pharmaceutical solutions are likewise ionic solutions. Understanding of the properties of the electrolytes is thus an important objective for this chapter. As shown in the text, these properties not only assist in developing pharmaceutical product but also affect the usage and pharmacological effects of the drug. The concepts of the activity and the activity coefficient are important in many pharmaceutical calculations, and this knowledge will assist the student in establishing a framework for the study of the solution properties of electrolytes in subsequent chapters.

VI. References

1. Lewis GN and Randall M: *Thermodynamics*. New York, McGraw-Hill, 1923, p. 255.
2. Lewis GN and Randall M: *Thermodynamics*. 2d ed. Revised by Pitzer KS and Brewer L. New York, McGraw-Hill, 1961.
3. Lewis GN and Randall M: *Thermodynamics*. New York, McGraw-Hill, 1923, p. 373.
4. Latimer WM: *The Oxidation States of the Elements and Their Potentials in Aqueous Solution*, 2d ed. Englewood Cliffs, NJ, Prentice-Hall, 1952.
5. Harned HS and Owen BB: *The Physical Chemistry of Electrolyte Solutions*, 3d ed. Princeton, NJ, Van Nostrand Reinhold, 1958.
6. Zografi G, Patel P, and Weiner NJ: *Pharm Sci.* 53: 545, 1964.

VII. Homework Problems

1. Search for and insert information in the blank spaces.

Name	Formula	Acid or Base or Salt	*i*	*q*
Sodium chloride	NaCl	Salt	2	1
Glucose	______	______	______	______
Calcium chloride	______	______	______	______
Sulfuric acid	______	______	______	______
Aluminum sulfate	______	______	______	______
Sodium calcium phosphate	______	______	______	______
Sodium dihydrogen phosphate	______	______	______	______
Sodium monohydrogen phosphate	______	______	______	______
Glycine	______	______	______	______
Morphine	______	______	______	______
Morphine sulfate	______	______	______	______
Sodium bicarbonate	______	______	______	______
Cefazolin sodium	______	______	______	______
Acetaminophen	______	______	______	______
Penicillin G	______	______	______	______
Penicillin GK	______	______	______	______
Potassium citrate	______	______	______	______

2. Calculate how many grams (g) of zinc chloride ($ZnCl_2$) are to be used to prepare 5 L of a mouthwash containing 0.1% of $ZnCl_2$.
3. A pharmacist is asked to prepare a solution containing 10 million units (U) of penicillin K per 20 mL. How many units of the drug will 0.50 mL of the solution contain?
4. How many milligrams (mg) of a drug should be used to prepare 5 L of an 0.01% solution of the drug?
5. To fill the following prescription, how many grams of zinc sulfate are needed?

Zinc sulfate (cryst.)	½%
Purified water qs	60 mL

6. (*a*) If 2.5 mEq of calcium (Ca^{2+}) is ordered to be dispensed to a patient, calculate the amount in milligrams (mg) of calcium chloride dihydrate needed (mol wt of $CaCl_2 \bullet 2H_2O = 147$) to prepare the above solution. (*b*) If $CaCl_2 \bullet 2H_2O$ is unavailable but $CaCl_2$ anhydrous is available (mol wt $CaCl_2$ anhydrous = 111), what would be the necessary amount of the anhydrous form to provide 2.5 mEq?
7. A physician's prescription for a patient weighing 110 lb calls for 500 mL of a sterile injectable solution containing 0.25 mEq of potassium chloride (KCl) per kilogram of body weight. How many milliliters of a sterile solution containing 50 mEq of KCl/10 mL should be used to prepare this order?
8. How many grams of sodium bicarbonate ($NaHCO_3$, mol wt = 84) are needed to provide 25 mEq of the bicarbonate ion?
9. Five milliliters of lithium carbonate (Li_2CO_3, mol wt = 74) syrup contains the equivalent of 8 mEq of Li^+. Calculate in milligrams the amount of Li_2CO_5 in each 5 mL dose of the syrup.
10. How many milliequivalents of Mg^{2+} ion are in 1 teaspoonful (5 mL) of a 2% solution of $MgCl_2$ (mol wt = 95.3)?
11. How many grams of K_2SO_4 (mol wt = 174) are needed to prepare a 240 mL solution containing 1 mEq/mL of K^+?
12. A solution of sucrose (mol wt of 342) is prepared by dissolving 0.5 g in 100 g of water. Compute (*a*) the weight percent, (*b*) the molality, and (*c*) the mole fraction of sucrose and of water in the solution.
13. An aqueous solution of glycerin, 7.00% by weight, is prepared. The solution is found to have a density of 1.0149 g/cm^3 at 20°C. The molecular weight of glycerin is 92.0473. What are the molarity and molality of glycerin in this solution?
14. What is the van't Hoff *i* factor for an acetic acid solution having a degree of dissociation of 3%?
15. Calculate the osmolality of a solution containing 0.9 g of NaCl (mol wt = 58.5) in 100 g of water.
16. What is the osmolarity of a solution that contains 0.02 *M* $CaCl_2$, 0.02 *M* NaCl, and 0.005 *M* dextrose?
17. What is the normality of a 25.0 mL solution of hydrochloric acid that neutralizes 20.0 mL of a 0.50 *N* sodium hydroxide solution?
18. How many grams of Na_2SO_4 (mol wt of 142) are required to make 1.2 L of an 0.5 *N* solution?
19. What is the number of equivalents per mole, or *q* value, for HCl, Na_2HPO_4, $Ba(OH)_2$, and $Fe_2(SO_4)_3$?
20. (*a*) What are the *q* values for the sodium, aluminum, and sulfate content, respectively, in the anhydrous $NaAl(SO_4)_2$ (mol wt = 242)? (*b*) Calculate the milliequivalents of aluminum content in 0.5 g of this salt.
21. If normal human plasma contains about 3 mEq/L of the hydrogen phosphate ion HPO_4^{2-}, how many milligrams of dibasic potassium phosphate, K_2HPO_4 (mol wt of 174), per liter of solution should be used to supply the needed HPO_4^{2-} for an electrolyte replacement in the hospital?
22. A solution contains 0.05 *M* $AlCl_3$ and 0.2 *M* Na_2HPO_4. What is the ionic strength of this solution?

23. What is the ionic strength of a solution containing 0.03 *M* NaH_2PO_4, 0.01 *M* Na_2HPO_4, 0.1 *M* NaCl, and 0.005 *M* glucose?
24. A solution contains 0.003 *M* sodium phenobarbital, 0.20 *M* sodium acetate, and 0.30 *M* acetic acid. Acetic acid is a weak acid that has a degree of dissociation of 0.008 in this solution. What is the ionic strength of the solution?
25. What is the *ionic activity coefficient* for Ca^{2+} in a solution containing 0.005 *M* $CaCl_2$ and 0.145 *M* NaCl?

    $$\log \gamma_i = -0.509 Z_i^2 \mu^{1/2} / (1 + \mu^{1/2})$$

26. Compute the mean ionic activity coefficient of 0.01 *M* sodium diphenylhydantoin in an aqueous solution containing 0.01 *m* KCl at 25°C.
27. What is the mean ionic activity coefficient of epinephrine HCl in a solution containing 0.05 *M* of the drug and 0.05 *M* KCl?
28. (*a*) What concentration of $CaCl_2$ should be added to an 0.02 *M* solution of neomycin sulfate to produce an ionic strength of 0.09? (*b*) Calculate the mean ionic activity and mean ionic activity coefficient for 0.02 *M* neomycin sulfate at an ionic strength of 0.09 and 25°C.

Colligative Properties and Isotonic Solutions

CHAPTER 2

The ingredients information given to consumers by the maker of a sterile eyedrop contains the substances listed in the box below. This information is probably overlooked by most consumers, but perhaps not by students who are learning the principles of physical pharmacy. Why are these substances, excluding the active ingredient tetrahydrozoline HCl, necessary for this formulation? And what are the quantities or concentrations of these added compounds? We shall answer these questions at the end of this chapter.

Formulation of a Sterile Eyedrop

Tetrahydrozoline HCl (0.05%)
Purified water
Sodium chloride
Boric acid
Sodium borate
Benzalkonium chloride (0.01%)
Edetate disodium (0.1%)

Pharmaceutical dosage forms contain nonmedicinally active agents, commonly referred to as *pharmaceutical excipients*. These agents are used for a variety of purposes, including maintaining the tonicity of the body fluids and achieving a desired drug delivery, designed to provide efficacious, nontoxic, and aesthetically appealing medications. This chapter presents an overview of common dosage forms based on drug delivery considerations and the properties of drugs. The focus of discussion is then placed on solutions and the solution properties that allow the dosage form to be compatible with the biological system. There are four properties of solutions that depend on the nature and the mole fraction of the solvent, but not on any of the properties of the solutes. They are known as the *colligative properties*. As we shall see, these properties play an important role in pharmaceutical solution preparations because, by the dependence on the number of particles of the solutes, they provide a method for determining this number from a measured value of one of the colligative properties. This datum then allows the quantity of each solute (or ingredient) to be determined for the preparation of an isotonic solution.

CHAPTER OUTLINE

OBJECTIVES

1. Understand the various types of pharmaceutical dosage forms.
2. Demonstrate an understanding of colligative properties of solutions and their application in the determination of the molecular weights of drugs.
3. Predict colligative property change based on the amount of drug present and its type (electrolytes, nonelectrolyte, or weak electrolyte).
4. Perform accurate calculations for the preparation of isotonic solutions, using methods derived from the principles of colligative properties of solutions.

I. Pharmaceutical Dosage Forms and Drug Delivery Considerations

A *pharmaceutical dosage form* is a preparation that functions as a vehicle for the administration of medication in a measured amount. Dosage forms contain various agents that are medicinally inactive, often referred to as the pharmaceutical excipients. It is these agents and the choice of dosage form that result in the development of efficacious and safe pharmaceutical products, and it is through these agents and forms that a desired drug delivery is achieved to improve the drug's therapeutic effect. Thus, it is clear that the dosage form is a determining factor of drug efficacy, and that generically or chemically equivalent drugs may not necessarily be bioequivalent because of dosage form variations. The most commonly used method of drug delivery is through either a solid or a liquid formulation. The principles involved in such a formulation closely parallel the chemical properties of drugs in solutions. Thus, as an introduction to pharmaceutical formulation, a brief discussion of the solid and solution dosage forms is provided below; more detailed discussion is given in later chapters.

Solid Dosage Forms

It is as effective as it is natural that most drugs can be delivered using oral dosage forms that include solutions, coarse dispersions (suspensions and emulsions), and solid forms. The basic strategy in dosage form design is to achieve the desired drug absorption pattern through the control of drug release from the dosage form to the biological fluid at the site of absorption. Solid dosage forms including tablets and capsules can be made for *immediate release* or *controlled release* of the drug. In the conventional immediate-release dosage forms, tablets or granules containing the drug are prepared with a wetting agent to allow rapid contact with water. The rate of drug dissolution from the dosage form in the gastrointestinal (GI) tract usually follows Fick's law of diffusion, a kinetic process that predicts the rate of drug release based on the solubility of the drug and the particle size of the drug material. It is well established that drug release from the dosage form in the GI tract gives a positive correlation with the drug's bioavailability, as indicated by the plasma concentration–time curve, and its measurable biological activity. The aqueous solubility of a drug is thus a key factor in formulation considerations, regardless of the state (liquid, solid, etc.) of the dosage form. Also note that the absorption of drugs in various segments of the GI tract is taken up by the hepatic portal vein that perfuses the liver. Oral delivery of drug is thus subjected to the first-pass hepatic metabolic effect. There are, however, small tablets designed for sublingual absorption, which bypass the GI tract for fast action. These tablets, such as those of nitroglycerin, are flat and oval shaped, and they dissolve rapidly when placed beneath the tongue.

The term *controlled release* represents a broad concept of dosage form design, with the intention to bring a more specific drug delivery when compared to conventional approaches. In solid dosage forms, both the *delayed-release* and the *extended-release* products have been met with great preference for their use as therapeutic products. The enteric coated aspirin tablet, e.g., is a delayed-release product which has an acid-resistant coating that prevents drug release in the gastric fluid, so that the drug release is delayed until it reaches the intestinal fluid, which has an alkaline pH. In comparison, the omeprazole delayed-release capsules consist of enteric coated granules that are acid-labile, allowing the drug to be released in the stomach for the treatment of duodenal ulcer. The extended-release dosage form is a system that can be used to reduce the dosing frequency of a drug compared to the use of a conventional (immediate-release) dosage form. Many drugs with relatively high solubility in water are short-acting and require multiple daily dosing to achieve the desired therapeutic results. When the dosing schedule is not followed, the resulting plasma–concentration curve may reflect a less than optimum drug therapy, as indicated by concentrations that either exceed the minimum toxic level or fall below the minimum therapeutic level. As illustrated in **Figure 2-1,** for an immediate-release dosage form, multiple doses at prescribed time intervals are usually required to achieve a steady-state plasma concentration. If a dose is missed, there will be a delay in achieving the desired plasma level. The extended-release product typically provides an immediate release of drug, which promptly produces the desired therapeutic effect, followed by a gradual and continual release of additional amounts of drug to maintain the effect over a predetermined time. Such a dosage form enhances patient compliance and is especially applicable to drugs used for the treatment of chronic conditions. The proprietary extended-release dosage forms have been developed using a number of pharmaceutical techniques including particle coating, as in the formulation of metoprolol, and the hydrophilic eroding matrix, as in the formulation of quinidine sulfate and morphine sulfate products. It is worth noting that a hydrophilic matrix made from the use of a hydrophilic polymer, such as hydroxypropyl methylcellulose, works as a barrier for drug release in two ways. In gastric fluid, upon wetting, the hydrophilic matrix forms a gel layer around the surface of the tablet, which increases in thickness with time as water permeates. Drug is released from tablet via diffusion through the gel layer. As the polymer becomes fully hydrated, it is eroded from the tablet core, allowing more drug release from the tablet. In this design, the rate of drug release is controlled by the processes of diffusion and tablet erosion.

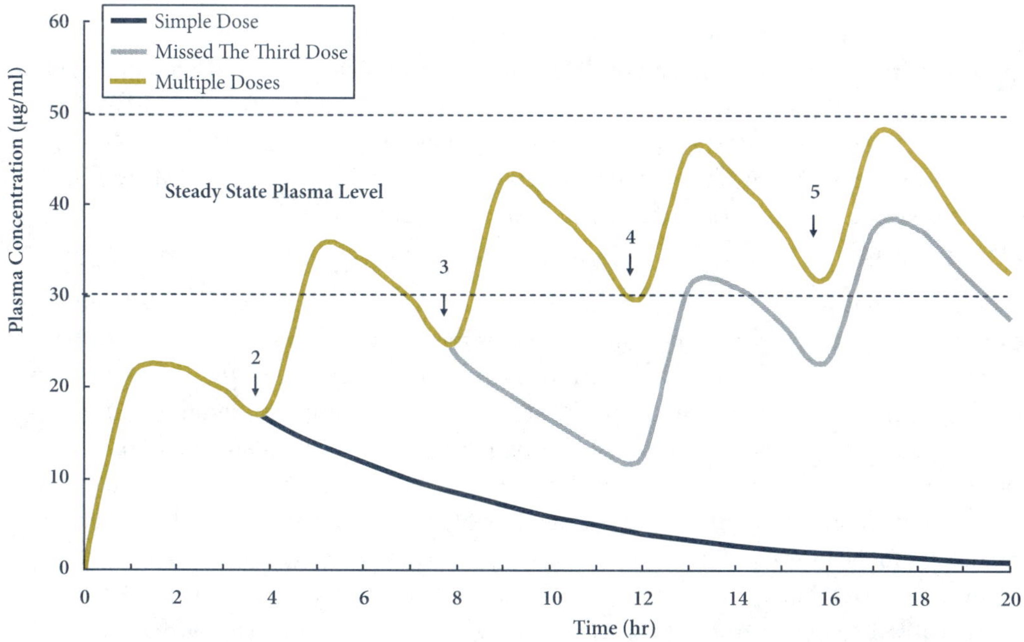

Figure 2-1 Plasma drug concentration versus time profiles: (*A*) a single oral dose, (*B*) multiple oral doses, and (*C*) the result of missing third dose in the multidosing regimen.

Solution Dosage Forms

The term *solution* is usually used to indicate a true solution, which is defined as a mixture of two or more components that form a homogeneous system in which the components are dispersed at the molecular level. In comparison, coarse dispersions, such as pharmaceutical suspensions and emulsions, show distinct separation of phases due to the presence of particles or liquid droplets with diameters greater than 500 nm. These are known as the *polyphasic systems*. Between true solution and the polyphasic system lies the colloidal dispersion, which contains particles in sizes of 1–500 nm. Certain colloidal dispersions may be classified as a true solution or a heterogeneous system depending on the concentrations and molecular aggregations of the dispersed phase. For example, many amphiphilic compounds, which are of pharmaceutical importance, form aggregates of molecules or ions of relatively small size and mass in an aqueous medium. At low concentrations they exist in true solutions, but at sufficiently high concentration, these molecules or ions associate to form micelles, known as *micellar colloids*.

The aqueous solution, which is applicable to nearly all routes of drug delivery except the intrapulmonary system, is much more versatile than the solids as a drug delivery system. There are, however, serious challenges in the development of a solution dosage form due to the poor solubility and chemical instability of many drugs in the aqueous system and the sterility requirement of solutions used for parenteral drug delivery. The solubility property of a drug affects not only the quantity of the drug that can be incorporated into a dosage form, but also the drug's bioavailability and biological activity (detailed discussion of drug solubility is given later). For oral drug delivery, the solubility concern may be partially overcome by using mixed solvent systems containing ethanol and/or propylene glycol in water, or pharmaceutical emulsions that enhance the solubility of water-insoluble drugs. As a historical note, the Sumerian clay tablets of the third millennium BC (University Museum, University of Pennsylvania) have shown us that *beer* was frequently used for the dispersion of pulverized seeds, herbs, and roots of medicinal plants. One suspects that the use of small alcohols to enhance the solubility of organic compounds was well known then, and that the mixed solvent system is, perhaps, the oldest known dosage form for the delivery of medicinal agents.

The most common reactions leading to drug degradation in solutions is the hydrolysis of organic acid derivatives. Hydrolysis is further subjected to specific acid and/or base catalysis, thus making pH an important factor in understanding the stability issue when formulating a solution dosage form. For example, procaine, an ester of *p*-amino benzoic acid and diethylaminoethanol, is notoriously unstable in alkaline pH due to the specific base-catalyzed hydrolysis. The maximum stability of the drug occurs in the pH range of 3.5–4.5. Hence, for the formulation of a solution, procaine hydrochloride, which is soluble in an acidic environment, is usually used. Many oral liquids are also made as reconstituted suspensions to circumvent problems associated with drug stability in solutions.

An important consideration for the preparation of pharmaceutical solutions intended for delivery of drugs through the ocular and parenteral routes is the compatibility of the solution with the biological fluids. The nature of blood serum and interstitial fluids reveals that the environment in which cells and tissue are bathed is an electrolyte solution made up largely of sodium chloride. The normal functioning of the cells demands that the composition and the total number of molecules and ions of these fluids be relatively constant. Although regulatory mechanisms exist to maintain this constancy, it can be disrupted by disease states or by the administration of solution that is incompatible with the biological fluid. Some solution properties, such as the osmotic pressure, depend only on the total number of molecules and ions, but not on the chemical nature of the constituents. It is these properties that are seen to provide a balance between intracellular and extracellular fluids and hence are the focus of discussion for this chapter.

II. Colligative Properties of Solutions

In the discussion of the colligative properties of solutions, it is important to realize that these properties depend on the chemical nature of the solvent and its mole fraction in the solution, but not on any of the properties of the solute. The solvent-specific properties for the liquid solution system include the liquid–vapor phase equilibrium, commonly indicated by vapor pressure, and osmosis, a phenomenon of solvent migration across a semipermeable membrane that allows only the solvent but not the solute molecules to pass through. The latter is measured as the osmotic pressure. To provide clarity to the description of these phenomena, the colligative properties are discussed first in nonelectrolyte solutions and then in electrolyte solutions, using a two-component system.

Vapor Pressures of Solutions

The liquid–vapor equilibrium of a solution can be best understood using the concept of *ideal* solution. It is known from *Dalton's law* for ideal gases that the total pressure of a gaseous solution is equal to the sum of the pressures of the components based on the kinetic molecular theory of noninteracting molecules. As liquids exist only because of molecular interactions, no such "ideal" liquid solutions can be expected in the same sense as an ideal gas solution. Some solutions, however, behave in a simple way and may be considered as ideal solutions. The classical example of a nearly ideal solution is the benzene–toluene system **(Figure 2-2),** which shows that, in equilibrium, the total vapor pressure and the partial vapor pressure for each component are linearly related to the composition of the components expressed in mole fractions.[1] This linear relationship for each component, which is the primary characteristic of an ideal solution, can be written as

$$P_a = X_a P_a^o \qquad P_b = X_b P_b^o \qquad \text{(Raoult's law)}$$

$$\text{and } P = P_a + P_b \qquad \text{(Dalton's law)} \qquad (2\text{-}1)$$

where P_a and P_b are the partial vapor pressures of components *a* and *b* above a solution, X_a and X_b are the mole fractions of *a* and *b*, P_a^o and P_b^o are the original vapor pressures of the pure components *a* and *b*, and *P* is the total vapor pressure of the solution. Solutions that obey Equations (2-1) and have vapor pressure diagrams similar to Figure 2-2 are said to conform to *Raoult's law*. Other systems such as carbon tetrachloride–silicon tetrachloride and chlorobenzene–bromobenzene also show similar and simple behavior. This has led to the generalization that *simplicity* (or ideality) of solution behavior can be expected from components that are similar in *molecular size* and in *intermolecular interactions*. These stipulations imply that the energy required to break the *a–a*, *b–b*, and *a–b* interactions is the same or similar, therefore resulting in zero heat of mixing, and the solution volume is the sum of the component volumes.

The vapor pressure–composition diagrams for nonideal solutions are usually classified as having either a minimum or a maximum in the total vapor pressure–composition curve, compared to the predicted total vapor pressure curve using Raoult's law **(Figure 2-3).** The chloroform–acetone system, e.g., exhibits lowered total vapor pressure compared to the sum of the vapor pressures of the two components.[2] A simple explanation of this phenomenon is that the intermolecular interaction, through hydrogen bonding between the carbonyl group of acetone and the slightly acidic hydrogen of chloroform,

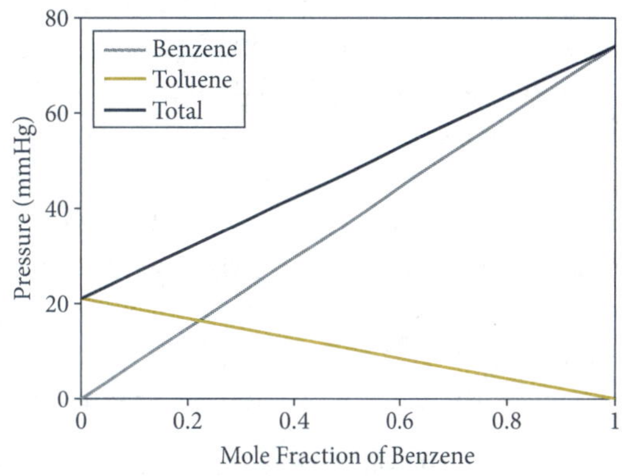

Figure 2-2 The partial and total vapor pressures for the nearly ideal solution of benzene and toluene at 20°C. Data from: B. Bell and T. Wright, *J. Phys. Chem.* 35:129, 1900.

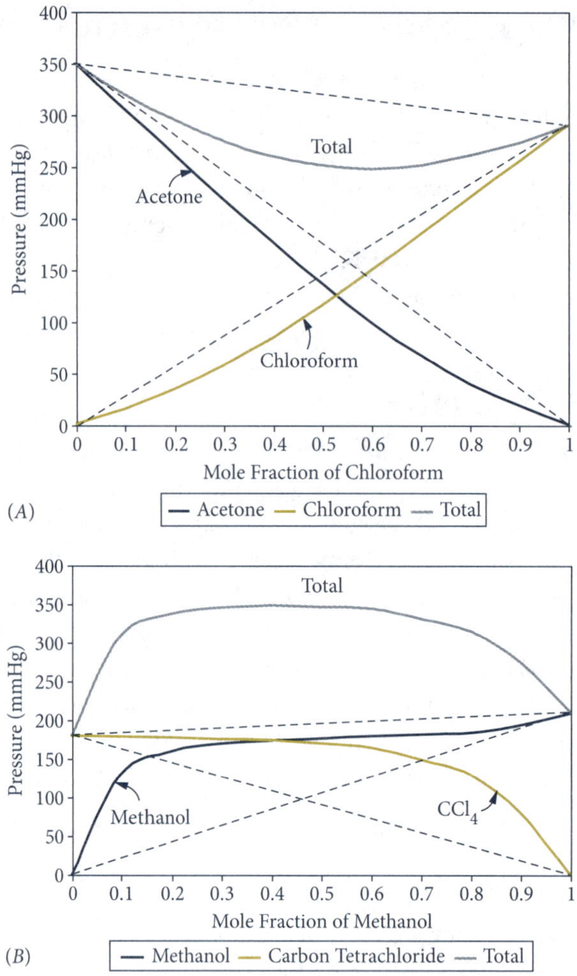

Figure 2-3 Total vapor pressure curves of nonideal solutions: (*A*) the chloroform–acetone system and (*B*) the carbon tetrachloride–methanol system at 35°C.

(*A*) Adapted from: J. von Zawidzki, *Z. Physik. Chem.* 35:129, 1900. (*B*) Adapted from: J. Timmermans, *Physico-chemical Constants of Binary Systems*, vol. 2, Interscience, New York, 1959.

$(CH_3)_2C{=}O\cdots H{-}C(Cl)_3$, is stronger than the interactions between acetone or chloroform molecules in their pure states. In such cases, heat is evolved from the solution upon mixing and thus results in a negative heat (enthalpy) of mixing. Qualitatively, one might also expect that the intermolecular interaction in solution would tend to restrict the motion of the molecules, thus giving the system less entropy than in the ideal case. Solutions that show a maximum in their total vapor pressure, such as in the carbon tetrachloride–methanol system,[3] are frequently those containing a component that is itself associated, as are small alcohols and water. In the carbon tetrachloride–methanol system, e.g., energy is required to break up some the self-association of methanol molecules, thus resulting in a positive heat of mixing. Because heat is added to the system, this enthalpy produces a free energy effect that leads to a higher total vapor pressure than in the ideal situation. These qualitative interpretations have been well tested by thermodynamic principles.

Studies of the vapor pressure–composition relationships of nonelectrolyte solutions have shown that both the concentration and the volatility of the solute contribute to solution nonideality. However, even for volatile solutes, the vapor pressure of the solvent near the two composition limits, i.e., in dilute solutions, tends to follow ideal solution behavior. In summary, an *ideal solution* is characterized by a zero heat of mixing, a solution volume that is the sum of the component volumes, and a vapor pressure–composition curve that obeys Raoult's law. Thus, in general, a solution of a nonvolatile solute in dilute concentrations may be taken as an ideal solution.

Vapor Pressure Lowering

According to Raoult's law, the partial vapor pressure of the solvent of an ideal solution is equal to the product of the mole fraction of the solvent and its vapor pressure in the pure state. For dilute solution containing a nonvolatile solute, by which the solution is deemed ideal, the partial vapor pressure of the solute P_b approaches zero. Equation (2-1) then becomes

$$P = P_a = X_a P_a^o$$

When the mole fraction of the solvent is expressed in terms of the mole fraction of the solute ($X_a = 1 - X_b$), the above equation gives

$$P = P_a^o (1 - X_b)$$

or $$P_a^o - P_a = \Delta P = P_a^o X_b \qquad (2\text{-}2)$$

The lowering of the vapor pressure, expressed as $P_a^o - P_a$, or ΔP, is thus seen, for dilute solutions, to depend only on the mole fraction of the solute and is, therefore, one of the colligative properties. It will be recalled that the mole fraction of the solute is related to the molality of solute by the equation $X_2 = m/(m + 55.5)$. Hence, for aqueous solution the vapor pressure lowering can be calculated directly using the molal concentration (m) according to the following equation:

$$\Delta P = mP_a^o/(m + 55.5) \qquad (2\text{-}3)$$

For dilute solutions where $m << 55.5$, Equation (2-3) becomes $\Delta P = mP_a^o / 55.5$.

Example 2-1: In an ideal solution containing two liquid components *a* and *b*, the mole fraction of component *a* (X_a) is 0.7. Calculate the total vapor pressure of the solution and the partial vapor pressure of the two components. The vapor pressures of pure components *a* and *b* are 22.3 and 74.7 mmHg at 20°C, respectively.

Solution: From Raoult's law (Equations (2-1)),

$$P_b = 74.7[0.3] = 22.41\ \text{mmHg}$$

$$P_a = 22.3[0.7] = 15.61\ \text{mmHg}$$

$$P = P_a + P_b = 22.41 + 15.61 = 38.02\ \text{mmHg}$$

Example 2-2: Calculate the vapor pressure lowering of a solution containing 50 g of dextrose (mol wt = 180) in 1000 g of water. The vapor pressure of water is 23.77 mmHg at 25°C.

Solution: Molality = 50 × 1000/180 × 1000 = 0.2778 mol/kg

Using Equation (2-3),

$$\Delta P = mP_a^o/(m + 55.5)$$

$$= 0.2778 \times 23.77 / (0.2778 + 55.5)$$

$$= 0.12\ \text{mmHg}$$

Boiling Point Elevation

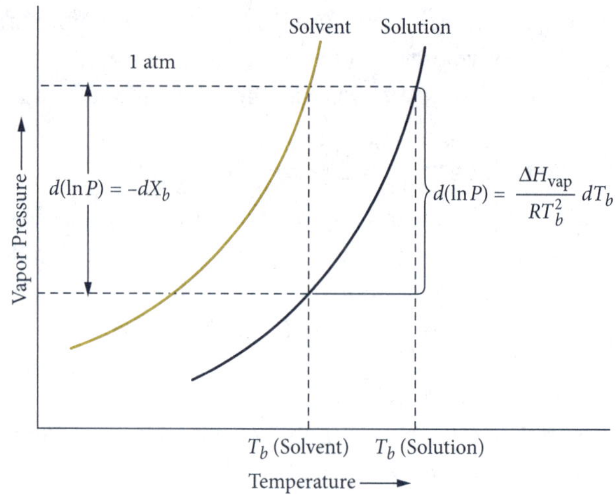

Figure 2-4 Thermodynamic expressions of vapor pressure and temperature changes in the region of the boiling point.
Adapted from: G. Barrow, *Physical Chemistry*, 2nd ed., McGraw-Hill Inc., New York, 1966.

The boiling point of a liquid is the temperature at which the vapor pressure of the liquid is equal to the external, usually atmospheric, pressure. Consider a solvent with a temperature at or near its boiling point. The addition of a nonvolatile solute, which according to Raoult's law must lower the vapor pressure of the pure solvent, thus will prevent the solution from boiling until the solution is heated to a higher temperature, at which the vapor pressure lowering by the solute is compensated by an increase in vapor pressure due to the increase in temperature. This results in a boiling point elevation. A thermodynamic explanation of the effect of solute concentration on the boiling point change may be derived from the consideration of the vapor pressure–temperature relationship coupled with the vapor pressure lowering phenomenon. The vapor pressure lowering equation $P_a^o - P_a = P_a^o X_b$ or $(P_a^o - P_a) / P_a^o = X_b$ indicates that at or near the boiling point, the addition of an infinitesimal amount of solute dX_b will result in an infinitesimal drop of vapor pressure expressed as dP/P, that is,

$$dP/P = d(\ln P) = -dX_b \tag{2-4}$$

This relationship is illustrated in **Figure 2-4**. To reach the external pressure and boiling point for a solution, the decrease in the logarithm of the vapor pressure due to the solute shown in Equation (2-4) must be counterbalanced by an increase of the same quantity through a temperature increase. Hence,

$$d(\ln P)_{solute} = -d(\ln P)_{temp} \tag{2-5}$$

The thermodynamic expression of the temperature dependence of vapor pressure is known as the *Clausius–Clapeyron relationship*, which shows that the change of vapor pressure as a function of temperature dP/dT is equal to the molar heat of vaporization ΔH_{vap} of the solution divided by the volume of the vapor V_{vap} and temperature:

$$dP/dT = \Delta H_{vap}/V_{vap}T \qquad \text{for ideal gas:} \qquad V_{vap} = RT/P$$

Assuming ideal gas conditions for the vapor, the term $d(\ln P)_{temp}$ can then be written as

$$d(\ln P)_{temp} = \frac{\Delta H_{vap}}{RT^2} dT \tag{2-6}$$

For our discussion, T is the boiling point (T_b); therefore, the combination of Equations (2-4), (2-5), and (2-6) gives the following relation:

$$dT_b = \frac{RT_b^2}{\Delta H_{vap}} dX_b \tag{2-7}$$

In Equation (2-7), dT_b is the boiling point elevation caused by dX_b solute, and R is the gas constant. For diluted solutions, the heat of vaporization for the solution is nearly identical to that of the pure solvent and is a *constant*. The boiling point elevation is therefore independent of all properties of the solute except its mole fraction in the solution. Thus, the boiling point elevation is another colligative property. The derivation of Equation (2-7) can also be achieved using a well-established thermodynamic concept that at equilibrium between two phases, such as the liquid–vapor system, the *chemical potential* μ, or partial molar free energy, of the solvent in the solution is equal to the partial molar free energy of the vapor.

For dilute solutions, the relationship between mole fraction and molality shows that

X_b = (molality of solute) (mol wt of solvent) / 1000

The common form of Equation (2-7) can thus be written as

$$\Delta T_b = \frac{RT_b^2}{\Delta H_{vap}} X_b = \left(\frac{RT_b^2\ (\text{mol wt of solvent})}{\Delta H_{vap}\ (1000)}\right) m \tag{2-8}$$

Here ΔT_b is the boiling point elevation; the expression in parentheses is known as the boiling point elevation or the ebullioscopic constant, generally noted as K_b. Thus,

$$\Delta T_b = K_b m \tag{2-9}$$

The calculated and observed values of K_b for a number of solvents are given in **Table 2-1**. Using Equation (2-8), Example 2-3 will show that for aqueous solutions, K_b has a calculated value of 0.513 deg-kg/mol.

Example 2-3: For water, T_b = 100°C, and ΔH_{vap} = 9720 cal/mol, what is the ebullioscopic constant for this solvent (mol wt = 18.02; R = 1.987 cal/mol-deg)?

Solution: Based on Equation (2-8),

$K_b = 1.987 \times (373.2)^2 \times 18.02 / 9720 \times 1000$

$= 0.513$ deg-kg/mol

Example 2-4: What is the boiling point elevation of a solution containing 50 g of dextrose (mol wt = 180.16) in 1000 g of water?

Solution: Using the value of K_b calculated above and Equation (2-9),

$\Delta T_b = 0.513 \times 50/180.16 = 0.142$°C

Table 2-1 Molal Boiling Point Elevation and Freezing Point Depression Constants at 1 atm Pressure

Solvent	T_b, °C	K_b, deg-kg/mL	T_f, °C	K_f, deg-kg/mol
Water	100.0	0.51	0.00	1.86
Benzene	80.1	2.53	5.50	5.12
Acetic acid	118.0	2.93	16.60	3.90
Ethanol	78.4	1.22		
Cyclohexane			6.50	20.00

Example 2-5: Calculate the concentration of dextrose (mol wt = 180.16), in % wt/wt expression, in a solution that produces a boiling point elevation of 0.222°C. The K_b of water is 0.513 deg-kg/mol.

Solution:

Molality of dextrose = $\Delta T_b/K_b$ = 0.222/0.513 = 0.433 mol/kg

Wt of dextrose = molality × mol wt = 0.433 × 180.16 = 78.01 g

% of dextrose in solution = 78.01 /1078 = 0.0724, or 7.24% wt/wt[†]

[†]% wt/wt = $wt_2 \times 100 / (wt_1 + wt_2)$, where 1 and 2 denote solvent and solute, respectively. For the current question, wt_1 = 1000 g; wt_2 =78.01 g.

Freezing Point Depression

The normal freezing point is the temperature at which the solid and liquid have equal vapor pressures when they are subjected to an open pressure of 1 atm. An important fact in freezing point depression is that the solid phase can also exert vapor pressure, which decreases with decreasing temperature, and this vapor pressure is unaffected by the solute in the solution, implying that the cooling of the solution will lead to the formation of the pure solid solvent rather than a solid solution. One may view the lowering of the vapor pressure of the solvent by the presence of solute as an extension of the ranges of pressure and temperature for which the liquid phase can exist. At the freezing point temperature of the pure solvent, the vapor pressure of the solution is obviously lower than that of the solid phase; i.e., the solid and liquid vapor pressures are not in equilibrium, and the system exhibits free energy that favors the liquid phase. At a temperature lower than the freezing point of the pure solvent, however, the vapor pressure of the solution will be lowered, in addition to the solute effect, by the lowering of temperature to that of the solid phase, thus reestablishing the equilibrium between solid and liquid, at which the solution freezes to yield the solid solvent.[4] This vapor pressure diagram for a solvent and solution near the freezing point at a total pressure of 1 atm is illustrated in **Figure 2-5**.

Consider points *A* and *B* in Figure 2-5, which represent the freezing points of the pure solvent and solution, respectively. The change of vapor pressure of the solid, based on the previously mentioned Clausius–Clapeyron equation, occurs via the heat of sublimation, that is, $d(\ln P)_{\text{sublimation}} = (\Delta H_{\text{sub}}/RT_f^2)\, dT_f$, with T_f being the freezing point of the pure solvent. The change of vapor pressure for the solution consists of first the lowering of vapor pressure by the solute, that is, $d(\ln P)_{\text{solute}} = -dX_b$, and then a temperature-dependent change as described in the previous section, that is, $d(\ln P)_{\text{temp}} = (\Delta H_{\text{vap}}/RT_f^2)\, dT_f$. Thus, at equilibrium,

$$d(\ln P)_{\text{sublimation}} = d(\ln P)_{\text{solute}} + d(\ln P)_{\text{temp}}$$

Together, these terms give

$$\frac{\Delta H_{\text{sub}} - \Delta H_{\text{vap}}}{RT_f^2}\, dT_f = -dX_b$$

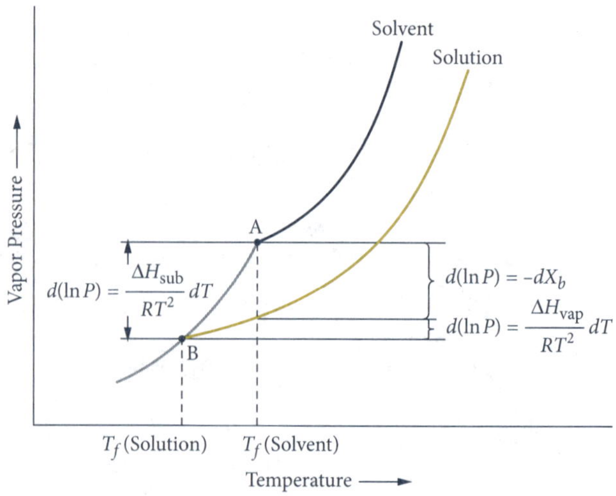

Figure 2-5 Vapor pressure diagram for a solvent and solution near the freezing point at a total pressure of 1 atm.
Adapted from: G. Barrow, *Physical Chemistry*, 2nd ed., McGraw-Hill Inc., New York, 1966.

The terms ΔH_{sub} and ΔH_{vap} can be combined to give the heat of fusion (ΔH_f) in that

$$\Delta H_f = \Delta H_{sub} - \Delta H_{vap}$$

Thus,

$$\frac{\Delta H_f}{RT_f^2} dT_f = -dX_b$$

or $$dT_f = -\frac{RT_f^2}{\Delta H_f} dX_b \tag{2-10}$$

Because the freezing point depression dT_f depends only on the properties of the solvent and the mole fraction of the solute, Equation (2-10) attests to the fact that the freezing point depression is a colligative property. The negative sign in Equation (2-10) indicates a lowering of the freezing point. The common form of Equation (2-10) is

$$\Delta T_f = \left(\frac{RT_f^2 \text{ (mol wt of solvent)}}{1000\ \Delta H_f}\right) m = K_f m \tag{2-11}$$

where ΔT_f is a positive value. The expression in parentheses is called the *freezing point depression* or *cryoscopic constant* (K_f), which can be calculated based on the molecular weight, heat of fusion, and freezing point of the pure solvent (see Example 2-6). For aqueous solutions, K_f = 1.86 deg-kg/mol.

Example 2-6: What is the K_f value for water?

Solution: From the *Handbook of Chemistry and Physics*, T_f = 0°C or 273.2 K and ΔH_f = 1437 cal/mol. Using R = 1.987 cal/mol-deg and mol wt of 18.02,

$$K_{f,\text{water}} = 1.987 \times (273.2)^2 \times 18.02 / 1000 \times 1437$$
$$= 1.860 \text{ deg-kg/mol}$$

Example 2-7: Calculate the freezing point depression of a solution containing 50 g dextrose (mol wt = 180.16) in 1000 g of water.

Solution: $\Delta T_f = K_f m$ = 1.86(50/180.16) = 0.516°C

Osmotic Pressure

The phenomenon of osmosis depends on the existence of semipermeable membranes characterized by the fact that only one of the components of a solution is allowed to pass through the membrane. Cellophane and a number of animal and protein membranes, e.g., are permeable to water but not higher-molecular-weight compounds. The mechanism by which a semipermeable membrane may operate varies. In some cases the membrane seems to act simply as a mechanical sieve, letting small molecules such as water through but preventing the passage of larger molecules. Other membranes do not pass or reject molecules based on size, but exhibit chemical properties that lead to the passage of one component but not others. An example of such a semipermeable membrane is the palladium foil, which is permeable to hydrogen but not to nitrogen and other gases based on the fact that hydrogen, but not other gases, dissolves and dissociates at the palladium surface and reunites into molecules after passage through the solid lattice. In any

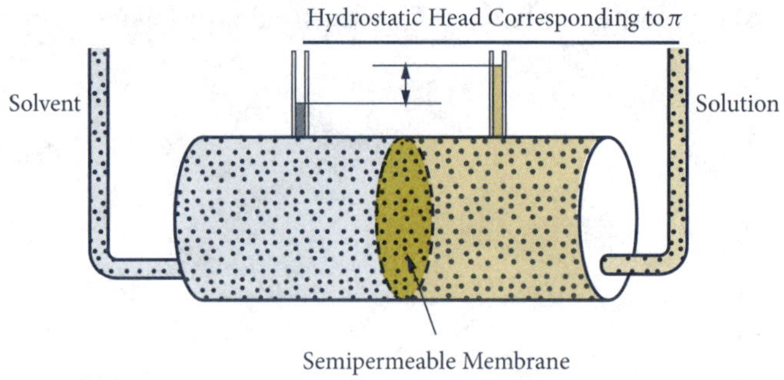

Figure 2-6 The schematic osmotic pressure apparatus.
Adapted from: R. M. Fuoss and D. J. Mead, *J. Phys. Chem.* 47:59, 1943.

case, it is important to point out that as long as a membrane is available that will pass the solvent but not the solute, osmosis can be studied, and the process by which osmosis is accomplished is immaterial.

In a two-chamber system containing the solvent and a solution separated by a semipermeable membrane, there is a natural tendency for the solvent to flow from the pure solvent chamber through the membrane into the solution chamber, and this tendency can be opposed by applying pressure to the solution chamber. As shown in the schematic osmotic pressure apparatus (**Figure 2-6**) of Fuoss and Mead,[5] this balancing pressure is indicated by the hydrostatic head that corresponds to the pressure at equilibrium, and it is called the *osmotic pressure* π.

Is osmotic pressure a colligative property? Before this question is answered, there is, perhaps, a need for a small digression to introduce an important thermodynamic concept on chemical equilibrium. The term *free energy change* (ΔG) is a measure of the useful work that might be obtained from a process at constant temperature and pressure, in that a decrease in free energy of this process (that is, ΔG is negative) indicates a tendency of the process to proceed spontaneously. When the free energy change reaches zero, the system is at equilibrium. If ΔG is positive, the process tends to proceed spontaneously in the opposite direction. The relation of free energy to equilibrium can be seen from the following examples. Consider an ideal gas undergoing change from state 1 with a pressure of P_1 to state 2 with a pressure P_2 at constant temperature. The partial differentiation of free energy G with respect to P at constant temperature is equal to the volume V of the gas based on the gas law. One can write $dG = V\,dP$, as the temperature is constant.

For an ideal gas, P and V are related by the ideal gas law, and the integration of the equation $dG = V\,dP$ gives

$$G_2 - G_1 = nRT \ln(P_2/P_1)$$

If we define state 1 as a standard state, that is, $G_1 = G^o$ at 25°C and 1 atm, then $P_1 = 1$ atm, and subscript 2 can be dropped from P_2. The molar free energy for this gas at any state is then

$$G = G^o + RT \ln P \tag{2-12}$$

Now, we further consider a reaction involving gases A, B, C, and D according to the following reaction

$$\mathrm{A + B \rightarrow C + D}$$

The equilibrium constant K for this reaction can be obtained by measuring the pressure of each reactant and product at equilibrium, using the equation

$$K = (P_C P_D / P_A P_B)_{\text{equilibrium}}$$

Based on Equation (2-12), one can write the free energy for each gas as

$$G_A = G_A^o + RT \ln P_A \qquad G_B = G_B^o + RT \ln P_B$$
$$G_C = G_C^o + RT \ln P_C \qquad G_D = G_D^o + RT \ln P_D$$

The free energy change for the reaction can now be calculated as

$$\Delta G = G_{products} - G_{reactants} = \Delta G^o + RT \ln(P_C P_D / P_A P_B)$$

At equilibrium, $\Delta G = 0$, thus,

$$\Delta G^o = -RT \ln K \tag{2-13}$$

Equation (2-13), which relates the standard free energy change to the logarithm of the equilibrium constant, represents one of the *most important results of thermodynamics*. The obvious value of the equation is that it allows the calculation of not only the direction in which a reaction will proceed but also the equilibrium state that the reacting system will finally attain.

With the discussion given above, we can now ascertain the thermodynamic basis of the osmotic pressure. The free energy of the solvent in the solution is less than the free energy of the solvent in pure solvent because of solute-induced vapor pressure lowering. Therefore, there is a spontaneous tendency for the solvent to move from the relatively high free energy state of pure solvent to the relatively low free energy state of solution. This tendency is balanced by increasing the free energy of the solution by subjecting it to an externally applied pressure. The free energy lowering that results from the addition of solute is given in terms of vapor pressure lowering from P^o to P; hence

$$\Delta G = \ RT \ln(P/P^o)$$

It is this free energy decrease that is balanced by the effect of the applied pressure. As has been mentioned, the dependency of free energy on pressure at constant temperature is the volume, that is, $dG/dP = V$, or $dG = V\,dP$. Because liquids are quite incompressible, the volume of solvent in the solution can be assumed to be a constant. Thus, the free energy per mole of solvent due to the applied osmotic pressure is πv (π is the osmotic pressure; v is the volume of 1 mol of solvent, or molar volume); the above equation can then be written as

$$\pi v = -RT \ln(P/P^o) \tag{2-14}$$

From Raoult's law, $P/P^o = X_a$, and for a two-component system, $X_a = 1 - X_b$. Thus,

$$\pi v = -RT \ln X_a = -RT \ln(1 - X_b) \tag{2-15}$$

This important thermodynamic result shows that the osmotic pressure is a function of the molar volume of the solvent, the temperature, and the concentration of the solution. It is therefore a colligative property.

Mathematically, one recalls that

$$-\ln(1 - X_b) = X_b + \tfrac{1}{2}X_b^2 + \cdots \approx X_b$$

The limiting value of $-\ln(1 - X_b)$ for a dilute solution is X_b. Also for dilute solutions, X_b approaches the value of the mole ratio of the solute over the solvent, i.e.,

$$X_b = n_b / (n_a + n_b) \approx n_b/n_a$$

With these relations, Equation (2-15) may be rewritten as

$$\pi v = RTX_b \qquad \text{or} \qquad \pi v n_a = RTn_b$$

The product of v and n_a gives the volume of the solvent V; hence,

$$\pi V_{\text{solvent}} = RTn_b$$

Two approximations can be made for the above expression. For aqueous solutions, water has a density of 1 g/mL. If the density of the solution is not significantly different from that of water, that is, V = kilograms of solvent, the above equation can be written as

$$\pi = n_b RT/V = mRT \tag{2-16}$$

The second approximation is that for dilute solutions; the contribution to the solution volume by the solute is negligible. In this case, the volume of the solvent is equal to the volume of the solution, thus

$$\pi = MRT \tag{2-17}$$

Equation (2-17) was first derived by van't Hoff in 1887.[6] The similarity of this expression to the ideal gas law led van't Hoff and others to the idea that the nature of the osmotic pressure may arise from a particle bombardment process. For osmotic pressure calculations, T is in kelvins (K), V is in liters, and R has a value of 0.082 L-atm/deg.

Example 2-8: Calculate the osmotic pressure of a 0.2 m solution of sucrose (mol wt = 342) at 20°C using Equations (2-14), (2-16), and (2-17). The solution has a vapor pressure of 17.475 mmHg and a density of 1.029 g/mL. The molar volume for water is 18.04 mL/mol (0.01804 L/mol), and the vapor pressure of pure water at 20°C is 17.542 mmHg.

Solution: (*a*) Using Equation (2-14), $\pi v = -RT \ln(P/P^o)$.

$$\pi = -0.082 \times 293.2 \ln(17.475/17.542) / 0.01804 = 5.10 \text{ atm}$$

(*b*) Using Equation (2-16),

$$\pi = mRT = 0.2 \times 0.082 \times 293.2 = 4.81 \text{ atm}^{\dagger}$$

(*c*) Using Equation (2-17), the solution contains 68.4 g of sucrose in 1000 g of water; thus the total wt of the solution is 1068.4 g. The density of the solution is 1.029 g/mL. Hence the volume of the solution is V = 1068.4 / 1.029 = 1038 mL.

$$\pi = MRT = 68.4 \times 1000 \times 0.082 \times 293.2 / 342 \times 1038$$
$$= 4.63 \text{ atm}^{\dagger}$$

† *Note*: The observed osmotic pressure for this solution is 5.06 atm, indicating that both approximations [Equations (2-16) and (2-17)] underestimate the osmotic pressure of the solution.

Colligative Properties of Electrolytes

It was recognized by Jacobus van't Hoff that the electrolyte colligative behavior could conveniently be obtained by modifying the colligative property equations for nonelectrolytes with a factor, known as the van't Hoff i factor. As discussed earlier, this factor derives from the dissociation of

Table 2-2 Degree of Dissociation for Hydrochloric Acid at 25°C

Concentration N	Λ, mho-cm²/Eq	α	$i\,[= 1 + \alpha(2 - 1)]$
0	(426.16)	1.0	
0.001	421.36	0.99	1.99
0.005	415.80	0.98	1.98
0.01	412.00	0.97	1.97
0.05	399.09	0.94	1.94
0.10	391.32	0.92	1.92

Table 2-3 Expressions of Colligative Properties

Colligative Property	Equation (Unit)	Constant for Aqueous System
Vapor pressure lowering	$\Delta P = imP^o\,/\,(m + 55.5)^{\dagger}$	P^o: constant at a given temperature
Boiling point elevation	$\Delta T_b = imK_b$ (°C)	$K_b = 0.513$ deg-kg/mol
Freezing point depression	$\Delta T_f = imK_f$ (°C)	$K_f = 1.860$ deg-kg/mol
Osmotic pressure	$\pi = imRT$ (atm)	$R = 0.082$ L-atm/mol-deg

† If $m << 55.5$, $\Delta P = imP^o/55.5$; the unit of vapor pressure is mmHg (torr).

electrolytes into ions, with i equal to the number of ions generated per molecule. Experimentally, i values can be determined via measurement of the solution equivalent conductance Λ, which, when compared to the equivalent conductance of solution at infinite dilution Λ_o, gives the degree of dissociation α, $\alpha = \Lambda/\Lambda_o$. With the value of α, i can then be determined. An example of this determination is shown in **Table 2-2**. These data indicate that for strong electrolytes, such as hydrochloric acid, in dilute solutions, there is a nearly complete ionization.

In summary, the colligative behavior of solutes applies to both nonelectrolyte and electrolyte solutions. **Table 2-3** summarizes the equations for the determination of the colligative properties. The concentration dependency of the colligative properties can now be attributed to the osmolality rather than the molality of the solution. Osmolality is equal to the value of i times molality. For electrolytes, i is the number of ions generated per molecule, and for nonelectrolytes i may be taken as 1. For weak electrolytes, i may be calculated via determination of the degree of ionization, when necessary. It should be mentioned that osmolality is a solution property, which, in solutions containing more than one solute, is equal to the sum of osmolalities of all solutes.

Example 2-9: The osmotic pressure of a dilute solution of KNO_3 in water is 357 mmHg when measured against water at 25°C. What would be the vapor pressure at 25°C (the vapor pressure of pure water is 23.756 mmHg at this temperature), the boiling point, and freezing point of the solution?

Solution: The common factor for all colligative properties is the osmolality of the solution. From the information of the osmotic pressure†

$$im = \pi/RT = 357\,/\,760 \times 0.082 \times 298.2 = 0.0192\ \text{osmol/L}$$

Thus,

$$\Delta P = imP^o\,/\,(im + 55.5) = 0.0192 \times 23.756\,/\,55.5 = 0.008\ \text{mmHg}$$

$P_{solution} = P^o - \Delta P = 23.756 - 0.008 = 23.748$ mmHg

$\Delta T_b = imK_b = 0.0192 \times 0.513 = 0.01$°C

The boiling point of the solution will be 100.01°C.

$\Delta T_f = imK_f = 0.0192 \times 1.86 = 0.036$°C

The freezing point of this solution will be –0.036°C.

[†]The osmotic pressure has a unit of atm; 1 atm = 760 mmHg.

Application of Colligative Properties

The colligative behavior of solutes in solution is an important concept that must be recognized in the preparation of pharmaceutical solutions for parenteral use or for delivery of drugs to soft tissues. This application is discussed in the next section. The principal use of the colligative concept in chemistry is to determine the molecular weights, based on the fact that for a nonelectrolyte

m = wt of drug × 1000 / (mol wt of drug) (wt of solvent)

The determination of the concentration, molality, depends on not only the accuracy of measurement of the colligative property but also the sensitivity that the method provides for such a determination. This is especially true in the determination of compounds with large molecular weights. To maintain dilute solution conditions, the solutions that can be prepared may exhibit insufficient molalities to produce a measurable effect, as can be seen from the calculations shown in Example 2-10.

Example 2-10: A new peptide drug has an estimated molecular weight of about 10,000 daltons. For accurate determination of the molecular weight, which one of the colligative properties would provide the best sensitivity for such a measurement using a solution containing 1 g of the drug in 100 g of water at 25°C? The density of the solution is 1.01 g/mL. The vapor pressure of pure water at 25°C is 23.77 mmHg. The density of mercury is 13.5462 g/mL.

Solution: Estimated molality for this drug = 1 × 1000 / 10,000 × 100
= 0.001 m

$\Delta P = imP^o / 55.5 = 0.001 \times 23.77 / 55.5 = 0.0004$ mmHg

$\Delta T_b = imK_b = 0.001 \times 0.513 = 0.0005$°C

$\Delta T_f = imK_f = 0.001 \times 1.860 = 0.0019$°C

$\pi = imRT = 0.001 \times 0.082 \times 298.2 = 0.0245$ atm[†]

The results show that the osmotic pressure measurement is most sensitive for the determination of molecular weights of macromolecules.

[†]0.0245 atm is equal to 18.58 mmHg or 249.2 mm solution based on the following conversion factors: 1 atm = 760 mmHg (or torr) and mm solution = mmHg × $d_{Hg} / d_{solution}$.

Although several devices exist, the determination of the boiling point elevation remains unpopular. The principal difficulty in accurately determining the boiling point elevation stems from the fact that it is the temperature of the boiling liquid and not the temperature of the refluxing vapor that must be measured. It is, therefore, necessary to arrange the apparatus so that the thermometer is drenched with representative samples of the solution and is not at the condensing vapor. As a result, it is difficult to obtain high precision with the measurement of boiling point elevation. The freezing point depression can usually be measured much more easily and accurately than can the boiling point elevation. The fact that the value of K_f, in the aqueous system, is more than 3 times that of K_b indicates that the freezing point depression method has a greater sensitivity than boiling point elevation for the determination of concentrations and molecular weights. Since the introduction of the Beckmann method, where the freezing point is determined by immersing the solution in a bath fixed at temperature several degrees below the expected freezing point of the solution, followed by temperature measurement of the cooling solution at the solid–solution equilibrium, new temperature-sensing devices have been introduced for freezing point determinations with great precision. Modern osmometers using the freezing point depression concept allow determination of the concentration as low as a few milliosmoles per kilogram of water using microliter-size samples. These instruments are ideal for molecular weight determinations, clinical use involving measurements of biological fluids, and formulations of pharmaceutical products.

The advancement of membrane technology has also led to the development of membrane osmometers for precise measurement of osmotic pressure. The principal use of osmotic pressure measurements is in the determination of the molecular weight of macromolecules such as pharmaceutical polymers and proteins. Solutions of high-molecular-weight compounds will have low-molecular concentrations even though they may be quite concentrated in terms of the weight of the solute. That the osmotic pressure produced by these solutions can be accurately measured makes it the most suitable of the colligative properties for the study of these compounds. It is recalled that Equation (2-16) is an approximation, which, for convenience, can be easily converted to the following expression using the definition of molality:

$$\pi / C = RT / \text{mol wt of solute}$$

where C is the concentration of solute in grams per milliliter. This approximation is only valid and accurate when the solution is at infinite dilution. One can achieve this by measuring π/C as a function of C and extrapolating the results to infinite dilution, so that the value of π/C at zero concentration C can be determined for the calculation of the molecular weight.[7] This application is shown in Example 2–11.

Example 2-11: The following table shows the osmotic pressure of polyisobutylene solutions in cyclohexane and benzene at 25°C.[7] What is the molecular weight of this compound?

Concentration (g/mL)	π/C (atm-mL/g)†	
	In Benzene	**In Cyclohexane**
0.0200	0.104	0.585
0.0150	0.101	0.440
0.0100	0.099	0.30
0.0050	0.098	0.18

† Calculated from the data of P. J. Flory, *J. Am. Chem. Soc.* 65:373, 1943.

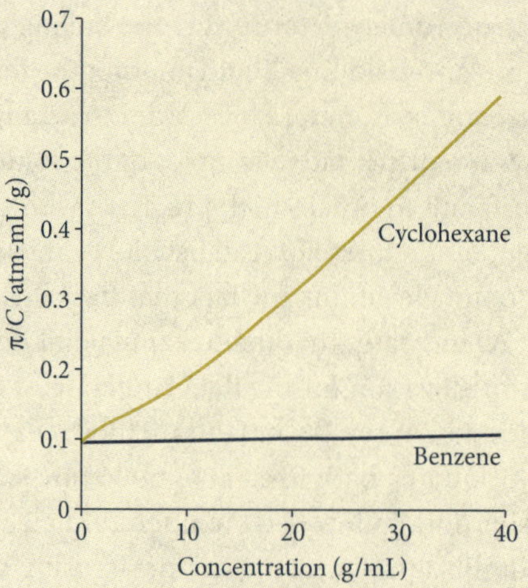

Figure 2-7 Determination of the limiting value of $RT/(\pi/C)$ for the molecular weight calculation in (*A*) benzene and (*B*) cyclohexane.

Solution: The plots of π/C versus C for both systems should yield the same limiting value when extrapolated to zero concentration (see **Figure 2-7**). From these plots, π/C at zero concentration is determined to be 0.097 atm-mL/g.

$$\text{Mol wt of polyisobutylene} = \lim_{C \to 0} RT/(\pi/C)$$
$$= 82.06 \times 298.2/0.097^{\dagger}$$
$$= 252{,}270$$

† Because C is expressed in grams per millimeter, R = 82.06 atm-mL/deg

III. Isotonic Solutions

Across the animal kingdom, the body fluids of all creatures are remarkably constant in their total osmolality, and the major component of the extracellular fluids is sodium chloride (NaCl). The body fluids have an osmotic pressure identical to that of an 0.9% solution of sodium chloride. This solution, being iso-osmotic with the biological fluids, is often referred to as an *isotonic solution*. However, the term *isotonic* implies that the solution does not produce a change in cellular constituents in the physiological system. Iso-osmoticity, in contrast, is a term used for any two liquids that have identical osmotic pressure (or other colligative properties). For instance, a solution of boric acid that is iso-osmotic with blood is not isotonic because it produces hemolysis of erythrocytes due to the ability of boric acid, regardless of its concentration, to cross the red blood cell membranes. Thus, isotonicity relates to the physiological compatibility of a solution, whereas iso-osmoticity only partially does so. Nevertheless, in pharmaceutical preparations, one can minimize cell damage by making the solutions iso-osmotic to body fluids, and thus they are referred to as isotonic solutions. Solutions with an osmotic pressure less than that of biological fluids are called *hypotonic solutions*, and those with a larger osmotic pressure are called *hypertonic solutions*.

It is well established that solutions for parenteral use or for ophthalmic and nasal applications should have the same osmoticity with that of body fluid to prevent cell or tissue damage.

Experiments have shown that when erythrocytes were introduced into a hypertonic solution (for example, 5% NaCl solution), osmosis occurred in which water from intracellular space passed through the cell membrane into the saline solution, resulting in a shrinkage of the red blood cells. This process is called *crenation*. In contrast, when erythrocytes were suspended in water, a hypotonic liquid, the extracellular water penetrated the cell membranes into the erythrocytes, producing a swelling effect and cell leakage of hemoglobin. This process is called *hemolysis*. In comparison, solutions such as normal saline solution (0.9% sodium chloride) and the solution of 5% dextrose (D5W), which are iso-osmotic to the body fluids, do not result in cell damage as described above. Hence, they are termed isotonic solutions.

Preparation of Isotonic Solutions

As a liquid drug delivery system, drugs must be prepared in a solution that is isotonic to the body fluid. This requires that a certain tonicity agent be added so that the total osmotic pressure is the same as the body fluid. Sodium chloride and dextrose are typical agents for the formulation of injectable, ophthalmic, and nasal solutions. Other compounds such as sodium acetate and boric acid have also been used as a tonicity agent. As mentioned before, boric acid can cause erythrocyte damage and is therefore not a choice for systemic drug delivery. But in ophthalmic preparations, it has been found that a buffer of alkaline pH is desirable, as most drugs used in ophthalmic preparations are weak acids, and the eye, through flow of tears, can tolerate a greater deviation from physiological pH toward alkalinity (i.e., with less irritation) than toward the acidic range. For these reasons, boric acid and its salt, sodium borate, have been used as tonicity agents for isotonic ophthalmic solutions.

For convenience, rather than actively measuring the colligative properties, a number of isotonic parameters have been defined and measured for various drugs based on the colligative concept. Because these are experimental values, which have already taken account of the solution nonideality, they can be used to calculate the amount of each ingredient needed for isotonic preparations with accuracy. These parameters include the sodium chloride equivalent (E), *freezing point depression of a 1% drug solution* ($D_{1\%}$ or $\Delta T_{f,\,1\%}$), and the *modified freezing point depression constant* L_{iso} at isotonic condition. Still, there are other expressions that aid in the calculation of isotonic requirement. For example, a *volume factor V*, defined as the milliliters of water required per gram of drug used, can also be used to make an isotonic solution. A list of these values for drugs that are included in this chapter is shown in **Table 2-4**. More extensive lists of these values may be found in standard pharmaceutical reference books.[8]

Sodium Chloride Equivalent (*E*) Method

The most basic guideline for the preparation of an isotonic solution is that an 0.9%, or 9 mg/mL, solution of NaCl is isotonic with body fluids. Both the body fluid and this 0.9% NaCl solution (known as normal saline) produce a freezing point depression of 0.52°C. Thus, in an isotonic preparation using sodium chloride to adjust the tonicity, one can calculate the amount A of NaCl needed in an equal volume of normal saline without the drug and convert the weight of a drug to an equivalent weight of sodium chloride B using the sodium chloride equivalent E value of the drug. The amount of NaCl needed for this preparation can then be determined to be the difference between A and B. The sodium chloride equivalent E is defined as the equivalent weight to sodium chloride from a unit weight of the drug. For example, if a drug has an E value of 0.12, then 1 g of the drug in a solution will contribute to the same osmolality as that of 0.12 g of NaCl. Based on the colligative property, E can be defined as

$$E_{drug} = \frac{(i_{drug})\,(\text{mol wt}_{NaCl})}{(i_{NaCl})\,(\text{mol wt}_{drug})} \qquad (2\text{-}18)$$

Table 2-4 Parameters for Isotonic Preparations†

Compound	Mol Wt	E	$D_{1\%}$	L_{iso}
Antipyrine	188.2	0.17	0.10	1.9
Atropine sulfate	694.8	0.13	0.07	5.3
Boric acid	61.8	0.50	0.29	3.5
Calcium chloride ($2H_2O$)	147.0	0.51	0.30	4.4
Chlorobutanol	177.5	0.24	0.14	2.5
Cocaine HCl	339.8	0.16	0.09	3.2
Dextrose anhydrous	180.2	0.18	0.10	
Dextrose ($1H_2O$)	198.2	0.16	0.09	1.9
Ephedrine HCl	201.7	0.30	0.18	3.6
Ephedrine sulfate	428.5	0.23	0.14	5.8
Epinephrine HCl	219.7	0.29	0.17	3.7
Homatropine HBr	356.3	0.17	0.10	3.6
Magnesium sulfate ($7H_2O$)	246.5	0.17	0.10	2.5
Metycaine HCl	292.8	0.20	0.12	3.4
Morphine HCl	375.8	0.15	0.09	3.3
Morphine sulfate	758.8	0.14	0.08	6.2
Naphazoline HCl	246.7	0.27	0.16	3.3
Neostigmine bromide	303.2	0.22	0.11	3.2
Penicillin G potassium	372.5	0.18	0.11	3.9
Phenacaine HCl	352.9	0.20	0.11	3.3
Physostigmine sulfate	648.5	0.13	0.08	5.0
Pilocarpine HCl	244.8	0.24	0.14	
Potassium chloride	74.5	0.76	0.45	3.3
Potassium iodide	166.0	0.34	0.20	3.3
Procaine HCl	272.8	0.21	0.12	3.3
Silver nitrate	169.9	0.33	0.19	3.3
Sodium borate ($10H_2O$)	381.4	0.42	0.25	9.4
Sodium chloride	58.5	1	0.58	3.4
Sodium nitrate	85.0	0.68	0.39	3.4
Tetracaine HCl	300.8	0.18	0.11	3.2
Zinc sulfate ($7H_2O$)	287.6	0.15	0.09	2.5

† Data represent values for 1% drug solution, taken from *Remington's Pharmaceutical Sciences*, 15th ed., Easton, PA, Mack Publishing Co., 1975, pp. 1408–1412.

Equation (2-18) is useful for the calculation of the E value based on the molecular weight of the drug and its ionization characteristic. For example, atropine sulfate has a molecular weight of 694.8 and an i value of 3, whereas NaCl has a molecular weight of 58.5 and an i value of 2; the calculated E value for atropine sulfate is thus $3 \times 58.5 / 2 \times 694.8 = 0.13$, which is identical to the observed value.

The calculations involved in the sodium chloride equivalent method can be summarized in simple steps as follows:

1. Determine the amount of NaCl in normal saline in a volume equal to that of the prescription order.

   $A = 9\ \text{mg/mL} \times \text{volume of Rx}$

2. Calculate the equivalent weights to NaCl B for all drug ingredients.

B = mg of drug × E_{drug}

Repeat the calculation for all drugs and express the values as $B_1, B_2, \ldots$

3. Calculate amount of NaCl needed for the prescription order C.

$C = A - B_1 - B_2 - \ldots$

Example 2-12: Calculate the amount of NaCl needed to fill the following Rx.

Rx Zinc sulfate 120 mg ($E = 0.16$)

Antipyrine 650 mg ($E = 0.17$)

NaCl qs

Distilled water qsad 60 mL

Sig: Isotonic solution for right eye, bid

Solution: The total volume of Rx is 60 mL. Thus,

$A = 9.0 \times 60 = 540.0$ mg

For zinc sulfate: $B_1 = 120 \times 0.16 = 19.2$ mg

For antipyrine: $B_2 = 650 \times 0.17 = 110.5$ mg

Amount of NaCl needed:

$C = A - B_1 - B_2 = 540.0 - 19.2 - 110.5 = 410.3$ mg

Answer: The amount of NaCl needed for this prescription is 410.3 mg.

As an important reminder, because the amount of NaCl in A is expressed in milligrams, all weights in subsequent calculations must also be in milligrams. A prescription may be written in different ways so that additional calculations may be required to arrive at the correct answer. Calculations involved in the use of an alternative tonicity agent based on the sodium chloride equivalent method are illustrated in Example 2-13. Here, the amount of the alternative agent D is calculated as the value of the amount of NaCl that would be needed, divided by the E value of the alternative tonicity agent.

Example 2-13: Show how you would prepare the following prescription.

Rx	Chlorobutanol	0.5%†	($E = 0.18$)
	Ephedrine HCl	1.0%	($E = 0.29$)
	Dextrose qs		($E = 0.16$)
	Distilled water qs	50 mL	
	Mft: Isotonic solution		
	Sig: As nose drops, u.d.		

Solution: Amount of NaCl in equal volume of normal saline is

$A = 9\,\text{mg/mL} \times 50\,\text{mL} = 450\,\text{mg}$

Equivalent weight from drugs:

$B_1 = 250\,\text{mg} \times 0.18 = 45\,\text{mg}$

$B_2 = 500\,\text{mg} \times 0.29 = 145\,\text{mg}$

Amount of NaCl that would be needed:

$C = 450 - 45 - 145 = 260\,\text{mg}$

Amount of dextrose (alternative tonicity agent) needed:

$D = 260\,\text{mg} / 0.16 = 1625\,\text{mg}$

Answer: Weigh out 250 mg of chlorobutanol, 500 mg of ephedrine HCl, and 1625 mg of dextrose; dissolve the ingredients in distilled water, and qs to 50 mL.

†0.5% or 1% in 50 mL gives a drug weight of 0.25 or 0.5 g, or 250 or 500 mg, respectively.

Often the preparation of an isotonic solution is made by using an isotonic (may be buffered) vehicle. Calculations involved in the use of an isotonic vehicle are shown in Example 2-14.

Example 2-14: How would you prepare the following prescriptions?

Rx 1	Procaine hydrochloride	0.25 g	($E = 0.22$)
	Purified water qs	50 mL	
	Mft: Isotonic with sodium chloride		
Rx 2	Procaine hydrochloride	0.25 g	($E = 0.22$)
	Sterile saline (0.9%) qs		
	Purified water qsad	50 mL	
	Mft: Isotonic solution		

Solution: For Rx 1,

Amount of NaCl needed $= 9 \times 50 - 250 \times 0.22$

$= 395\,\text{mg}$

For Rx 2, the amount of NaCl needed is the same as in Rx 1, but must be supplied by the normal saline solution. The volume of normal saline (NS) that contains 395 mg of NaCl is

$V_{NS} = 395\,\text{mg} / (9\,\text{mg/mL}) = 43.89\,\text{mL}$

Thus, to prepare Rx 2, dissolve 0.25 g of procaine HCl in 43.89 mL of normal saline and add purified water to 50 mL.

The $D_{1\%}$ Method

$D_{1\%}$ is the same expression as $\Delta T_{f,1\%}$ in other textbooks, which represents the freezing point depression caused by a drug when the solution strength is 1% wt/v. This value, when divided by K_f, gives the osmolality or osmolarity of a 1% drug solution. It will be recalled that for dilute solutions, the difference between osmolality and osmolarity is small, and they may be used interchangeably for isotonic preparations. The requirement for an isotonic solution is to exhibit a freezing point depression of 0.52°C. Thus, using D to express the freezing point depression, one can see that in the final prepared solution

$$D_{\text{tonicity agent}} = 0.52°\text{C} - D_{\text{drug1}} - D_{\text{drug2}} - \cdots$$

The freezing point depression of a drug at a prescribed strength can be determined from the $D_{1\%}$ value using the following relationship:

$$D_{\text{drug}} = \frac{D_{1\%} \times \text{wt of drug (g)} \times 100}{V_{\text{Rx}}}$$

If more than one drug is present in the solution, repeat calculations are needed for all drugs. With these values, the freezing point depression to be made up by the tonicity agent can then be determined. Using sodium chloride as the tonicity agent, it can be seen that the amount of NaCl needed is

$$\text{Wt}_{\text{NaCl}} = \frac{D_{\text{tonicity agent}}}{0.52} \times 9\,\text{mg/mL} \times V_{\text{Rx}} \tag{2-19}$$

In Equation (2-19), the calculated weight of NaCl has a unit of milligrams. The use of the $D_{1\%}$ value in isotonic preparation is shown in Example 2-15.

Example 2-15: Calculate the amount of sodium chloride needed to make 60 mL of an isotonic solution containing 0.3 g of atropine sulfate ($D_{1\%} = 0.075°\text{C}$).

Solution: $D_{\text{drug}} = 0.075 \times 0.3 \times 100 / 60 = 0.0375°$

$D_{\text{NaCl}} = 0.52 - 0.0375 = 0.4825°$

$\text{Wt}_{\text{NaCl}} = 0.4825 \times 9 \times 60 / 0.52 = 501.1\,\text{mg}$

The $D_{1\%}$ value can also be used to determine the volume of water needed to make an isotonic solution containing a given weight of the drug, when an isotonic vehicle is used. It is readily seen from the definition of $D_{1\%}$ that the percentage strength of a drug that is isotonic is equal to the value of $0.52°/D_{1\%}$. The volume of water required to make this percentage strength can thus be calculated using the following relationship:

$$V_{\text{water}} = \frac{D_{1\%} \times \text{wt of drug (g)}}{0.52} \times 100$$

The above equation is very useful in the preparation of solutions using a buffered isotonic vehicle, as Example 2-16 indicates.

Example 2-16: How would you prepare the following prescription?

Rx	Atropine sulfate	0.3 g	($D_{1\%} = 0.075°$)
	Sterile preserved water qs	60 mL	
	Mft: Isotonic with Sørensen's isotonic buffer (pH 6.8)		
	Sig: u.d.		

Solution: % of drug solution that is isotonic = (0.52 / 0.075)%

= 6.93%

Sterile preserved water needed: $V_{water} = 0.3 \times 100 / 6.93 = 4.33$ mL

Answer: Weigh out 0.3 g of atropine sulfate, dissolve the drug in 4.33 mL of sterile preserved water, and qs to 60 mL with buffered isotonic vehicle.

The L_{iso} Method

The quantity of L_{iso} is defined as the value of iK_f when the molar or molal concentration of a drug produces a freezing point depression of 0.52°C. For example, the 0.9% solution of NaCl is isotonic with body fluids and has a molar concentration of 0.154 *M*. Using the freezing point depression equation shown in Table 2-3,

$$L_{iso} = 0.52 / 0.154 = 3.38$$

Because L_{iso} is an experimental value, it measures the nonideality or the effective *i* value of a strong electrolyte or the partial ionization of a weak electrolyte at a concentration that is isotonic with the body fluid. For nonelectrolytes, L_{iso} is approximately the same as K_f. In isotonic preparations, the L_{iso} value is used to determine the freezing point depression of the drug using Equation (2-20). As can be seen, this equation allows the determination of freezing point depression based on the molal concentration of the drug, without having to consider the van't Hoff *i* factor.

$$\Delta T_f = L_{iso}\, m \tag{2-20}$$

The adjustment of tonicity using a tonicity agent can then be calculated using the same equation for the tonicity agent, or using the method described in the $D_{1\%}$ method, as illustrated in Example 2-17.

Example 2-17: Calculate the amount of NaCl needed to prepare the following order.

		L_{iso}	mol wt
Procaine hydrochloride	1%	3.4	272.8
Make isotonic with NaCl		3.4	58.5
Sterile water qs	500 mL		

Solution: The freezing point depression of the 1% procaine HCl is

$$\Delta T_{f,\,drug} = 3.4 \times 1 \times 1000 / 272.8 \times 100 = 0.125°C$$

$$D_{NaCl} = 0.52 - 0.125 = 0.395°C$$

Equation (2-20) can also be used to determine the concentration of NaCl needed by letting

$$\Delta T_{f,\,NaCl} = L_{iso} M_{NaCl}$$

Thus, $M = 0.395 / 3.4 = 0.1162\,M$.

$$Wt_{NaCl} = 0.1162 \times 58.5 \times 500 / 1000 = 3.40\text{ g}$$

Alternatively, the amount of NaCl needed can be determined using Equation (2-19):

$$Wt_{NaCl} = \frac{D_{NaCl}}{0.52} \times 9\,\text{mg/mL} \times V_{Rx}$$

$$= 0.395 \times 9 \times 500 / 0.52 = 3418\,\text{mg or } 3.42\,\text{g}$$

Now we can answer the questions posed at the beginning of this chapter. The active ingredient of the sterile eyedrops, tetrahydrozoline HCl, is a topical ocular vasoconstrictor used to alleviate local swelling and congestion. Ophthalmic solutions contain preservatives (such as benzalkonium chloride and edetate disodium) to prevent contaminations from microorganisms, and they are buffered isotonic solutions. The boric acid–sodium borate system is to provide a buffered solution with alkaline pH, which has been shown to cause little or no pain or damage to the ocular system. Studies have shown that the strength of a buffer solution, i.e., the buffer capacity, plays an important role in the preparation of ophthalmic solutions. Although the pH and buffer phenomena will be discussed later, it is clear that at relatively low buffer capacity, the eyedrops can be easily neutralized to physiological pH by the lacrimal fluid and are therefore more compatible with the ocular system. A possible formulation of the eyedrop is given in Example 2-18. Here, the quantities of boric acid and sodium borate are chosen to yield a pH 9 solution with a buffer capacity of about 0.01, which is well below the buffer capacity of the physiological fluids (~0.028 – 0.031) such as the lacrimal fluid. This solution is made isotonic using sodium chloride as the tonicity agent.

Example 2-18: Determine the amount of sodium chloride needed for the preparation of the following isotonic solution.

Tetrahydrozoline HCl	0.05%	$E = 0.22$
Benzalkonium chloride	0.01%	$E = 0.16$
Edetate disodium	0.1%	$E = 0.23$
Boric acid	0.05 g	$E = 0.50$
Sodium borate ($Na_2B_4O_7 \cdot 10H_2O$)	0.40 g	$E = 0.42$
NaCl gs		
Purified water qsad	100 mL	

Solution: Based on the sodium chloride equivalent method,
Sodium chloride equivalent weight from drugs

$$= 50 \times 0.22 + 10 \times 0.16 + 100 \times 0.23 + 50 \times 0.50 + 400 \times 0.42$$

$$= 228.6\,\text{mg}$$

Amount of NaCl needed = $9 \times 100 - 228.6 = 671.4$ mg

IV. Chapter Summary

This chapter presents the concept of using iso-osmoticity in pharmaceutical preparations to prevent cell and tissue damage caused by drug delivery alone. However, not all pharmaceutical solutions are iso-osmotic with the biological fluid, as many solutions for infusion are, out of necessity, hypertonic. Such solutions must be delivered via alternative routes to overcome the adverse osmotic effects. Osmoticity may also play a role in oral drug delivery. Oral medicines that exhibit high osmolalities due to mixed use of drugs or undiluted calcium lactate solution have been shown to cause necrotizing enterocolitis in neonatal patients. This chapter has also provided an overview of the pharmaceutical dosage forms with emphasis on solutions. The expected learning outcomes for this chapter are to understand the physical chemical theories of the colligative properties from which the iso-osmoticity concept is derived and to use the methods of the colligative properties to determine accurately the contents of an isotonic solution.

V. References

1. Bell R and Wright TJ. *Phys Chem.* 31:1884, 1927.
2. von Zawisdzki J. *Z Physik Chem.* 35:129, 1900.
3. Timmermans J. Physico-chemical Constants of Binary Systems, vol 2. New York, Interscience Publishers, Inc., 1959.
4. Barrow G. *Physical Chemistry*, 2nd ed. New York, McGraw-Hill Inc., 1966.
5. Fuoss RM and Meas DJ. *J Phys Chem.* 47:59, 1943.
6. van't Hoff JH. *Z Physik Chem.* 1:481–508, 1887.
7. Flory PJ. *J Am Chem Soc.* 65:373, 1943.
8. *Remington's Pharmaceutical Sciences.* 15th ed., Easton, PA, Mack Publishing Co, 1975, pp. 1408–1412.

VI. Homework Problems

1. What is the concentration in milliosmoles per liter of $MgSO_4 \cdot 7H_2O$ (mol wt = 246.47) in a solution containing 65 g of the drug per liter of solution?
2. What is the vapor pressure at 100°C of a solution containing 1.68 g of sucrose (mol wt = 342.30) and 15.6 g of water (mol wt = 18.02)?
3. The freezing point lowering of a solution containing 1.00 g of an unknown drug and 100 g of water is 0.573°C at 25°C. (*a*) What is the molecular weight of this drug? (*b*) What is the boiling point of the solution? (*c*) What is the osmotic pressure of the solution?
4. A solution containing 0.2223 g of benzanthine penicillin G in 1000 g of benzene has a freezing point of 0.00124° below that of the pure solvent (5.5°C). What is the molecular weight of this drug? The K_f of benzene = 5.10 deg-kg/mol.
5. (*a*) Calculate the freezing point depression of 1 g of methylcellulose (mol wt of 26,000 g/mol) dissolved in 100 g of water. (*b*) Compute the osmotic pressure of this solution at 20°C. Express the result in millimeters of solution. The density of mercury at 20°C is 13.5462 g/mL; the density of the solution is 1 g/mL.
6. Compute the freezing point depression of a solution containing 0.20% wt/v glucose (mol wt of 180) and 0.5% NaCl (mol wt of 58.5).
7. The freezing point of blood is –0.52°C. (*a*) What is the osmotic pressure of blood at 25°C? (*b*) What is the vapor pressure lowering of blood at this temperature? The vapor pressure of pure water at 25°C is 23.82 mmHg.
8. A solution of sucrose with a concentration of 1.0 *m* (molality) has a measured osmotic pressure of 24.8 atm at 0°C. What is the van't Hoff *i* factor for sucrose at this concentration?
9. The ΔT_f of a solution containing 4.00 g of methapyrilene HCl (mol wt = 297.85) in 100 mL of solution was 0.423. What is the van't Hoff *i* factor?
10. The vapor pressure of water at 25°C is 23.8 torr (mmHg). Compute the lowering of the vapor pressure of water when 25 g of $CaCl_2$ (mol wt = 111 g/mol) is added to 100 g of water.

11. The *E* value for $MgSO_4 \cdot 7H_2O$ is 0.17. What is the *E* value for the anhydrous salt?
For Problems 12–15, use the *E* values from Table 2-4.

12. How many milligrams of NaCl are needed to fill the following prescriptions?

Rx 1: Ephedrine sulfate 260 mg
NaCl qs
Distilled water qsad 30 mL
Mft: Isotonic
Sig: Use as directed

Rx 2: Procaine HCl 1%
NaCl qs
Distilled water qsad 100 mL
Mft: Isotonic

13. How many grams of boric acid are needed to fill the following prescription?

Rx Atropine sulfate 1%
Distilled water qsad 30 mL
Mft: Isotonic with boric acid
Sig: gtts. iv o.d.

14. Calculate the amount of dextrose anhydrous needed to fill the following prescription.

Rx Tetracaine HCl 1%
Dextrose anhydrous qs
Distilled water qsad 60 mL
Mft: Isotonic solution
Sig: gtts iv in each nostril qid

15. How would you prepare the following prescription?

Rx Ephedrine HCl 1.0%
Chlorobutanol 0.5%
D50W qs
Distilled water qsad 30 mL
Mft: Isotonic
Sig: Use as nose drops, u.d.

16. Calculate the amount of distilled water needed and explain how you would fill this prescription. (The 1.9% boric acid is an isotonic vehicle.)

Rx Epinephrine HCl 0.5% ($D_{1\%} = 0.16°$)
$ZnSO_4$ 0.3% ($D_{1\%} = 0.0086°$)
Distilled water qs
Boric acid, 1.9% qsad 30 mL
Mft: Isotonic solution

17. How many grams of sodium nitrate are needed to make 100 mL of an isotonic solution of silver nitrate with a strength of 1:1000?

18. The 1% boric acid has a freezing point depression of 0.29°C. How many milligrams of NaCl are needed to make 100 mL of a 1% boric acid isotonic solution?

19. (*a*) Using the L_{iso}, E, and the $D_{1\%}$ methods, calculate the amount of sodium chloride or boric acid needed to fill the following prescriptions.

(*a*)

Rx 1	L_{iso}	**Mol Wt**	E	$D_{1\%}$, °C
Ephedrine HCl 0.5 g	3.4	201.7	0.30	0.17
Purified water qs 100 mL				
NaCl qs to make isotonic	3.4	58.5		0.58

(*b*)

Rx 2	L_{iso}	**Mol Wt**	E	$D_{1\%}$, °C
Ephedrine sulfate 0.5 g	4.3	428.5	0.23	0.11
NaCl qs	3.4	58.5		0.58
Purified water qsad 50 mL				
Make isotonic solution				

(c)

Rx 3	L_{iso}	**Mol Wt**	E	$D_{1\%}$, °C
Epinephrine HCl 1%	3.4	219.7	0.29	0.17
Scopolamine HBr 0.5%	3.4	438.3	0.12	0.07
NaCl qs	3.4	58.5	0.58	
Purified water qsad 60 mL				
Make isotonic				

(*d*)

Rx 4	E	$D_{1\%}$, C
Tetracaine HCl 0.1 g	0.18	0.11
Zinc sulfate 0.05 g	0.15	0.086
Boric acid qs	0.52	0.29
Purified water qsad 30 mL		

CHAPTER 3

Acid–Base Equilibrium and Buffered Solutions

The term pH, which is perhaps the most used term in the drug literature, refers to the hydrogen ion activity in an aqueous solution, expressed in a logarithm scale ($pH = -\log \gamma_{H^+}[H_3O^+]$). It is through this term that many biological processes are understood, and it is based on this term that the pharmacological activities of many drugs may be altered by chemical and/or pharmaceutical methods. The discussion of acid–base phenomena, in which the pH is at the center stage, appears in books of nearly all disciplines of the pharmaceutical and biomedical sciences, in somewhat condensed illustrations. In most of the discussions, however, the basic chemical theories and solution properties that regulate the acid–base equilibrium are not presented. The fact that these theories work remarkably well in predicting the experimental pH suggests that they should be closely and collectively considered in dealing with pH-related issues. Thus, the goal of this chapter is to present the acid–base phenomena as they arise from the chemical principles, so that students can have a clear understanding of the phenomena rather than rely on named equations that can be memorized but not understood. Also discussed in this chapter is the role of acid–base equilibrium in mediating biological processes, drug properties, and pharmaceutical development.

CHAPTER OUTLINE

OBJECTIVES

1. Understand the ionization of water and its role in acid–base equilibrium.
2. Describe the Lewis and the Brønsted–Lowry theories on acids and bases as well as the structural characteristics of organic acid and base drugs.
3. Derive the equilibrium expressions of the acid–base reactions and their acidity and basicity constants.
4. Apply knowledge of the ionic properties of solutions to determine the hydronium ion activity.
5. Derive the pH (Henderson–Hasselbalch) equation.
6. Predict the solution pH.
7. Show full knowledge of the buffer systems and buffer capacity as well as their applications in the biological and pharmaceutical systems.
8. Be able to prepare a buffered solution based on pH, buffer capacity, and ionic strength requirements.

I. Ionization of Water and the pH Phenomenon

The Hydronium Ion

Water is one of the most versatile molecules on Earth by virtue of the fact that it produces a proton that combines with a water molecule to form the hydronium ion (H_3O^+). The concentration of this ion in pure water is 10^{-7} *M* at 25°C. This concentration, which appears to be small in number, is in fact within the range of those concentrations of the biological substances and of drug concentrations found in the physiological system. Thus, just as the proton can bind to a water molecule, biological and drug molecules can be protonated or deprotonated depending on the properties of the drug and the conditions that regulate the hydronium ion concentration in the aqueous solution. Although the hydronium ion effects are extensively discussed in subsequent sections, it is important to note at the onset that in the physiological system, molecules such as proteins and enzymes are designed so that their activities are based on the hydronium ion concentration. When a drug molecule that is capable of accepting or donating a proton is introduced into this system, it must also exist in a form dictated by the hydronium ion concentration.

Ionization of Water

Based on chemical equilibrium, the ionization of water and its equilibrium constant can be written as

$$H_2O + H_2O = H_3O^+ + OH^-$$

$$K = [H_3O^+][OH^-] / [H_2O]^2$$

Here, because the concentrations of the hydronium and hydroxide ions are much smaller than the concentration of water, $[H_2O]$ is essentially a constant. The equilibrium constant for the ionization of water is then defined as K_w, according to the following equation:

$$K_w = [H_3O^+][OH^-] = 1 \times 10^{-14}$$

In pure water, $K_w = 1.008 \times 10^{-14}$ at 25°C, and the hydronium ion and hydroxide ion concentrations are equal and have a value of 10^{-7} *M*.

In the human body the hydronium ion concentration ranges from $10^{-0.985}$ *M* in the gastric fluid to $10^{-7.523}$ *M* in the pancreatic juice. One can see the inconvenience of expressing such a wide range of concentrations. This was in fact noted by scientists in the early 1900s, and it led to the introduction of a logarithm scale by Sørenson in 1909,[1] through which the concentration of the hydronium ion was expressed using the term pH, defined as the positive number of the power when the concentration is expressed in base 10, that is,

$$pH = -\log [H_3O^+] \tag{3-1}$$

In a similar fashion, the concentration of the hydroxide ion and the constant K_w can be defined as pOH and pK_w in that

$$pOH = -\log [OH^-] \qquad pK_w = -\log K_w$$

With these designations, the equilibrium of water can be written as

$$pK_w = pH + pOH = 14 \tag{3-2}$$

The aqueous system is thus seen to have a pH range from 0 to 14. The activity, or the effective concentration, of an ion depends on the ionic strength of the solution (refer to the Debye–Hückel theory). With this consideration, the pH of a solution is further defined according to Equation (3-3):

$$pH = -\log a_{H^+} = -\log \gamma_{H^+}[H_3O^+] = -\log [H_3O^+] - \log \gamma_{H^+} \tag{3-3}$$

Example 3-1: Calculate the pH of an 0.05 *M* HCl in water, assuming this strong acid is completely ionized, using Equations (3-1) and (3-3).

Solution: Equation (3-1) gives

$$pH = -\log 0.05 = 1.30$$

Equation (3-3) gives

$$pH = -\log 0.05 - \frac{-0.5091 \times (0.05)^{1/2}}{1 + (0.05)^{1/2}} = 1.39$$

II. Chemical Theories on Acids and Bases

Brønsted–Lowry Acid–Base Theory

The addition of a solute to water can change the ionization equilibrium of water if the solute molecule has a dissociable hydrogen that would increase the hydronium ion concentration, or a functional group that would accept a proton to decrease the hydronium ion concentration of the solution. This is the basis of the *Brønsted–Lowry acid–base theory,*[2] which shows that in a solution, the solute and the solvent interact with each other by acting as an acid–base pair, and this interaction involves the transfer of a proton from an acid to a base. This concept can be seen from the following chemical interactions.

$$\underset{\text{Base}_1}{NH_3} + \underset{\text{Acid}_2}{H_2O} \leftrightarrows \underset{\text{Acid}_1}{NH_4^+} + \underset{\text{Base}_2}{OH^-}$$

$$\underset{\text{Acid}_1}{CH_3COOH} + \underset{\text{Base}_2}{H_2O} \leftrightarrows \underset{\text{Acid}_2}{H_3O^+} + \underset{\text{Base}_1}{CH_3COO^-}$$

In the ammonia solution, ammonia is a weak base whereas water is a weak acid. This interaction leads to the formation of the ammonium ion, which is the conjugate acid of ammonia, and the hydroxide ion, which is the conjugate base of water. In the acetic acid solution, water is now acting as a base. Its interaction with acetic acid leads to the formation of the acetate ion, which is the conjugate base of acetic acid. *Acid-base conjugation* is the key concept of the Brønsted-Lowry theory that demonstrates the proton transfer process in acid-base chemistry. An interesting observation from the study of the relative strengths of various Brønsted acids and bases is that the strongest acids (or bases) have the weakest conjugate bases (or acids). This is another way of saying that if a proton is anxious to leave the molecule, the proton is not likely to come back and reattach itself to the site from which it departed, under the same conditions. It should be pointed out that in the aqueous system, water itself acts as an acid–base pair in the generation of the hydronium and hydroxide ions. Thus, to preserve the equilibrium maintained by K_w, the increase in the hydronium ion concentration brought about by the addition of an acid (a proton donor) must be accompanied by a decrease in the hydroxide ion concentration, and vice versa if the added solute is a base (see Example 3-2). The acid–base phenomena can thus be viewed as a system in which a solute may alter the ionization equilibrium of water to exhibit a certain hydronium ion concentration (or pH), but it is the pH of the solution that dictates in what form the solute may exist.

Example 3-2: If a weak acid is added to water, resulting in a change of pH from 7.0 to 5.0, what are the hydroxide ion concentrations before and after the addition of the weak acid?

Solution: Before addition of the weak acid

$$\text{pOH} = 14 - 7 = 7$$

$$[\text{OH}^-] = \text{antilog}(-\text{pOH}) = \text{antilog}(-7) = 1 \times 10^{-7}\,M$$

After addition of the weak acid

$$\text{pOH} = \text{p}K_w - \text{pH} = 14 - 5.0 = 9.0$$

$$[\text{OH}^-] = \text{antilog}(-9) = 1 \times 10^{-9}\,M$$

One should also view the acid–base phenomena as being solvent-dependent. For example, nitric acid is a strong acid in water but only a weak acid in methanol or ethanol. The organic carboxylic acids (RCOOH) appear to be strong acids when reacting with the base NH_3. In aqueous solution, however, they have incomplete dissociation and behave as weak acids. When treated with HCl or sulfuric acid, these compounds, in fact, behave as bases. It is also worth noting that when water, as a solute, is dissolved in sulfuric acid, H_3O^+ and HSO_4^- ions are generated. Because water has taken away a proton from sulfuric acid, the solution is thus more basic than sulfuric acid. One may argue that the H_3O^+ formed is acidic, but it is obviously not as acidic as the sulfuric acid molecules that have been consumed by water.

Lewis Acids and Bases

At about the same time as the Brønsted–Lowry theory was introduced in 1923, G. N. Lewis[3] defined the acid–base reaction as involving the donation of a pair of electrons from the base to the acid. The acidity of a compound is thus the measured ability of a compound to accept an electron pair from a donor known as the *Lewis base.* There are three classes of *Lewis acids* that are of interest. The first class consists of compounds having *less than a full octet of electrons*, such as the boron (III) compounds. It is interesting to point out that boric acid, an important pharmaceutical agent, is not a Brønsted acid, as it was treated in the early literature. Neither the proton nor the hydroxyl group from boric acid, $B(OH)_3$, is dissociated in water. Instead, boric acid acts as a Lewis acid according to the following reaction:

$(OH)_3B + :OH_2 \rightleftarrows B(OH)_4^- + H^+$

Boric acid Tetrahydroborate

In relatively high concentrations (≥ 0.025 *M*) and alkaline pH (7–10), the tetrahydroborate ions aggregate through the borate ester (—B—O—B—) linkage to form the tetraborate ions ($B_4O_7^{2-}$), which are the anions of sodium borate found in the mineral borax.

Metal ions, except those of the alkali group, are often regarded as the second class of Lewis acids. These ions are strongly hydrated in solution. Using the ferric ion as an example and a noncommittal formula for the hydration number, the acidity of $Fe(H_2O)_x^{3+}$ can be seen from the following reaction:

$$Fe(H_2O)_x^{3+} + H_2O \rightleftarrows Fe(H_2O)_{x-1}^{2+} + H_3O^+$$

The acidity of the ferric ion ($K = 6 \times 10^{-3}$) is in fact about the same as that of phosphoric acid (H_3PO_4) and is known to play a role in the physiological buffer system. Compounds having double bonds, excluding those of the carbon—carbon linkage, are the third class of Lewis acids. In the reaction below, it can be seen that the dissolved CO_2 in an aqueous solution is a Lewis acid, which, by accepting an electron pair from the donor hydroxide ion, yields the bicarbonate. The carbonic acid–bicarbonate equilibrium is one of the most important buffer systems in the biological fluids.

$$O=C=O + :OH^- \rightarrow [\,O=C=O\,] \rightarrow O=C-O^-$$

$$\qquad\qquad\qquad\qquad \uparrow \qquad\qquad\qquad |$$

$$\qquad\qquad\qquad\qquad :OH^- \qquad\qquad OH$$

III. The Acid–Base Equilibrium

The Acidity and Basicity Constants

The equilibrium of a chemical reaction based on concentration considerations is the state at which the rate of the forward reaction is equal to the rate of the reverse reaction in a closed system, so that no further net changes of the reactant and product concentrations will take place; i.e., the process of chemical reaction is now absent. According to the molecular collision theory, for a reaction given in the following chemical equation

$$aA + bB \rightleftarrows cC + dD$$

the rate of the forward and reverse reactions can be written as

$$R_f = k_f\,[A]^a[B]^b \qquad R_r = k_r[C]^c[D]^d$$

where R is the reaction rate, f and r denote forward and reverse processes, respectively, and k_f and k_r are the rate constants for the forward and reverse reactions, respectively. Because at equilibrium, $k_f[A]^a[B]^b = k_r[C]^c[D]^d$, it follows that

$$K = k_f\,/\,k_r = [C]^c[D]^d\,/\,[A]^a[B]^b \qquad (3\text{-}4)$$

where K is the equilibrium constant and the concentrations in brackets are expressed in molarity. For convenience, the need for the use of activity rather than concentration in equilibrium expressions is postponed for now until the ionic strength effect on equilibrium is discussed.

Using HA to represent a weak acid with one dissociable proton and B to represent a weak base, the Brønsted–Lowry acid–base phenomena in an aqueous solution can be easily expressed by the following equations:

$$HA + H_2O = H_3O^+ + A^- \quad (3\text{-}5)$$

$$B + H_2O = OH^- + BH^+ \quad (3\text{-}6)$$

In the above equations, it is recalled that A^- is the conjugate base of HA, whereas BH^+ is the conjugate acid of B. Assuming that the weak acid being considered is acetic acid, then A^- is the acetate. One can certainly make a solution using sodium acetate to study the acid–base phenomenon of acetic acid, but in this case, the reactant is A^-, and the acid–base equilibrium should be expressed as

$$A^- + H_2O = OH^- + HA \quad (3\text{-}7)$$

The same case can be made for the conjugate acid of a weak base, such as the use of ephedrine hydrochloride (BH^+) to replace ephedrine (B), in that

$$BH^+ + H_2O = H_3O^+ + B$$

Consider the acid–base reaction given in Equation (3-5). The equilibrium constant of the weak acid HA can be expressed according to Equation (3-4) as

$$K = [H_3O^+][A^-] / [HA]\,[H_2O]$$

Because in an aqueous solution, water is always in large excess compared to the concentration of the solute, that is, $[H_2O]$ is a constant, it is convenient to express the equilibrium constant as $K[H_2O]$. With this approach, the equilibrium can be rewritten as

$$K_a = K[H_2O] = [H_3O^+][A^-] / [HA] \quad (3\text{-}8)$$

where the equilibrium constant K_a is now seen as the hydronium ion concentration of the solution multiplied by the ratio of the dissociated base to the remaining concentration of the acid. For this reason, K_a is called the acidity constant. For comparison of the acid strength of various compounds, larger values of K_a correspond to stronger acids and greater degrees of ionization. The acidity constant, as can be seen from Equation (3-8), has a unit of molarity, and the value of K_a for a weak acid is always smaller than the concentration of $[H_3O^+]$ that the acid generates. For example, if an acid undergoes a 10% dissociation according to Equation (3-5), then $K_a = [H_3O^+]/9$. As the hydronium ion concentration is preferably expressed in pH, the acidity constant can also be expressed in a logarithm scale known as the pK_a, that is, $pK_a = -\log K_a$.

Equation (3-8) is the most important equation in acid–base chemistry, from which all aspects of the acid–base phenomena can be understood. However, we shall postpone the discussion of the use of Equation (3-8) for now and further establish the relationship of the acid and its conjugate base in equilibrium expressions.

Based on similar considerations, the equilibrium given in Equation (3-7) can be shown to yield a basicity constant K_b for the base A^-, according to the following equation:

$$K_b = [OH^-][HA] / [A^-] \quad (3\text{-}9)$$

As can be seen, whereas K_a is expressed in the generation of hydronium ions by the acid, K_b is associated with the production of the hydroxide ions by the base. Because we are examining the same acid–base system using Equations (3-8) and (3-9), it is clear that

$$K_aK_b = ([H_3O^+][A^-] / [HA])\,([OH^-][HA] / [A^-])$$

The result of the above equation is that

$$K_aK_b = [H_3O^+][OH^-] = K_w = 1 \times 10^{-14} \qquad \text{(at 25°C)}$$

or, by further defining $K_b = -\log K_b$,

$$pK_a + pK_b = pK_w = 14 \quad (3\text{-}10)$$

There are two important points to be made concerning Equation (3-10). First, the addition of a weak acid or weak base can be viewed as a process to shift the equilibrium of water because a weak acid increases the hydronium ion concentration, whereas a weak base increases the hydroxide ion concentration. Second, the pK_a of a weak acid and the pK_b of its conjugate base indicate the same acid–base equilibrium, and they are numerically interchangeable according to Equation (3-10). The same is true for the acid–base equilibrium initiated by a weak base drug. For example, one can deduce the acid–base property of ephedrine using the pK_b value of the drug, but one can also indicate the same process using the pK_a value of ephedrine HCl. For convenience, it is customary for most reference books to express all acid and base constants in pK_a values, as is also the format of this book when these values are listed (see **Table 3-1**). The use of pK_a for all acids and bases also allows easier assessment of drug properties in solutions, based on the simple relationship that if the pH of a solution is higher than the pK_a, the majority of the molecules of a weak acid or weak base will exist in the base form.

Table 3-1 Weak Acids and Weak Bases and Their Acidity and Basicity Constants at 25°C

A. Weak Acid (Functional Group)	**Mol Wt**	K_a	pK_a
Acetaminophen (ArOH; Ar: aromatic)	151.16	3.09×10^{-10}	9.51
Acetic acid (—COOH)	60.05	1.75×10^{-5}	4.76
Acetylsalicylic acid (—COOH)	180.15	3.27×10^{-4}	3.49
p-Aminobenzoic acid (—NH_3^+; —COOH)	137.13	K_1 3.16×10^{-3} K_2 1.35×10^{-5}	2.50 4.87
Amobarbital (cyclic ureide)	226.27	1.15×10^{-8}	7.94
Ascorbic acid (the enolic group at C_3 and C_2)	176.12	K_1 5.0×10^{-5} K_2 2.51×10^{-12}	4.3 11.6
Barbital (cyclic ureide)	184.19	3.71×10^{-8}	7.43
Barbituric acid (in base, it forms the aromatic barbiturate ion)	128.09	9.77×10^{-5}	4.01
Benzoic acid (—COOH)	122.12	6.30×10^{-5}	4.20
Benzyl penicillin (—COOH)	334.38	1.74×10^{-3}	2.76
Boric acid ($B(OH)_3 + H_2O \rightarrow B(OH)_4^- + H^+$)	61.84	5.8×10^{-10}	9.24
Citric acid (triprotic carboxylic acid; $H_3C_6H_5O_7$; $H_2C_6H_5O_7^-$; $HC_6H_5O_7^{2-}$)	192.12	K_1 7.4×10^{-4} K_2 1.73×10^{-5} K_3 4.0×10^{-7}	3.13 4.76 6.40
Glycine (zwitterions; —COOH; —NH_3^+)	75.07	K_1 4.5×10^{-3} K_2 1.7×10^{-10}	2.35 9.78
Methylparaben (ArOH)	152.14	4.0×10^{-9}	8.4
Monochloroacetic acid (—COOH)	94.50	1.40×10^{-3}	2.86
Penicillin V (—COOH)	350.38	1.86×10^{-3}	2.73
Pentobarbital (cyclic ureide)	226.28	1.0×10^{-8}	8.0
Phenobarbital (cyclic ureide)	232.23	3.9×10^{-8}	7.41
Phenol (ArOH)	95.12	1.0×10^{-10}	10.0
Phenytoin (imide)	252.26	7.9×10^{-9}	8.1

(Continues)

Table 3-1 (*Continued*)

A. Weak Acid (Functional Group)	Mol Wt	K_a	pK_a
Phosphoric acid (triprotic, H_3PO_4, $H_2PO_4^-$; HPO_4^{2-})	98.02	K_1 7.1×10^{-3} K_2 6.2×10^{-8} K_3 4.5×10^{-13}	2.15 7.21 12.35
Salicylic acid (—COOH)	138.12	1.06×10^{-3}	2.97
Succinic acid (diprotic; $HO_2CC_2H_4COOH$; $HO_2CC_2H_4CO_2^-$)	118.09	K_1 6.4×10^{-5} K_2 2.3×10^{-6}	4.19 5.63
Sulfacetamide (sulfonamide; —SO_2—NH—)	214.24	1.35×10^{-6}	5.87
Sulfadiazine (sulfonamide)	250.28	3.3×10^{-7}	6.48
Sulfamerazine (sulfonamide)	264.30	8.7×10^{-8}	7.06
Sulfapyridine (sulfonamide)	249.29	3.6×10^{-9}	8.44
Sulfathiazole (sulfonamide)	255.32	7.6×10^{-8}	7.12
Sulfisomidine (sulfonamide)	278.34	3.4×10^{-8}	7.47
Sulfisoxazole (sulfonamide)	267.30	1.0×10^{-5}	5.00
Tetracycline HCl (zwitterions)	480.9	K_1 5.01×10^{-4} K_2 2.09×10^{-8} K_3 2.04×10^{-10}	3.30 7.68 9.69
Trichloroacetic acid (—COOH)	163.40	1.3×10^{-1}	0.89

B. Weak Base (Functional Groups)	Mol Wt	K_b	pK_b	pK_a of Conjugate Acid
Acetanilide (aniline; Ar—NH—)	135.16	4.1×10^{-14}	13.39	0.61
Ammonia (NH_3)	35.05	1.74×10^{-5}	4.76	9.24
Apomorphine (tertiary amine)	267.31	1.0×10^{-7}	7.00	7.00
Atropine (tertiary amine)	289.4	4.5×10^{-5}	4.35	9.65
Benzocaine (Ar—NH_2)	165.19	6.0×10^{-12}	11.22	2.78
Cocaine (tertiary amine)	303.35	2.6×10^{-6}	5.59	8.41
Codeine (tertiary amine)	299.36	1.6×10^{-6}	5.8	8.2
Ephedrine (—NH—)	165.23	2.3×10^{-5}	4.64	9.36
Epinephrine (—NH—; catechol)	183.20	K_1 7.9×10^{-5} K_2 3.2×10^{-6}	4.1 5.5	9.9 8.5
Erythromycin (tertiary amine)	733.92	6.3×10^{-6}	5.2	8.8
Ethylenediamine (diamine)	60.10	K_1 7.1×10^{-8} K_2 8.32×10^{-5}	7.15 4.08	6.85 9.92
Morphine (tertiary amine)	285.33	7.4×10^{-7}	6.13	7.87
Nalorphine (tertiary amine)	311.37	6.3×10^{-7}	6.2	7.8
Papaverine (pyridine)	339.39	8×10^{-9}	8.1	5.9
Physostigmine (tertiary amines)	275.34	K_1 7.6×10^{-7} K_2 5.7×10^{-13}	6.12 12.24	7.88 1.76
Pilocarpine (imidazole)	208.25	K_1 7×10^{-8} K_2 2×10^{-13}	7.2 12.7	6.8 1.3
Procaine (tertiary amine)	236.30	7×10^{-6}	5.2	8.8

B. Weak Base (Functional Groups)	Mol Wt	K_b	pK_b	pK_a of Conjugate Acid
Quinacrine dihydrochloride (amines)	472.88	1×10^{-6}	6.0	8.0
Quinine (tertiary amine, pyridine)	324.41	K_1 1×10^{-6} K_2 1.3×10^{-10}	6.0 9.89	8.00 4.11
Reserpine (tertiary amine)	608	4×10^{-8}	7.4	6.6
Scopolamine (tertiary amine)	303.35	1.6×10^{-6}	5.8	8.2
Strychnine (tertiary amine)	334.40	K_1 1×10^{-6} K_2 2×10^{-12}	6.0 11.7	8.0 2.3
Theobromine (—N=C—OH; purine)	180.17	K_1 7.76×10^{-7} K_2 4.8×10^{-14}	6.11 13.3	7.89 0.7
Theophylline (imidazole nitrogens)	180.17	K_1 1.58×10^{-9} K_2 5.0×10^{-14}	8.88 5.20	13.3 0.7
Tolbutamide (sulfonylurea)	270.34	2.0×10^{-9}	8.70	5.30

Example 3-3: The pK_a value listed for the conjugate acid of ephedrine is 9.36. Calculate the pK_b and the basicity constant for this drug.

Solution: From Equation (3-10)

$$pK_b = 14 - pK_a = 14 - 9.36 = 4.64$$

$$K_b = \text{antilog}(-4.64) = 2.29 \times 10^{-5}$$

Alternatively,

$$K_a = \text{antilog}(-9.36) = 4.37 \times 10^{-10}$$

$$K_b = K_w/K_a = 1 \times 10^{-14}/\ 4.37 \times 10^{-10} = 2.29 \times 10^{-5}$$

Organic Weak Acids and Weak Bases

Because the majority of the organic medicinal agents can be classified as weak acids and weak bases, it is useful to examine the structural characteristics of these molecules that make up their weak acidic and basic properties. This information should also aid students in identifying the weak acids and bases and appreciating the role of acid–base chemistry in mediating drug activities. A list of drugs and their acid–base functional groups, along with their pK_a values, is given in Table 3-1. In general, organic acids consist of functional groups that contain the oxygen or sulfur atoms, and in cases where a proton is dissociable, a nitrogen group. The classes of compounds that exhibit acid properties, with pK_a ranges in parentheses, include phenols (8–11), carboxylic acids (4–5), imides and barbiturates (7–10), thiols (8–10), and sulfonamides (5–9). The aromatic system plays a role in acid–base equilibrium in that the phenolic hydrogen is dissociable in water owing to the *resonance effect* of the aromatic ring, which stabilizes the anion formed after releasing the proton. In comparison, aliphatic alcohols are not acidic because of the absence of the resonance effect. The effect of the aromatic system on the basicity of amines, however, is opposite to its effect on the acidity, because a positive charge, resulting from protonation, cannot be delocalized into the aromatic ring. Hence, anilines are very weak, if any, in basicity compared to the aliphatic amines. The strength of an acid can also be enhanced by an *inductive effect* brought about by electron-withdrawing group(s) adjacent to the acid moiety. For example, the acidities of the chloroacetic acids can be readily seen to follow this order because of the electronegativity of the chlorine atom(s):

$$(Cl)_3C\text{—}COOH > (Cl)_2CH\text{—}COOH > ClCH_2\text{—}COOH > CH_3\text{—}COOH$$

The imide hydrogen (—CONHCO—) is dissociable because the anion formed after ionization is stabilized by the resonance delocalization of the negative charge among the electron-withdrawing oxygen and nitrogen atoms. This group is common to the anticonvulsant drugs including phenytoin, barbiturates, and glutarimides. The barbiturates are cyclic ureides. An interesting case is the acidity of barbituric acid compared to the acidities of the barbitals where the hydrogens at the C5 position of barbituric acid are substituted with larger groups. Barbituric acid is a much stronger acid ($pK_a = 4.01$) than the barbitals because of the keto-enol tautomerization that leads to the formation of a stable, complete aromatic ion after losing a proton, known as the barbiturate ion (see reactions below). In 5,5-disubstituted barbitals, the anion formed after losing a proton is stabilized through the imide group without aromatic stabilization, thus exhibiting weaker acidity ($pK_a = 7.43$). Unlike the disubstituted barbitals, barbituric acid does not possess hypnotic-sedative activity, which is due primarily to its low pK_a (4.01) in that at physiological pH (7.4) this compound is in the inactive ionic form.

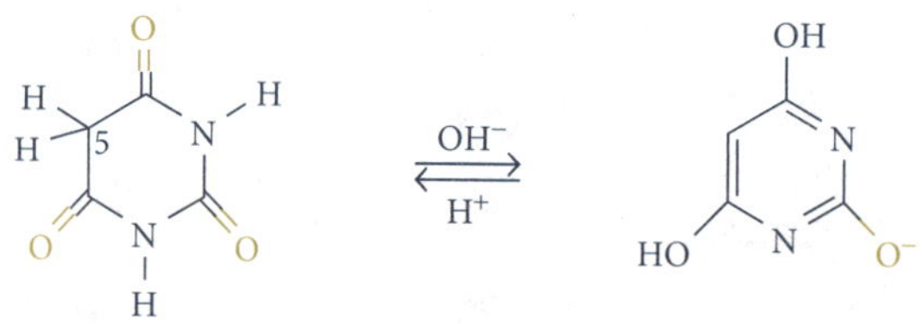

Barbituric acid ($pK_a = 4.01$) Barbiturate ion (aromatic)

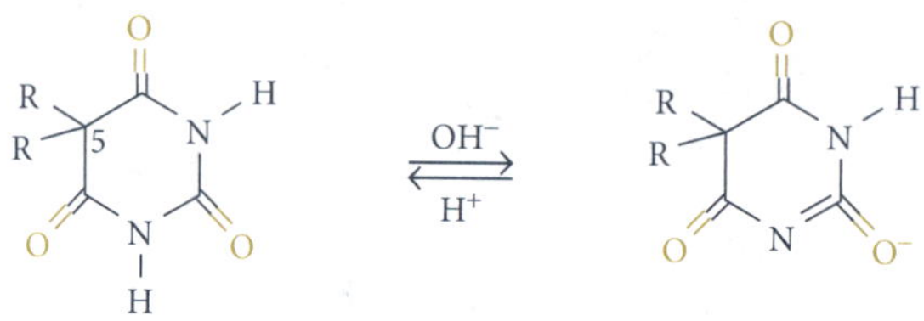

5,5-Diethylbarbituric acid ($pK_a = 7.43$) ($R = \text{—}CH_2CH_3$) Barbiturate ion (non-aromatic)

Most organic bases are primary and substituted amines. With a pK_a (of the protonated conjugate acid) in the range of 9–11, these compounds are predominantly positively charged in physiological solutions (pH = 7.4). Heterocyclic nitrogen compounds containing the pyridine or imidazole ring are also weak bases with pK_a in the range of 5–7. The protonated imidazole group of histidine, e.g., has a pK_a of 6.04. The heterocyclic bases of the nucleic acids are either pyrimidine or purine derivatives. The latter contains a fused pyrimidine and imidazole ring system. The nucleic bases contain multiple acid–base groups, which collectively determine their acid–base property at physiological pH. In cytosine, e.g., the protonated amino group ($\text{—}NH_3^+$) has a pK_a of 4.5. The basicity of the pyrimidine nitrogen (N_1) allows tautomerization of the —N═C—OH group to the keto form, making the hydrogen considerably less acidic ($pK_a = 12.2$) than the typical phenolic hydrogen. For guanine, the pK_a of the protonated amino group is 3.3, whereas the $\text{—}N_1\text{═}C_6\text{—}OH$ has a pK_a of 9.5. These data show that at physiological pH, both bases are noncharged and exist in the tautomeric forms that are necessary for their hydrogen bonding in the DNA molecules.

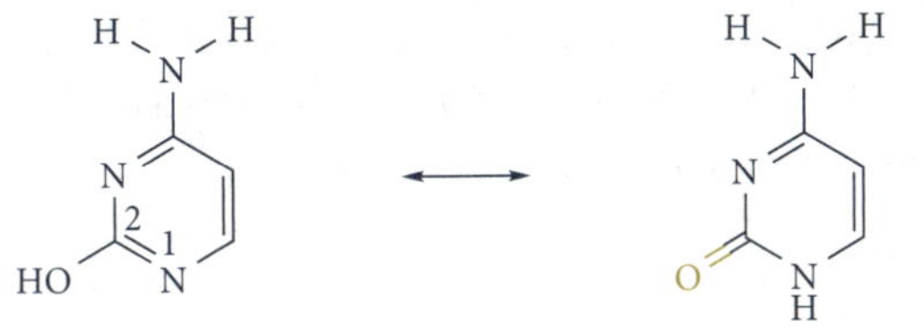

Cytosine (pK_a: 4.5, 12.2) Tautomer

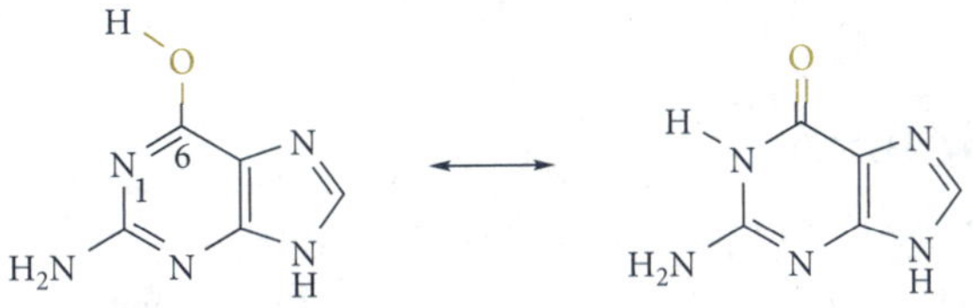

Guanine (pK_a: 3.3, 9.5, 12.3) Tautomer

The combination of both the acidic and basic properties is the makeup of the amphoteric characteristics of the amino acids, peptides, and proteins. The amino acid contains an α-amino group adjacent to the carboxylic moiety, which under physiological pH is deprotonated at the carboxylic group and protonated at the amino group, forming the zwitterions. The acid and base properties allow these molecules to be condensed into peptides and proteins. Their metabolism is also crucial for the de novo synthesis of the heterocyclic bases of the nucleic acids. With the basic knowledge of the acid–base properties of drugs, we now turn our attention to the pH phenomenon.

The pH of a Weak Acid or Weak Base Solution

The immediate application of the acid–base equilibrium is to predict the pH of a drug solution, as this is an important factor to be considered for pharmacological studies and for the development of a pharmaceutical solution. It is well recognized that for strong acids (for example, HCl, H_2SO_4, and HNO_3) and strong bases (for example, NaOH or KOH), the hydronium ion concentration can be directly seen from the concentration used and can be converted to pH, as these compounds dissociate completely in the aqueous solution. The pH of the solution of a weak acid or base, however, is not immediately apparent, nor is the pH produced by a salt (a product of acid–base reaction) of strong base and weak acid, weak base and strong acid, or weak base and weak acid. This is so because the hydronium ion concentration in a weak acid or weak base solution depends on the acidity or basicity constant that describes the partial dissociation of the proton at equilibrium, as shown in Equations (3-8) and (3-9).

The acidity or basicity constant of a drug is determined experimentally by using various methods that are briefly discussed in later sections. With the knowledge of this constant, the pH of a weak acid or weak base solution can be determined based on the equilibrium shown in Equation (3-8) or (3-9). In a solution containing a single acid (HA), the concentration of H_3O^+ is identical to that of A^-, and the concentration of HA remaining in solution will be $C_a - [H_3O^+]$, where C_a is the total (or initial) concentration of the drug. Thus, by applying Equation (3-8), one obtains

$$K_a = [H_3O^+]^2 / (C_a - [H_3O^+])$$

With known values of K_a and C_a, the above equation can be solved to yield the hydronium ion concentration without stipulations. But for a weak acid with a low degree of dissociation, the condition that $C_a >> [H_3O^+]$ can be met at relatively high concentrations of the drug. In such cases,

$$[H_3O^+] = (K_a C_a)^{1/2} \qquad (3\text{-}11)$$

This equation allows one to calculate the hydronium ion concentration in a weak acid solution, which can then be converted to pH. A similar equation can be derived for a solution containing a weak base, which is given in Equation (3-12)

$$[OH^-] = (K_b C_b)^{1/2} \tag{3-12}$$

where C_b is the concentration of the weak base. The use of Equations (3-11) and (3-12) for pH calculations is illustrated in Example 3-4.

The pH of Salt Solutions

In practical considerations, the salt of a strong base and weak acid, such as sodium acetate (which ionizes to yield the acetate ion), is a weak base. Likewise, the salt of a weak base and strong acid is a weak acid. For these salts, their pH can be determined by using Equations (3-11) and (3-12). It is important to point out, however, that in the calculation of pH of salt solutions, the ionic strength effect on the hydronium ion activity should be considered and the pH is defined as the negative logarithm of the hydrogen ion activity, i.e.,

$$pH = -\log a_{H^+} = -\log \gamma_{H^+}[H_3O^+] = -\log [H_3O^+] - \log \gamma_{H^+}$$

The use of Equations (3-11) and (3-12) for pH calculation of salt solutions is shown in Example 3-5.

Example 3-4: Calculate the pH of the solution containing (*a*) 0.01 *M* acetic acid ($K_a = 1.75 \times 10^{-5}$) and (*b*) 0.01 *M* procaine ($K_b = 7 \times 10^{-6}$).

Solution: (*a*) Acetic acid is a weak acid; thus,

$$[H_3O^+] = (K_a C_a)^{1/2} = (1.75 \times 10^{-5} \times 0.01)^{1/2}$$
$$= 0.418 \times 10^{-3} M$$
$$pH = -\log [H_3O^+] = -\log (0.418 \times 10^{-3}) = 3.38^{\dagger}$$

(*b*) Procaine is a base, so that

$$[OH^-] = (K_b C_b)^{1/2} = (7 \times 10^{-6} \times 0.01)^{1/2}$$
$$= 2.65 \times 10^{-4} M$$
$$pH = 14 - pOH = 14 + \log (2.65 \times 10^{-4}) = 14 - 3.58$$
$$= 10.42$$

†*Note*: The calculated pH value using the equation $K_a = [H_3O^+]^2 / (C_a - [H_3O^+])$, that is, $[H_3O^+] = -\frac{1}{2}\{K_a - (K_a^2 + 4K_a C_a)^{1/2}\}$, is 3.39.

Example 3-5: Calculate the pH of a solution containing (*a*) 0.01 *M* sodium acetate ($K_a = 1.75 \times 10^{-5}$) and (*b*) 0.01 *M* procaine HCl (K_b of procaine $= 7 \times 10^{-6}$).

Solution: (*a*) Sodium acetate is a weak base, so that

$$K_b = 1 \times 10^{-14} / 1.75 \times 10^{-5} = 0.57 \times 10^{-9}$$
$$[OH^-] = (K_b C_b)^{1/2} = (0.57 \times 10^{-9} \times 0.01)^{1/2} = 0.239 \times 10^{-5} M$$
$$[H_3O^+] = 1 \times 10^{-14} / 0.239 \times 10^{-5} = 4.184 \times 10^{-9} M$$

Because the solution has an ionic strength of 0.01,

$$\log \gamma_{H^+} = -0.5091(0.01)^{1/2} = -0.05$$

Thus,

$$pH = -\log \gamma_{H^+}[H_3O^+] = -\log [H_3O^+] - \log \gamma_{H^+}$$
$$= -\log (4.184 \times 10^{-9}) - (-0.05) = 8.43$$

(*b*) Procaine HCl is a weak acid:

$$K_a = 1 \times 10^{-14}/7 \times 10^{-6} = 0.1428 \times 10^{-8}$$
$$[H_3O^+] = (K_a C_a)^{1/2} = (0.1428 \times 10^{-8} \times 0.01)^{1/2}$$
$$= 0.38 \times 10^{-5} M$$

This solution also has an ionic strength of 0.01, as shown above, $\log \gamma_{H^+} = -0.05$. Hence

$$pH = -\log [H_3O^+] - \log \gamma_{H^+} = -\log (0.38 \times 10^{-5}) + 0.05$$
$$= 5.47$$

Note: If the ionic strength is greater than 0.01, $\log \gamma_{H^+}$ should be calculated using the equation $\log \gamma_i = -0.5091\, Z_i^2\, \mu^{1/2}/(1 + \mu^{1/2})$.

Salts of Weak Acid and Weak Base

The addition of a salt to water can change the pH in two ways. The first is the ionic strength effect, as mentioned above, which applies to all salt solutions. Salts from a strong acid and strong base, such as NaCl, do not produce a net change of the hydronium ion or hydroxide ion concentration; hence, their effect on pH is attributed to changes in the ionic activity of the hydronium ion. In solutions containing a salt of weak acid and weak base, however, dual equilibria from both species exist. This can be readily illustrated using the example of ammonium acetate, which, as shown in the following equations, involves acid dissociation from acetic acid (HAc) and the ammonium ion (NH_4^+):

$$HAc + H_2O = H_3O^+ + Ac^- \qquad K_{a,1} = [H_3O^+][Ac^-] / [HAc]$$
$$NH_4^+ + H_2O = H_3O^+ + NH_3 \qquad K_{a,2} = [H_3O^+][NH_3] / [NH_4^+]$$

Combining the two K_a expressions gives

$$K_{a,1}K_{a,2} = [H_3O^+]^2[Ac^-][NH_3] / [HAc][NH_4^+]$$

Because Ac^- and NH_4^+ come from the same compound, they should have the same initial concentration. Thus, in equilibrium, $[HAc] + [Ac^-] = [NH_4^+] + [NH_3]$. If the equilibrium condition is such that the proton gained by Ac^- to form HAc is equal to the proton lost by NH_4^+ to form NH_3, then $[HAc] = [NH_3]$ and $[Ac^-] = [NH_4^+]$. This condition is valid because water is a weaker acid than NH_4^+ and a weaker base than HAc^-, or else the reaction between HAc and NH_3 to form NH_4Ac would have not occurred. With this adjustment, the combined expression of the two equilibrium processes is thus simplified to

$$K_{a,1}K_{a,2} = [H_3O^+]^2$$

or $[H_3O^+] = (K_{a,1} \times K_{a,2})^{1/2}$ (3-13)

The K_a values for acetic acid and NH_4^+ are 1.75×10^{-5} and 5.75×10^{-10}, respectively. Calculations using Equation (3-13) lead to a pH of 7.00 for the ammonium acetate solution. It is also worth noting that the pK_a values for these two systems are 4.76 and 9.24, respectively. At pH 7.0, as we shall discuss in the next section, 99.5% of the salt will remain as the ionic species (Ac^- and NH_4^+). This also suggests that the concentration of Ac^- is practically equal to that of NH_4^+ at equilibrium, as very small amounts of these ions are converted to the neutral species.

The pH of Ampholytes

The acid–base behavior of ammonium acetate is in some way an analogue to that of an ampholyte that contains a base group and an acid moiety. For example, glycine, an α-amino acid, is protonated at low pH ($^+NH_3CH_2CO_2H$), a zwitterion ($^+NH_3CH_2CO_2^-$) at sufficiently high pH due to the dissociation of the carboxylic proton, and an anion ($NH_2CH_2CO_2^-$) at high pH due to the dissociation of the —NH_3^+ proton. The acid–base equilibrium can be written as

$$K_1 = [H_3O^+][^+NH_3CH_2CO_2^-] / [^+NH_3CH_2CO_2H]$$

$$K_2 = [H_3O^+][NH_2CH_2CO_2^-] / [^+NH_3CH_2CO_2^-]$$

When these two equilibrium steps are combined,

$$K_1K_2 = [H_3O^+]^2[NH_2CH_2CO_2^-] / [^+NH_3CH_2CO_2H]$$

or $[H_3O^+]^2 = K_1K_2\ [^+NH_3CH_2CO_2H] / [NH_2CH_2CO_2^-]$

At the condition that the concentration of the positively charged species is equal to that of the negatively charged species,

$$[H_3O^+] = (K_1K_2)^{1/2} \qquad (3\text{-}14)$$

For glycine, $K_1 = 4.5 \times 10^{-3}$ (pK_1 = 2.35) and $K_2 = 1.7 \times 10^{-10}$ (pK_2 = 9.77). These values lead to a calculated pH of 6.06 using Equation (3-14). It is important to point out that at pH 6.06, glycine exists predominantly in the form of the zwitterions; i.e., less than 0.02% of the compound is in the cationic or anionic form. Hence this pH is called the *isoelectric point*, commonly known as the pI value. It is also the most stable pH for a glycine solution in water, where no other acid or base is present. The pI value is a constant that describes the acid–base properties of amino acids, peptides, and proteins.

IV. The Henderson–Hasselbalch Equation

The basic concept of the acid–base equilibrium is demonstrated by Equation (3-8), i.e.,

$$K_a = [H_3O^+][A^-] / [HA]$$

where HA represents a weak acid and A^- is the conjugate base. Because both pH and pK_a are expressed in logarithmic scale, it would be fruitful to change the above equation by taking the logarithm on both sides of the equation. This gives

$$\log K_a = \log [H_3O^+] + \log ([A^-]/[HA])$$

By definition, $\log K_a = -\text{p}K_a$, and $\log [H_3O^+] = -\text{pH}$; thus,

$$\text{pH} = \text{p}K_a + \log\frac{[A^-]}{[HA]} \qquad (3\text{-}15)$$

As a historical note, the acid–base equilibrium of Equation (3-8) was described by L. J. Henderson in 1908[4] for his study of the strength of carbonic acid as a buffer to preserve neutrality, *before* the Brønsted–Lowry theory of 1923. The Henderson equation was later rewritten in logarithmic terms, as in Equation (3-15), by K. A. Hasselbalch in 1917 in his study of acidosis.[5] Equation (3-15) is thus known as the *Henderson–Hasselbalch equation*. This equation is considerably more useful than Equation (3-8) in that Equation (3-15) allows (1) the preparation of drug solutions at a desired pH using both the neutral and the salt forms of a drug, (2) the determination of the percentage of the neutral or ionic form of a weak acid or weak base drug at a given pH, and (3) the determination of the pK_a of an acid or base.

Determination of pH

Equation (3-15) shows that a drug solution can be made to exhibit a specific pH by using both the acid and the conjugate base. Because of the use of salt, it is necessary that Equation (3-15) be modified to indicate the ionic activity of the conjugate base. Thus,

$$\text{pH} = \text{p}K_a + \frac{\log \gamma_{A^-} [A^-]}{[HA]} = \text{p}K_a + \log\frac{[A^-]}{[HA]} + \log \gamma_{A^-}$$

[HA] is a neutral species, and its activity coefficient may be considered to be 1. Because

$$\log \gamma_{A^-} = -0.5091(-1)^2 \mu^{1/2} / (1 + \mu^{1/2})$$

it follows that

$$\text{pH} = \text{p}K_a + \log\frac{[A^-]}{[HA]} - \frac{0.5091\mu^{1/2}}{1 + \mu^{1/2}} \tag{3-16}$$

For a weak base (B), the conjugate acid (BH^+) is in the salt form, and the above equation becomes

$$\text{pH} = \text{p}K_a + \log\frac{[B]}{[BH^+]} + \frac{0.5091\mu^{1/2}}{1 + \mu^{1/2}} \tag{3-17}$$

Equations (3-16) and (3-17) are derived based on the condition that only one proton is dissociated in the acid–base equilibrium. The use of Equation (3-16) for the determination of solution pH is illustrated in Example 3-6.

Example 3-6: A buffered solution was made to contain 0.04 *M* of sodium acetate and 0.01 *M* of acetic acid ($pK_a = 4.76$). What is the pH of this solution?

Solution: $\mu = [(0.04(1)^2 + 0.04(-1)^2] / 2 = 0.04$

Using Equation (3-17),

$$\text{pH} = 4.76 + \log(0.04/0.01) - 0.5091(0.04)^{1/2} / [1 + (0.04)^{1/2}]$$

$$= 4.76 + 0.60 - 0.08 = 5.28$$

As previously mentioned, pH plays an important role in mediating the drug's solubility and stability. A number of weak bases, such as morphine, cocaine, and procaine, have been found to be stable only in acidic solutions. The pH for these drugs is usually controlled using buffered solutions. In cases where the desired pH is within 1.5 pH units of the pK_a of a drug, solution can be made using the acid and base forms of the drug, which in itself acts as a buffer system. For example, pilocarpine, a cholinergic agent used in ophthalmic solutions to reduce intraocular pressure, undergoes degradation through base-catalyzed hydrolysis and epimerization, but is stable in solutions of pH 6.0 and lower. The pK_a of the conjugate acid of pilocarpine is 6.80; hence, it is possible to prepare a stable pilocarpine solution (at pH below 6.0) using pilocarpine and pilocarpine HCl, according to Equation (3-17) (see Example 3-7).

Example 3-7: How would you prepare 100 mL of a pilocarpine solution with a pH of 5.8, a total drug concentration of 0.02 *M*, and an ionic strength of 0.02? If needed, use NaCl to make up the ionic strength. Molecular weights of pilocarpine and pilocarpine HCl are 208.3 and 244.8, respectively. The pK_a of pilocarpine HCl is 6.80.

Solution: (*a*) Calculating [B] and [BH^+] by using Equation (3-17) gives

$$\log([B]/[BH^+]) = 5.8 - 6.80 - 0.5091(0.02)^{1/2} / [1 + (0.02)^{1/2}]$$

$$= 5.8 - 6.80 - 0.06 = -1.06$$

$[B]/[BH^+] = 0.087$ or $[B] = 0.087[BH^+]$

Total drug concentration = $[B] + [BH^+] = 0.02\,M$

Substituting $0.087[BH^+]$ for [B] gives

$0.087[BH^+] + [BH^+] = 0.02$ or $[BH^+](1 + 0.087) = 0.02\,M$

Hence,

$[BH^+] = 0.02/1.087 = 0.0184\,M$

$[B] = 0.02 - 0.0184 = 0.0016\,M$

For 100 mL:

Wt of pilocarpine = $0.0016 \times 208.3 \times 100/1000$

$= 0.033$ g

Wt of pilocarpine HCl = $0.0184 \times 244.8 \times 100/1000$

$= 0.450$ g

(*b*) The ionic strength of the solution is 0.02.

($\mu_{BH^+} = 0.0184$)

Because [BH^+] is 0.0184 *M*, the concentration of NaCl needed to make up the ionic strength is 0.0016 *M* or 0.009 g/100 mL.

($\mu_{NaCl} = 0.0016$)

Answer: Dissolve 0.033 g of pilocarpine, 0.450 g of pilocarpine HCl, and 0.009 g NaCl in purified water and qs to 100 mL.

Percentage of Drug in Acid or Base Form

With given values of pH and pK_a, the ratio $[A^-]/[HA]$ can be determined using Equation (3-16). The percentage of the neutral acid (HA) in solution can then be calculated by letting $[A^-]/[HA] = r$, and

$$\%HA = \frac{[HA]}{[HA] + [A^-]} \times 100 = \frac{1}{1 + r} \times 100\% \qquad (3\text{-}18)$$

For a solution containing a free base (B), Equation (3-17) may be used to determine the ratio of $[B]/[BH^+]$. The percentage of free base is then determined using the following expression:

$$\%B = \frac{[B]}{[B] + [BH^+]} \times 100 = \frac{r}{1 + r} \times 100\% \qquad (3\text{-}19)$$

where $r = [B]/[BH^+]$. A sample calculation of the existence of a weak acid drug with an assigned pK_a of 6.0, at different pH, is shown in Example 3-8. These data show that when the pH is equal to pK_a, that is, $[A^-] = [HA]$, 50% of the drug will exist in the neutral form or ionic form. As the pH increases, %HA decreases. At a pH that is 2 units above pK_a, 99% of the drug will exist in the ionized (conjugate base) form. A lower pH compared to the pK_a value favors the existence of the free acid (HA) following the same pattern.

Example 3-8: Calculate the percent of the acid and base form of a weak acid drug in a dilute solution of varying pH from 3.0 to 9.0. This weak acid has a pK_a of 6.0. The ionic strength effect for this dilute solution is negligible.

Solution: At pH 7.0, according to Equation (3-16),

$\log([A^-]/[HA]) = 7 - 6 = 1$ $\quad r = [A^-]/[HA] = 10$

Thus,

$\%HA = 100/(1 + 10) = 9.09\%$

$\%A^- = 100\% - \%[HA] = 90.91\%$

Complete calculations over the pH range yield these data:

pH	$\%A^-$	%HA
3.0	0.10	99.90
4.0	0.99	99.01
5.0	9.09	90.91
6.0	50.00	50.00
7.0	90.91	9.09
8.0	99.01	0.99
9.0	99.90	0.10

The neutral form of an acid or base drug is often pharmacologically active, whereas the ionic form is not, because of the ability of the neutral form, which is lipid-soluble, to interact with the biological membranes. The Henderson–Hasselbalch equation is therefore quite useful in estimating the percentage of drug that is biologically active. This can be seen from the calculations shown in Example 3-9.

Example 3-9: Calculate the percentage of free acid for (*a*) phenobarbital ($pK_a = 7.40$) and (*b*) hexobarbital ($pK_a = 8.4$) at physiological conditions (pH =7.4; $\mu = 0.16$).

Solution: (*a*) Using Equation (3-16),

$\log([A^-]/[HA]) = 7.4 - 7.4 + 0.15 = 0$

$r = [A^-]/[HA] = 1.40$ $\quad \%HA = 100/(1 + 1.40) = 41.7\%$

(*b*) $\log([A^-]/[HA]) = 7.4 - 8.4 + 0.15 = -0.85$

$r = [A^-]/[HA] = 0.14$ $\quad \%HA = 100/(1 + 0.14) = 87.7\%$

Observation: Hexobarbital, with an *N*-methyl substitution, is a weaker acid than phenobarbital, which is thus largely in the free acid, nonionized lipid-soluble form (87.7%) at physiological pH. This drug, when compared to barbitals without the *N*-methyl substitution (~pK_a 7.4–7.6), readily enters the central nervous system and rapidly equilibrates into peripheral fatty acid stores. As a result, it has a shorter onset and duration of action.

Determination of pK_a

The pK_a value of a weak acid is commonly determined via pH titration, in which the acid solution of a fixed concentration is titrated with small increment (usually the smallest measurable volume) of a strong base of standardized concentration, and the pH of the solution is measured after each increment of base. A curve of pH versus the concentration of the strong base can then be constructed. Because the addition of base also results in an increase in the ionic strength of the solution, which affects the system according to Equation (3-16), the *y* axis of the titration curve can be modified to represent pH – log γ_{A^-}. As an example, the pH titration curve of 0.05 *M* boric acid using NaOH is shown in **Figure 3-1**; the experimental data[6] is shown in **Table 3-2**. As with all pH titrations, the plot of Figure 3-1 gives a sigmoidal curve, with the inflection point occurring at the half point of the titration, i.e., when the concentration of the added base is equal to one-half of the acid concentration. The pK_a value can then be determined as pH – log γ_{A^-} at the inflection point. The reason for the sigmoidal shaped curve is that near or within ~1.5 pH units of the pK_a value, pH is a function of log [A$^-$]/[HA], and the added base is consumed by the acid to form A$^-$, thus resulting in a smaller change in pH compared to the pH change produced by the same amount of base in a system without the presence of an acid.

Depending on experimental conditions, the determination of the inflection point can be difficult. A simple method for the determination of pK_a is to perform a linear plot of pH – log γ_{A^-} versus log ([A$^-$]/[HA]), according to a rearranged expression of Equation (3-16):

$$\text{pH} - \log \gamma_{A^-} = pK_a + \log([A^-]/[HA])$$

where $\log \gamma_{A^-} = -0.5091\mu^{1/2}/(1 + \mu^{1/2})$. Here, from the straight-line plot, pK_a is determined as the value of pH – log γ_{A^-} at the point where log ([A$^-$]/[HA]) is zero. For the titration of boric acid with sodium hydroxide, the experimental and calculated data are given in Table 3-2. The plot of pH – log γ_{A^-} versus log ([A$^-$]/[HA]) yields a straight line (see Figure 3-1) that corresponds to a pK_a value of 9.24 for boric acid.

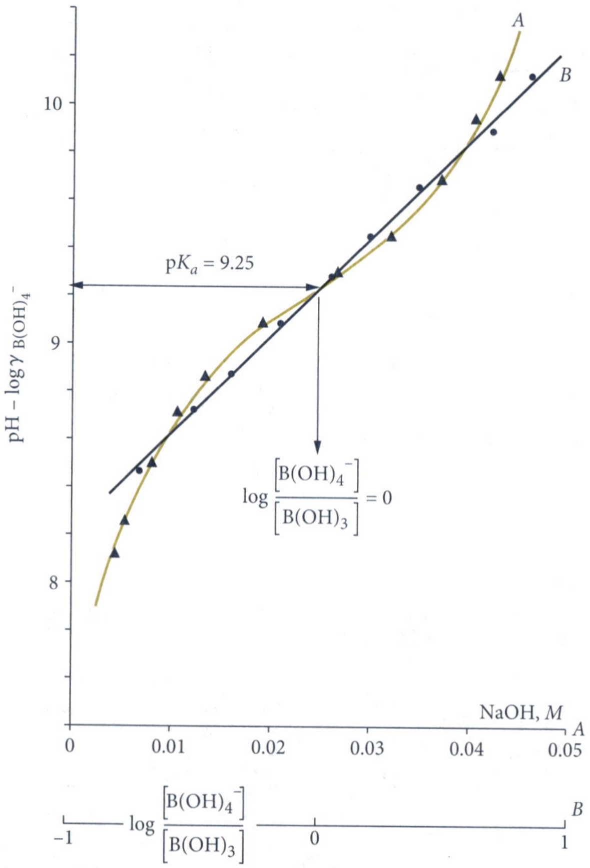

Figure 3-1 Determination of pK_a of boric acid by pH titration: (*A*) Plot of pH – log $\gamma_{[B(OH)_4^-]}$ as a function of the concentration of NaOH. (*B*) Plot of pH – log $\gamma_{B(OH)_4^-}$ versus log {[*B*(OH)$_4^-$]/[*B*(OH)$_3$]}.

Table 3-2 Data for the Determination of pK_a of Boric Acid Shown in Figure 3-1

Equilibrium: $B(OH)_3 + H_2O = B(OH)_4^- + H_3O^+$
Acid Base

$$pH = pK_a + \log([\text{base}]/[\text{acid}]) + \log \gamma_{\text{base}}$$

In solution containing 0.05 *M* boric acid, 0.05 *M* KCl, and added NaOH:

pH†	NaOH,† *M*	μ	$-\log \gamma_{\text{base}}$	$pH - \log \gamma_{\text{base}}$	log ([base]/[acid])‡
8.00	0.0039	0.054	0.095	8.10	−1.073
8.20	0.0060	0.056	0.097	8.30	−0.865
8.40	0.0086	0.059	0.099	8.50	−0.683
8.60	0.0118	0.062	0.101	8.70	−0.510
8.80	0.0158	0.066	0.103	8.90	−0.335
9.00	0.0208	0.071	0.107	9.11	−0.147
9.20	0.0264	0.076	0.110	9.31	0.049
9.40	0.0321	0.082	0.113	9.51	0.254
9.60	0.0369	0.087	0.116	9.72	0.450
9.80	0.0406	0.091	0.118	9.92	0.635
10.00	0.0437	0.094	0.119	10.12	0.841

†Data from: USP (27)/NF (22), 2004, U.S. Pharmacopeial Convention, Inc., Rockville, MD, pp. 2724–2725.
‡The ratio of [base]/[acid] is calculated as [NaOH]/(0.05 − [NaOH]).

V. Buffered Solutions

What Constitutes a Buffered System?

From the preceding section, we have gained, through the use of the Henderson–Hasselbalch equation, several useful observations of the acid–base phenomena. First, one can make a solution having a desired pH by using both the acid and its conjugate base at predetermined concentrations. Second, in a system containing a weak acid and its conjugate base, the change of pH by the addition of a base (or acid) in the region near the pK_a is considerably less than in regions outside of this pK_a zone. This is so because at pH near the pK_a, acid–base equilibrium of the weak acid exists, and the added base or acid is absorbed through the change in the base/acid ratio. Because the change in pH is not a function of this ratio, but a function of its logarithmic value, the effect of the added base (or acid) on pH is thus suppressed. Hence, the pH near the pK_a (within ±1.5 pH units) is known as the buffer zone; the weak acid and its conjugate base are the buffer agents; and the solution of a weak acid and its conjugated base, for the purpose of controlling pH against factors that cause pH changes, is the buffered solution. Although a drug may be formulated as a buffered solution by using its acid and base forms, as shown in Example 3-7, buffered solutions are usually vehicles for drug delivery and biological studies. They are primarily prepared using systems that are inert but compatible with the biological system. The commonly used buffer agents include, but are not limited to, the acetic acid–acetate, boric acid–borate, citric acid–citrate, and the monobasic phosphate–dibasic phosphate systems.

The Buffer Capacity

The Henderson–Hasselbalch equation is also known as the pH or buffer equation. It is clear from this equation that one can make a solution of a desired pH using different concentrations of the buffer agents, as long as the [base]/[acid] ratio is kept the same. For example, if solution A consists of 0.01 M acetic acid and 0.01 M sodium acetate and solution B consists of 0.05 M acetic acid and 0.05 M sodium acetate, the two solutions should have the same pH, excluding the ionic strength effect. But these two buffered solutions are not equivalent because if we add a base equivalent to 0.005 M in each solution, the change in pH in solution A (calculated as the change in log ([base]/[acid]) is 0.477, whereas the change in pH in solution B is 0.087. This shows that, in addition to the pH for which a buffer is prepared for, there is another important characteristic of a buffered solution, which is known as the *buffer capacity* or buffer strength. From the first glance at this property using the above example, it is seen that the buffer capacity is, at least, proportional to the concentration of the buffer agents used.

In the effective pH range of a buffer system containing [HA] and [A⁻], the change of pH by an added base (or acid) is measured by the change of [A⁻] and [HA]. Thus, the strength of a buffer, or the buffer capacity (designated as β), can be defined as

$$\beta = d[A^-]/dpH$$

With this designation, it can be shown that the differentiation of the buffer equation (Equation (3-16)) as a function of pH leads to the following expression[7]:

$$\beta = 2.303C_t \frac{K_a\,[H_3O^+]}{(K_a + [H_3O^+])^2} \tag{3-20}$$

where C_t is the total concentration of the buffer agents ($C_t = [A^-] + [HA]$). The buffer capacity has a unit of concentration, and this concentration is an indication of the amount of base needed to raise the solution pH by 1 pH unit.

It is important to point out that it is the buffer equation (Equation (3-16)) that specifies the ratio of the base to acid ($[A^-]/[HA]$) needed to obtain a desired solution pH, but it is the buffer capacity equation (Equation (3-20)) that fixes the total concentration of the buffer agents ($[A^-] + [HA]$) at a specific strength. Hence, both equations are necessary to prepare or understand the properties of a buffered solution. The use of these equations is shown in Examples 3-10 and 3-11.

Example 3-10: A buffered solution was prepared by first mixing 50 mL of 0.2 M acetic acid with 35 mL of 0.2 M NaOH and then diluting the solution to 200 mL with water. The final solution also contains 0.05 M NaCl. Acetic acid has a pK_a of 4.76. What are (*a*) the pH and (*b*) the buffer capacity of this solution?

Solution: It is necessary to know that the addition of NaOH converts acetic acid to sodium acetate. Thus, the concentration of the conjugate base in the final solution is

$$[A^-] = 35\,\text{mL} \times 0.2\,M / 200\,\text{mL} = 0.035\,M$$

The concentration of the weak acid is then

$$[HA] = (50 \times 0.2 - 35 \times 0.2) / 200 = 0.015\,M$$

Ionic strength (from both NaCl and sodium acetate):

$$\mu = [0.05(1)^2 + 0.05(-1)^2 + 0.035(1)^2 + 0.035(-1)^2]/2$$
$$= 0.085$$

(*a*) Calculation of solution pH using Equation (3-17):

$$pH = pK_a + \log\frac{[A^-]}{[HA]} - \frac{0.5091\,\mu^{1/2}}{1+\mu^{1/2}}$$

$$= 4.76 + \log 0.035/0.015 - 0.5091(0.085)^{1/2}/1 + (0.085)^{1/2}$$

$$= 4.76 + 0.37 - 0.12 = 5.01$$

(*b*) Calculation of buffer capacity using Equation (3-19): Convert pK_a and pH (calculated above) to K_a and $[H_3O^+]$:

$$K_a = 1.75 \times 10^{-5} \qquad [H_3O^+] = 0.98 \times 10^{-5} M$$

$$C_t = 0.035 + 0.015 = 0.05\,M$$

$$\beta = 2.303\,C_t\frac{K_a\,[H_3O^+]}{(K_a + [H_3O^+])^2}$$

$$= \frac{2.303 \times 0.05 \times 1.75 \times 10^{-5} \times 0.98 \times 10^{-5}}{(1.75 \times 10^{-5} + 0.98 \times 10^{-5})^2}$$

$$= 0.0265\,M$$

Equation (3-20) indicates that while the buffer capacity increases with increasing total concentration of the buffer agents C_t, it is also pH-dependent. A buffer system of a fixed concentration of C_t, such as the boric acid buffer shown in Figure 3-1, can be prepared at different pH values, but these buffers exhibit different buffer capacity as shown in **Figure 3-2**. At pH 8.0, the buffer strength is only about one-fifth of that at pH 9.2. The pH at which a buffer has the highest value in buffer capacity is equal to the pK_a of the buffer system. At this pH, Equation (3-20) becomes

$$\beta_{max} = 2.303C_t/4 = 0.576C_t$$

Thus, the basic criteria for selecting a buffer system include the determination whether the desired pH is within the effective range of the buffer system, which can be set as $pK_a \pm 1.5$ pH units or a tighter pH range. The use of boric acid ($pK_a = 9.24$) to make an acidic buffer, e.g., would not make sense in terms of its buffer capacity.

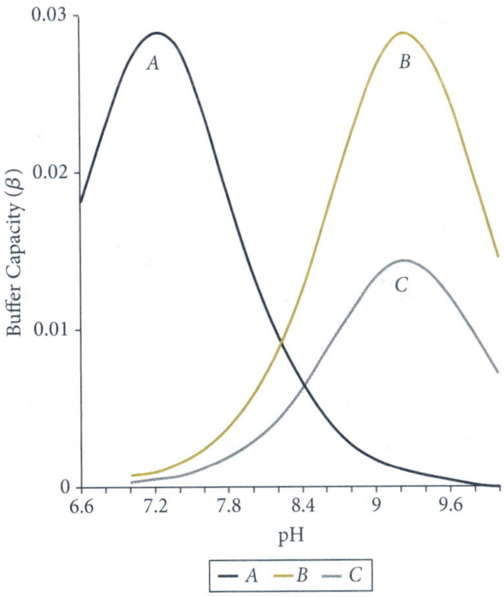

Figure 3-2 Concentration and pH dependency of buffer capacity: (*A*) 0.05 *M* phosphoric acid, 0.05 *M* KCl, and varying concentrations of NaOH; (*B*) 0.05 *M* boric acid, 0.05 *M* KCl, and varying concentrations of NaOH; (*C*) 0.025 *M* boric acid, 0.05 *M* KCl, and varying concentrations of NaOH.

Preparation of Buffered Solutions

It is always a good learning experience for students and researchers to prepare a buffered solution, particularly when the contents of the buffer play a role in deciding the experimental outcome or the use of this solution. The question of what should be included in a buffered solution can be answered based on the factors that affect the buffer's pH and the buffer capacity. The buffer system can be chosen based on its pK_a, as has been previously mentioned. It is also apparent that the pH of a solution is significantly affected by the solution's ionic strength; thus it is necessary to use a salt to fix the ionic strength of the buffered solution. For biological studies, e.g., because an 0.9% NaCl (0.154 *M*) solution is isotonic to the body fluid, the ionic strength of the body fluid is about 0.16. One can prepare a buffered solution using this value and NaCl to make up the required ionic strength. Hence, a basic buffered solution contains the buffer agents and a salt based on the specified pH, buffer capacity, and ionic strength. The amounts of these agents needed for a given volume of the solution can be determined using the following procedure:

1. Determine the $[A^-]/[HA]$ ratio of the buffer agents using the buffer equation.
2. Determine C_t, using the buffer capacity equation.
3. Solve $[A^-]$ and $[HA]$ from the results of steps 1 and 2.
4. Determine the ionic strength contribution from the buffer agents and the concentration of salt needed to make up the desired ionic strength.
5. Convert the molarities of HA, A^-, and the salt into weight expressions.

These calculations are shown in Example 3-11.

Example 3-11: Show how you would prepare 1 L of a buffered solution at pH 4.5, with a buffer capacity of 0.02 and an ionic strength of 0.05.

Solution: Assuming that the acetic acid–acetate buffer system is compatible with the delivery of a drug for which this buffer is used, you choose this buffer system because it has a pK_a of 4.76. You have also elected to use NaCl to make up the ionic strength.

1. Determine the $[A^-]/[HA]$ ratio, using Equation (3-16):

$$4.5 = 4.76 + \log[A^-]/[HA] - 0.5091(0.05)^{1/2} / [1 + (0.05)^{1/2}]$$

$$\log[A^-]/[HA] = 4.5 - 4.76 + 0.09 = -0.17$$

This calculation gives $[A^-]/[HA] = 0.676$

2. Determine C_t, using Equation (3-20):

$$K_a = 1.75 \times 10^{-5} \qquad [H_3O^+] = 3.16 \times 10^{-5}\,M$$

$$0.02 = 2.303C_t\,[1.75 \times 10^{-5} \times 3.16 \times 10^{-5} / (1.75 \times 10^{-5} + 3.16 \times 10^{-5})^2]$$

This calculation gives $C_t = [A^-] + [HA] = 0.038\,M$

3. Solve $[A^-]$ and $[HA]$.

Because $[A^-]/[HA] = 0.676$, it follows that $[A^-] = 0.676[HA]$

Thus, $[A^-] + [HA] = 0.676[HA] + [HA] = 0.038\,M$

$$[HA] = 0.0380/1.676 = 0.023\,M$$

$$[A^-] = C_t - [HA] = 0.038 - 0.023 = 0.015\,M$$

4. The ionic strength contribution from sodium acetate (A^-) is 0.015. The ionic strength of a salt with univalent ions, as in sodium acetate or sodium chloride, is equal to its molar concentration. Thus the concentration of NaCl needed is $0.05 - 0.015 = 0.035\,M$.

5. Amount of each ingredient needed:

Acetic acid (mol wt = 60): wt/L = 0.035 × 60 = 2.10 g/L

$NaCH_3CO_2$ (mol wt = 82): wt/L = 0.015 × 82 = 1.23 g/L

NaCl (mol wt = 58.5): wt/L = 0.035 × 58.5 = 2.05 g/L

Answer: Dissolve 2.10 g of acetic acid, 1.23 g of sodium acetate, and 2.05 g of sodium chloride in water in a 1000-mL volumetric flask, and dilute solution to mark with water.

The Phosphate Buffers

Phosphoric acid (H_3PO_4) is a triprotic weak acid that undergoes stepwise dissociation of its protons according to the following equilibrium:

$$H_3PO_4 + H_2O = H_3O^+ + H_2PO_4^- \qquad K_1 = 7.11 \times 10^{-3} \qquad pK_1 = 2.15$$
$$H_2PO_4^- + H_2O = H_3O^+ + HPO_4^{2-} \qquad K_2 = 6.17 \times 10^{-8} \qquad pK_2 = 7.21$$
$$HPO_4^{2-} + H_2O = H_3O^+ + PO_4^{3-} \qquad K_3 = 4.47 \times 10^{-13} \qquad pK_3 = 12.35$$

As can be seen from the acidity constants, the dissociation of the first proton by the acid is done more readily than the dissociation of the second and third protons. This is due to the negative inductive effect caused by a negative charge, in that, for the second equilibrium step, the acid form ($H_2PO_4^-$) already possesses a negative charge, and it is obviously more difficult for this ion to lose another proton. Hence, the step 2 equilibrium ($pK_2 = 7.21$) occurs around neutral pH, whereas step 3 equilibrium ($pK_3 = 12.35$) occurs only in strong alkaline solutions. In the biological system, phosphates are abundant as well as essential; the physiological pH dictates that the phosphates be present as $H_2PO_4^-$ and HPO_4^{2-}.

The buffer equation for the step 2 equilibrium, with the consideration of the ionic strength effect, is

$$\begin{aligned} pH &= pK_2 + \log \gamma_{2-}[HPO_4^{2-}] / \gamma_-[H_2PO_4^-] \\ &= pK_2 + \log [HPO_4^{2-}] / [H_2PO_4^-] + \log \frac{\gamma_{2-}}{\gamma_-} \end{aligned}$$

Here, because the acid and its conjugate base are both charged species, their activities are thus subjected to the ionic strength effect. It can be shown (see Example 3-12) that when the activity coefficients are converted to ionic strength based on the Debye–Hückel theory, the above equation yields the following expression:

$$pH = pK_2 + \log [HPO_4^{2-}] / [H_2PO_4^-] - 0.5091(3)\mu^{1/2} / (1 + \mu^{1/2}) \qquad (3\text{-}21)$$

The Debye–Hückel equation used in Equation (3-21) is considered applicable to solutions having an ionic strength of 0.1 or less. When this equation is used to predict the pH of phosphate buffers in the pH range of 5.8–7.6 and the ionic strength range of 0.07–0.14, the calculated pH is about −0.03 pH unit of the buffer pH (see Example 3-13 for calculations). This indicates that the ionic strength effect on hydrogen ion activity is an important consideration in pH calculations and in acid–base chemistry.

Example 3-12: What is the ionic strength effect on the acid–base equilibrium of phosphoric acid?

Solution: The ionic strength effect on ionic activity is

$$\log \gamma_i = -0.5091 Z_i^2\, \mu^{1/2} / 1 + \mu^{1/2}$$

1. The equilibrium between $H_2PO_4^-$ and H_3PO_4 consists of one charged species and $Z_i^2 = 1$; thus the pH equation can be written as

$$\begin{aligned} pH &= pK_1 + \log [H_2PO_4^-] / [H_3PO_4] + \log \gamma_- \\ &= pK_1 + \log [H_2PO_4^-] / [H_3PO_4] - 0.5091(1)\, \mu^{1/2} / 1 + \mu^{1/2} \end{aligned}$$

2. The equilibrium between HPO_4^{2-} and $H_2PO_4^-$ consists of two charged species, and the Z_i^2 are 4 and 1, respectively. The term $\log \gamma_{2-} / \gamma_-$ is then

$$\begin{aligned} \log \gamma_{2-} / \gamma_- &= 0.5091(2)^2 \mu^{1/2} / [1 + \mu^{1/2}] - 0.5091(1)^2 \mu^{1/2} / [1 + \mu^{1/2}] \\ &= 0.5091(3)\, \mu^{1/2} / 1 + \mu^{1/2} \end{aligned}$$

Thus, $pH = pK_2 + \log [HPO_4^{2-}] / [H_2PO_4^-] - 0.5091(3)\mu^{1/2}/[1 + \mu^{1/2}]$

3. For the third equilibrium the Z_i^2 for PO_4^{3-} and HPO_4^{2-} are 9 and 4, respectively. This would give

$$\log \gamma_{3-} / \gamma_{2-} = 0.5091\,(5)\, \mu^{1/2} / [1 + \mu^{1/2}]$$

and

$$pH = pK_3 + \log [PO_4^{3-}] / [HPO_4^{2-}] - 0.5091(5)\mu^{1/2} / [1 + \mu^{1/2}]$$

A general pH equation for polyprotic acids is

$$pH = pK_n + \log [B^{n-}] / [A^{(n-1)-}] - 0.5091(2n - 1)\mu^{1/2} / [1 + \mu^{1/2}]$$

where n is the nth proton involved in the equilibrium, $A^{(n-1)-}$ is the conjugate acid with $n - 1$ negative charges, and B^{n-} is the conjugated base with n negative charges.

Example 3-13: A buffered solution was prepared by first mixing 50 mL of 0.2 *M* KH_2PO_4 with 39.1 mL of 0.2 *M* NaOH and then diluting the solution to 200 mL with water. What are (*a*) the pH and (*b*) the buffer capacity for this solution?

Solution: The addition of NaOH converts $H_2PO_4^-$ to HPO_4^{2-}. Thus,

$$[HPO_4^-] = 39.1 \times 0.2/200 = 0.0391\, M$$

$$[H_2PO_4^{2-}] = 0.2\,(50 - 39.1)/200 = 0.0109\, M$$

$$\mu = [0.0391 \times 2(1)^2 + 0.0391(-2)^2 + 0.0109(1)^2 + 0.0109(-1)^2] / 2 = 0.1282$$

(*a*) Calculation of pH using Equation (3-21):

$$\begin{aligned} pH &= pK_2 + \log [HPO_4^{2-}] / [H_2PO_4^-] - 0.5091(3)\mu^{1/2} / (1 + \mu^{1/2}) \\ &= 7.21 + \log 0.0391/0.0109 - 0.5091(3)(0.1282)^{1/2}/(1 + (0.1282)^{1/2}) \\ &= 7.21 + 0.56 - 0.40 = 7.37^{\dagger} \end{aligned}$$

(*b*) Calculation of buffer capacity using Equation (3-19):

$$\beta = \frac{2.303 \times 0.05 \times 6.17 \times 10^{-8} \times 4.27 \times 10^{-8}}{(6.17 \times 10^{-8} + 4.27 \times 10^{-8})^2}$$

$$= 0.0278\,M$$

† The above formulation is the USP guideline for a pH 7.4 phosphate buffer.

Phosphate-Buffered Saline

The phosphates are suitable for the preparation of buffered solutions in the pH range of 5.8–8.0. A total concentration of 0.05 *M* yields a buffer capacity (as shown in Example 3-13) similar to that of the biological fluid. However, the amount of phosphate in these buffers well exceeds the phosphate concentration of the extracellular biological fluids. Hence, for biological studies, a buffered saline solution using the phosphate buffer system is often employed for routine collection and processing of cell and tissue samples. These solutions are known as phosphate-buffered saline (PBS). There are several formulas for the preparation of PBS. The basic solution contains NaCl, KCl, potassium or sodium monobasic phosphate, and sodium dibasic phosphate. Other compounds such as calcium chloride, magnesium sulfate, and glucose may be added for cell culture studies. It should be pointed out that some of the formulated PBS solutions, whether produced by commercial sources or reported in literature, are not isotonic with the body fluids; and even in the condition of iso-osmoticity, the phosphate content is usually much higher than that of the extracellular body fluids. Because these solutions are prepared to mimic the biological fluids, it is useful to compare the ionic compositions of some isotonic PBS solutions with those of the major body fluids. **Table 3-3** shows the ionic content, in milliequivalents per liter, of the extracellular, interstitial, and intracellular fluids and two PBS formulations. PBS_1 contains 137 m*M* of NaCl (8 g/L of solution), 2.68 m*M* of KCl (0.2 g/L), 1.47 m*M* of KH_2PO_4 (0.2 g/L), and 8.1 m*M* of Na_2HPO_4 (1.15 g/L); and PBS_2 contains 135 m*M* of NaCl, 1.3 m*M* of KCl, 0.5 m*M* of KH_2PO_4, and 3.2 m*M* of Na_2HPO_4 (pH = 7.4). Both solutions are Ca^{2+}-free and Mg^{2+}-free.

Table 3-3 Comparison of Ionic Composition (mEq/L) in Common PBS Solutions with Those of Major Body Fluids

Ion	Plasma†	Interstitial Fluid†	Intracellular Fluid†	PBS_1	PBS_2
Na^+	145	140	10	153	141.4
K^+	5	5	141	4.2	1.8
Ca^{2+}	5	3	—		
Mg^{2+}	3	2	58		
Cl^-	103	108	4	139	136.3
HCO_3^-	28	28	10		
Phosphate	4	4	75	18.2	6.9
Others	25	10	103		
pH	7.4	7.4	7.0	7.4	7.4
μ	0.163	0.153	0.215	0.165	0.150
β	0.004‡			0.005	0.002

† Data from: A. Guyton, *Textbook of Medical Physiology*, 5th ed., Philadelphia, W. B. Saunders Co., 1976.

‡Represents calculated buffer capacity of HCO_3^- and phosphates in fluid.

Table 3-3 shows that the intracellular fluid contains large quantities of potassium, phosphate, and magnesium. The distribution of electrolytes in the extracelluar fluid, however, is reversed and is characterized by the large presence of sodium, calcium, chloride, and bicarbonate, but small quantities of potassium and phosphate. When expressed in molar concentration rather than milliequivalents per liter, the plasma concentration of the phosphates is about 2.2 mmol/L. In comparison, the PBS solutions exhibit much higher phosphate contents (9.57 mmol/L for PBS_1 and 3.7 mmol/L for PBS_2). Because these solutions do not contain the bicarbonate, the higher phosphate concentration may be necessary to obtain an effective buffer capacity. But it should be mentioned that in the extracellular fluid, the phosphate system is not a significant buffer, and the combined buffer capacity from the phosphates and the bicarbonate systems is only about 0.004 *M* based on the data of Table 3-3. The preparation of PBS at phosphate concentrations consistent with that of the body fluid may be of value. PBS_2, which has a phosphate concentration much closer to that of the extracellular fluids, is designed for use in ELISA (enzyme-linked immunosorbent assay) determination of biological molecules. The ionic compositions given in Table 3-3 also show that the ionic strength of the intracellular fluid is much higher than that of the extracellular fluid, although many of these ions are protein bound.

VI. Buffers in Biological Systems

Plasma

The arterial blood normally has a pH of 7.45, whereas the venous blood has a pH of 7.35. This gives an average blood pH of 7.40. The pH of the venous blood is lower than that of the arterial blood because the venous blood picks up CO_2 at the tissue capillaries, which reacts with water to form carbonic acid (H_2CO_3). One can view the plasma, excluding proteins, as a saline solution buffered by the carbonic acid–bicarbonate and the phosphate buffer systems. But the preceding section has pointed out that the buffer capacities of these systems are relatively low, and they are insufficient to handle the amount of protons generated by the metabolically produced CO_2. What may be the buffer system to maintain the blood pH at its normal value? The answer to this question lies in the erythrocytes. Just as these cells are responsible for oxygen transport through their main content hemoglobin (Hb), they are also responsible for carrying and disposing of the metabolically produced CO_2 in transit between tissues and lungs. At the systemic capillary level, CO_2 produced by tissue cells continuously diffuses into the blood, where it is dissolved, bound to Hb, or converted to bicarbonate. About 30% of the CO_2 is bound to Hb at the globin portion of the molecule. The reduced form of Hb has a greater affinity toward CO_2 binding than oxygenated Hb. Thus, the protein molecule may be seen as a carrier that unloads oxygen at the tissue capillaries and picks up CO_2 on its return to the lungs, where the Hb-bound CO_2 is removed and released into alveolar spaces and the protein is reoxygenated. The majority of the CO_2 molecules (~60%), however, are converted to bicarbonate in the red blood cells. Carbon dioxide is a Lewis acid, which reacts with water to form carbonic acid, and the dissociation of carbonic acid leads to the generation of proton and the bicarbonate. This reaction occurs slowly in the plasma, but in the red blood cells, it occurs swiftly via the catalytic action of the erythrocyte enzyme carbonic anhydrase (*ca*). The proton thus produced is absorbed by hemoglobin, and its release from Hb in the pulmonary circulation facilitates the regeneration of CO_2 in the lungs. This carbonic acid/hemoglobin/bicarbonate buffer system is shown in **Figure 3-3**. The buffer capacity due to the erythrocytes is in the range of 0.025–0.031 *M*.[8]

Proteins are often excellent buffers, as these molecules contain both acidic and basic groups that can accept or donate a proton. Thus, plasma proteins may also contribute to the overall buffer capacity to maintain the normal blood pH.

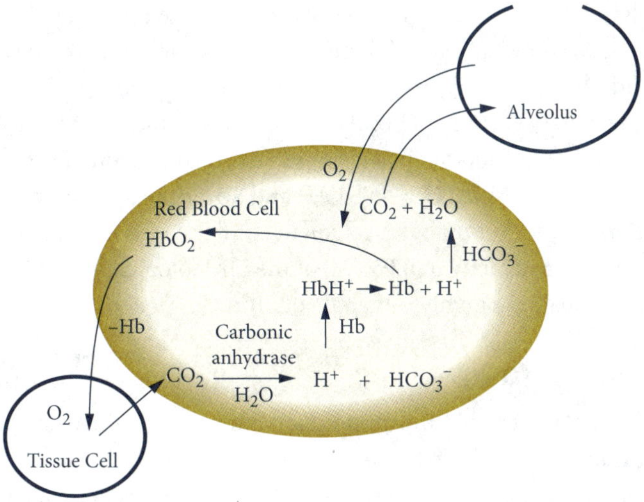

Figure 3-3 The hemoglobin–bicarbonate buffer system in blood.

Effect of pH Fluctuation on Body Chemistry

Life is compatible with only a narrow pH range of the body fluids. Acidosis exists when the blood pH falls below 7.35, whereas alkalosis occurs when the blood pH is above 7.45. Death occurs if the arterial pH falls outside the range of 6.8–8.0 for only a few seconds. The proton concentration has a marked effect on enzyme activity, as even slight deviations in H^+ can alter the shape and activity of protein molecules. Perhaps the most vulnerable of the organ systems is the nervous system. Acidosis causes a depression of the central nervous system (CNS) that leads to disorientation and, in severe cases, coma. Alkalosis produces hyperexcitability of first the peripheral and later the central nervous system. In less serious situations, CNS hyperexcitability is manifested as extreme nervousness. The change in H^+ concentration also influences K^+ levels in the body. In reabsorption of Na^+ from the filtrate, the renal tubular cells secret either K^+ or H^+ in exchange. There is an intimate relationship between secretion of K^+ and H^+ by the kidneys in that an increased rate of secretion of one ion is accompanied by a decreased rate of secretion of the other. At normal pH, the tubular cells secrete a preponderance of K^+ compared to H^+. When the body fluids are acidotic, protons are secreted in preference to K^+, thus resulting in the retention of potassium, which can affect cardiac function, among other detrimental consequences.

Urine

The urine pH has been found to be in the range of 4.5–7.8. Although the phosphates are not important buffer agents in the extracellular fluid, they contribute significantly to intracellular buffering, being rivaled only by the presence of plentiful intracellular proteins, and are solely responsible for regulating urine pH. Humans normally consume more phosphates than needed. The excess amount of phosphates is filtered through the kidneys and remains, without reabsorption, in the tubular fluid to be excluded. Thus, the phosphate system is an excellent buffer for urine as the latter is being formed in the tubular fluid. There is no other buffer system present in the tubular fluid.

Lacrimal Fluid

The aqueous component of the tear film contains water, electrolyte, and a large variety of (more than 90) proteins, peptides, and glycoproteins. The isotonicity of the tear fluid is the same as that of the plasma fluid, and its pH is about 7.4. Although the working buffering system(s) is (are) not clear, it is likely involving the presence of the many proteins. The presence of carbonic anhydrases, whose inhibition has been shown to cause blurred vision, also suggests the formation of the bicarbonate in the tear fluid. A common approach in ophthalmic drug delivery is to use solutions with sufficiently low buffer capacity that the pH of the ophthalmic vehicle can be instantaneously converted to the physiological condition by the tear fluid. The recommended vehicles for ophthalmic solutions include the 1.9% boric acid (C_t = 0.031 *M*) and Sørensen's phosphate-buffered solution (C_t = 0.067 *M*). The boric acid solution has a calculated buffer capacity of 0.001 *M*, whereas the phosphate buffer has a buffer capacity of 0.037 *M*, at the physiological pH of 7.4. The latter suggests that the lacrimal fluid, or tear, is a highly buffered solution.

Gastrointestinal Fluids

In humans, in the fasted state, the pH in the stomach after the administration of 250 mL of water is 1.2–7.4 (median 1.7). In the fed state, the pH in the stomach increases to about 6.4. The pH values in the duodenum and jejunum are 6.2–7.0 and 6.8, respectively, in the fasted state. The main buffer in the intestine is the sodium bicarbonate system, which has a concentration of about 6.7 m*M* in the fasted state.[9] The volume of the intestinal fluid is estimated to be about 600 mL.[10]

VII. Buffers in Pharmaceutical Development

In pharmaceutical testing, research, and development, buffered solutions are routinely used in (1) analytical procedures and pH calibrations, (2) dissolution testing of solid dosage forms, (3) preparation of isotonic solutions, and (4) the establishment of solubility and stability monographs of drugs and dosage forms. The USP official monographs for drug substances require that specific methods and standards be used to establish the identity and activity of a drug, and that, for successful pharmacopeial testing, the pH of a solution be controlled by the addition of buffered solutions. For this reason, the USP has established a number of standard buffer systems over the pH range of 1.2–10; see **Table 3-4**.

The phthalate and phosphate buffers are made using the potassium salt of the buffer agents. The hydrochloric acid buffer can be made in the pH range of 1.2–2.0 using varying concentrations of HCl (0.085 *M* for pH 1.2 and 0.008 *M* for pH 2.2). A strong acid (or a strong base) forms a buffer solution at low (or high) pH because the pH is expressed in the logarithmic scale. There is a natural buffer zone brought about because up to 99% neutralization of the strong acid by a base results in a change of pH of only up to 2 pH units, whereas a 100% neutralization yields a pH of 7. The buffer zones are pH 2 or below for a strong acid and pH 10 and above for a strong base.

Table 3-4 Standard Buffer Systems over the pH Range of 1.2–10

Buffer	pH	Buffer Agents (Concentration)
Hydrochloric acid	1.2–2.2	HCl (varying concentrations); KCl (0.05 *M*)
Acid phthalate	2.2–4.0	Phthalic acid/biphthalate (0.05 *M*)
Neutralized phthalate	4.2–5.8	Biphthalate/phthalate (0.05 *M*)
Acetate	4.1–5.5	Acetic acid/sodium acetate (0.05 *M*)
Phosphate	5.8–8.0	$H_2PO_4^-$ / HPO_4^{2-} (0.05 *M*)
Alkaline borate	8.0–10.0	$B(OH)_3/B(OH)_4^-$ (0.05 *M*); KCl (0.05 *M*)

Adapted from: USP (27)/NF (22), 2004, U.S. Pharmacopeial Convention, Inc., Rockville, MD, pp. 2724–2725.

The pH is a key factor for consideration in the preparation of pharmaceutical solutions. As discussed in detail in later chapters, both the solubility and the potential chemical degradation of the weak acid and weak base drugs are pH-dependent. Thus, pharmaceutical solutions should be buffered to maintain a desired pH to ensure the uniformity and stability of the drug and dosage form. When used in physiological systems, buffers are carefully chosen so as not to interfere adversely with the pharmacological activity of the medicament or the normal function of the biological system. The issue of whether a drug solution is compatible with the biological system as a result of pH differences can be viewed as a consideration of whether the buffered solution is easily changed to physiological conditions. Factors that play a role in this regard include (1) the buffer capacity of the pharmaceutical solution, (2) the buffer capacity of the biological fluid, and (3) the volume of the biological fluid versus the volume dose of the solution. These considerations can be illustrated by the use of buffers in ophthalmic solutions. Sørensen's phosphate-buffered solutions (pH 5.8–8.0) have been used for ophthalmic formulations, which contain a total buffer concentration of 0.067 *M* and added NaCl to render the solution isotonic. Boric acid solutions (1.9%) or its alkaline buffers are also isotonic vehicles for ophthalmic drug delivery. Studies have shown that tissue irritations caused by ophthalmic preparations result from large differences in pH between the solution and the lacrimal fluid. Sørensen's phosphate buffer, which has a buffer capacity of 0.039 at pH 7.4, was found to produce irritation in the eyes of some subjects when the pH was below 6.5 or greater than 8.0, but the acidic isotonic boric acid solution did not produce irritation in the same subjects because of its low buffer capacity ($\beta = 0.001$ at pH 7.4).[11] This suggests that although solutions should be sufficiently buffered, lower buffer concentration may be advantageous for the formulation of solutions to be delivered to soft tissues, especially in ophthalmic and nasal systems that have limited fluid volumes. In comparison, the pH and buffer capacity of solutions for injection into the blood are usually adequately handled by the physiological conditions due to the large volume of blood compared to the drug sample size.

VIII. Chapter Summary

The concept of the Debye–Hückel theory on ionic activity is quite important in dealing with pH and acid–base chemistry. For a phosphate-buffered solution, the difference in calculated pH using the Henderson–Hasselbalch equation with or without the ionic strength effect is about 0.43 pH unit at an ionic strength of 0.16. This difference is sufficient to produce errors in buffered solution preparations and a different view of the relative presence of the acid and base forms of a weak electrolyte in the solution. The modified pH Equations (3-16) and (3-21) using the Debye–Hückel concept are in fact quite accurate in predicting the solution pH. For monoprotic acids, such as the acetate buffer, Equation (3-16) overestimates the pH by about 0.03 in the pH range of 4.1–5.4 when compared to measured pH values. For the phosphate buffers in the pH range of 5.8–7.8, Equation (3-21) underestimates the pH by about 0.03. Thus, the significance of the ionic strength effect on hydrogen ion activity should not be lost when dealing with pH issues. To aid in calculations, pertinent equations for solving the homework problems are summarized in **Table 3-5**.

Table 3-5 Equations of Acid–Base Equilibrium

1. Properties of the ionic solution:
$\mu = (\Sigma C_i Z_i^2) / 2$
$\log \gamma_i = -0.5091 Z_i^2 \mu^{1/2} / (1 + \mu^{1/2})$
$\text{pH} = -\log a_{H^+} = -\log \gamma_{H^+}[H_3O^+] = -\log [H_3O^+] - \log \gamma_{H^+}$

(Continues)

Table 3-5 ***(Continued)***

2. pH and pK_a relationships:
Weak acids: $[H_3O^+] = (K_aC_a)^{1/2}$
Weak bases: $[OH^-] = (K_bC_b)^{1/2}\ (K_b = K_w/K_b)$
Zwitterions: $[H_3O^+] = (K_1K_2)^{1/2}$
Conjugated acid–base systems:
Weak acid: $pH = pK_a + \log[A^-]/[HA] - 0.5091\mu^{1/2} / (1 + \mu^{1/2})$
Weak base: $pH = pK_a + \log[B]/[BH^+] + 0.5091\mu^{1/2} / (1 + \mu^{1/2})$ $(pK_a = pK_w - pK_b)$
Phosphate: $pH = pK_2 + \log[HPO_4^{2-}] / [H_2PO_4^-] - 0.5091(3)\mu^{1/2} / (1 + \mu^{1/2})$
Percent of drug in acid or base form:
Weak acids: Let $[A^-]/[HA] = r$. Then
$\%HA = \frac{[HA]}{[HA] + [A^-]} \times 100 = \frac{1}{1 + r} \times 100\%$
Weak bases: Let $[B]/[BH^+] = r$. Then
$\%B = \frac{[B]}{[B] + [BH^+]} \times 100 = \frac{r}{1 + r} \times 100\%$
3. Buffer capacity:
$\beta = 2.303C_t\,[H_3O^+]\,(K_a) / ([H_3O^+] + K_a)^2$

IX. References

1. Sørensen SLP. *Biochem Z.* 21:131, 1909; also 22:352, 1909.
2. Brønsted JN. *Rec Trav Chim.* 42:718, 1923. Lowry TM. *J Chem Soc.* 123:848, 1923.
3. Lewis GN. *Valancy and the Structure of Atoms and Molecules.* New York, Reinhold, 1923; also see Luder WF and Zuffanti S. *Electronic Theory of Acids and Bases.* New York, Wiley, 1947.
4. Henderson LJ. *Am J Physiol.* 21:173–179, 1908.
5. Hasselbalch KA. *Biochem Z.* 78:112–144, 1917.
6. USP (27)/NF (22). Rockville, MD, U.S. Pharmacopeial Convention, Inc., 2004, pp. 2724–2725.
7. Van Slyke DD. *J Biol Chem.* 52:525, 1922. Also Spiro K. *Biochem Z.* 65:409–439, 1914.
8. Salenius P. *Scan J Clin Lab Invest.* 9:160, 1957. Ellison G. et al., *Clin Chem.* 4:453, 1958.
9. Yu LX. *Pharm Res.* 16:1883–1887, 1999.
10. Kalantzi L, Goumas K, Kalioras V, Abrahamsson B, Dressman JB, and Reppas C. *Pharm Res.* 23:165–176, 2006.
11. Martin FN and Mims JL. *Arch Ophthalmol.* 44:561, 1950.

X. Homework Problems

The pK_a or pK_b values of acid and base drugs can be found in Table 3-1.

1. What is the pH of the normal saline solution (0.9% NaCl in water)? (Mol wt = 58.5.)

2. Practice calculations involving pH and pOH:
   a. If the pH of a solution of a strong base is 8.75, what is its hydroxyl ion concentration? What is its hydrogen ion concentration?
   b. The solubility of phenobarbital in water at 25°C is 0.14% (wt/v). What is the pH of the saturated solution?
   c. If 15 mL of 0.02 *M* NaOH is added to 15 mL of 0.02 *M* acetic acid, what is the pH of the solution?
3. If 100 mL of 0.005 *M* sulfathiazole is mixed with 60 mL of 0.003 *M* sodium hydroxide, what is the pH of the mixture without considering the ionic strength effect? Sulfathiazole reacts in part with NaOH to give sodium sulfathiazole. The pK_a of sulfathiazole is 7.12.
4. (*a*) What is the mole percent of free phenobarbital in solution at pH 8.00? (*b*) What is the mole percent of free cocaine in solution at pH 8.00?
5. Compute the hydronium ion concentration and pH of an 0.001 *M* solution of acetic acid.
6. Calculate the pH of an 0.01 *M* solution of physostigmine at 25°C.
7. The sulfonamides can exist in the form of an ampholyte $^{+}NH_3C_6H_4SO_2NR^{-}$ in aqueous solution. The two acidity constants of sulfadiazine are $pK_1 = 2.1$ and $pK_2 = 6.5$. What is the isoelectric point for this drug?
8. Choline theophyllinate (Oxtriphylline) is a choline $[(CH_3)_3NCH_2CH_2OH]$ salt of theophylline $(C_7H_8N_4O_2)$, working as a bronchodilator. This drug is more soluble in water, better absorbed from the GI tract, and produces less gastric irritation than aminophylline, a complex of theophylline and ethylenediamine. Hence it is effective orally for the management of chronic obstructive lung diseases. It behaves as a weak base. A 1% solution of this drug (mol wt = 283.3) in water has a pH of 10.3. Calculate the pK_a of this drug and identify the conjugate acid and base in this system.
9. What is the pH of a sulfadiazine sodium solution containing 0.5 *M* of the drug in 1000 mL of solution?
10. When taken orally, sulfisomidine, $pK_a = 7.47$, exists as an 0.073 *M* aqueous solution in the upper intestinal tract where the pH is 5.83. Calculate the percent of sulfisomidine in the neutral form in the solution of the intestinal tract.
11. The pH of a 1:500 aqueous solution of ephedrine was determined with a pH meter and was found to be 10.70. Calculate the pK_b for ephedrine.
12. Benzylpenicillin has a pK_a of 2.76. If benzylpenicillin sodium (mol wt = 356.38) is used to make a 3% wt/v solution in the isotonic normal saline (0.9% NaCl, mol wt = 58.5), what is the pH of this solution?
13. What is the [base]/[acid] ratio of a boric acid solution buffered to pH 8.8, without considering the ionic strength effect?
14. (*a*) What is the pH of a solution consisting of 0.12 *M* NaH_2PO_4 and 0.08 *M* Na_2HPO_4 without considering the ionic strength effect? (*b*) What is the pH if the ionic strength effect is considered?
15. (*a*) What is the pH of an 0.1 *M* ascorbic acid (mol wt = 176.12; $pK_a = 4.3$)? (*b*) To raise the pH to 5.5 for injection purposes, what concentration of sodium bicarbonate is required to convert the acid to sodium ascorbate (assuming the total ionic strength of the solution is 0.1)? (*c*) What is the buffer capacity of the solution in (*b*)?
16. Your product research director asks you to prepare a buffered solution of pH 7.4 having a buffer capacity of 0.03 *M* and an ionic strength of 0.16. Choose a suitable buffer system and calculate the concentrations needed.

17. A titration is conducted beginning with 50 mL of 0.2 *N* acetic acid and adding (*a*) 10 mL, (*b*) 25 mL, (*c*) 50 mL, and (*d*) 50.1 mL of 0.2 *N* NaOH. What is the pH of the solution after each increment of base added?

Hint: $[A^-] = (V_{NaOH} \times 0.2)/V_{solution}$; $[HA] = ((50 - V_{NaOH}) \times 0.2)/V_{solution}$; $\mu = [A^-]$.

18. Calculate the percent of nonionized aminophylline ($pK_b = 5.0$, mol wt = 421.2) and its molar concentration after IV injection of 10 mL of an aqueous 2.5% solution at 25°C. The normal blood pH is 7.4, and the total blood volume is approximately 5 L.

19. If the normal human plasma contains 4 mEq/L of total phosphates, what is the total plasma phosphate concentration in mmol/L? In plasma, phosphate exists in two forms: $H_2PO_4^-$ and HPO_4^{2-}; the ionic strength is 0.16.

Hint: First, calculate the $[HPO_4^{2-}]/[H_2PO_4^-]$ ratio using the buffer equation. Second, use the following equation to determine millimoles from milliequivalents.

$$mEq/mL = [H_2PO_4^-] \times q_1 + [HPO_4^{2-}] \times q_2$$
where $q_1 = 1$ and $q_2 = 2$.

20. What is the buffer capacity of an 0.02 *M* pilocarpine solution at (*a*) pH 5.8 and (*b*) pH 7.4?

CHAPTER 4

Drug Solubility and Distribution in Immiscible Systems

In drug development, the traditional concept of selecting drug candidates based on potency is costly and often results in failure. Newer standards specify that a drug candidate not only needs to be active but also must exhibit "druglike" properties in solubility, permeability, metabolic stability, and transporter effects in order to be advanced to clinical development. In contrast, nondruglike molecules are those that cannot be easily developed into a drug product because of the poor quality of the properties mentioned above. The first of these properties is the solubility, which, along with permeability, is critically important in determining the drug's oral bioavailability. Indeed, poor solubility and poor permeability account for many pharmacokinetic failures. This has led to the establishment by the FDA of the Biopharmaceutical Classification System (BCS), intended to aid researchers to select suitable technology for drug discovery based on the drug's solubility and permeability.[1] This chapter discusses the physiochemical theories on solubility and partition phenomena, the current concept in improvement, and their relations to drug dissolution and absorption.

CHAPTER OUTLINE

OBJECTIVES

1. Understand the differences in kinetic and equilibrium solubility and the supersaturation phenomenon.
2. Understand the basic theories on drug solubility and intermolecular forces that govern the solute–solvent interactions and solvent classifications.
3. Predict drug solubility based on equilibrium expressions in solubility product and acid–base chemistry for strong and weak electrolytes.
4. Describe the various factors (temperature, salt, pH, cosolvency) that affect the solubility of a drug in pharmaceutical solutions and in biological fluids.
5. Understand the concept of solvent partition, molecular interactions, and the pharmacological implications.
6. Describe the octanol–water partition coefficient and its use in predicting the intrinsic solubility of organic molecules.
7. Know the role of drug solubility in drug discovery and development and be able to relate the basic theories of drug solubility to current strategies in solving drug delivery problems associated with practically insoluble drugs.

I. Solubility Expressions

Terminology

Solubility is the concentration of a saturated solution in which the dissolved solute is in equilibrium with its solid phase (in excess) at constant temperature. For nonelectrolytes and organic weak acids and weak bases in their free (nondissociated or nonprotonated) forms, the solubility is an equilibrium constant that describes an intrinsic property of the drug (which cannot be changed), and thus it is referred to as the *intrinsic solubility*. To establish the intrinsic solubility, it is essential to confirm, via a time-course study, that the equilibrium concentration is established with the specific solid form. The crystalline form of a compound has a large impact on its solubility. But the solid forms tend to transform into the most stable one; it is thus difficult experimentally to obtain the equilibrium solubility of a meta-stable form or the amorphous form.

In drug discovery tests, detailed studies to establish the intrinsic or the equilibrium solubility of a drug are not practical and can be postponed to a later time. Instead, the *apparent solubility* can be measured by setting a long incubation time (up to 24 h) of the drug in a solvent, with the intention to reach equilibrium.[2,3] The origin of the drug is not necessarily a powder, but can be a concentrated solution in a rich solvent such as DMSO (dimethyl sulfoxide). In the latter case, a DMSO sample is diluted with a solvent for which the solubility of the drug is to be determined; precipitation of drug occurs; and then the saturated concentrations can be measured as a function of incubation time. Sugano et al.[3] have demonstrated that the measured aqueous solubility of drugs using the DMSO stock is higher than the equilibrium solubility at shorter incubation time (10 min) but approaches the equilibrium solubility at an incubation time of 20 h. This establishes the apparent solubility as being similar to the equilibrium solubility but without equilibrium conformation. The DMSO method also allows one to measure the *kinetic solubility*, defined as the solubility measured at shorter incubation times (a few minutes to 1 or 2 h) following the precipitation of drug from the DMSO stock solution.[4] Many studies[3–5] have shown that the kinetic solubility is significantly higher than the equilibrium solubility, which has been attributed to the possible DMSO effect, differences in the solid forms in the precipitation, and the relatively short incubation time. Finally, the term *thermodynamic solubility* refers to solubility measured using a solid sample rather than a concentrated stock solution.

Supersaturation

A solution may be supersaturated—i.e., the drug concentration is higher than its equilibrium solubility—before the establishment of a solid–solution equilibrium. The kinetic solubility, as mentioned above, depends on the precipitation of the solute as the DMSO stock solution is diluted by the solvent and is a good example of supersaturated solutions. Other processes include the dissolution of salts, the meta-stable or amorphous form of drug, and solid dispersion and pH shift from the high-solubility region to the low-solubility region. The supersaturation will eventually settle down via precipitation to reach the equilibrium solubility. But the supersaturation process, which can be explained via thermodynamic principles, is of pharmaceutical significance. Their effects on drug formulation and activity are discussed in later sections.

Solubility Designations

The chemical definition of solubility is the saturated concentration, so that the traditional concentration terms such as molarity, molality, mole fraction, and percentage all apply, and they provide an accurate, quantitative account of the drug's property. But for semiquantitative assessment of drug solubility, the USP describes the solubility of drugs as the parts of a solvent needed to dissolve

Table 4-1 U.S. Pharmacopeial Designation of Solubility Ranges

Designation	Parts of Solvent/One Part of Solute	Solubility Range (g/mL)
Very soluble	< 1	> 1
Freely soluble	1–10	0.1–1.0
Soluble	10–30	0.03–0.1
Sparingly soluble	30–100	0.01–0.03
Slightly soluble	100–1000	0.001–0.01
Very slightly soluble	1000–10,000	0.0001–0.001
Practically insoluble	> 10,000	< 0.0001

one part of the solute with units in grams and/or milliliters, and the USP adopts a number of descriptive terms, such as soluble (1:10 to 1:30) and slightly soluble (1:100 to 1:1000), to designate the solubility ranges. For example, aspirin, which has a solubility of 1 g in 300 mL of water, is seen as slightly soluble, whereas calcium lactate (1 g in 20 mL) is *soluble* in water. The USP designation of solubility range is shown in **Table 4-1**.

It should be mentioned that even the slightly and very slightly soluble drugs, as classified by the USP designation, may be considered as "druglike" solubility for oral drug absorption. To take aspirin as an example, the normal dose is 325 mg. With a solubility of about 3.3 mg/mL, a gastrointestinal (GI) fluid of 600 mL[6] and a GI transit time of 3–4 h, the maximum absorbable amount of aspirin would exceed the actual dose even with a very poor absorption rate. It is the practically insoluble compounds that present a challenge in drug formulation. In the Biopharmaceutical Classification System, drugs are classified into high solubility–high permeability, low solubility–high permeability, high solubility–low permeability, and low solubility–low permeability classes.[1] Here, the solubility is defined as the volume of water required to dissolve the highest dose strength across the physiological pH range.

II. Theories on Solubility

Thermodynamic Concepts

Drug Solubility in Ideal Solution

Because most drugs are in solid form, this discussion is limited to the solubility of solid drugs in a liquid solvent. Without considering the chemical structural characteristics, the physical chemistry offers a theoretical estimation of the solubility of drugs based on their melting properties. The equilibrium between a solid and its saturated solution may be considered as a condensed system, where the gaseous phase need not be considered by the Gibbs phase rule:

$$F \text{ (degree of freedom)} = C \text{ (components)} - P \text{ (phases)} + 2$$

In this case, the two-component, two-phase system has a degree of freedom of 2, meaning that the equilibrium will be affected by both pressure and temperature. Because solubility is always measured at constant pressure (1 atm), it is thus clear that the change in solubility can be expressed by a concentration–temperature curve. For most compounds, the solubility increases with increasing temperature, but in a few cases, solubility actually decreases with increasing temperature. For example, at 32.38°C, $Na_2SO_4 \cdot 10H_2O \rightleftarrows Na_2SO_4 + 10H_2O$; as the compound loses its hydration, the solubility decreases with increasing temperature because of its negative heat of solution (ΔH_s). For compounds having a positive heat of solution (i.e., additional energy is required), solubility increases with increasing temperature.

The relationship between concentration and temperature at the solid–solution equilibrium can be readily seen from the freezing point depression concept. The formation of ice in an aqueous solution may be viewed as the result of a supersaturation of water, and thus a necessity to maintain the equilibrium between the solid and the solution. In solubility considerations, the presence of the solid drug in a solution is the result of the equilibrium between the solid and the saturated solution. In this light, the two systems differ only in the designation of the solute and solvent but describe a similar equilibrium process. Thus, with proper changes in notation for the solute and solvent, it can be shown that

$$\log X_2 = \frac{-\Delta H_f}{2.303R}\left(\frac{1}{T} - \frac{1}{T_o}\right) = \frac{-\Delta H_f}{2.303R}\,\frac{T_o - T}{TT_o} \qquad (4\text{-}1)$$

where X_2 is the solubility of the drug in mole fractions at temperature T; ΔH_f is the heat (or enthalpy) of fusion of the solute; R is the gas constant (= 1.987 cal/mol); and T_o is the melting point of the compound. Here, the solubility of a drug at temperature T, with the condition that $T < T_o$, can be calculated based on the molar heat of fusion and the melting point of the drug. Equation (4-1) suggests that the saturated concentration of the drug at a given temperature is the same in any solvent if the condition of ideal solution is met, because both the heat of fusion and the melting point are properties of the solute. Because it is a saturated solution, the condition for ideality is, of course, difficult to obtain. A few studies have shown that Equation (4-1) has validity but is limited to solutions where the solute and solvent exhibit similar chemical structures (see Example 4-1 for discussion). But studies have shown that if two compounds have similar ΔH_f values, a higher melting point corresponds to a lower solubility; and if the two compounds exhibit similar melting points, a lower ΔH_f results in a higher solubility. Equation (4-1) also indicates that there is a linear relationship between $\log X_2$ and $1/T$, with the slope of the plot equal to $-\Delta H_f/2.303R$. Studies have shown that this linear relationship does exist over a broad temperature range, but the slope does not appear to indicate the theoretical value.

Example 4-1: The melting point and molar heat of fusion for naphthalene are 80.2°C and 4540 cal/mol, respectively. Calculate the solubility of this compound at 20°C in an ideal solution.

Solution: Using Equation (4-1),

$$\log X_2 = -4540\,(353.2 - 293) \,/\, 2.303 \times 1.987 \times 293 \times 353.2$$

$$= -0.5771$$

$$X_2 = 0.265^{\dagger}$$

†*Observation*: The measured mole fraction solubility of naphthalene is 0.241 in benzene but is only 0.018 in methanol, indicating that the prediction of solubility using Equation (4-1) is quite reasonable in "like" solvent (benzene) but not in a nonideal solution owing to the structural difference between methanol and naphthalene.

Because of the linear relationship of $\log X_2$ versus $1/T$, Equation (4-1) may be rewritten as

$$\log S = \frac{-\Delta H_s}{2.303R}\left(\frac{1}{T}\right) + \text{constant}$$

$$\log \frac{S_2}{S_1} = \frac{\Delta H_s}{2.303R}\left(\frac{T_2 - T_1}{T_1 T_2}\right) \qquad (4\text{-}2)$$

Here, using S to represent solubility, S_1 and S_2 are the solubility of a drug at temperature T_1 and T_2, respectively, within the linear range. As mentioned above, the thermodynamic constant (ΔH) does not conform to the heat of fusion (ΔH_f) in nonideal solutions but may be viewed as the heat of solution (ΔH_s). Equation (4-2) shows that the solubility of a drug at a given temperature can be determined from its known solubility at another temperature if the heat of solution is known. But ΔH_s, unlike the heat of fusion, is not readily available, and it is likely that the heat of solution for a given drug may vary with different solvents. But the concept of the heat of solution is of interest. Like the heat of fusion, the heat of solution is a latent energy under isothermal conditions, which is compensated by a change in molar volume of the solute from the solid state to the liquid state. Studies of the temperature effect on solubility thus may aid in understanding of the solute–solvent interactions.

Solubility Prediction

The ability to predict solubility without, or with minimum, experimental data is a scientific challenge as well as a practical need for drug development work, as the measurement of solubility of large numbers of drug candidates is difficult and very time consuming. The significance of the thermodynamic approach is that the solubility of a drug can be expressed by fundamental chemical constants. For this reason, attempts to modify the thermodynamic concept of Equation (4-1) have been made by many studies. The general approach is that for nonideal solubility, Equation (4-1) may be modified by the addition of a $\log \gamma_2$ term (Equation (4-3)), where γ_2 is the activity coefficient of the solute.

$$-\log X_2 = \frac{\Delta H_f}{2.303R}\left(\frac{T_o - T}{TT_o}\right) + \log \gamma_2 \tag{4-3}$$

A number of studies by Scatchard and Hildebrand and Wood have shown that $\log \gamma_2$ is proportional to the work required to create a hole in the solvent, remove a molecule from the solute phase and deposit it in the solvent phase, and to the molecular volume of the solute as a supercooled liquid.[7,8] This led to the extended Hildebrand solubility approach,[9] which can be expressed as

$$\log \gamma_2 = (\delta_1^2 + \delta_2^2 - 2W)V_2 f_1^2/2.303RT$$

Here V_2 is the molar volume of the solute, f_1 is the molar volume fraction of the solvent defined as $X_1V_1/(X_1V_1 + X_2V_2)$, R is the gas constant, and T is the absolute temperature. The term δ is known as the *solubility parameter*, which is taken as the square root of energy needed to break the solvent–solvent or solute–solute interactions. The term W indicates the potential energy of the solute–solvent interaction. According to the extended Hildebrand approach, the $\log \gamma_2$ term accounts for both the van der Waals forces and residual, presumably stronger, forces in the solvent–solute interactions. The use of the Hildebrand approach for the prediction of solubility requires knowledge of the solubility parameters and the use of a simulated equation for the calculation of W. The system is applicable to polar and nonpolar solutes in single and mixed solvent systems.

In a different approach to the method described above, Yalkowsky and Valvani have derived equations for the prediction of the intrinsic equilibrium solubility[10] of organic molecules based on their melting points, entropies of fusion, and the octanol–water partition coefficients (K_{ow}). One of these equations is given below:

$$\log S_w = -\log K_{ow} - 1.11\,\frac{\Delta S_f(\text{MP} - 25)}{1364} + 0.54 \tag{4-4}$$

It can be seen that this equation is relatively simple and requires only the melting point (MP) and the calculated K_{ow} to determine the solubility of a nonelectrolyte drug. We postpone the discussion of this equation and its application in predicting solubility to a later section following the distribution phenomena.

Solubility and Particle Size

Although the particle size has been mostly discussed in terms of its effect on the dissolution rate of a drug powder, the physicochemical theory shows that particle size also affects solubility. Consider a pure substance existing in spherical particles with a radius r and a solubility S' and the same substance with a flat crystal surface with a solubility of S. The increase in free energy (dG) with respect to the change in moles of molecules from the flat surface to the spherical particle (dn) corresponds to an equilibrium shift from S to S' under ideal conditions, i.e.,

$$dG = dn\,RT\ln(S'/S)$$

The free energy change is equal to the surface tension (γ) times the change in surface area. The surface area (A) of a particle with radius r is $4\pi r^2$; therefore

$$dG = \gamma\,dA = \gamma\,d(4\pi r^2) = \gamma(8\pi r)\,dr$$

The molar volume of the solute (V) of the spherical particle is $V = 4\pi r^3/3n$, where n is the moles of molecules. Applying differentiation, we see that

$$dn = (4\pi r^2/V)\,dr$$

Combining the above equations gives

$$\log(S'/S) = 2\gamma V/2.303RTr \qquad (4\text{-}5)$$

Because the right-hand side of the equation always has a positive value, it specifies that S' must be greater than S. The log ratio of the solubility in fact increases with decreasing radius of the particle size.

Note that S' and S are the concentrations of the solute near their particle surface in a solid–solution equilibrium, not the equilibrium solubility of the drug. This particle size effect, however, can produce supersaturated solution. For example, the solubility of calcium sulfate at 18°C is 2.085 g/L. With a particle size of 0.3 μm, the solubility increases to 2.476 g/L. The particle size effect may be used to explain the fact that the previously mentioned kinetic solubility, as measured using the DMSO method, is usually significantly greater than the equilibrium solubility of the drug. As the drug from the DMSO stock solution is precipitated via solvent dilution, fine to very fine particles may be formed, and these particles would lead to a supersaturated solution that is significantly higher in concentration than the equilibrium solubility. The dissolution of the salt forms of drugs in media of different pH can also encounter conditions in which the drug may be rapidly precipitated as fine particles. In such cases, the particle size–mediated supersaturation is likely to have an effect on the dissolution rate. Indeed, it has been shown that the dissolution rate of nondisintegrating sodium tolbutamide pellet is significantly higher in 0.1 *N* HCl, where precipitation is likely to occur, than in a pH 7.2 buffer.[11]

Solute–Solvent Interactions

The chemical approach in understanding or predicting the solubility phenomena recognizes the intermolecular forces that govern the solvent–solvent, solute–solute, and solute–solvent interactions. Before we examine these forces, it is worth noting that the chemicals are diverse. They range from substances that have even covalent bonds throughout the molecule, as in hydrocarbons, to salts whose activity is completely dependent on their ability to separate into ions. In between the extremes are molecules with functional groups that show an uneven sharing of the pair of electrons by the bonding atoms. Thus, there is a degree of polarization (i.e., a charge separation) that can be assigned to each molecule, and through the concept of polarity, many of the solubility phenomena can be understood. Using this concept, some compounds are deemed polar, whereas other compounds may be said to be semipolar or nonpolar. The intermolecular forces that govern molecular cohesion (attraction of like molecules) and adhesion (attraction of different molecules) include van der Waals forces, hydrogen bonding, and electrostatic interactions. The ionization of weak or strong electrolytes, which involves the breaking of a coordinate covalent or ionic bond, is also part of the solubilization process.

Van der Waals Forces

If a chemical bond in a molecule is formed through uneven sharing of the pair of electrons because of the greater electronegativity of one atom compared to the other, this chemical bond will have a partial separation of positive and negative charges, and the compound is said to be a permanent dipole (a polar compound). The strength of the dipole is measured as the dipole moment μ, an electrostatic property that is directional from the positive to the negative charge centers. For a compound having several dipoles, the dipole moment depends on the symmetrical arrangement of the bonds. For example, chloroform ($CHCl_3$) exhibits a dipole moment of 1.05 debye (D) (10^{18} esu-cm), whereas carbon tetrachloride (CCl_4) has a dipole moment of zero. This is so because in the latter, the four C—Cl bonds, although individually they behave as a dipole, cancel one another through the tetrahedral structure. As pure compound, the dipole molecules may position themselves with neighboring molecules in such a way that the opposite charge centers point toward one another. This is known as the *dipole–dipole interaction* or Keesom force, which occurs readily between solvent molecules that exhibit permanent dipole. The dipole moment alone does not determine the polarity of a compound. Acetone, e.g., has a greater dipole moment than water, but water is a more polar solvent.

Many compounds, such CCl_4 and hydrocarbons, do exist in liquid form but without a permanent dipole. This suggests that another attractive force between the molecules exists, even though this force may be relatively small. Indeed, it has been shown that such a force can arise from electronic oscillation that produces a temporary polarization in one molecule, which in turn causes a temporary polarization of bonds in the neighboring molecules. This is known as the induced dipole–induced dipole interaction or the London force. By similar mechanism, a permanent dipole can also induce temporary polarization of nonpolar bonds of other molecules, which is known as the Debye force. Collectively, the Keesom, London, and Debye attractive forces are called the van der Waals forces, which are always involved in the solvent–solvent molecular interactions.

Hydrogen Bonds

If hydrogen is involved in a permanent dipole, it is partially, positively charged. The extreme of charge separation allows the hydrogen to leave the dipole as a proton, such as in the acid–base interactions. Even without complete charge separation, the partially charged hydrogen can interact with an electronegative group to form the hydrogen bond. Because the hydrogen is usually bound to a permanent dipole, the hydrogen bonding may be seen as a linkage of two electronegative atoms that normally would show a repulsive tendency toward each other. The hydrogen bond (bonding energy of 2 to 8 kcal/mol) is considerably weaker than the covalent bond (50 to 100 kcal/mol) and the ionic bond (over 100 kcal/mol). For this reason, hydrogen bonding interactions between molecules, such as those involved in biomolecular interactions and solubility phenomena, can readily occur and thus play a significant role in determining the biological activity of many molecules. It is well known that carboxylic acids form dimers through hydrogen bonding in a nonpolar environment. The tendency of forming dimers by acetic acid is so pronounced that it occurs even in the vapor state. Hydrogen bonding occurs intermolecularly as well as intramolecularly (**Figure 4-1**).

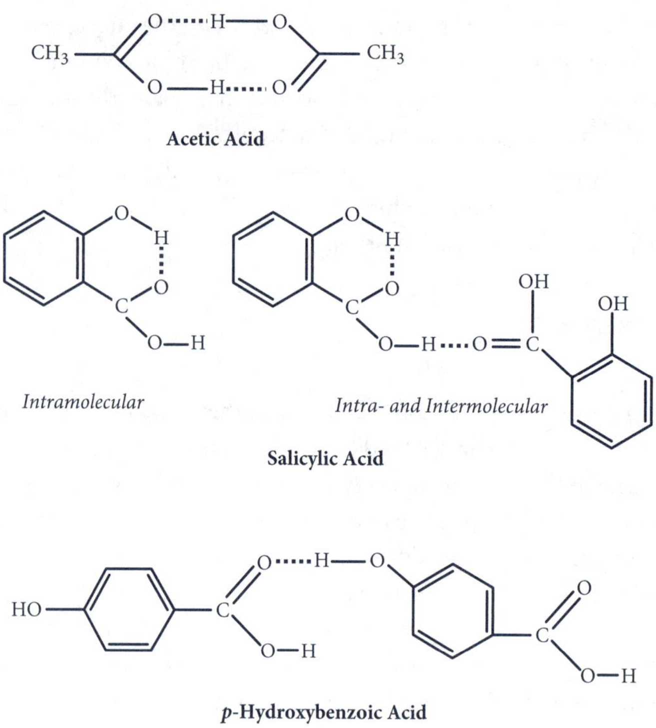

Figure 4-1 Hydrogen bonding in acetic acid, salicylic acid, and *p*-hydroxybenzoic acid.

For example, in salicylic acid (*o*-hydroxybenzoic acid), the structure is characterized by strong intramolecular hydrogen bonding, whereas in *p*-hydroxybenzoic acid (or *m*-hydroxybenzoic acid), only intermolecular hydrogen bonding is formed (Figure 4-1). As a result, salicylic acid is a much stronger acid ($pK_a = 3.0$) and is less soluble in water than the *p*-isomer ($pK_a = 4.5$). The *p*-isomer also has a higher melting point than salicylic acid due to its intermolecular hydrogen bonding. Pharmacologically, salicylic acid shows analgesic and antipyretic properties, whereas *m*- and *p*-hydroxybenzoic acids do not because of the hydrogen bonding effect.

Hydrogen bonding, to which the water molecule is both a hydrogen donor and a hydrogen acceptor, is inherently associated with the property of water. If one attempts to draw the structure of water through hydrogen bonding, one quickly comes to the conclusion that the number of possibilities is infinite. Without the versatility of hydrogen bonding, as in H_2S, water would not exist as a liquid in our life-sustaining temperature range. Many organic solvents can also serve as hydrogen donors or acceptors (or both) in their interactions with the solutes. Together with the van der Waals forces, these organic liquids are excellent solvents for solute molecules of a wide range of polarization properties. In addition, in a mixed solvent system, hydrogen bonding between the two solvent molecules can occur and can lead to altered solubility mechanism and outcome.

Solvation and Electrostatic Force

The separation of an electrostatic interaction between oppositely charged ions requires a solvent with a high dipole moment and the orientation of the solvent molecules to pull the charged ions apart from one another. This process is called the solvation, and when water is used as a solvent, it is the hydration. The solvation process is analogous to the thermodynamic concept that work must be done in order to create a "hole" among solvent molecules to allow the solute to get in. The necessity of solvation for the ionization of weak electrolytes is discussed in a later section. A second requirement for the separation of ions is to prevent or reduce the attractive force between the oppositely charged ions and, therefore, their reunion. In more precise terms, it has been shown that one solvent can do a better job than the other of reducing the electrostatic attractive force, due to a property called the dielectric constant (ε) in which ε is inversely proportional to the electrostatic force between two oppositely charged ions:

$$F = \frac{1}{\varepsilon}\frac{e_+e_-}{r^2} \tag{4-6}$$

Here F is the attractive force, e_+ and e_- are electric charges of the ions, r is the distance between the ions, and ε is the dielectric constant. The ionization of weak and strong electrolytes does occur in some organic solvents including the alcohols, acetone, and aniline, but the degree of ionization is relatively low because of their low dielectric constants. The dielectric constant is related to the dipole moment and the polarization of the solvent molecule. The mathematical relationship does not indicate a linear change of dielectric constant with changes in dipole moment, but in general, a higher dipole moment corresponds to a higher dielectric constant among the commonly used solvents.

Classification of Solvents

Based on the intermolecular forces described above, solvents have been classified as polar, semipolar, and nonpolar. Clearly if the chemical property of a solute allows certain intermolecular force to occur with a solvent molecule, dissolution of the solute in this solvent will take place. Hence, solutes can have similar designations to match the solvent action. In addition, it is always a goal for scientists to develop quantitative relationships, in this case, of the solubility with some measurable parameters. For this reason, classification of solvents has also been based on the dielectric constants of the solvents. These classifications are shown in **Table 4-2**.

Polar Solvents

Polar solvents are those that exhibit strong dipolar bonds and hydrogen bonding property. Water, as a polar solvent, induces ionization of weak and strong electrolytes and mixes freely with low-molecular-weight alcohols, sugars, and polyhydroxyl compounds. In addition, water dissolves

Table 4-2 Classification of Solvents

Polarity	Solvent	Dipole Moment (debye)†	Dielectric Constant (20°C)
Polar	Water	1.85	80
Semipolar	Glycerin		46
	Propylene glycol		41
	Methyl alcohol		33
	Ethyl alcohol		25
	Acetone	2.80	21
	Aniline	1.51	7.0
Nonpolar	Chloroform	1.05	5.0
	Ethyl ether	1.14	4.3
	Octyl alcohol		3.4
	Benzene	0	2.2
	Carbon tetrachloride	0	2.2

†1 Debye = 1×10^{-18} esu-cm.

ketones, aldehydes, acids, amines, and other compounds, via hydrogen bonding, serving as either a hydrogen donor or a hydrogen acceptor. The solubility of the organic compounds depends, to a large extent, on the ratio of the polar to nonpolar groups of the solute. As the nonpolar structure expands, the solubility in water decreases. Straight chain alcohols, aldehydes, ketones, and acids with more than four or five carbons are only slightly soluble in water, because the long chain structure prevents the entry of the solute into the hydrogen-bonded structure of water (less solvation). In contrast, the branch-chained 1-butyl alcohol, $(CH_3)_3COH$, is completely miscible with water whereas *n*-butanol is not, because of more extended solvation of the former.

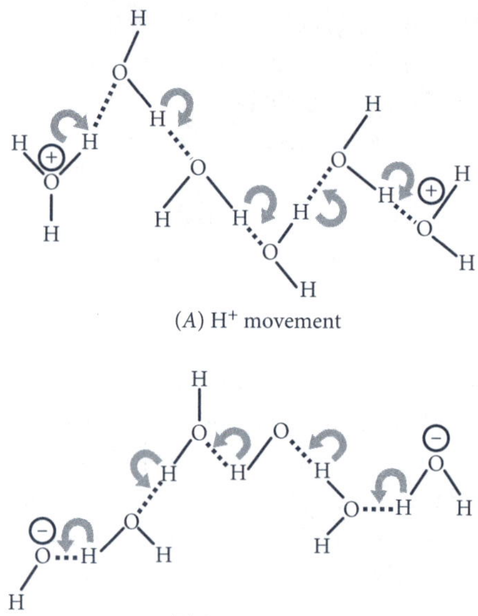

Figure 4-2 Movement of (*A*) H^+ and (*B*) OH^- by the Grotthuss mechanism.

The use of dielectric constant as a solvent polarity indicator actually places emphasis of the solvent classification on the ionization of molecules, because the dielectric constant directly relates to the stability of the ions. As mentioned earlier, solvation is necessary for the separation of ions. This can be seen from the Grotthuss mechanism, through which the unusually large equivalent conductance and ion mobility measured for H^+ and OH^- in water, compared to other ions, was attributed to the hydration-mediated movement of the ions (**Figure 4-2**). Similarly, the waterlike conductivity of H^+ also occurs in small alcohols, which have the hydroxyl group, but not in acetone. The reason is that although acetone can bind a proton, $(CH_3)_2C{=}OH^+$, it lacks the hydroxyl group needed for the movement of H^+ via the Grotthuss mechanism. This shows that alcohols may exhibit waterlike activity, whereas other solvents do not.

Semipolar and Nonpolar Solvents

Solvents that exhibit strong dipole but do not have a strong hydrogen bonding activity are semipolar solvents. In comparison, the nonpolar solvents, such as chloroform, benzene, hexane, and vegetable and mineral oils, are solvents that have low or little dipolar character. They are immiscible with water. The semipolar solvents are capable of dissolving both polar and nonpolar substances through permanent and induced dipoles as well as hydrogen bonding as a hydrogen acceptor or donor. Hence, they can serve as a medium for the preparation of a three-component homogeneous system containing polar and nonpolar solvents. Acetone, e.g., will increase the solubility of ether in water, resulting in a water–acetone–ether cosolvent system. This is of special value in analytical procedures, such as chromatography, where the analysis of compounds requires the separation of these compounds according to their polarity characteristics.

Henry's Law

The solubility of a gas in liquid represents the phase equilibrium between the vapor pressure of the gas and the concentration of the gas in solution. In such a system, the change in concentration may be described via pressure–concentration and temperature–concentration relationships. In general, the solubility of a gas decreases with increasing temperature. In contrast, the change in gas concentration in solution under isothermal conditions follows Henry's law, which states that in dilute solution, the partial vapor pressure of a solute (P_2) is proportional to the mole ratio of the solute (n_2) to that of the solvent (n_1) in solution, that is, $P_2 = k(n_2/n_1)$. Henry's law may be written in different forms with different proportional constants. If the dissolved gas V_2 is expressed in milliliters and the solvent volume is V_1 mL, then

$$V_2/V_1 = kP_2/P_t \qquad (4\text{-}7)$$

In this expression, P_2 is the partial vapor pressure of the gas, P_t is the total vapor pressure, and k is known as the solubility coefficient. Equation (4-7) is quite useful for the estimation of gas content in water at constant and different temperature conditions (see Example 4-2 for calculations).

Example 4-2: At 20°C, the vapor pressure of water is 17.5 mmHg, and the solubility coefficients for N_2, O_2, and CO_2 are 0.0154, 0.0310, and 0.8780, respectively. Assume the air contents of these gases are N_2, 79%; O_2, 20.96%; and CO_2, 0.04%. Calculate the gas content in 100 mL of water, which is well bubbled with air, at 20°C and 1 atm pressure.†

Solution: Vapor pressure from air = 760 – 17.5 = 742.5 mmHg

Partial pressures:

$P_{N_2} = 742.5 \times 0.79 = 586.6$ mmHg

$P_{O_2} = 742.5 \times 0.2096 = 155.6$ mmHg

$P_{CO_2} = 742.5 \times 0.0004 = 0.297$ mmHg

$V_{N_2} = kV_{water}P/P_t = 0.0154 \times 100 \times 586.6 / 760 = 1.188$ mL

$V_{O_2} = 0.0310 \times 100 \times 155.6 / 760 = 0.635$ mL

$V_{CO_2} = 0.878 \times 100 \times 0.297 / 760 = 0.034$ mL

Total air gases in water = 1.188 + 0.635 + 0.034 = 1.857 mL

% air gases in water:

N_2: 1.188/1.857 = 63.97%

O_2: 0.635/1.857 = 34.20%

CO_2: 0.034/1.857 = 1.83%

†For temperature effect, try similar calculations at 50°C and 1 atm pressure using the following data:

	Solubility Coefficient			
	0°C	20°C	50°C	100°C
H_2	0.0215	0.0182	0.0161	0.0161
N_2	0.0239	0.0154	0.0109	0.0095
O_2	0.0489	0.0310	0.0209	0.0170
CO_2	1.713	0.878	0.436	—
NH_3	1170	700	360	90

Notice that from the information given in Example 4-2, the solubility coefficients for CO_2 and NH_3 are very large compared to those of the other gases. This is so because CO_2 forms carbonic acid, whereas NH_3 forms the ammonium ion, in solutions. Gases dissolved in a solution are frequently liberated when an electrolyte (e.g., sodium chloride) is added to the solution. This is so because the added salt competes with the gas for solvation by the water molecules. Nonelectrolytes such as sucrose or glucose can produce the same effect. This phenomenon is called salting out.

The above discussion shows that the solubility of a gas in liquid is affected by the pressure, temperature, salt, and possible chemical reactions of the gas in solution. The pharmaceutical solutions of gases in water include those of hydrochloric acid, carbon dioxide, and ammonia, all of which undergo interactions with water in the formation of acids and base.

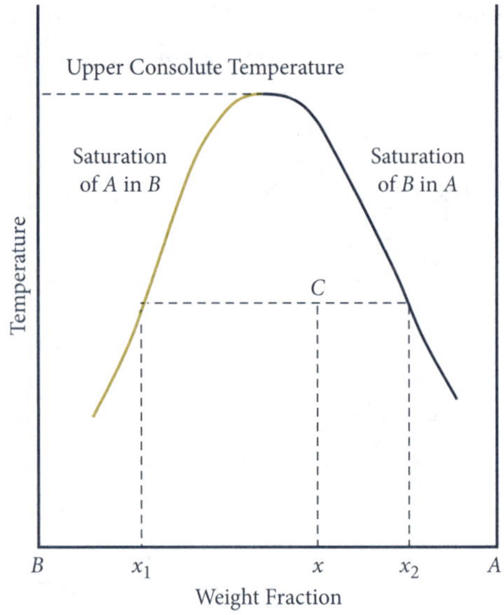

Figure 4-3 Temperature and composition effects on solubility and phase separation of a binary liquid–liquid system.

Solubility of Liquids in Liquids and Cosolvency

Miscibility and Phase Separation

The miscibility of two liquids depends largely on the intermolecular forces that govern the solubility of one compound in another, as previously discussed. Two liquids, such as water and ethanol, can be completely miscible with each other at any composition in the temperature range of interest. But in many systems, such as the mixing of water with organic liquids or oily substances in pharmaceutical preparations, the two liquids are only partially miscible, indicating that at a certain composition of the two liquids, the mixing can result in a homogeneous solution, yet, at other compositions, separated liquid phases may be present. This phenomenon can be readily explained using a phase diagram, which demonstrates not only the temperature-dependent mutual solubility of these liquids but also the contents of the separated phases in any given formulation.

Consider a binary system containing liquids A and B such that the solubility of both A in B and B in A increases with increasing temperature (this temperature effect is most common among binary liquid systems). At a given temperature, if the composition of liquid A (which also defines the composition of liquid B), expressed in percent w/w, is below the solubility of A in B or greater than the composition that indicates the solubility of B in A, then the two liquids will form a homogeneous solution. In between the range, however, phase separation will occur at equilibrium, and the separated phases will have a saturated concentration of A in B and B in A. This phenomenon is illustrated in **Figure 4-3** by a temperature–composition phase diagram, where the solid curve represents saturated solutions of A in B (left) and B in A (right) at different temperatures. This curve forms a composition boundary, within which two liquid phases exist. As the temperature increases, both solubility concentrations increase until they reach the maximum point at which their compositions become identical. The temperature at the maximum of the curve is known as the critical solution temperature or *upper consolute temperature*; i.e., above this temperature, the two liquids become completely miscible at any compositions.

The phase diagram of Figure 4-3 also allows one to determine the amount of each liquid in the separated phases at any point within the phase separation boundary. At point *C* (of Figure 4-3), e.g., where the composition of A is *x*, the weight ratio of liquid phase 1 (A in B) and phase 2 (B in A) can be determined by

$$w_1/w_2 = (x_2 - x) / (x - x_1) \quad (4\text{-}8)$$

where w_1 is the total weight in phase 1, w_2 is the total weight in phase 2, x_1 is the composition of A that corresponds to the solubility of A in B, and x_2 is the composition of A that corresponds to the solubility of B in A. Note that x is the initial weight percent of A, but not the composition of any of the two liquid phases (see Example 4-3 for the application of Equation (4-8)).

Example 4-3: The binary liquid–liquid system containing phenol (A) and water (B) shows a temperature–composition diagram similar to that of Figure 4-3. At 30°C, the solubility of phenol in water is 8% w/w, whereas the solubility of water in phenol corresponds to 70% w/w of phenol. If a formulation is made at 30°C to contain 40 g of phenol and 60 g of water, is this formulation a homogeneous solution? If not, calculate the amounts of water and phenol in each liquid phase.

Solution: At 40% phenol, the formulation greatly exceeds the solubility of phenol in water but has an insufficient amount of phenol to dissolve the amount of water. Hence, this system must exist in two liquid phases.

Calculation: The weight ratio of the two-liquid phase is

$$w_1/w_2 = (x_2 - x) / (x - x_1) = (0.7 - 0.4) / (0.4 - 0.08) = 0.938$$

or $w_1 = w_2 \times 0.938$

The total weight of the formulation is 100 g; that is, $w_1 + w_2 = 100$ g. Thus,
$w_2 = 100 / 1.938 = 51.61$ g $\quad w_1 = 100 - 51.61 = 48.39$ g

Answer: Liquid phase 1: concentration: 8% phenol

$wt_{phenol} = 0.08 \times 48.39 = 3.87$ g $\quad wt_{water} = 48.39 \times 0.92 = 44.52$ g

Liquid phase 2: concentration: 70% phenol

$wt_{phenol} = 51.61 \times 0.7 = 36.13$ g $\quad wt_{water} = 51.61 \times 0.3 = 15.48$ g

In some liquid–liquid systems, such as the water–triethylamine mixture, the mutual solubility decreases with increasing temperature, thus exhibiting a lower consolute temperature. A few systems, such as the water–nicotine equilibrium, can also exhibit both lower and upper consolute temperatures, thus forming a wheel-like boundary of the phase separation equilibrium. This behavior of increased mutual solubility at lower temperature is not normally expected but may be attributed to certain interactions between the components that can be effective at lower temperatures.

Cosolvent Systems

Water is the solvent of choice in pharmaceutical preparations, but it may be ineffective for several reasons including the limited aqueous solubility of many drugs and excipients, chemical stability, and sterility. A number of small alcohols and polyhydroxyl liquids have been found to be biocompatible and may be used to produce a cosolvent system with water to overcome the solubility and chemical stability problems. Most frequently ethanol is used to enhance the solubility of alkaloids, glycosides, essential oils, resins, and many drugs; glycerin and propylene glycol are cosolvents for salts, vegetable acids, enzymes (pepsin), some natural products, carbohydrates, and gums with some preservative activity; and for external applications, isopropanol is widely used in the preparation of lotions and liniments.

The alcohols have a lower dielectric constant and exhibit greater affinity toward dissolving neutral compounds than water. It is postulated that the solubility of a drug in a mixed solvent system may be described based on the changes in dielectric constant, which may be taken to be the percentage or mole fraction mean of those of the two solvents, i.e.,

$$\varepsilon_{\text{mixture}} = X_1\varepsilon_1 + X_2\varepsilon_2$$
$$\varepsilon_{\text{mixture}} = (\%)_1\varepsilon_1 + (\%)_2\varepsilon_2 \quad (4\text{-}9)$$

Studies have shown that the prediction of solubility based on the above concept works quite well for the solubility of salts, but not for nonelectrolytes. This is understandable because the dielectric constant, as mentioned earlier, measures the ionic stability by virture of the fact that it is inversely proportional to the electrostatic attractive force between ions. But what constitutes the dielectric property of a mixed solvent remains largely unknown.

It is well recognized that hydrogen bonding is a critical feature of polar and some semipolar solvents. In fact, in a mixed system containing an alcohol and water, hydrogen bonding between the alcohol and water molecules is not avoidable. The miscibility of a solvent with water thus depends largely on the hydrogen bonding activity. To test this concept, Zia et al.[12] reported a dielectric constant profile of a cosolvent system containing water and dimethyl isosorbide (DMI) and the effect of the cosolvency on the solubility of some steroid drugs. DMI contains two cyclic ether linkages (its structure can be seen in **Figure 4-4**) and is completely miscible with water. The ability of DMI to act as a hydrogen acceptor was verified using methanol as a hydrogen donor and NMR techniques. As can be seen from Figure 4-4, the dielectric constant profile of water and DMI shows a strong negative deviation from the relationship given in Equation (4-9). Going from low to high water concentration, the addition of water up to a mole fraction of 0.5 (1 : 1 water/DMI ratio) did little to increase the dielectric constant of the solution despite the fact that water has a dielectric constant of 80, whereas DMI has a value of 6.5. Further increase in water concentration resulted in a sigmoidal curve in the region where the mole ratio of water/DMI is 2. Although there are no stoichiometric relationships established, these data indicate that association of water molecules to DMI occurs at both ether linkages and that the dielectric constant reflects the associated species rather than a mixture of two solvent molecules. This is supported by the solubility data. DMI is a much better solvent than water for the steroids (prednisone, dexamethasone, and prednisolone). Interestingly, however, the maximum solubility for these drugs occurred not in the pure DMI solvent but in the region where hydrogen bonding between water and DMI took place. It is worth noting that when DMI is made a cosolvent with polyethylene glycol 400 (PEG), no hydrogen bonding activity was expected because of the rather large molecule of PEG, and the data showed a linear increase in prednisolone solubility with a linear decrease in dielectric constant (**Figure 4-5**). These data show that in a cosolvent system, the structural change of the solvent system due to interactions among the solvent components plays an important role in determining solubility. One might even view the water-associated DMI as a solvent different from DMI

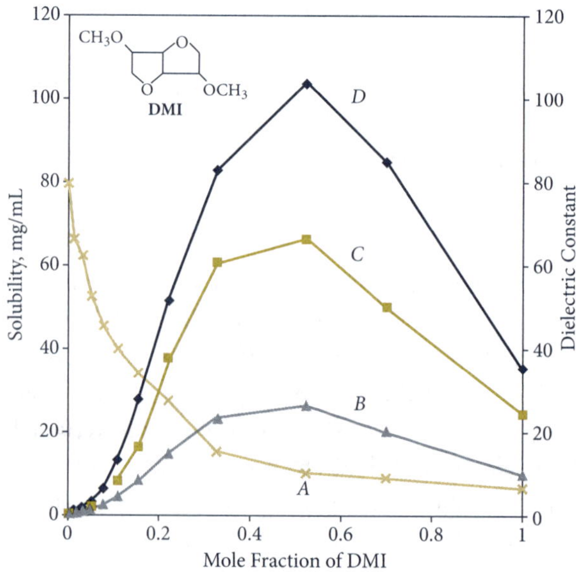

Figure 4-4 Dielectric constant profile (*A*) of the water–dimethyl isosorbide (DMI) cosolvent and steroid solubility (*B*, prednisone; *C*, dexamethasone; *D*, prednisolone).

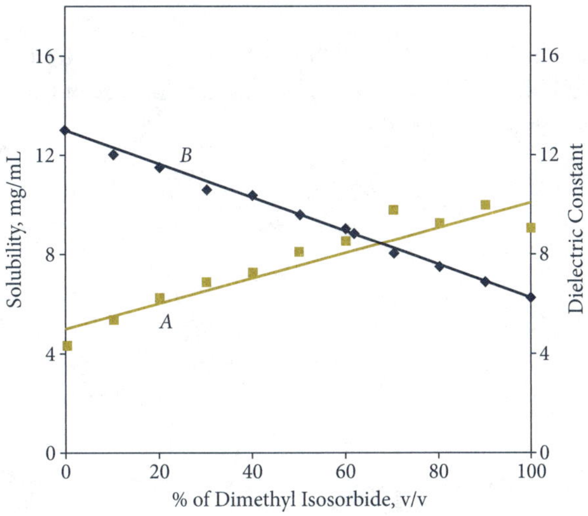

Figure 4-5 Linear relationships of increasing solubility of prednisolone (*A*) with decreasing dielectric constant (*B*) in the DMI–PEG cosolvent.

alone. The dielectric constant appears to be a useful parameter for the determination of solvent–solvent interactions.

III. Solubility of Strong and Weak Electrolytes

Solubility Product of Strong Electrolytes

Solubility Product

Strong electrolytes may be only slightly soluble, but they undergo complete ionization when dissolved in water. Thus, the equilibrium between a solid and its saturated solution for a strong electrolyte, using AgCl as an example, may be expressed as follows:

$$AgCl_{solid} \rightleftarrows Ag^+ + Cl^-$$

The equilibrium constant can be written as

$$K\,[AgCl_{solid}] = [Ag^+][Cl^-] = K_{sp} \qquad (4\text{-}10)$$

The K_{sp} (*solubility product*) designation stems from the fact that the solubility of AgCl is equal to $[Ag^+]$ or $[Cl^-]$ under complete ionization, so that $K_{sp} = S \times S$, where S stands for solubility. The K_{sp} for AgCl is 1.25×10^{-10}, hence the solubility of silver chloride is $(1.25 \times 10^{-10})^{1/2}$, or $1.12 \times 10^{-5}\,M$. This calculation is valid for a solution containing only the dissociated ions due to their small concentrations. In a solution where other ions may be present, or the ionic strength of the solution is sufficiently high, Equation (4-10) should be modified to

$$K_{sp} = [Ag^+][Cl^-]\,\gamma^2_{\pm} \quad \text{or} \quad S = (K_{sp})^{1/2}/\gamma_{\pm} \qquad (4\text{-}11)$$

The solubility expression of a salt is based on its chemical formula. For example, the ionization and K_{sp} for calcium hydroxide, $Ca(OH)_2$, is

$$Ca(OH)_2 \rightarrow Ca^{2+} + 2OH^- \quad \text{and} \quad K_{sp} = \gamma_{\pm}^{3}\,[Ca^{2+}][OH^-]^2$$

Because the solubility is equal to $[Ca^{2+}]$, $K_{sp} = 4S^3\,\gamma_{\pm}^{3}$.

Example 4-4: (*a*) The solubility product of calcium carbonate, found in drinking water, is 9×10^{-9}: what is the solubility of this salt? (*b*) What is the solubility of $CaCO_3$ in water if 0.20 *M* NaCl is added to the solution?

Solution: (*a*) $K_{sp} = [Ca^{2+}][CO_3^{2-}] = S^2 = 9 \times 10^{-9}$

$$S = 9.49 \times 10^{-5}\ M$$

(*b*) From the *Debye–Hückel theory*,

$$\log \gamma_{\pm} = -0.509 \times 4 \times (0.2)^{1/2} / [1 + (0.2)^{1/2}] = -0.6292$$

$$\gamma_{\pm} = 0.235$$

$$K_{sp} = [Ca^{2+}][CO_3^{2-}]\ \gamma_{\pm}^2 = S^2\ \gamma_{\pm}^2$$

or

$$S = K_{sp}^{1/2} / \gamma_{\pm} = 9.49 \times 10^{-5} / 0.235 = 4.04 \times 10^{-4}\ M$$

Observation: Compared to (*a*), the solubility of $CaCO_3$ is increased in the presence of NaCl.

Common Ion Effect

The alteration of the solubility of a salt occurs frequently when the ions common to those of the salt are present in the solution. The common ions drive the equilibrium toward non-ionization, thus resulting in a substantial decrease in the solubility of the salt. This effect can be seen from Example 4-5.

Example 4-5: What is the solubility of silver chromate (Ag_2CrO_4) (*a*) alone, (*b*) in the presence of 0.04 *M* silver nitrate, and (*c*) in the presence of 0.04 *M* K_2CrO_4, excluding the ionic strength effect? The K_{sp} of silver chromate is 2×10^{-12}.

Solution: (*a*) Alone: $K_{sp} = [Ag^+]^2[CrO_4^{2-}] = (2S)^2(S) = 4S^3$

$$S = (K_{sp}/4)^{1/3} = (2 \times 10^{-12}/4)^{1/3} = 7.94 \times 10^{-5}\ M$$

(*b*) In the presence of 0.04 *M* silver nitrate,

$$K_{sp} = [2S + 0.04]^2 S = 0.0016S \qquad (S \text{ is taken to be} << 0.04\ M)$$

$$S = K_{sp} / 0.0016 = 1.25 \times 10^{-9}\ M$$

(*c*) In the presence of 0.04 *M* potassium chromate,

$$K_{sp} = [2S]^2(0.04 + S) = 0.16S^2 \qquad (S << 0.04\ M)$$

$$S = (K_{sp} / 0.16)^{1/2} = 3.54 \times 10^{-6}\ M$$

The K_{sp}-regulated solubility is not limited to inorganic salts. The weak acids and weak bases are often made into salts to enhance their solubility. At first glance, it seems that they should be freely soluble in water, but the solubility of these salts depends on their solubility product and is subject to common ion effect (see Example 4-6). In the pharmaceutical and biological fluids, the frequently encountered ions at relatively high concentrations are Na^+, Cl^-, phosphate, citrate, HCO_3^-, etc. All these ions may serve to limit the solubility of a weak acid or weak base drug. In addition, the original salt form of a drug does not necessarily indicate the solubility in solution that contains other ions. For example, in a phosphate buffer, the solubility of an ionic species is likely determined by the K_{sp} of the phosphate salt.

Example 4-6: Morphine HCl · $3H_2O$ (mol wt = 375.85) has a reported solubility of about 1 g in 18 mL of water. (*a*) What is K_{sp} for morphine hydrochloride ($\gamma_\pm$ is about 0.75 for this solution)? (*b*) What is the solubility of this drug in 0.154 *M* NaCl, assuming the final solution has a $\gamma_\pm$ of about 0.70?

Solution: (*a*) Molarity of drug = 1 × 1000 / 375.85 × 18 = 0.1478 *M*

$$K_{sp} = S^2\gamma^2_\pm = (0.1478 \times 0.75)^2 = 0.0123$$

(*b*) $K_{sp}/\gamma_\pm = S\,(S + 0.154) \qquad S^2 + 0.154S - K_{sp}/\gamma_\pm = 0$

$$S = \frac{-0.154 + [(0.154)^2 + 4K_{sp}/\gamma_\pm]^{1/2}}{2} = 0.0763\,M$$

This solubility is equivalent to 1 g in 34 mL of water.

Solubility of Weak Electrolytes

The pH is the principal factor that controls the solubility of weak electrolytes. It is recalled that for a weak acid (HA)

$$\text{pH} = \text{p}K_a + \log\frac{[\text{A}^-]}{[\text{HA}]} - \frac{0.5091\mu^{1/2}}{1+\mu^{1/2}}$$

In a saturated solution, the concentration of HA will reach a maximum value equal to the intrinsic solubility of the undissociated acid (S_o). At a given pH, [HA] is in equilibrium with $[\text{A}^-]$; hence, the total concentration of the dissolved drug S_t is

$$S_t = [\text{HA}]_{\text{saturated}} + [\text{A}^-] = S_o + [\text{A}^-]$$

With this relationship, it can be seen that

$$\text{pH} = \text{p}K_a + \log\frac{S_t - S_o}{S_o} - \frac{0.5091\mu^{1/2}}{1+\mu^{1/2}} \qquad (4\text{-}12)$$

Equation (4-12) shows that the equilibrium between the solid and the saturated solution will shift toward higher solubility at higher pH, as more dissolved drug molecules are needed to maintain the intrinsic solubility S_o and to provide increased concentration of $[\text{A}^-]$ for the pH increase.

Similarly, for a weak base (B), the intrinsic solubility of the free base (B) does not change with pH, which may be designated as S_o, but the total solubility of the drug S_t increases with decreasing pH due to increases in $[\text{BH}^+]$ in acidic solution. Using the pH equation and the relation $S_t = S_o + [\text{BH}^+]$, it can be shown that

$$\text{pH} = \text{p}K_a + \log\frac{S_o}{S_t - S_o} + \frac{0.5091\mu^{1/2}}{1+\mu^{1/2}} \qquad (4\text{-}13)$$

In both Equations (4-12) and (4-13), S_t is the maximum concentration of the drug that can be dissolved at a given pH. Examples 4-7 and 4-8 will show that the pH condition is critical for the preparation of a weak acid or weak base drug solution.

Example 4-7: What is the minimum† pH below which barbital will begin to precipitate from a 1.5% solution of sodium barbital (mol wt = 206.2)? The solubility of barbital is 0.0048 *M*, and $K_a = 1.23 \times 10^{-8}$.

Solution: Molar concentration = 1.5 × 1000 / 206.2 × 100 = 0.0727 *M*, which gives an ionic strength of 0.0727. From the K_a value, $pK_a = 7.91$. Thus, using Equation (4-12),

$$\begin{aligned} pH &= 7.91 + \log[(0.0727 - 0.0048)/0.0048] \\ &\quad - 0.5091(0.0727)^{1/2}/[1 + (0.0727)^{1/2}] \\ &= 7.91 + 1.15 - 0.11 = 8.95 \end{aligned}$$

Answer: Precipitation of the acid occurs at pH below 8.95.

†The calculated pH in the above example is sometimes referred to as pH_p, the threshold pH to maintain a given total concentration.

Example 4-8: What is the highest pH allowed† to prepare a 1% morphine solution? (Mol wt of drug = 285.35; $S_o = 6 \times 10^{-4}\,M$; pK_b of morphine = 6.17.)

Solution: $S_t = 1 \times 1000/285.35 \times 100 = 0.035\,M$; $S_o = 0.0006\,M$

$$\begin{aligned} pH &= 14 - 6.13 + \log[0.0006/(0.035 - 0.0006)] \\ &\quad + 0.5091(0.035)^{1/2}/[1 + (0.035)^{1/2}] \\ &= 7.87 - 1.76 + 0.08 = 6.19 \end{aligned}$$

†The calculated pH in the above example is sometimes referred to as pH_p, the threshold pH to maintain a given total concentration.

The pH-Solubility Profile

The maximum pH effect on the solubility of a weak acid or weak base may result in as high as a 10,000-fold change of the intrinsic solubility of the undissociated drug. This corresponds to a change in pH by 4 pH units above the pK_a of a weak acid, or below the pK_a of a weak base, where the drug is 99.99% ionized. But the maximum solubility of a drug in the ionic form is limited by its K_{sp}, which could significantly change the maximum pH effect. If the solution or the relevant biological fluid contains a common ion, the solubility of the drug and the pH effect can be further reduced. For a solubility product–limited ion solubility of a 1 : 1 salt,

$$S_{ion} = K_{sp}^{1/2}/\gamma_{\pm}$$

the maximum pH effect may be written as

$$pH_{max} = pK_a + \log[K_{sp}^{1/2}/S_o] \text{ (weak acid)}$$

or $$pH_{max} = pK_a + \log[S_o/K_{sp}^{1/2}] \text{ (weak base)} \quad (4\text{-}14)$$

Using morphine as an example, the changes in the logarithm of total solubility S_t as a function of pH, known as the *pH–solubility profile*, are illustrated in **Figure 4-6**. Here the intrinsic solubility of morphine is taken to be 0.17 mg/mL, whereas the ionic solubility is taken to be 55.5 mg/mL of morphine $HCl \cdot 3H_2O$[13] with a calculated K_{sp} of 0.0123. These numbers are not to be taken as

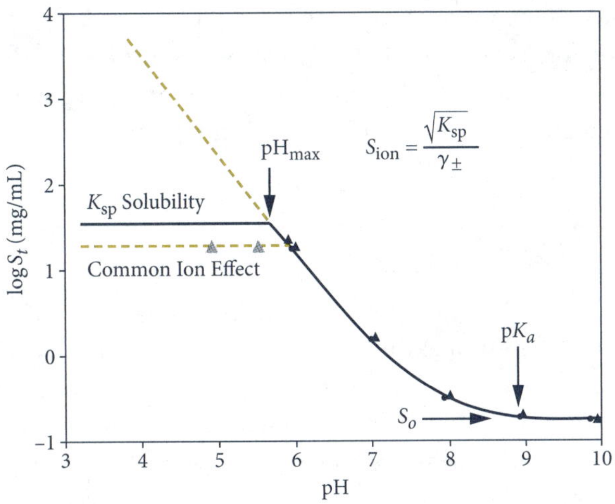

Figure 4-6 The pH- and K_{sp}-dependent solubility of a weak base in the absence (circle) and presence (triangle) of 0.1 *M* NaCl. Data are calculated using the approximate solubility of morphine and morphine HCL and Equations (4-11), (4-13), and (4-14).

precise experimental values. Figure 4-6 shows that the solubility of a weak base (or weak acid) is regulated by the pH and the solubility product. The effective pH range is between pK_a and pH_{max}, and the latter can be determined using Equation (4-14). The figure also shows that in the presence of a common ion, the effective pH range is narrowed and the total solubility is decreased. The pH–solubility profile is very useful for the study of drug dissolution and drug absorption in the GI tract, as the pH, as well as the presence of common ions, varies at different GI positions.

IV. Distribution Phenomena

The Distribution Law

Partition Coefficient

Consider a binary liquid–liquid system, in which the two liquids are largely immiscible. If a solute is added to this system and it is vigorously shaken, each liquid phase is expected to contain certain amount of the solute after the phases are separated and equilibrium is reestablished. The thermodynamic definition of equilibrium is that the chemical potential, or partial molar free energy, required to produce a C_1 concentration of solute in phase 1 and that required to produce a C_2 concentration in phase 2 become equal, so that no further changes in concentrations can be expected. The chemical potential for the two phases can be written as

$$\mu_1 = \mu_1^o + RT \ln \gamma_1 C_1$$
$$\mu_2 = \mu_2^o + RT \ln \gamma_2 C_2$$

At equilibrium, $\mu_1 = \mu_2$, and

$$\mu_2^o - \mu_1^o + RT \ln (\gamma_2 C_2/\gamma_1 C_1)$$

Because the standard chemical potentials are constants under constant pressure, the activity ratio of the two phases must be a constant, that is, $\gamma_2 C_2/\gamma_1 C_1 = K$. In dilute solutions, the activity coefficient may be considered to be 1; hence,

$$K = C_2/C_1 \tag{4-15}$$

Equation (4-15) is known as the *distribution* or *partition law*, where K is called the *partition coefficient*. The condition for Equation (4-15) to be true is that the chemical identities of the solute in phases 1 and 2 must be the same. For example, a weak acid may exist in an aqueous solution as HA and A^-, but when partitioned into an organic solvent, it can exist as HA but not A^-. In this case, $K = [HA]_{organic}/[HA]_{water}$.

Apparent Partition Coefficient

The distribution of a solute in two immiscible liquids depends on both the chemical nature of the solute and the liquid phases. The primary interest in drug research involves, of course, the aqueous phase, in which a weak acid or weak base may exist in both the neutral and the ionic forms. In the organic, or oil, layer, these solutes often undergo self-association into dimers or complexation with other molecules. It has been shown that some organic solvents such as 1-octanol contain an appreciable amount of water at equilibrium, which significantly reduces the tendency of weak acids in dimerization. In such a system, the distribution phenomena may be described in the following diagram for a weak acid drug:

Organic phase	HA
	⇅
Water phase	HA + A^-

The partition occurs through HA, and the concentration ratio of the two phases is

$$\frac{C_o}{C_w} = \frac{[HA]_o}{[HA]_w + [A^-]}$$

Substituting $K_a[HA]/[H_3O^+]$ for $[A^-]$ (acid–base equilibrium), it can be shown that

$$\frac{C_o}{C_w} = \frac{[HA]_o}{[HA]_w(1 + K_a/[H_3O^+])} = \frac{K[H_3O^+]}{K_a + [H_3O^+]} = K' \quad (4\text{-}16)$$

In Equation (4-16), the partition coefficient K is equal to $[HA]_o/[HA]_w$ as previously defined; the concentration ratio of the organic to water phases (C_o/C_w) will be a constant if the aqueous solution is buffered at a given pH. This constant is known as the *apparent partition coefficient* (K'). In experimental studies, the partition coefficient K of a weak acid may be determined using acidified water (solution with pH 2–3 units below its pK_a to prevent ionization) or using buffered solutions at different pH, through which both K and K' are determined using Equation (4-16).

Molecular Association

The nonpolar organic solvents such as benzene, hexane, and carbon tetrachloride can serve as an inert medium for the study of interactions between polar or semipolar substances. On the other hand, interactions by the solutes, such as the self-association of the carboxylic acids, also reduce their overall polarity, thus allowing the solute to partition into the organic phase. The distribution phenomenon of a weak acid between acidified water and a nonpolar solvent can be seen from the following diagram:

Organic phase	nHA ⇄ (HA)n
	⇅
Water phase	HA

Here n is the number of molecules involved in the association in the organic phase, and this molecular interaction may be expressed by its dissociation constant K_d:

$$K_d = [HA]^n/[(HA)n]$$

From this, it can be seen that $[HA]_o = K_d^{1/n}\,[(HA)n])^{1/n}$. In the organic phase, the total drug concentration is C_o. If all molecules participated in association, i.e., the amount of single molecules in the organic phase is negligible, then $C_o = [(HA)n]$. In the aqueous layer, $C_w = [HA]_w$. The partition coefficient ($K = [HA]_o/[HA]_w$) can then be written as

$$K / K_d^{1/n} = C_o^{1/n} / [HA]_w \quad \text{or} \quad K'' = C_o^{1/n} / C_w \qquad (4\text{-}17)$$

Equation (4-17) shows that under molecular association, the *n*th root of C_o divided by C_w is a constant (K''), whereas C_o/C_w is not. Many studies, including the one given in Example 4-9, have shown that carboxylic acids form dimers ($n = 2$) in a nonpolar environment.

Example 4-9: Explain the distribution data (first two columns) of acetic acid in carbon tetrachloride and water at 25°C.

Conc. in CCl_4	Conc. in Water	C_o / C_w	$C_o^{1/2} / C_w$	$C_o^{1/3} / C_w$
0.0096	0.684	0.0140	0.143	0.311
0.0187	1.021	0.0183	0.132	0.260
0.0460	1.691	0.0272	0.127	0.212

Answer: According to the calculated values shown in columns 3–5, C_o/C_w is not a constant, nor is $C_o^{1/3}/C_w$. But $C_o^{1/2}/C_w$ approximates a constant, indicating the acetic acid forms dimers in CCl_4 (see Figure 4-1 for the hydrogen bonding feature).

Solvent Extraction

In analytical and industrial procedures, solvent extraction is the most powerful tool for the separation, isolation, and purification of drug molecules. In general, weak electrolytes are converted to non-ionized species via pH adjustment before extraction. As a convenience, the partition coefficient for solvent extraction is defined as follows:

$$K = \text{concentration in original solvent / concentration in extracting solvent}$$
$$= (w_1 / V_1) / [(w_t - w_1) / V_2]$$

Hence, the amount of drug that remains in the original solvent after one extraction, w_1, is

$$w_1 = \frac{w_t KV_1}{KV_1 + V_2}$$

where w_t is the original amount of drug, V_1 is the volume of the original solvent, and V_2 is the volume of the extracting solvent.

For multiple extractions using the same volume of extracting solvent each time, the amount of drug remaining in the original solvent (w_n) after the *n*th extraction is

$$w_n = w_t\,[KV_1 / (KV_1 + V_2)]^n \qquad (4\text{-}18)$$

The use of Equation (4-18) is illustrated in Example 4-10.

Example 4-10: An aqueous solution contains 1.2 g of a drug in 100 mL of solution. (*a*) If the drug was extracted using 100 mL of chloroform, how many grams of the drug remain in the aqueous layer? The drug is known to have an *o/w* partition coefficient (C_o/C_w) of 5.0. (*b*) If the extraction was carried out 4 times each with 25 mL chloroform, what would be the amount of drug remaining in the aqueous solution?

Solution: (*a*) Because water is the original solvent, $K = C_w / C_o = 0.2$. Using Equation (4-18), let $n = 1$,

$$w_1 = 1.2(0.2 \times 100) / (0.2 \times 100 + 100) = 0.2\,\text{g}$$

(*b*) Let $n = 4$ and $V_2 = 25\,\text{mL}$,

$$w_4 = 1.2[(0.2 \times 100)/(0.2 \times 100 + 25)]^4 = 0.0468\,\text{g}$$

Observation: Multiple extractions are more efficient in removing the solute and use less solvent compared to single extraction using a larger volume.

Partition Coefficients and Drug Solubility

Significance of Partition Coefficient

In comparison to the polarity designation for the solvent, the partition coefficient is a measurement of the lipophilicity of a solute. There is no more important parameter than lipophilicity in the quantitation of biological responses. Historically, partition coefficients were first correlated with the biological activity of hypnotic and narcotic drugs by Overton[14] and Meyer.[15] Since then, various mathematical models have been developed for the establishment of *quantitative structure–activity relationships* (QSARs) that include drug permeability, in vivo transport of xenobiotics through aqueous and lipid compartments,[16] drug binding, molecular structures and connectivity, liquid chromatography, and the aqueous solubility of organic drugs. The partition coefficient is an additive and constitutive property, which can be calculated with reasonable accuracy using published methods.[17, 18] Detailed discussion of all these relationships is beyond the scope of this book. Instead, we examine the nature of the partitioning process and its application in the prediction of the aqueous solubility of organic compounds.

The Octanol–Water System

Although the partition coefficient may be measured in any binary liquid system displaying some immiscibility, Leo et al.[19] have pointed out a convincing rationale for the use of the *octanol–water system*. 1-Octanol, having a polar head and a hydrophobic alkyl chain, resembles the lipids of biological membranes. A wider range of compounds is soluble in octanol compared to hydrocarbons such as cyclohexane and isooctane. The solubility of water in octanol is 2.3 *M*, or 0.27 in mole fraction. This relatively high concentration of water allows the transfer of hydrated molecules from the aqueous to the organic phase without breaking of hydrogen bonds or solvation and reduces the tendency of drug molecules to self-association. In contrast, the solubility of octanol in water is 0.0045 *M*, which is small and negligible, allowing easier solubility calculations and predictions. Hydrocarbon solvents are generally associated with molecular associations, which yield partition coefficients that do not correspond to the drug solubility.[20] Given its tendency to allow the existence of drug in one species in both phases, the octanol–water system is ideal for measuring the hydrophobicity of drugs. This system has served as the basis for various theoretical predictions of partition coefficient using chemical structural parameters such as the *hydrophobic substituent constant* π and the *hydrophobic fragmental constant* f and provided useful relationships between the biological activity and partition coefficient.

Solubility and Partition Coefficient

It is now clear that the solubility of a solid drug depends on two separable properties. The first property is the energy involved in breaking the crystal lattices as described in Equation (4-1). This process depends on the melting point and the heat of fusion of the solid solute. The second property deals with intermolecular cohesion of solute–solute and solvent–solvent molecules and the adhesion between solute and solvent molecules. The Scatchard–Hildebrand equation[7, 8] shows the work that must be done to achieve solubility; other studies[10, 21] have taken a different approach, in that the intermolecular interactions may be treated as the solubility of a liquid in liquid that can be explained by the partition phenomenon using the octanol–water system.

The relationship between the partition coefficient and solubility may be seen from the following discussion. For the distribution of a liquid solute in two immiscible liquid phases, if one selects the pure solute as the standard state, then the activity that yields the chemical potential, following Raoult's law, is the mole fraction multiplied by its activity coefficient. At equilibrium, the chemical potentials of the two phases are identical; hence,

$$X_o\,\gamma_o = X_w\,\gamma_w \tag{4-19}$$

where X_o and γ_o are the respective mole fraction and activity coefficient of the solute in the octanol phase, and X_w and γ_w are the same designated parameters in the water phase. If the partition coefficient K_{ow} is expressed as the ratio of the mole fractions, as used by Yalkowsky and Valvani,[10] then

$$K_{ow} = X_o/X_w = \gamma_w/\gamma_o$$

$$\text{or } \log K_{ow} = \log \gamma_w - \log \gamma_o \tag{4-20}$$

Chiou et al.[21] have shown that when K_{ow} is expressed in molar concentration ratio, Equation (4-18) can be rewritten as

$$K_{ow} = C_o/C_w = \gamma^*_w V^*_w/\gamma^*_o V^*_o$$

where V_o and V_w are the molar volumes of the octanol and water phases, respectively, and the asterisk indicates equilibrium condition rather than pure solvents.

It is recalled that the ideal solubility of a solid, given in Equation (4-1), was modified for the nonideal solution using the term $\log \gamma_2$ in the extended Hildebrand approach (Equation (4-2)). This term was added to account for the intermolecular interactions. Equation (4-20) suggests that these interactions can be quantified by the partition coefficient. Letting $\Delta S_f = \Delta H_f/T_o$, with MP as the melting point, and with the temperature of solubility determination to be 25°C, Yalkowsky and Valvani showed that Equation (4-1) can be modified to

$$\begin{aligned} \log X_w &= \frac{-\Delta S_f}{1364}(\text{MP} - 25) - \log \gamma_w \\ &= -\Delta S_f(\text{MP} - 25)/(1364) - \log K_{ow} - \log \gamma_o \end{aligned} \tag{4-21}$$

They chose to use the entropy rather than the heat of fusion, because the former is more easily understood and predicted for rigid nonelectrolyte molecules. The significance of the above equation lies in the use of $\log K_{ow}$, also known as $\log P$, to estimate the aqueous solubility of nonelectrolytes. The term $\log \gamma_o$ is largely unknown. It is suggested that $\gamma_o = 1$ if the solubility of the drug in octanol follows ideal behavior. Nevertheless, the term $\log \gamma_o$ is not as important, because the actual use of Equation (4-21) involves calculation of the solubility of a very large number of compounds that have observed solubility data, so that more refined equations are generated through linear regression analysis. For example, Equation (4-4), where the mole fraction solubility of Equation (4-21) is now converted to the conventional molar solubility, was shown to predict the solubility of 167 organic nonelectrolytes within 0.5 log unit of the observed value.

$$\log S_{\text{int}} = -\log K_{ow} - 1.11\,\frac{\Delta S_f\,(\text{MP} - 25)}{1364} + 0.54$$

$$n = 167 \qquad r = 0.994 \quad r^2 = 0.988 \qquad s = 0.242 \tag{4-4}$$

The theory that $\log \gamma_w$ represents the logarithm of the mole fraction solubility of organic liquids was also tested by Yalkowsky and Valvani. They showed that

$$-\log \gamma_w = -1.08 \log K_{ow} - 1.04$$

$$n = 417 \qquad r = 0.946 \qquad s = 0.356$$

Similar results that K_{ow} may be used to predict solubility of organic liquids were also reported by Chiou et al.[21] Yalkowsky et al.[22] have also established a relation between the partition coefficient and the relative solubility of a drug in the two phases in that

$$\log K_{ow} \,/\, \log (S_o/S_w) = 1.027$$

The nearly unit value of the above relationship indicates that the partition coefficient is, in fact, the ratio of the solubilities of the drug in the octanol and water phases.

As the theory of the partition coefficient was more closely tested with larger databases, a general solubility equation was proposed by Jain and Yalkowsky,[23]

$$\log S_w = 0.5 - 0.01(\text{MP} - 25) - \log K_{ow} \tag{4-22}$$

where S_w is the molar aqueous solubility and MP is the melting point. If the solute is a liquid at 25°C, the term MP − 25 is set to zero. This equation was developed based on the assumptions that (1) ΔS_f is 56.5 J/deg-mol for nonassociating compounds, (2) $K_{ow} = S_o/S_w$, (3) complete miscibility of a solute with octanol corresponds to a mole fraction solubility of 0.5 or a molar solubility of 3.15, and (4) the melting point of the solute does not change in the presence of water. It has been shown to have a strong applicability in predicting the solubility of a very large number of organic molecules, with solubility range over 15 orders of magnitude[24] (see **Figure 4-7**). Some calculations using Equations (4-1), (4-4), and (4-22) can be seen from Example 4-11.

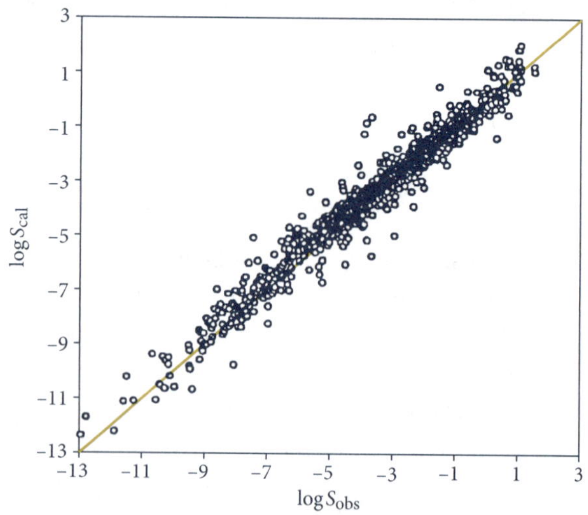

Figure 4-7 Predicted $\log S_w$ using the general solubility equation versus experimental $\log S_w$, $n = 1026$.
Reprinted from: *Chemosphere*, Vol 48, Issue 5, Yingqing Ran, Yan He, Gang Yang, Jennifer L.H. Johnson, Samuel H. Yalkowsky, Estimation of aqueous solubility of organic compounds by using the general solubility equation, Pages 487–509, Copyright 2002, with permission from Elsevier.

Example 4-11: Using the data given in **Table 4-3**, calculate the solubility of (*a*) warfarin† and (*b*) methanol† in water at 25°C using Equations (4-1), (4-4), and (4-22).

Solution: (*a*) Warfarin:

MP = 161°C, $\log K_{ow} = 2.89$ (calculated)

For consistency, Equation (4-1) can be converted to indicate molar solubility as follows:

$$\log S_w = -\Delta S_f (\text{MP} - 25)/(1364) + 1.744$$

According to the general solubility equation assumption,

$$\Delta S_f = 56.5 \text{ J/deg-mol} = 56.5/4.184 = 13.50 \text{ cal/deg-mol}$$

Using Equation (4-1),

$$-\log S_w = -13.5\,(161 - 25)/1364 + 1.744$$
$$= -1.346 + 1.7442 = 0.3983 \qquad (S_w = 2.5\,M)$$

Using Equation (4-4),

$$\log S_w = -2.89 - 1.11 \times 1.346 + 0.54 = -3.84$$

$(S_w = 1.4 \times 10^{-4} M)$

Using Equation (4-22): $\log S_w = 0.5 - 0.01(161 - 25) - 2.89 = -3.75$

$(S_w = 1.78 \times 10^{-4} M)$

(*b*) Methanol: for liquid, let MP – 25 be zero, $\log K_{ow} = -0.76$.

Table 4-3 Solubility and Melting Point Data of Some Organic Compounds

Compound	MP, °C	Calc. $\log K_{ow}$	$\log S_{w,obs}$
Decachlorobiphenyl	304	9.92	−11.89
Benzo[*a*]pyrene	178	6.12	−8.25
Ibuprofen	76	3.68	−3.76
Digitoxin	256	3.05	−5.28
Warfarin	161	2.89	−3.89
Lidocaine	67	1.95	−1.76
Prednisone	234	1.62	−3.48
Codeine	155	0.98	−1.52
Cimetidine	142	0.35	−1.35
Antipyrene	111	0.20	−0.56
Methanol	−98	−0.76	1.56
D-Mannitol	168	−2.05	0.07

Data from: Ran et al., *Chemosphere*, 48:487–509 (2002).

Using Equation (4-4),

$\log S_w = -(-0.76) + 0.54 = 1.30 \qquad (S_w = 19.95\,M)$

Using Equation (4-22),

$\log S_w = 0.5 - (-0.76) = 1.26 \qquad (S_w = 18.2\,M)$

†The observed $\log S_w$ value is −3.89 ($S_w = 1.29 \times 10^{-4}\,M$) for warfarin and 1.56 ($S_w = 31.62\,M$) for methanol.

V. Enhancement of Drug Solubility

In light of the difficulties of using conventional formulation techniques for drug product development involving poorly water-soluble drugs, scientists have continuously attempted new approaches that either improve the solubility of the drug or provide novel delivery methods to overcome the solubility problems. These approaches include the use of polymeric compounds, such as the cyclodextrins,[25] surfactant materials,[26, 27] and the pro-drug approach[28] to improve solubility; and delivery strategies using solid dispersions,[29] lipid-based formulation,[27] pH modifiers,[30, 31] and nanoparticle-based drug delivery.[32, 33] A brief description of these approaches is given below, whereas the physical chemistry of these methods is discussed in later chapters as they relate to the subject of interest. There are, however, excellent reviews (as indicated by the citation in each subject) of these topics in the literature that provide the rationale and methodology on how improved drug solubility and absorption is achieved.

Cyclodextrins are cyclic oligosaccharides that contain a number of glucose monomers (6–8 units) forming a toroid-shaped structure. The interior of the toroids is not hydrophobic but is considerably less hydrophilic than the bulk aqueous environment. Practically insoluble drugs can form inclusion complexes with cyclodextrin as either monomers or small aggregates. This leads to increased drug solubility. Interactions of lipophilic drugs with phospholipids and synthetic surfactants have long been used to improve drug solubility through the formation of micelles, liposomes, and microemulsions. The lipid-based formulations have been shown to also improve oral drug absorption through enhanced membrane permeability due to lipid–membrane interactions. The prediction of drug solubility in lipid vehicles depends on a number of factors involving the interfacial effects as well as the microstructure of the lipid vehicle. A number of models with varying degrees of sophistication have been shown to be useful in predicting drug solubility based on the chemical characteristics of the drug, lipid, oil, and solvent used. There is a mutual effect of the water–lipid equilibrium in that while the lipid extracts the drug from the aqueous system through partition, water alters lipid solubility by changing lipid organization in the microstructure. The pro-drug approach has been recommended as a viable approach in the early drug discovery process, as some of the most successful drugs are pro-drugs. With a better understanding of the active-transport processes of a drug at the cell membranes, a pro-drug may be designed to improve the drug's solubility and bioavailability.

Lipophilic drug may be dissolved in hydrophilic polymeric carrier as a solid dispersion. This strategy removes the crystallinity barrier and produces very fine particles that lead to supersaturated solution. The application of this concept in drug formulation depends on the physiochemical properties and the stability of the carrier systems. The same is also true for lipid-based formulations such as liposomes and microemulsions, where product stability is of primary importance. Although solid dispersion offers the advantage of supersaturated solubility for drug dissolution, this process is also pH-dependent for acid and base drugs. The inclusion of a pH modifier in the solid dispersion can lead to changed microenvironmental pH, ionization of drug, interaction between drug and polymer, and thus an altered drug dissolution rate. Studies have shown that in immediate-release formulations using the salt form of the drug, a pH modifier that results in precipitation of the drug enhances dissolution. In contrast, the pH modifiers can be used in controlled-release dosage forms to diminish the release rate, such as by increasing the microenvironmental pH for a weak base. Nanosuspensions are not—and are more viscous than—true solutions, but evidence suggests that nanoparticles have the ability to interact with complex cellular matrix and result in drug absorption that is significantly different from those of microparticle preparations. This difference, as shown in studies of some ophthalmic preparations, is manifested by the enhancement in the rate and extent of drug absorption and the duration of the drug effect. Our understanding of the properties of nanoparticles is incomplete, and it is only in the past few years that nanoscience, which is anticipated to play a key role in current and future drug delivery research, has been applied to the formulation of water-insoluble drugs.

VI. Chapter Summary

This chapter describes the physicochemical principles that govern the solubility of a drug. Although the theories appear to be easy, it is actually complicated and requires a breadth of knowledge when these theories are applied to solve drug formulation problems. Solubility is an important issue in drug development as well as in extemporaneous pharmaceutical compounding, and this requires a clear understanding of theories on the solubilization process. As outlined in this chapter, the measurement of drug solubility of sparingly soluble compounds can be notoriously difficult. Although this problem is somewhat alleviated through the development of high-throughput methods, prediction of solubility can be used for screening of drug candidates in drug development studies. Thus, methods for the prediction of drug solubility are of importance despite the fact that the predicted solubility may be 2- to 10-fold different from that of the observed value. It should be mentioned that there are many models for the prediction of a drug's aqueous solubility. These methods utilize the chemical structural characteristics and predict the solubility using fragment-based and descriptor-based methods[34, 35] with various statistical techniques. The K_{ow}-based solubility prediction is presented here as it relates to the physicochemical principles discussed in this chapter.

VII. References

1. Dahan A, Miller JM, and Amidon GL. *AAPS J.* 11:740–746, 2009.
2. Obata K, Sugano K, Machida M, and Aso Y. *Drug Dev Ind Pharm.* 30:181, 2004.
3. Sugano K, Kato T, Suzuki K, Keiko K, Sujaku T, and Mano T. *J Pharm Sci.* 95:2115–2122, 2006.
4. Sugano K, Okazaki A, Sugimoto S, Tavornvipas S, Omura A, and Mano T. *Drug Metab Pharmacokinet.* 22:225–254, 2007.
5. Sugaya Y, Yoshiba T, Kajima T, and Ishihama Y. *Yakugaku Zasshi.* 122:237–246, 2002.
6. Yu LX. *Pharm Res.* 16:1883–1887, 1999.
7. Scatchard G. *Chem Rev.* 8:321, 1931.
8. Hildebrand JH and Wood SE. *J Chem Phys.* 1:817, 1933.
9. Martin A, Newburge J, and Adjei A. *J Pharm Sci.* 68:487, 1980; also Martin A, Paruta AN, and Adjei A. *J Pharm Sci.* 70:1115–1120, 1981; Martin A, Wu PL, and Velasques T. *J Pharm Sci.* 74:277–282, 1985.
10. Yalkowsky SH and Valvani SC. *J Pharm Sci.* 69:912–922, 1980.
11. Banker GS and Rhodes CT. *Modern Pharmaceutics*, New York, Marcel Dekker, 1979, p 164.
12. Zia H, Ma JKH, O'Donnell JP, and Luzzi LA. *Pharm Res.* 8:502–504, 1991.

13. Swinyard EA in *Remington's Pharmaceutical Sciences,* 5th ed., Easton, PA, Mack Publishing Co., 1975, pp 1037–1039.
14. Overton E. *Z. Physik Chem.* 22:189–209, 1897.
15. Meyer H. *Arch Exper Pathol Pharmakol.* 42:109–118, 1899.
16. Penniston JT, Beckett L, Bentley DL, and Hansch C. *Mol Pharmacol.* 5:333–341, 1969.
17. Rekker RF. *The Hydrophobic Fragmental Constant.* Amsterdam, Elsevier, 1977.
18. Hansch C and Leo A. *J Org Chem.* 32:2583–2586, 1967.
19. Leo A, Hansch C, and Elkins D. *Chem Rev.* 71:525–616, 1971.
20. Dearden JC. *Environ Health Perspect.* 61:203–228, 1985.
21. Chiou CT, Schmedding DW, and Manes M. *Environ Sci Technol.* 16:4–10, 1982.
22. Yalkowsky SH, Valvani SC, and Roseman TJ. *J Pharm Sci.* 72:866–870, 1983.
23. Jain N and Yalkowsky SH. *I Pharm Sci.* 90:234–253, 2000.
24. Ran Y, He Y, Yang G, Johnson JLH, and Yalkowskey SH. *Chemosphere.* 48:487–509, 2002.
25. Loftsson T. *Pharmazie.* 65:404–407, 2010.
26. Rane SS and Anderson BD. *Adv Drug Deliv Rev.* 60:638–656, 2008.
27. Fricker G, Kromp T, Wendel A, et al. *Pharm Res.* 27:1469–1486, 2010.
28. Hsieh PW, Hung CF, and Fang JY. *Curr Pharm Des.* 15:2236–2250, 2009.
29. Janssens S and Van den Mooter G. *J Pharm Pharmacol.* 61:1571–1586, 2009.
30. Badawy SI and Hussain MA. *J Pharm Sci.* 96:948–959, 2007.
31. Bassi P and Kaur G. *Expert Opin Drug Deliv.* 7:845–857, 2010.
32. Kassem MA, Abdel Rahman AA, Ghorab MM, Ahmed MB, and Khalil RM. *Int I Pharm.* 340:126–133, 2007.
33. Merisko-Liversidge EM and Liversidge GG. *Toxicol Pathol.* 36:43–48, 2008.
34. Du-Cuny L, Huwyler J, Wiese M, and Kansy M. *Eur J Med Chem.* 43:501–512, 2008.
35. Wang J, Hou T, and Xu X. *J Chem Inf Model.* 49:571–581, 2009.

VIII. Homework Problems

1. The solubility of $Ba(OH)_2 \cdot 8H_2O$ in water at two temperatures was reported as follows:

Temperature (°C)	0.0	20.0
Molal solubility S	0.0974	0.227

Calculate: (*a*) the heat of solution ΔH_{soln}, using data obtained at 0 and 20°C, and (*b*) the solubility of barium hydroxide octahydrate at 30°C in water.

2. (*a*) If the solubility product of silver chromate is 2×10^{-12} at 25°C, what is the solubility in moles per liter of silver chromate? (*b*) If 0.05 *M* potassium chromate is added to the solution, what is the solubility of silver chromate?

3. Brequinar sodium dissociates as brequinar$^-$ and Na^+. Its solubility product $K_{sp} = 0.0502$. Compute (*a*) the solubility of this compound without the ionic strength effect, (*b*) the solubility with the ionic strength effect (using mean activity coefficient), and (*c*) the solubility after the addition of an 0.05 *M* solution of KCl.

4. What is the pH_p of a 2% solution of sodium phenobarbital in a hydroalcoholic solution containing 15% by volume of alcohol? The solubility of phenobarbital in 15% alcohol is 0.22%. The pK_a of phenobarbital in this solution is 7.60. The molecular weight of sodium phenobarbital is 254.22 g/mol and that of phenobarbital is 232.23 g/mol.

5. The minimum pH required for complete solubility of sodium phenobarbital in a 3% solution using an alcohol–water mixed solvent system is as follows:

% Alcohol	10	20	30	40
pH_p	8.73	8.63	8.55	8.02

Explain why pH_p is lowered when the alcohol content increases?

6. The molar solubility of codeine S_o in water at 25°C is approximately 0.0279 mol/L; the pK_a of the conjugate acid of codeine is 8.21 at 25°C; and the molecular weight of codeine phosphate (USP) is 406.37. Calculate the pH_p required for complete solubility of 60 mg of codeine phosphate in 5 mL solution.
7. If a container of pure water is shaken in the air, the water will dissolve atmospheric carbon dioxide until the dissolved gas reaches the solubility of CO_2, 1×10^{-5} mol/L. The acidity constant K_1 of carbonic acid is 4.0×10^{-7}. What would be the pH of water saturated with CO_2?
8. (*a*) Calculate the solubility of sulfisoxazole ($K_a = 7.6 \times 10^{-6}$) in an aqueous buffer having a pH of 5.12 at 25°C; the aqueous solubility of non-ionized drug is 0.15 g/L. (*b*) Using the equation below, calculate the solubility of the drug at pH 5.12 when 3.0% Tween 80 is included in the solution (assuming that only the non-ionized drug is partitioned into the micelles, with $K = 79$).

$$S_{t,\ \text{surfactant soln}} = [\text{HA}]_w \left(1 + qK + \frac{K_a}{[\text{H}_3\text{O}^+]}\right)$$

$$q = \frac{\text{Volume of Surfactant}}{\text{Volume of Aqueous Soln.}}$$

9. (*a*) If 0.15 g of succinic acid in 100 mL of ether is shaken with a 10 mL portion of water, how much succinic acid is left in the ether layer? The partition coefficient K = (conc. in ether)/(conc. in water) = 0.125 at 25°C. (*b*) How much succinic acid is left in the ether when the ether phase is extracted with an additional 10 mL of water? (*c*) How much succinic acid is left in the ether after four extractions, each with 10 mL of water?
10. How much benzoic acid, $K_a = 6.3 \times 10^{-5}$, will remain undissociated in the aqueous phase of a 50% oil–water emulsion if the initial concentration of benzoic acid is 0.5%? The aqueous phase is buffered at pH 5.0 and the *o*/*w* partition coefficient = 5.33. Assume that benzoic acid remains as a monomer in the oil phase.
11. The distribution of salicylic acid between CCl_4 and acidified water was shown to be as follows:

C_o, mol/L	C_w, mol/L
0.009	0.065
0.023	0.104
0.058	0.165

Determine the appropriate partition coefficient and explain the partition phenomena.

12. The solubility of a substance is 1 g in 3 mL of water. When 5 g is dissolved in 15 mL of water, the volume of the solution is 16.8 mL. How many grams of the substance and how many milliliters of water should be used to make 200 mL of a saturated solution?
13. A saturated solution of potassium iodide contains 100 g of KI in each 100 mL of saturated solution. The density of the solution is 1.70 g/mL. What is the solubility of KI?
14. Using the data given in Table 4-3, calculate the aqueous solubility of ibuprofen, cimetidine, and prednisone at 25°C using Equations (4-1), (4-4), and (4-22).
15. If a drug has $\log K_{ow} = 1$ and a solubility of 0.1 *M* in octanol, what is the aqueous solubility of this drug?

CHAPTER 5

Molecular Interactions of Drugs

Chemical interactions that are readily reversible play an important role in the molecular recognition processes of drugs and macromolecules in the biological system. Most drugs, e.g., are bound to plasma proteins after absorption. The resulting *protein binding* may then act as a transport system that controls the drug's metabolism, action, and excretion. The binding of the drug at a receptor site, usually a component of the cell that, when activated, initiates a chain of events leading to an observable response, either enhances or inhibits this response by blocking the binding of the active substrate. This process must also be initiated in some fashion by the formation as well as the nature of the drug–receptor complex. In addition, it may be recalled that drug solubility and drug stability are the two key factors in drug formulation considerations. Recent advancement in molecular interaction research has shown that through alteration of the microenvironment of drugs using molecules of unique structures, both the solubility and the stability of aqueous labile drugs can be greatly enhanced. This approach has become increasingly popular for the development of new drug products. The understanding of the molecular recognition processes of drugs and biological macromolecules requires a detailed characterization of the structural and quantitative aspects of the complexation of drugs with pharmaceutical and biological molecules. Quantitative assessment of molecular interactions is of particular importance, as it provides the fundamental know-how for the development of structure-based molecular design strategies. This chapter provides a general discussion of the theories and methods for the determination of molecular interactions, with emphasis on metal ion complexation, drug–polymer interactions, inclusion complexes, and protein binding phenomena.

CHAPTER OUTLINE

OBJECTIVES

1. Understand the intermolecular forces involved and the complex types in molecular complexation of organic molecules.
2. Understand and recognize commonly occurring reactive species and their potential effects on pharmaceutical and biological systems.
3. Describe the Fenton and Fenton-like reactions.
4. Describe the theories of metal complexation and methods of determination of stability constants.
5. Describe chelation and chelating agents.
6. Describe the structural characteristics of cyclodextrins, the inclusion complexes, and their pharmaceutical significance.
7. Understand the theories and methods used in the determination of drug–protein binding.
8. Perform quantitative assessment of the drug–protein binding effect, and discuss its importance in drug interactions and distribution.

I. Forces of Molecular Interaction and Reactive Species

Complexation of Organic Molecules

The intermolecular forces that govern molecular interactions involve ionic, electron pair sharing, and non-ionic interactions through hydrogen bonding, dipole–dipole, induced dipole, and hydrophobic forces. The type of chemical interactions based on their bonding strength is illustrated in **Table 5-1**. It is readily seen that the formation of covalent bonds requires relatively very high energy. Most drugs do not possess functional groups of the type that would lead to ready formation of the strong and essentially irreversible covalent bonds between drug and biological molecules. However, for certain drugs, relatively long-lasting or irreversible effects occur, and they are designed as such for eliciting their pharmacological effects. For example, many alkylating agents, such as nitrogen mustards and doxorubicin, are used in cancer chemotherapy. These drugs act by formation of covalent bonds and active intermediates that alkylate and link together proteins or nucleic acids, thus preventing their normal participation in cell division. The antibacterial action of the penicillins also derives from covalent bonding by acylation of the bacterial cell-wall constituents. Discussion of covalent drug actions is not the intention of this chapter, and it is of interest to point out that for most drugs, it is desirable that the drug effects be reversible.

Table 5-1 Types of Molecular Interaction

Bonding Type	Bond Strength (kcal/mol)	Bond Length (Å)	Type of Complex
Covalent	40–140	0.75–1.8	Drug–polymer conjugates
Reinforced ionic	10		Drug–receptor complex
Ionic	5		Organic ion pair
Hydrogen	1–7	1.9	$R{-}O{-}H \cdots O{=}C\langle$
Ion–dipole	1–7	3–5	Coordination compounds
Charge transfer			Charge-transfer complex
Dipole–dipole	0.5–2		
London force	0.5–1		Molecular dispersion
Hydrophobic	1	10–30	Drug–protein, drug–polymer, and inclusion complexes

Reinforced Ionic Interaction

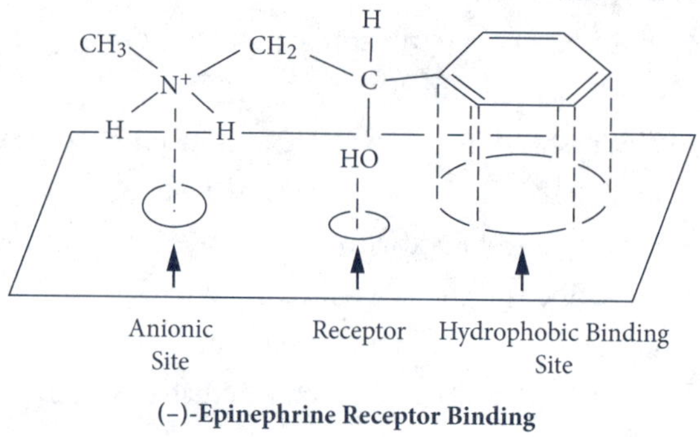

Figure 5-1 Binding of (–)-epinephrine to adrenergic receptor through ion pairing, hydrogen bonding, and hydrophobic force (the (+)-optical isomer, whose hydroxyl group is oriented away from the receptor site, does not have hydrogen bonding and is thus less pharmacologically active).

By virtue of their structural specificity, organic molecules can form complexes with other compounds through hydrogen bonds; ionic bonds; ion–dipole, dipole–dipole, and induced dipole interactions; and hydrophobic forces. Ionization of carboxylic acid and amino weak bases at appropriate pH and the quaternary ammonium groups at any pH are the sources of potential ionic interactions. In compounds containing functional groups such as the carbonyl, ester, amide, and nitrile, the electronegativity of the oxygen and nitrogen relative to the carbon atom leads to unsymmetrical distribution of the electron pair (dipole), which is then capable of forming weak bonds with ions (ion–dipole) or other dipoles (dipole–dipole). It is likely that many of the organic complexations involve multiple forces of interaction. One of the key functions of the hydrogen bonding is to provide an increased stability of the molecular complexation. Although many organic complexes are very weak in bonding energies (approximately less than 5 kcal/mol), organic ion pairs coupled with hydrogen bonding and hydrophobic interactions, known as the *reinforced ionic bond*, have been shown to play an important role in drug–receptor binding. The adrenergic receptor, e.g., has long been shown to exhibit three binding regions.[1] They are (1) a flat surface providing binding to an aromatic ring, (2) a cavity into which the hydroxyl group can be attached to the receptor surface, and (3) an anionic site that binds to the protonated amine. This receptor binding, however, is stereoselective with respect to one of the optical isomers of the drug. An interesting example is (–)-epinephrine, which shows strong binding to the adrenergic receptor through all three binding groups (**Figure 5-1**). In the case of (+)-epinephrine, however, the hydrogen bonding is not involved in the binding because, upon binding to the receptor, the hydroxyl group of the (+)-isomer is oriented away from the receptor site. Consequently, the (–)-isomer is 12–15 times more active as a vasoconstrictor than the (+)-isomer of epinephrine. Other studies[2] have shown that the interaction of dopaminergic agonists with human dopamine D2A receptor can be explained using a similar model that includes hydrogen bonding between the phenolic hydrogen of the agonist ligand and the receptor, ion-pair interaction, and the aromatic moieties around the anionic site that stabilize the ion-pair formation through hydrophobic interactions.

Hydrophobic Bonding

Hydrophobic bonding is one of the more important forces of molecular interaction because it affects the action of nearly all drugs through its role in drug absorption, plasma protein binding, and drug–receptor interactions. Proteins contain nonpolar regions, made up, in part, by amino acid residues with aliphatic chain and aromatic moieties, which cannot be solvated by water. As a consequence, the water molecules in the nonpolar region may associate through hydrogen bonds to form quasi-crystalline structures and produce a higher degree of order than water molecules in the bulk phase. If two nonpolar regions (from the protein and a drug) came close together, these regions would be shielded to a greater extent by interacting water molecules. The process may involve the collapse of the quasi-crystalline water structures of the isolated nonpolar regions, which produces a gain in entropy. The gain in free energy achieved through a decrease in the ordered state of many water molecules in turn stabilizes the close contact of the associated nonpolar regions. This association is called *hydrophobic bonding*.

Note that the term hydrophobic interaction does not refer to any of the weak forces, although they may be involved in the interaction, but shows a hydrophobic microenvironment at the binding site. In fact, most organic molecular interactions, even between ionic species, tend to form a more hydrophobic environment at the site of interaction. The role of hydrophobic interaction in regulating the biological fate of a drug may be described as follows. The hydrophobicity of a compound is closely related to the drug's aqueous solubility and its partition into nonpolar phases. Thus, hydrophobic bonding, but not the structural specifics of the drug, determines the rate and extent of drug absorption and tissue distribution. In the blood, however, a greater degree of structural specificity of a drug is required for its interaction with the plasma proteins, which involves hydrophobic as well as other interactive forces. This indicates that structural considerations may be used to modify the drug–protein interactions, but many drugs may bind to the same site of a protein. In comparison to protein binding, drug interaction with a biological receptor is highly structure-specific, whereas hydrophobic interaction is involved in stabilizing the drug–receptor complex.

Hydrogen Bonding and Biological Action of Drugs

Hydrogen bonding plays an important role in stabilizing the secondary and tertiary structures of proteins and nucleic acids. Reagents that are capable of breaking hydrogen bonds denature the protein. Although the relative importance of the hydrogen bond in drug action is difficult to assess, a few examples have shown that hydrogen bonding does correlate with the drug's biological property. For example, both phenol and benzoic acid exhibit antibacterial activities. In comparison of salicylic acid (*o*-hydroxybenzoic acid) to *p*-hydroxybenzoic acid, it is seen that the former, which exhibits intramolecular hydrogen bonding, is a much stronger acid ($pK_a = 3.0$) and shows higher lipid solubility and bactericidal action than *p*-hydroxybenzoic acid ($pK_a = 4.5$), which forms intermolecular hydrogen bond (**Figure 5-2**). Note that through the intramolecular hydrogen bond, salicylic acid has the phenolic group masked, but functions as an antibacterial agent as benzoic acid through the carboxylic group, whereas *p*-hydroxybenzoic acid must form intermolecular hydrogen bonds leading to higher self-association, thereby lowering its antibacterial effect. In the case of the esters of salicylic acid and *p*-hydroxybenzoic acid, however, the opposite effect in bactericidal activity is observed. Methyl salicylate is without significant antibacterial effect due to the masking of its phenolic hydrogen by intramolecular hydrogen bonding and the loss of the carboxylic proton (Figure 5-2), but the methyl ester of *p*-hydroxybenzoic acid is a very useful preservative. Although the methyl and other alkyl esters of *p*-hydroxybenzoic acid may associate

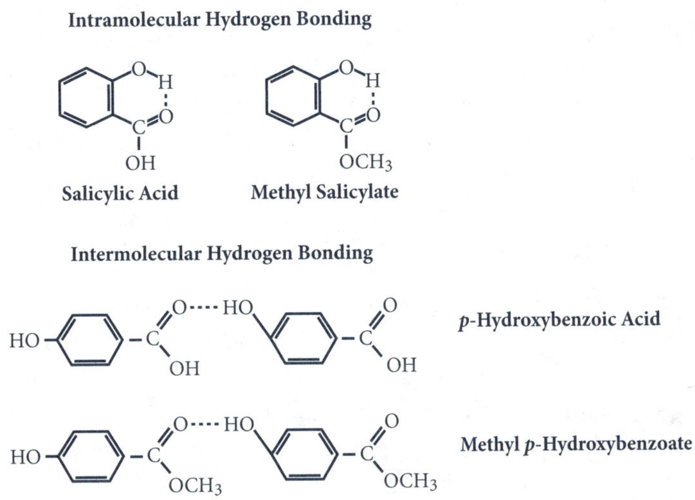

Figure 5-2 Inter- and intramolecular hydrogen bonding in salicylic acid, methyl salicylate, *p*-hydroxybenzoic acid, and methyl *p*-hydroxybenzoate.

through intermolecular hydrogen bonds, the partition coefficient and the antibacterial activity data suggested otherwise, as the alkyl esters of *p*-hydroxybenzoic acid may function as substituted phenols in their bactericidal effect. These examples show that either the phenolic or the carboxylic proton is required for their antibacterial effect, and that these molecules (salicylic acid and the alkyl esters of *p*-hydroxybenzoic acid) may first attach themselves to the site of action through the formation of a hydrogen bond, without which they become ineffective.

Charge-Transfer Complexation

The *charge-transfer* (CT) *complexes* are formed between molecules that act as electron pair donors and acceptors, respectively. This type of complexation occurs mainly by sharing π electrons that are known to be more polarizable than the sigma (single) bond electrons. Aromatic compounds, in which the π electrons are delocalized in the ring system through the resonance effect, are most capable of charge-transfer interactions. Compounds such as benzene and toluene are electron pair donors. But many polynitro (or polychloro) aromatic hydrocarbons, such as trinitrobenzene and picric acid, where the strong electron withdrawing effect of the nitro groups renders the ring more able to accept a negative charge, act as electron pair acceptors. It is well-known that picric acid, 2, 4, 6-trinitrophenol, forms charge-transfer complexes with many polynuclear aromatic hydrocarbons. A well-known CT complex in pharmaceutical use is butesin picrate, a yellow, water-insoluble powder that consists of two molecules of butyl *p*-aminobenzoate with one molecule of picric acid. This complex, by combining the antiseptic effect of picric acid and the antibacterial action of butesin, is used as a local anesthetic for burns and painful skin irritations.

The charge-transfer interaction has also been described as involving weak forces through dipole-induced dipole, dipole–dipole, or ionic interactions by a process similar to that of the Lewis acid–base interaction, indicating that different theories exist regarding the bonding mechanism of the charge-transfer complexation. But the formation of a CT complex can be easily identified using absorption spectroscopic methods. The ultraviolet/visible spectroscopy can be used to detect chromophors of a molecule that contain excitatory electron pairs to produce an absorption spectrum. When a molecule is excited with an energy source, the energy absorbed results in a transition of the electron pair from the bonding orbital (for example, a π orbital) to the excited state antibonding orbital (π^*) and is displayed as an absorption band at a given wavelength. The energy associated with the CT π–π^* transition for the electron pair, which is already in an excited state, will be less than that of the donor or acceptor alone. As a result, the spectrum will display an absorption band, known as the charge-transfer band, at a wavelength that is longer than that of the donor or acceptor alone. The CT band usually appears as a broad and intense band, with the absorbance quantitatively proportional to the formation of the CT complex. Many CT complexes exhibit colored solution, and their CT bands appear in the visible light wavelengths. A classical example of a CT complex is formed between iodine (I_2), the electron pair acceptor, and starch, which gives an intense purple color.

Drug–Polymer Interaction

A variety of polymeric compounds have been used in pharmaceutical preparations either as excipients for specific purposes related to the formulation or for direct use to modify drug properties, dissolution, and rate of drug release from dosage forms. Molecular interactions between drugs and polymer may involve any of multiple interactive forces listed in Table 5-1. It is to be recognized that most drugs may bind to polymeric compounds. The hydrophilic polymers such as polyethylene glycols, sodium carboxymethylcellulose, and polyvinylpyrrolidone K30 may be used to enhance drug solubility in solutions or drug dissolution from solid dosage forms. Sodium carboxymethylcellulose, e.g., will interact with a variety of drugs including quinine, procaine, caffeine, *N*, *N*-dimethylacetamide, sodium *p*-aminobenzoate, sodium salicylate, and *γ*-butyrolactone, all of which interactions result in increased dissolution rate. Interaction of drugs with certain polyethers such as carbowaxes, pluronics, and Tweens, in contrast, have been shown to cause formulation incompatibilities manifested by precipitation, flocculation, diminished absorption, loss of drug activity, and other undesired physical and chemical changes.[3]

The formation of drug–polymer complexes through ionic interactions, which ensures high binding affinities, has proved to be very effective for the development of controlled-release formulations. Studies have shown that the delivery of a cationic drug, such as doxorubicin, may be achieved using anionic polymers such as polyacrylates and *γ*-polyglutamic acid[4, 5] for pH-dependent release of drug, whereas chitosan, a cationic polymer carrier, has been used for the delivery of polyanionic small interfering RNA molecules and other drugs.[6, 7] The drug–polymer interactions via complexation, microsphere, and nanopreparations and covalent conjugation for drug delivery purposes are discussed in later chapters.

Chemistry of Some Reactive Species

The Hydrogen and Hydroxide Ions

Because the hydrogen ion is unavoidable in all aqueous systems, it is of interest to emphasize the importance of this ion in mediating molecular interactions in the pharmaceutical and biological systems. As a positively charged ion, the proton participates in many reactions and serves as a catalyst to facilitate these reactions. The most noted reactions, which are the main cause of drug instability in aqueous solutions, are the specific acid-catalyzed hydrolysis of organic acid derivatives in which the rate-limiting step is the conversion of the protonated reactant to the protonated product. Similarly, the hydroxide ion also catalyzes these reactions, which are known as the specific base catalysis, in which the conversion of deprotonated reactant to the deprotonated product is the rate-limiting step. The reaction rate catalyzed by proton or hydroxide can be several orders of magnitude of that of the uncatalyzed reactions. This makes pH the most important parameter in pharmaceutical solution formulations.

It is recalled that the ion mobility of the proton, due to its hydration and the Grotthuss mechanism, is unusually fast compared to other cations. In comparison, our knowledge on the fast transport and hydration properties of the hydroxide ion, which also plays an important role in many chemical and biological processes, is far from complete. Recent studies showed that the hydroxide ions may in fact form interchangeable hydration complexes, particularly the hypercoordinated $OH^-(H_2O)_4$ species and tricoordinated $OH^-(H_2O)_3$, the hydration complexes of OH^- can form a transient hydrogen bond between the H atom of the OH^- and a neighboring water molecule.[8] This process may allow fast transport of hydroxide ions in water in a mechanism similar to that of the hydrogen ion.

The hydrogen ion concentration (pH) plays a major role in mediating the chemical and biological activities of drugs and macromolecules. In most cases, weak acids and weak bases in their neutral forms have been regarded as the active compounds. This may be due to the fact that the drug action takes place inside the cells or within cell membrane, where molecules must gain entrance to the cell in the undissociated form. After reaching the site of action, they may then function as ions. In this case, the biological activity of the drug resembles the typical sigmoidal pH curves. Some compounds, however, show increased biological activity with increasing degree of ionization. Because of the difficulty for ions to penetrate membranes, it is likely that compounds of this type exert their effect on the outside of the cells. Examples of ionic active drugs are the aminoacridines, whose antibacterial actions depend on at least 60% ionization at 37°C or 75% ionization at 20°C at physiological pH.[9]

Most biological processes, including events in subcelluar organelles, are pH dependent. This reflects the importance of the local pH on all processes in the cell. The hydrogen ions are known to cause acidic/basic unfolding and pH-dependent stability of proteins.[10, 11] Changes in pH can also trigger formation of amyloid fibers and aggregation and altered protein–protein, protein–substrate, and protein–membrane associations.[12–14] There is likely a correlation between the function or activity of the protein and its structural stability, as both may be affected by the pH of the local environment. Indeed, studies by Warwicker and coworkers[15, 16] have shown a good correlation between the pH of maximal stability of monomeric proteins and the characteristic pH of the subcellular organelles. There is a constraint on pH-dependent protein stability, in relation to the local pH, in that the protein shows minimum pH dependence in the pH region in which the protein is most stable and active. This may be brought about by adaptation of amino acid residues with appropriate ionization characteristics (pKas) in various positions of the protein structure. In another study, Talley and Alexov[17] examined the pH dependency of protein activity or function and its structural stability toward a particular subcellular environment using the literature results on 310 proteins. They found a strong correlation between optimum pH for stability and the optimum pH for activity, where the optimum pH was taken to be either a maximal pH or a pH interval as reported in the literature (see **Figure 5-3**). This correlation was illustrated by the counts of protein that exhibit a calculated difference between the optimum pH for activity and the corresponding optimum pH for stability. If the two pH values are identical, the difference is zero, that is, the optimum pH is the same for both activity and stability.

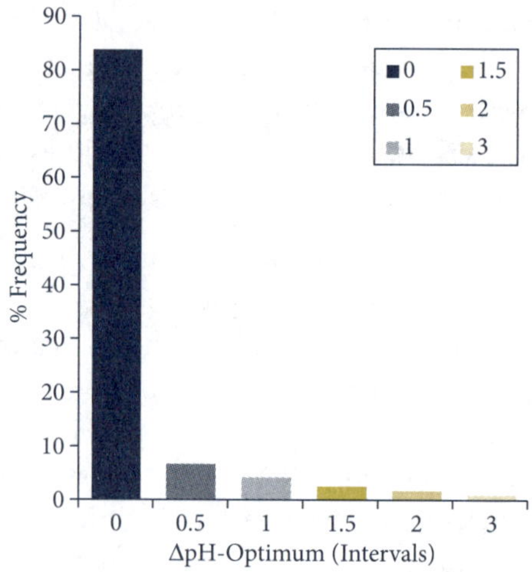

Figure 5-3 Correlation of the optimum pH for activity and optimum pH for stability of 310 proteins (median = 0.0, variance = 0.65, SE = 0.05, data points = 310).
Reproduced from: Talley K, Alexov E. On the pH-optimum of activity and stability of proteins. *Proteins: Structure, Function and Bioinformatics.* 2010;78(12):2699–2706.

This study establishes that for a given protein in its natural (wild-type) sequence and fold, the optimum pH values for activity and stability will most likely be the same. It suggests that a protein may evolve toward the pH of a particular subcellular organelle, where the hydrogen ion plays a key role in regulating the protein's structural integrity and activity.

Metal Oxides

With the advancement of nanosciences, metal oxide nanoparticles are being engineered for chemical and industrial processes and may also find their way into medicinal and pharmaceutical applications. Attachment of biological molecules to the particle surface, e.g., may aid in the diagnosis of diseases and/or delivery of pharmaceutical agents. Studies of surface chemistry of metal oxides have provided some interesting phenomena with respect to the effect of hydration on surface adsorption of organic molecules.[18, 19] The metal oxide surfaces are usually hydrated or hydroxylated under ambient conditions, which can serve as a proton donor to adsorbed molecules. The titanium dioxide (TiO_2) surface, e.g., consists of rows of fivefold-coordinated Ti atoms separated by rows of twofold-coordinated, bridge-bonded oxygen atoms. It becomes hydroxylated when some of the oxygen atoms are removed and replaced by water. It has been shown that organic molecules such as carboxylic acids and catechol, an aromatic compound with two adjacent hydroxyl groups ($C_6H_4(OH)_2$), can bond to the surface through oxygen–titanium linkages. These compounds can be used as anchoring species for molecular attachment to particle surface. In the case of the catechol, it forms a bidentate catecholate with Ti atoms of adjacent rows where the protons released from the catechol are captured by the surface to form additional hydroxyl groups.

Using scanning tunnel microscopy, Diebold and coworkers[19] showed that the surface-bound catechol can regain the protons and become mobilized. The transfer of hydrogen from the surface hydroxyls to the catecholate substantially lowers the activation barrier for the rotational motion, thus allowing the detached molecule to roll over to the next lattice, where the molecule regains the catecholate linkage by transferring again the hydrogens to the TiO_2 surface. This shows a dynamic process of molecular diffusivity across the particle surface, which may aid in the understanding of the molecular assembly and the catalytic properties of the metal oxide nanoparticles.

Oxygen Radicals and Metal Ions

A free radical may be defined as any species that possesses one or more unpaired electrons.[20] Under this definition, most transition metals and the oxygen molecule itself are free radicals. Oxygen has two unpaired electrons, each located in a different π^* antibonding orbital. These two electrons have the same spin quantum number, and so if O_2 attempts to oxidize another molecule by accepting a pair of electrons from it, both new electrons must be of parallel spin so as to fit into the two unpaired π^* orbitals. This results in a slow oxidation process, as O_2 must accept its electrons one at a time when it reacts with nonradical species. The transition metals, which are found at the active site of many oxidases and oxygenases, can accept and donate single electrons without spin restriction. Hence, they are reactive in redox reactions and can generate *reactive oxygen species* (ROS).

If a single electron is accepted by the ground state O_2, the product is called superoxide anion (O_2^-), which is formed virtually in all aerobic cells. The important sources of superoxide are the phagocytes, such as neutrophils, monocytes, macrophages, and eosinophils, as they undergo respiratory burst in the generation of ROS upon phagocytosis of foreign particles or immune complexes. The addition of a second electron to superoxide yields the peroxide ion, which will be immediately protonated to give hydrogen peroxide in aqueous solution. This process is known as the desmutation of superoxide, as indicated in the following overall reaction:

$$2O_2^- + 2H^+ \rightarrow H_2O_2 + O_2$$

Homolytic fission of H_2O_2 gives two hydroxyl radicals, $^{\bullet}OH$, which can be achieved by heat or ionizing radiation. But the generation of the hydroxyl radical occurs readily in a mixture of H_2O_2 and ion(II) salts, and this was first observed by Fenton in 1894.

$$Fe^{2+} + H_2O_2 \rightarrow Fe^{3+} + {}^{\bullet}OH + OH^- \quad (5\text{-}1)$$

There are multiple reactions associated with the *Fenton reaction*, such as

$$Fe^{3+} + H_2O_2 \rightarrow Fe^{2+} + O_2^- + H^+$$

$${}^{\bullet}OH + H_2O_2 \rightarrow H_2O + H^+ + O_2^-$$

$$O_2^- + Fe^{3+} \rightarrow Fe^{2+} + O_2$$

Thus, a simple mixture of an iron salt and H_2O_2 can provoke a whole series of radical reactions. Similar to the action of Fe(II), copper(I) ions also react with H_2O_2 to produce hydroxyl radicals and, in fact, show a much greater rate constant than that of the Fe(II) salts:

$$Cu^+ + H_2O_2 \rightarrow Cu^{2+} + {}^{\bullet}OH + OH^- \quad (5\text{-}2)$$

The hydroxyl radical reacts with extremely high rate constants with almost every type of molecule found in living cells. These reactions include (1) hydrogen atom abstraction that leads to the formation of organic free radicals, (2) addition (hydroxylation) to aromatic ring structures such as to the purine and pyrimidine bases of DNA, and (3) electron transfer to produce inorganic radicals (such as the carbonate radical, $CO_3^{\bullet -}$). In the living systems, if both H_2O_2 and Cu(I) or Fe(II) ions are present, the hydroxyl radicals will form and react immediately with whatever molecules are in their vicinity. This can lead to oxidative tissue damage and/or the generation of secondary radicals of variable reactivity. Metal ions other than iron and copper have not been shown to exhibit Fenton-like reactions. This makes the iron and copper ions culpable for metal ion–induced oxidative stress and diseases.

Inflammatory diseases are associated with abnormal phagocytic activity and superoxide- and hydroxyl radical–mediated tissue damage. In rheumatoid arthritis, the oxidative stress is accompanied by abnormalities in body iron metabolism, manifested by decreased total iron content in blood but increased deposition of iron proteins in the synovium of the joints.[21] It seems likely that the altered distribution of body iron potentiates inflammation by promoting hydroxyl radical formation at the synovial membranes. In animal studies, it has been shown that desferrioxamine, a specific iron chelator, while inducing acute inflammation, suppresses the chronic inflammatory responses.[22] In cancer, increased oxygen radical generation can lead to DNA damage and is thus potentially carcinogenic, but there is little indication that failed protection against radicals in body defense is related to the origin of human cancer. One of the most likely places for oxidative stress is the human brain, which uses about 20% of the oxygen consumed. The human cerebrospinal fluid contains high levels of antioxidants that include, among others, ascorbic acid, which is acquired through dietary intake, and carnosine, which is synthesized in the olfactory bulbs of the brain. Carnosine, β-alanyl-L-histidine, can act against oxidative stress by scavenging ROS and by chelation of copper ions.[23] Both copper and iron have been linked to neurodegenerative diseases that may benefit from chelation therapies.[24–26]

II. Metal Ion Complexation

Coordination Bonds in Metal Complexes

Coordination Number

The term complexes in inorganic chemistry refers to mainly coordination compounds of metal ions, simply known as metal complexes, which either exist as solid forms that decompose in solution or produce complex ions when in solution. For example, students will keenly remember $Ag(NH_3)_2^+$ from qualitative analysis as being the complex formed when silver chloride is dissolved in excess ammonia. The classical *Werner's theory* on coordination chemistry states that metal ions exhibit primary (ionizable) and secondary (non-ionizable) valences, where the latter indicate the *coordination number*. The secondary valences may be satisfied by anions or neutral molecules (positive ions do present sometimes, but rarely), known as ligands, arranged spatially around the metal ion in a linear or bent chain, tetrahedral or square planar, or octahedral configuration that corresponds to the coordination number of 2, 4, or 6, respectively. This theory has provided the basis for the understanding of the formation of metal complexes. The coordination number of various metal ions is given in **Table 5-2**. The atoms of small atomic volume have the lower coordination number, which is in line with the theory that the coordinating agents or ligands must "cover" the metal ion.

Table 5-2 Coordination Numbers of Metal Ions

Mo^{3+}	8
Cr^{3+}, Fe^{3+}, Fe^{2+}, Co^{3+}, Ni^{3+}, Mn^{3+}, Al^{3+}, Au^{3+}, Pd^{4+}, Pt^{4+}	6
Ni^{2+}, Pd^{2+}, Pt^{2+}, Cu^{2+}, Zn^{2+}, Cd^{2+}, Hg^{2+}	4
Cu^+, Ag^+, Au^+	2

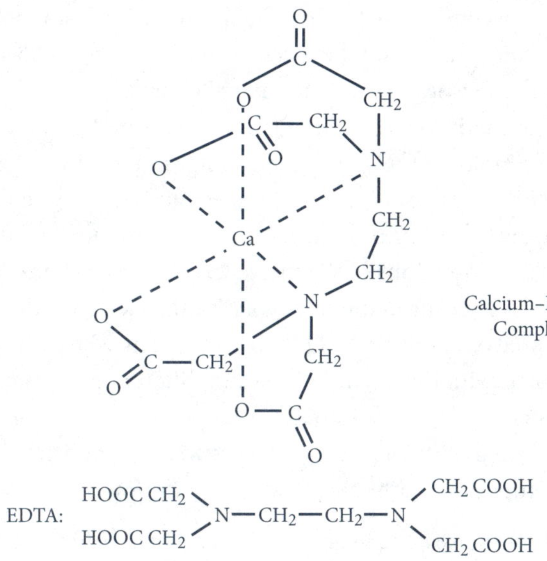

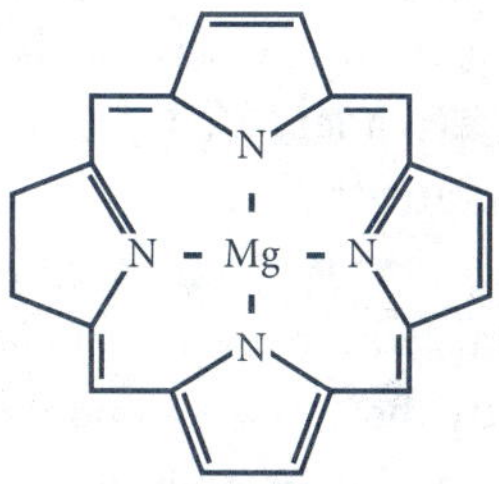

Magnesium–Chlorophyll Complex (Ring System Only)

Figure 5-4 Calcium complex of the anion of EDTA and the ring system of chlorophyll for the chelation of magnesium. (Stable complexes of alkaline–earth metals are confined to cyclic structures.)

In general, metal ions in the highest valence state form the most stable complex. For ions having the same charge, the smaller ions tend to form more stable complexes than the larger ones. Across the periodic table, the most stable metal complexes are formed by the ions of group VIII transition elements (Fe, Co, Ni, Pd, Pt). The strength and desire to form coordination compounds decrease from group VIII in both directions. No cases of coordination compounds have been observed for group IA elements. The alkaline earth metals (group IIA) may form stable complexes only if the atom becomes incorporated into a cyclic structure. Indeed, in the case of Ca^{2+}, formation of stable complexes is confined exclusively to cyclic structure as in the calcium–ethylenediaminetetraacetic acid (EDTA) complex. The five ring structures of this complex accounts for its very unusual stability (**Figure 5-4**). The most noted complex of Mg^{2+} is chlorophyll of the plant kingdom, which rivals the significance of hemoglobin in the mammalian system where the central atom of the heme is iron. In chlorophyll, the magnesium atom is surrounded by four nitrogens in a large organic ring system, called the *porphyrin group* (Figure 5-4). The coplanar porphyrin system is such a powerful coordinator that it is able to hold the magnesium atom tightly, even though the direction characteristics of the four Mg—N bonds are not what would be expected for an alkaline–earth metal complex.

The Ligand Field Effects

Although the bonding in metal complexes has been described via molecular orbital hybridization that implies covalent bonding (e.g., the Co—N bonds in $Co(NH_3)_6^{3+}$ were said to involve d^2sp^3 hybridization as in SF_6), there are inconsistencies to this approach. For example, studies of the magnetic properties showed that $CrCl_6^{3-}$ and $CoCl_6^{3-}$ were predominantly covalent, but $FeCl_6^{3-}$ was predominantly ionic; yet iron lies between chromium and cobalt in the periodic table. In the *ligand field theory*, the properties of transition metal complexes may be simply considered as arising from electrostatic attraction or ion–dipole interactions between the metal ion and the ligands. This immediately accounts for the octahedral configuration associated with coordination number of 6 and the tetrahedral configuration assumed by most tetracovalent complexes, because these highly symmetrical layouts allow minimum repulsion among the ligands. The ligand field theory allows for additional considerations of the interaction between the central ion and the ligands. The positive charges of the central ion may polarize the electron clouds associated with the ligands to produce some degree of covalency, and their *d* electrons will try to move out of the way of the electron cloud associated with the ligand. Moreover, different ligands may impart a different ligand field strength that splits the *d* orbitals into low-energy and high-energy groups, where the *d* electrons will select the low-energy orbitals either alone or in electron pairs. This would lead to the formation of two types of complexes of different electron configurations.

By way of the octahedral complexes, the ligand field effects may be described as follows. In a three-dimensional coordination, the five *d* orbitals of a transition metal may be divided into two groups: the first three (d_{xy}, d_{xz}, d_{yz}) lying along the "diagonals" between the axes and the other two (d_{y2}, d_{x2-z2}) lying directly *on the axes* (readers are referred to texts of inorganic chemistry for details). If the six ligands coordinate octahedrally along the axial directions, the *d* electrons of the metal ion will choose to occupy the three diagonal orbitals to avoid the electron cloud of the ligands, rather than the two axial orbitals where repulsion will be maximum. Electrons going into the *diagonals* will have lower energy than those going into the axial orbitals. The greater the strength of the ligand field, the greater will be the energy difference between the two groups of orbitals. As demonstrated in spectroscopic studies, the *d* electrons in a complex may be excited from the low-energy orbitals to the high-energy orbitals by absorption of visible (vis) or ultraviolet (uv) light, and the energy difference between the two orbital groups corresponds to the wavelength of the uv/vis absorption band. There is a spectrochemical series of the ligands, which indicates an order of ligand field strength induced by their complexation with the metal ions. The spectrochemical series is $CN^- > NO_2^- > NH_3 > NCS^- > F^- > OH^- > Cl^- > Br^- > I^-$. As can be seen, the ligand field set up by cyano or nitro groups will be much stronger than those of the hydroxide and halides.

The layout of *d* electrons of the metal ion in a complex depends on the ligand field. If the field is weak, the electron configuration of the metal atom will be the same as that of the free ion, i.e., with maximum permitted number of unpaired *d* electrons. This is known as the spin-free complex. If the field is strong, where the energy separation of the two orbital groups is high, it will be more favorable for the electrons to pair up in the lower energy level, resulting in spin-paired complexes. The distribution of *d* electrons in octahedral complexes for a number of transition metals is shown in **Table 5-3**.

This table is quite useful and offers a number of observations that have been proved through experimental studies. With only three *d* electrons, the choice for a spin-paired complex is not available to Cr^{3+}. But for metal ions that have more than three *d*-orbital electrons, both types of complex can be formed. Thus, Fe^{3+} will form spin-free complexes with water or halides but spin-paired complex with CN^-. The Cr^{3+} complexes, whose low-energy *d* orbitals are spin-free and half occupied, and the spin-paired complexes of Co^{3+}, which have a stable configuration and no electrons in the high-energy orbitals, are some of the most stable metal complexes. The spin-free complex of Cr^{2+} and the spin-paired complex of Co^{2+} both have one electron in the high-energy orbital beyond a very stable configuration, indicating that these complexes are highly susceptible to oxidation. Finally, it can be seen that the octahedral complexes of Ni^{2+} and Cu^{2+} would be relatively unstable, because when formed, electrons would have to occupy the high-energy *d* orbitals.

Table 5-3 The *d* Electron Configuration in Spin-Free and Spin-Paired Octahedral Complexes

	Spin-Free (Weak Field)					Spin-Paired (Strong Field)				
Metal Ion	d_{xy}	d_{xz}	d_{yz}	d_{y2}	d_{x2-z2}	d_{xy}	d_{xz}	d_{yz}	d_{y2}	d_{x2-z2}
Cr^{3+}	*†	*	*	—	—	*	*	*	—	—
Mn^{3+} (Cr^{2+})	*	*	*	*	—	**‡	*	*	—	—
Fe^{3+} (Mn^{2+})	*	*	*	*	*	**	**	*	—	—
Co^{3+} (Fe^{2+})	**	*	*	*	*	**	**	**	—	—
Co^{2+}	**	**	*	*	*	**	**	**	*	—
Ni^{2+}	**	**	**	*	*	**	**	**	*	*
Cu^{2+}	**	**	**	**	*	**	**	**	**	*

†Indicates single (one asterisk) *d* electron in designated *d* orbital.
‡Indicates paired (two asterisks) *d* electrons in designated *d* orbital.

Indeed, octahedral complexes for these ions are rare, and those that exist are distorted octahedra with a pair of the trans groups lying significantly farther from the central atom. Ni^{2+} and Cu^{2+} form, by far, square planar complexes.

Chelates and Chelating Agents

Metal complexes can be made to contain a ligand that occupies two or more coordination positions on the central atom. For example, Cu^{2+} ions form $Cu(NH_3)_4^{2+}$ with ammonia but $Cu(ethylenediamine)_2^{2+}$ with ethylenediamine ($H_2NCH_2CH_2NH_2$). The two complexes have the same coordination number of 4, but the latter consists only of two ethylenediamine molecules. The name *chelate*, applied to such a structure, stemmed from the Greek Chele, or "claw". Ethylenediamine and others (such as the amino acids) having two coordinating groups per molecule are said to be bidentate, meaning "two teeth." More complicated chelating agents may have as many as six donor atoms and are named accordingly. For example, EDTA, which locks Ca^{2+} into a stable complex (Figure 5-4) despite the metal's tendency of not participating in complexation, is a sexadentate chelating agent (a six-toothed clawing sequestrator). Likewise, the porphyrin group of chlorophyll may be said to be quadridentate.

Among the divalent cations, Pd^{2+}, Cu^{2+}, and Ni^{2+} have the highest tendency of chelation, which may be related to their high secondary ionization potentials. The formation of cyclic structures enhances complex stability. It might be said that whereas one ring is good, several rings will be better, as in the calcium–EDTA complex. The most stable ring structures in chelation are the five- or six-member rings. If the complexation results in a conjugated double bond system, the stability of the complex will be further enhanced through the resonance effect. One such example is the formation of a six-member ring complex between Cu^{2+} and the carbonyls of acetylacetone (CH_3—CO—CH_2—CO—CH_3), which is stabilized by resonance structures. The complexation is facilitated by the tautomerization of the compound from the keto to the enol form. Without this capability, as in 4-hydroxy-2-pentanone (CH_3—CHOH—CH_2—CO—CH_3), there is no chelation. The β-diketones exhibit greater enol content than that of ketocarboxylates. In ketones, such as acetone, the enol form is virtually insignificant.

Studies have shown that the copper, iron, and zinc ions are involved in Alzheimer's disease, where the formation of Cu and Zn complexes with the peptide amyloid-beta was detected in Alzheimer's disease but not in healthy conditions.[24] There is compelling evidence that alteration in copper homeostasis can lead to abnormal protein behavior and aggregation and, as previously discussed, oxidative stress through generation of reactive oxygen species (ROS). Hence, it is of interest to look further into the formation of copper complexes. Transition metal ions in the biological systems exist primarily in bound forms to amino acids, peptides, and proteins. Cu(II) is well known for its complexation with histidine[27–29] to form the Cu(II)(histidine)$_2$ complexes. The adult human body contains about 80 mg of copper. In plasma, there is an exchangeable pool of copper, in which the metal ion is bound to serum albumin and α_2-macroglobulin,[28] which contains a histidine- and cysteine-rich region. Studies have shown that plasma albumin also forms the albumin–copper–histidine tertiary complex,[29] and either the copper-bound proteins or the copper–histidine complexes may be responsible for the delivery of copper to cells. The histidine complex of copper also plays a role in control of Cu(II) binding to DNA.[30] Renewed interest has emerged on the studies of Cu(II)–peptide complexes to probe the role of copper in neurodegenerative processes[25] and to search for chelating agents for potential therapeutic effect.[26] The drug captopril, an angiotensin-converting enzyme inhibitor, has been shown to provide protection against ROS-mediated damage through copper binding. The action involves the oxidation of the sulfhydryl (—SH) group of captopril (CpSH) by Cu(II), which then leads to the formation of Cu(I) complex with CpSSCp (dimer of captopril with a disulfide linkage).[31] It is suggested that this copper(I) chelation may play a major role in captopril's ROS scavenging effect. Some polyphenols, such as curcumin and phloretin, have well-described neuroprotective properties and exhibit a 1,3-dicarbonyl enol feature as that of the acetylacetone, which, as shown earlier, forms stable complex with Cu(II). Studies by LoPachin et al.[32] have shown that the 1,3-dicarbonyl compounds provide substantial protection to cells from hydrogen peroxide–induced toxicity in a cellular model of oxidative stress, and they suggest that these compounds, such as acetylacetone and 2-acetylcyclopentanone, may be a new class of neuroprotectants through radical scavenging and metal ion chelation.

Equilibrium Considerations and Stability Constants

Depending on the coordination number of the metal ion, quantitative treatment of the equilibrium expressions for the stepwise complexation can be mathematically complicated. If, e.g., six of the same ligand are bound to a metal ion, there will be six formation constants. For convenience, we first consider the complexation of a metal ion (M), such as Cu(II) that has a coordination number of 4, with a bidentate ligand (A). The following equilibrium steps can be expected:

$$\begin{aligned} \mathrm{M} + \mathrm{A} &= \mathrm{MA} \qquad & K_1 &= [\mathrm{MA}]/[\mathrm{M}][\mathrm{A}] \\ \mathrm{MA} + \mathrm{A} &= \mathrm{MA_2} \qquad & K_2 &= [\mathrm{MA_2}]/[\mathrm{MA}][\mathrm{A}] \end{aligned} \tag{5-3}$$

where K_1 and K_2 are the formation or *stability constants* of the stepwise complexes. The combination of the above equations gives

$$\beta = K_1K_2 = [\mathrm{MA_2}]/[\mathrm{M}][\mathrm{A}]^2$$

where β is the overall consecutive stability constant for the formation of the most stable or end product. Quantitative treatment of the equilibrium expressions may be made by defining a function $\bar{n}$ as the *total bound concentration of the ligand per total concentration of the metal ion* in solution. It can be seen that in a given solution, the total bound ligand concentration is [MA] + 2[MA$_2$], whereas the total concentration of the metal ion is [M] + [MA] + [MA$_2$]. Thus,

$$\bar{n} = \frac{[\mathrm{MA}] + 2[\mathrm{MA_2}]}{[\mathrm{M}] + [\mathrm{MA}] + [\mathrm{MA_2}]}$$

Applying the equilibrium expressions given in Equation (5-3), $\bar{n}$ can be rewritten as

$$\bar{n} = \frac{K_1[\mathrm{A}] + 2K_1K_2[\mathrm{A}]^2}{1 + K_1[\mathrm{A}] + K_1K_2[\mathrm{A}]^2}$$

The above equation can be rearranged to give

$$\frac{\bar{n}}{(2-\bar{n})\,[A]^2} = K_1K_2 + K_1\frac{1-\bar{n}}{(2-\bar{n})\,[A]} \tag{5-4}$$

Equation (5-4) can be used directly for the determination of the stability constants of K_1 and K_2 if both $\bar{n}$ and the free ligand concentration [A] are determined experimentally. The plot of $\bar{n}/[(2-\bar{n})[A]^2]$ versus $(1-\bar{n})/[(2-\bar{n})[A]]$ will yield a straight line with a slope of K_1 and a *y* axis intercept of K_1K_2.

A second look at Equation (5-4) shows that at $\bar{n} = 1$,

$$K_1K_2 = 1/[A]^2 \qquad \text{or} \qquad \log K_1K_2 = -2\log[A] = 2p[A]$$

This allows the determination of the overall constant K_1K_2 using $p[A]$ at $\bar{n} = 1$. Equation (5-4) also indicated that the individual constants may be approximated at certain free ligand concentrations. Because K_1 is usually greater than K_2 and $1/[A]$ is much smaller than K_2, at lower values of $\bar{n}$, Equation (5-4) may be written as

$$\frac{\bar{n}}{(2-\bar{n})\,[A]} = K_1\frac{1-\bar{n}}{2-\bar{n}}$$

It follows that at $\bar{n} = 0.5$, $1/[A] = K_1$, or $p[A] = \log K_1$. A similar approximation can be made that at $\bar{n} = 1.5$, $p[A] = \log K_2$.

Considerable difficulty arises in the treatment of equilibrium data if more than two steps are involved in the equilibrium process, but a number of methods are available in the literature.[33–35] The most convenient approach is known as the modified Scatchard method,[34, 35] in which a function Q is defined as $Q = \bar{n}/[(N-\bar{n})[A]]$, or

$$\log Q = \frac{\log \bar{n}}{N-\bar{n}} + p[A] \tag{5-5}$$

where $\bar{n}$ is the total bound concentration of the ligand per metal ion concentration, N is the maximum number of ligands, and $p[A] = -\log[A]$. The $\log Q$ function is very useful for the determination of stability constants of multiple equilibrium steps. If $N = 2$, as in the Cu(II)–bidentate system discussed above, Equation (5-5) will show that $\log Q = p[A]$ at $\bar{n} = 1$. We already know that at $\bar{n} = 1$, $p[A] = ½ \log K_1K_2$. Hence, $\log Q$ is a function of the free ligand concentration that is related to the formation constants and through which the individual stability constants can be determined by using the approximation method described above. Let us consider the formation of an octahedral complex between Co^{3+} and ammonia, where $N = 6$ and the function $\bar{n}$ can be written as

$$\bar{n} = \frac{K_1[A] + 2K_1K_2[A]^2 + \cdots + 6K_1K_2K_3K_4K_5K_6[A]^6}{1 + K_1[A] + K_1K_2[A]^2 + \cdots + K_1K_2K_3K_4K_5K_6[A]^6}$$

If we further define a series of "intrinsic constants" (*I*'s) in that

$$I_1 = K_1/6 \qquad I_2 = 2K_2/5 \qquad I_3 = 3K_3/4 \qquad I_4 = 4K_4/3 \qquad I_5 = 5K_5/2 \qquad I_6 = 6K_6$$

then the plot of $\log Q$ versus $\bar{n}$ will have limiting intercepts that equal $\log I_1$ and $\log I_6$ at $n = 0$ and 6, respectively. The values of $\log K_1$ and $\log K_6$ can then be calculated from the definition of the intrinsic constants. The plot of $\log Q$ versus $\bar{n}$ also allows the determination of the free ligand concentrations at specific $\bar{n}$ values. Based on the approximation method, the values of $p[A]$ at $\bar{n} = 1.5$, 2.5, 3.5, and 4.5 can then be taken to be the values of $\log K_2$, $\log K_3$, $\log K_4$, and $\log K_5$, respectively.

Methods of Determination

The pH Titration

Metal complexation with amino acids and peptides involves changes in pH and proton ionization characteristics. The pH titration method not only is reliable for such measurements but also provides additional information regarding the metal complexes and the catalytic role of the metal in compound stability. This method will be illustrated via a study of the interaction of Cu(II) with ampicillin, which is an α-amino amide derivative that possesses a protonated amino group at the C-10 position (**Figure 5-5**). Cu(II) and other metal ions have been shown to promote hydrolysis of peptides such as glycylglycine in acidic conditions but inhibit the hydrolysis in basic solutions. The catalytic effect of Cu(II) is due to the binding of the metal to the α-amino and carbonyl groups of the ligand. Polarization of the carbonyl group by Cu(II) promotes nucleophilic attack of the carbonyl by water or hydroxide ion. The inhibitory effect of Cu(II) on peptide hydrolysis at higher pH is due to the cupric ion–mediated ionization of the amide hydrogen through the formation of a deprotonated complex that is catalytically inactive. This Cu(II)-promoted ionization also occurs in its complexation with ampicillin (see Figure 5-5), which can be visualized by a color change of the solution, when it happens, from blue to violet.

The pH titration studies can be carried out in solutions of controlled ionic strength, and the initial solution pH may be lowered to an appropriate point with standardized HCl solution prior to titration by standardized NaOH solution. Titration curves can be generated for a given concentration of the ligand in the absence and presence of the metal ion at predetermined ligand/metal concentration ratios. The results of such titration curves for ampicillin (0.0050 *M*) in the absence and presence of 0.0025 *M* $CuCl_2$ are shown in **Figure 5-6**. It can be seen that the titration of ampicillin requires the addition of 1 mol of base per mole of ampicillin, with a measured pK_a of 7.25 (dissociation of hydrogen from the protonated amino group). Titration in the presence of Cu(II) requires the addition of 2 mol of base per mole of ligand, indicating the ionization of a second proton. Titration of other penicillins lacking the amide linkage, such as benzylpenicillin, did not show dissociable protons.

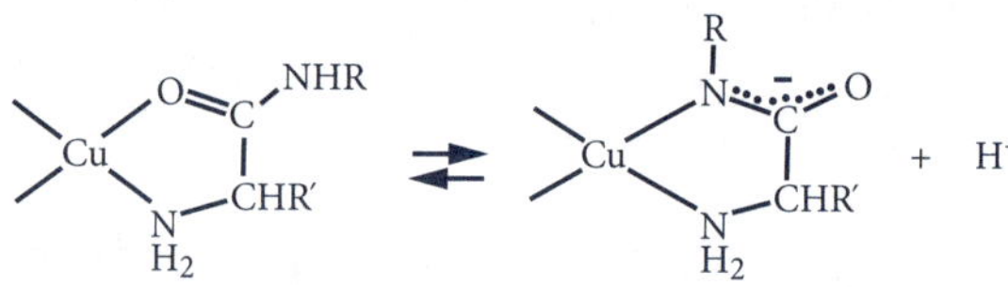

Figure 5-5 Ampicillin and cupric ion–mediated ionization of amide hydrogen.

The stoichiometry of Cu(II)–ampicillin complex was assessed in this way. The amount of base needed to titrate the copper–ampicillin solution to pH 10 was about 4 mol of base per mole of copper when the ampicillin/metal ion ratio is 2 : 1. When this ratio was increased to 5 : 1 and 7 : 1, then 7 and 9 mol of base per mole of metal ion were needed to reach the same pH. This indicates the formation of a 1 : 2 Cu(II)–ampicillin complex. **Figure 5-7** shows the µv/vis absorption spectra of the copper–ampicillin complexation as a function of pH. As pH increases, the spectrum shifted toward shorter wavelength (a blue shift) with increased absorbance, which indicates a switch

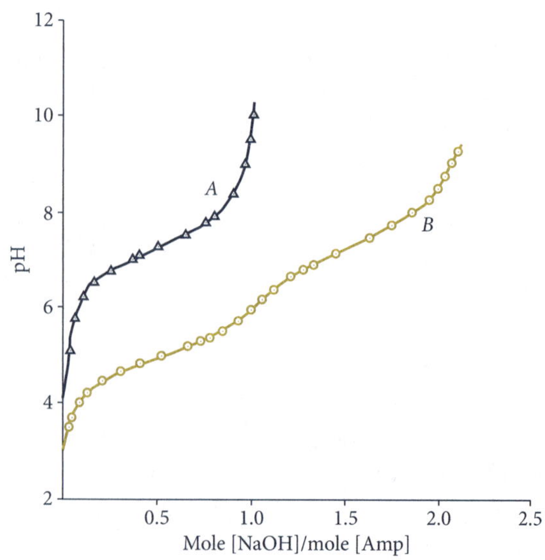

Figure 5-6 The pH titration curves of 0.005 *M* ampicillin in the absence and presence of 0.0025 *M* $CuCl_2$.

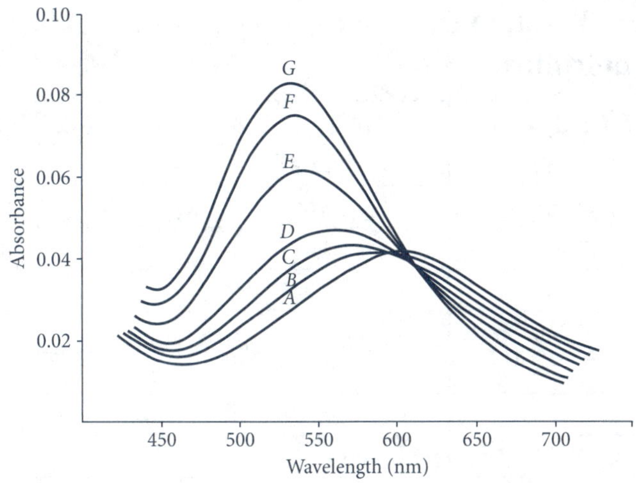

Figure 5-7 Absorption spectra of Cu(II)–ampicillin complexation at different solution pH: (*A*) 5.9, (*B*) 6.5, (*C*) 7.0, (*D*) 7.9, (*E*) 10.0, (*F*) 10.4, and (*G*) 10.6.

of bonding from the carbonyl to the amide nitrogen[36] as a result of cupric ion–promoted ionization of the amide hydrogen illustrated in Figure 5-5.

Determination of Stability and Ionization Constants

The equilibrium of the Cu(II)–ampicillin complexation is represented by Equation (5-4). To determine the value of $\bar{n}$ and the free ligand concentration, the difference in NaOH concentrations used between solutions with and without Cu(II) at the same pH can be taken as the bound concentration of the ligand. Hence, the values of $\bar{n}$ and the free concentration of the ligand, designated as HA^-, can be obtained by using Equations (5-6) and (5-7):

$$\bar{n} = \Delta[B]/C_M = ([B]_2 - [B]_1)/C_M \qquad (5\text{-}6)$$

$$[HA^-] = K_a(C_{Am} - \Delta[B])/[H_3O^+] \qquad (5\text{-}7)$$

Here, $\Delta[B]$ is the difference in NaOH used to titrate the Cu(II)-containing solution ($[B]_2$) and Cu(II)-free solution ($[B]_1$) to the same pH; C_M and C_{Am} are the initial concentrations of Cu(II) and ampicillin, respectively; and K_a is the acidity constant for the ionization of the protonated amino proton. Because ampicillin has two dissociable protons toward copper binding, it is designated as H_2A. The free or nonbound ampicillin is designated as HA^-, which relates to C_{Am} according to the acid–base equilibrium of Equation (5-7). Note that the negative charge in HA^- comes from the dissociated carboxylic group that is not involved in the complexation. The data generated for the Cu(II)–ampicillin complexation are partially given in **Table 5-4**, with which the stability constants can be determined by using Equation (5-4) as previously described.

The ionization of the protonated amino hydrogen of ampicillin due to Cu(II) binding may occur at a lower pH than the ionization of this proton in solution containing only ampicillin, due to the catalytic effect of the metal ion. This can be studied by defining a function M[35] in that $M = ([H_3O^+]\ \Delta[B]/C_M)/(2 - \Delta[B]/C_M)$. By letting $h = \Delta[B]/C_M$, one obtains

$$M = (h[H_3O^+])/(2 - h)$$

or

$$pM = -\log[(h[H_3O^+])/(2 - h)] \qquad (5\text{-}8)$$

Table 5-4 The pH Titration Data on the Complexation of 0.0025 *M* $CuCl_2$ with 0.005 *M* Ampicillin at 25°C

pH	$\bar{n}$ (Δ[B]/C_M)	[HA^-],† 10^{-6} *M*	*Q* (*n*/(2 – *n*)[HA^-]), 10^5 M^{-1}
3.6	0.050	1.092	0.235
3.8	0.085	1.693	0.262
4.0	0.140	2.615	0.288
4.2	0.230	3.943	0.330
4.4	0.360	5.793	0.379
4.6	0.490	8.457	0.384
4.7	0.615	9.735	0.456
4.8	0.705	11.451	0.475
5.0	0.970	14.479	0.650
5.1	1.100	16.015	0.763
5.2	1.270	16.289	1.068
5.3	1.415	16.447	1.471
5.4	1.530	16.518	1.971
5.5	1.620	16.693	2.554
5.6	1.701	16.869	3.372
5.7	1.750	17.572	3.984
5.8	1.790	18.451	4.620

†Calculated using Equation (5-7); K_a for the ionization of the protonated amine in ampicillin is 5.623 × 10^{-8} (pK_a = 7.25).[37]

The term *h* represents the mean number of protons dissociated per molecule of Cu(II) complex. The pK_a values of the amino hydrogen of the two ligands can be designated as pK_1 and pK_1'. With this approach a plot of p*M* versus *h* should extrapolate to pK_1 + log 2 as *h* approaches zero, and to pK_1' – log 2 as *h* approaches 2. Likewise, the pK_a values corresponding to the dissociation of the amide hydrogen can be designated as pK_2 and pK_2' and determined at a higher pH region using Equation (5-8).

A summary of the stability and ionization constants determined for the complexation of Cu(II) with ampicillin is given in **Table 5-5**. These results show that the pH titration method can yield very detailed reaction mechanisms for the complexation phenomena. Cu(II) binds to ampicillin at the side chain rather than to the ring system as observed for other penicillins. The formation of $Cu(H_2A)^{2+}$ complex occurs in acidic pH. The coordination involves the C-10 amino and the C-9 carbonyl groups. Binding of Cu(II) promotes the ionization of both the protonated amino and the amide hydrogens. Cu(II) significantly lowered the pK_a of the protonated amino group from 7.25 to 4.86 and 5.11. The p*K* values for the ionization of the amide hydrogen of copper-bound ligands are 6.98 and 7.43, respectively, indicating that a significant switch of the coordination bonds from the carbonyl to the amide nitrogen begins to take place around neutral pH in the Cu(II)–ampicillin complex.

Other Methods of Molecular Interaction Studies

The determination of binding stoichiometry and constants depends on the use of appropriate methods to measure the concentrations of bound and free species in the system. Various analytical techniques exist for such studies. The measurement of bound drug concentration can be achieved either by monitoring specific physicochemical property changes due to the complexation using spectroscopy methods, NMR technique, and potentiometric analysis, or by using separation

Table 5-5 Ionization and Stability Constants of Cu(II)–Ampicillin Complexation at 25°C

Reaction	Stability Constant	Ionization
Ampicillin (H_2A) (0.0050 *M*): Dissociation of protonated amino hydrogen: $H_2A + H_2O = HA^- + H_3O^+$		$pK_a = 7.25$
Ampicillin (0.0050 *M*) + $CuCl_2$ (0.0025 *M*): $Cu^{2+} + 2H_2A = Cu(H_2A)2^{2+}$	$\log \beta = 5.12^{\dagger}$	
Dissociation of protonated amino hydrogen: $Cu^{2+} + H_2A = Cu(HA)^+ + H^+$ $Cu(HA)^+ + H_2A = Cu(HA)_2 + H^+$	 $\log K_1 = 5.06$ $\log K_2 = 4.59$	 $pK_1 = 4.86$ $pK_1' = 5.11$
Dissociation of amide hydrogen: $Cu(HA)_2 + H_2O = Cu(HA)(A)^- + H_3O^+$ $Cu(HA)(A)^- + H_3O = Cu(A)_2^{2-} + H_3O^+$		 $pK_2 = 6.98$ $pK_2' = 7.43$

†Calculated based on the combined stability and ionization constants: $\beta = K_1K_2K_a^2/K_1K_1'$.

H_2A: Ampicillin with two dissociable protons; HA^-: Ampicillin ion after dissociation of ammonium proton; A_2^-: Ampicillin ion after dissociation of both ammonium and amide protons.

techniques such as chromatography, dialysis, solvent extraction, and affinity capillary electrophoresis to differentiate bound and free drug concentrations. Readers may refer to texts of analytical chemistry for detailed methodologies. Metal complexation with charged organic molecules often leads to the formation of water-insoluble complexes. Solvent extraction, which is commonly used to remove either the metal ion or the ligands from solutions, is an effective method for metal complexation studies. With proper equilibrium considerations and the partition theories described earlier, solvent extraction methods are very useful for the determination of the stoichiometry as well as the stability constants of metal complexes.[38]

III. Cyclodextrins and the Inclusion Complexes

Drug–Cyclodextrin Complexation

Inclusion complexes are formed between interacting molecules in which a guest molecule is entrapped in a host molecule through unique molecular architecture of the host. Such complexation depends largely on the molecular structure and size and, to a lesser extent, mechanisms of chemical interactions. It has been shown, e.g., that compounds such as urea or hydroquinone can crystallize into a channel-like or cagelike structure that permits the enclosure of certain small molecules but occludes others based on structure and size.[39] These complexations have been shown to be useful for the separation of long-chain hydrocarbons or optical isomers. More significantly, the formation of inclusion complexes in solutions using starch and starch derivatives has received great attention in various pharmaceutical applications. The well-known starch–iodine solution is a channel-type complex consisting of iodine molecules entrapped within spirals of the glucose residues. Starch can also be converted to *cyclodextrins* (CDs), known as the Schardinger sugars, by cyclodextrin glycosyltransferases.[40] These molecules exist as toroids in solution and are capable of forming inclusion complexes with lipophilic compounds. In 2009, research from the laboratory of Brown and Goldstein[41] showed that cyclodextrin may be used to remove cholesterol from lysosomes in Niemann–Pick Type C disease, a lysosomal storage disorder that causes progressive deterioration of the nervous system and dementia. Numerous studies have followed showing that hydroxypropyl-beta-cyclodextrin (HP-β-CD), a currently FDA approved investigational new drug, enhances the aqueous solubility of lipophilic compounds through the formation of inclusion complexes and plays an important role in cholesterol metabolism. To date, there are more than

20 marketed drugs that contain CDs,[42] and more publications are emerging each year that illustrate the use of CDs for drug formulation and delivery.

Structure of Cyclodextrins

The chemistry and structure of the naturally occurring cyclodextrins (CDs) have been well characterized since the mid-1970s.[43] Typical CDs are constituted by 6-, 7-, and 8-glucopyranoside units, designated respectively as α-, β-, and γ-CDs, arranged as a toroid in which the larger and smaller openings are lined with secondary and primary hydroxyl groups, respectively (see **Figure 5-8**). Due to the presence of the hydrophilic hydroxyl groups, CDs are in general water-soluble, but the interior of the toroid is relatively hydrophobic compared to the solvent environment and is able to host a hydrophobic drug, forming an inclusion complex. As a result, hydrophilic CDs have been used to increase the aqueous solubility of lipophilic drugs. Although chemical interactions do play a role, the formation of the inclusion complex depends largely on the cavity size of the CD in relation to the molecular size of the guest molecule. The internal diameters of the α-, β-, and γ-CD are about 5, 6, and 8 Å, respectively, which makes the β- and γ-CDs more useful in pharmaceutical applications owing to their greater capacity to accommodate larger drug molecules. With the progressive development of CD-based formulation, synthetic derivatives of CDs have been made and classified as hydrophilic, hydrophobic, and ionic CDs. These compounds exhibit multifunctional characteristics and are being tested in various pharmaceutical developments.

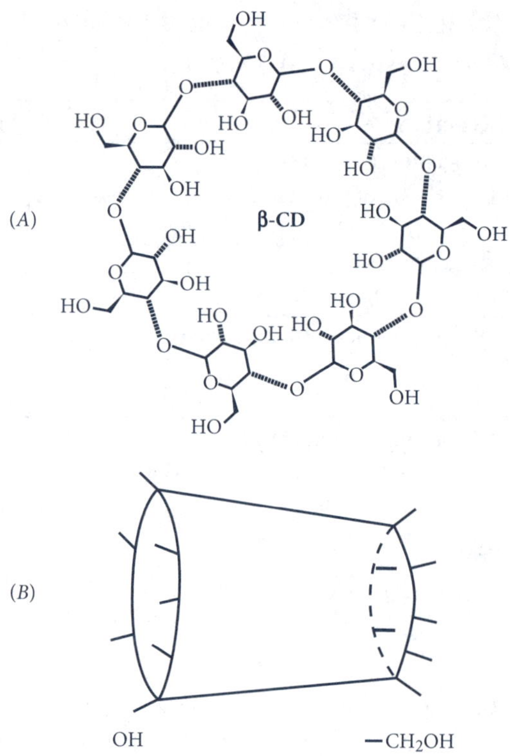

Figure 5-8 (*A*) β-Cyclodextrin and (*B*) its truncated cone-shaped structure.

Equilibrium and Binding Studies

The simplest and most frequent stoichiometry of drug A–CD complexation is the formation of a 1 : 1, A˙CD, complex, although the formation of a 1 : 2 complex (A˙CD_2) is not uncommon. In studies of the econazole/β-CD complexation, which forms mainly 1 : 1 complex, the formation of a 2 : 3 complex has also been reported.[44] The chemical equilibrium for the formation of a 1 : 1 complex between drug A and CD is illustrated in Equation (5-9):

$$\begin{aligned} &A + CD \rightleftarrows A^{\cdot}CD \\ &K_{11} = [A^{\cdot}CD]/[A][CD] \end{aligned} \quad (5\text{-}9)$$

where K_{11} is the binding constant and [A], [CD], and [A˙CD] are the concentrations of free drug, free CD, and bound drug, respectively. For the formation of a 1 : 2 complex,

$$\begin{aligned} &A^{\cdot}CD + CD \rightleftarrows A^{\cdot}CD_2 \\ &K_{12} = [A^{\cdot}CD_2]/[A^{\cdot}CD][CD] \end{aligned} \quad (5\text{-}10)$$

where K_{12} is the binding constant for the formation of the 1 : 2 complex.

Various analytical techniques exist for drug binding studies. The very property of the solubility enhancement by CD has led to the Higuchi–Connors *phase solubility method*,[45] which allows the determination of bound drug through measurements of total drug solubility as a function of CD and the intrinsic solubility of the drug. In this method, the intrinsic solubility of the drug S_o is essentially equal to [A] in a saturated solution, whereas the total solubility in the presence of CD, S_t, is equal to $[A] + [A{\cdot}CD] + [A{\cdot}CD_2]$, according to Equations (5-9) and (5-10). Hence, it can be seen that

$$S_t - S_o = [A{\cdot}CD] + [A{\cdot}CD_2]$$

and
$$\frac{S_t - S_o}{S_o} = \frac{[A{\cdot}CD]}{[A]} + \frac{[A{\cdot}CD_2]}{[A]}$$

$$= K_{11}[CD] + K_{11}K_{12}[CD]^2 \qquad (5\text{-}11)$$

The binding studies can be carried out at the condition where the concentration of cyclodextrin is in large excess compared to the drug concentration. In this case, [CD] can be taken as the value of the added CD concentration, C_{CD}. For a system that involves the formation of mainly a 1:1 complex, the plot of $(S_t - S_o)/S_o$ versus C_{CD} should yield a straight line with the slope equal to K_{11}. Alternatively, linear regression analysis of Equation (5-11) allows the determination of both K_{11} and K_{12}.

The formation of drug–cyclodextrin inclusion complexes depends largely on the cavity size and functional groups of the cyclodextrins and their interaction with other pharmaceutical agents. As new CDs are being developed, drug binding studies play an important role in characterizing the CD properties and their potential use for specific drug formulation purposes. This calls for methods that can be used for routine studies. Chen et al.[46] reported a phase distribution method designed for high-throughput determination of drug–CD binding constants, which offers the advantage of saving time and drug materials in comparison to the solubility measurements. In this method, drug (econozole or miconozole) of known concentration was embedded in a polymer film (2.5 µL) of poly(vinyl chloride) and dioctyl sebacate at a 1:2 ratio at the bottom of the wells of a 96-well microplate. CD-containing aqueous buffers (200 µL) of varying pH were then manually dispensed over the films, and the plates were covered by adhesive sealing films and incubated in a shaker at 25°C until it reached the predetermined equilibrium time (~ 4 h). Drug concentration in the supernatant from each well was then determined using a high performance liquid chromatographic method, from which the distribution of drug between the aqueous and polymer film phases was calculated as

$$D = C_{eq}/(C_t - C_{eq})\,Q$$

Here, C_{eq} and C_t are the drug concentrations in the aqueous phase at equilibrium and if the drug in film is totally extracted into the aqueous phase, respectively, and Q is the phase ratio (aqueous over polymer film). Under experimental conditions that the distribution phenomenon is limited to the neutral drug, the drug concentration in film is in large excess compared to its aqueous solubility, and the added CD concentration C_{CD} is in large excess of drug concentration in aqueous solution, it can be shown that

$$(D - D_o)/D_o = K_{11}[CD] + K_{11}K_{12}[CD]^2$$

$$= K_{11}C_{CD} + K_{11}K_{12}(C_{CD})^2 \qquad (5\text{-}12)$$

where D and D_o are the distribution constants of drug between the aqueous and film phases in the presence and absence of CD, respectively. Equation (5-12) is essentially identical to

Equation (5-11), but allows the determination of binding constants with a time-saving protocol that uses less experimental materials compared to the phase solubility method.

Binding Characteristics

The results of various binding studies have provided valuable insight into the formation of inclusion complexes by cyclodextrins. Binding of drugs to CD may be limited by the cavity size of the cyclodextrin and the hydrophobicity of the drug and the cyclodextrin molecules. Drugs such as mitomycin C and indomethacin have been shown to be too large to be placed entirely into the cavity of β-cyclodextrin.[47, 48] The ^{1}H NMR studies of aspirin binding to CD by Loftsson et al.[49] have also shown that the phenyl group is completely included into the cavity of β-CD, but the ester group stands somewhat outside the cavity. It has been proposed that the β-CD cavity can hold five to seven water molecules, which corresponds to a molar volume similar to that of benzene in water ($\sim 83 \times 10^{-6}\, m^3\, mol^{-1}$).[50] The interaction of aspirin with β-CD, as revealed by ultrasonic relaxation studies reported by Fukahori et al.,[51] results in a replacement of about five water molecules from the CD cavity, which is in agreement with the molecular volume data.

The above studies also showed that there is a 10-fold difference in binding constants between the inclusion of the neutral and ionized aspirin to β-CD. Interestingly, both the neutral and ionized aspirin showed the same rate of inclusion into the β-CD cavity, but the rate of the reverse from the inclusion for the ionized aspirin is 10-fold greater than that of the neutral aspirin molecule, indicating that a charged species is not stable in the hydrophobic environment of the CD cavity. In the study by Chen et al.,[46] the binding constants for the inclusion of econozole into a number of CDs were reported (see **Table 5-6**). They showed that the β-cyclodextrins, such as β-CD and HP-β-CD, generally exhibit higher binding constants than α-CD, and that the 2,6-di-*O*-methyl substitution of β-CD greatly enhanced the inclusion capacity of the cyclodextrin for econozole, indicating that increased size and hydrophobicity of the CD cavity result in increased formation of the inclusion complex with lipophilic drug. It is also interesting to note that the binding of econozole, a weak base, to CD is significantly diminished in acidic solution where the drug is in the cationic form.

Cyclodextrins as Pharmaceutical Agents

Owing to their broad applicability to pharmaceutical development, there is a globalized interest in cyclodextrin-related science and technology. Cyclodextrins, both natural and substituted, have been shown to exhibit different properties suitable for various pharmaceutical applications.

Table 5-6 The Binding Affinities of β-Cyclodextrins toward Econazole in pH 7.4 Phosphate Buffer at 25°C

Cyclodextrin (Formula; Mol Wt)	K_{11}, $10^3\,M^{-1}$	K_{12}, M^{-1}
α-CD ($C_{36}H_{60}O_{30}$; 972.84)	1.78 ± 0.30	256 ± 44
β-CD ($C_{42}H_{70}O_{35}$; 1134.98)	4.08 ± 0.50	47.6 ± 12.1
HE-β-CD (1480)†	3.98 ± 0.13	4.9 ± 0.5
HP-β-CD (1580)†	3.90 ± 0.22	10.0 ± 1.9
DM-β-CD ($C_{56}H_{98}O_{35}$; 1331)†	29.3 ± 2.2	57.7 ± 8.7
TM-β-CD ($C_{63}H_{112}O_{35}$; 1429.54)†	0.66 ± 0.04	53.9 ± 3.7

†HE-β-CD: hydroxyethyl-β-cyclodextrin, randomly substituted. HP-β-CD: hydroxypropyl-β-cyclodextrin, randomly substituted. DM-β-CD: 2,6-di-*O*-methyl-β-cyclodextrin, randomly substituted. TM-β-CD: heptakis-2,3,6-tri-*O*-methyl-β-cyclodextrin.

Data from: Chen Z, Lu D, and Weber SG. *J. Pharm. Sci.*, 2009;98:229–238.

The hydrophilic CDs are being used to enhance the solubility and bioavailability of drugs that are poorly soluble in water. The aqueous solubility of retinoic acid, e.g., increases from 0.5 to 160 mg/L via the formation of inclusion complex with *β*-CD.[52] Because solubility is a key parameter that controls the rate of dissolution of drugs from solid dosage forms, incorporation of CD in solid formulations has been shown to enhance the rate of drug dissolution[53] and thus their absorption into the blood circulation. Our understanding of CD-mediated increase in drug solubility is not yet complete. For example, studies by Faucci and Mura[54] showed that the use of hydrophilic polymers, such as sodium carboxymethylcellulose and PEG 6000, in combination with CD resulted in an enhancement of naproxen solubility that is greater than either drug–polymer or drug–CD binary system alone. The results suggest a synergistic effect between CD and the polymer on drug solubility, where the latter enhances the binding of naproxen to the cyclodextrins.

The effect of CD on drug stability stems from the concept that the chemically labile group of the drug may be embedded in the CD cavity and thus be protected from the aqueous environment. This has been demonstrated by Beckers et al.[55] in the inclusion complex of mitomycin C with *γ*-CD, where the aziridine ring is protected from degradation in acidic solution. It should be pointed out that for stability applications, the size of the CD cavity is of importance, as many drugs are only partially included in the *β*-cyclodextrins. The cavity size–dependent binding between drugs and CD also allows for the development of methods for enantiomer separations using CD as a chiral selector. Using econozole and miconazole, studies have shown that *β*-CD, HP-*β*-CD, and TM-*β*-CD all form enantioselective inclusion complexes with the drugs where the inclusion occurs through the phenyl ring closer to the azo group.[56]

Synthetic substitutions of the natural cyclodextrins have led to CD derivatives of different properties. The water solubility of cyclodextrins may be enhanced by random methylation of the primary and secondary hydroxyl groups, which reduces the intra- and intermolecular hydrogen bonding and allows for increased interaction with the water molecule. Limited methylation, as in the formation of 2,6-di-*O*-methyl-*β*-CD, also enhances the binding constant of CD with drug. The water-soluble methylated *β*-CD is also known to form soluble inclusion complexes with cholesterol and provide more efficient removal of cholesterol than *β*-CD in cell culture. Excessive methylation, however, as in heptakis-2,3,6-tri-*O*-methyl-*β*-CD, decreases its capacity to form the inclusion complex.[46]

The current literature shows a broad range of interests and approaches in using the cyclodextrins for pharmaceutical development. These approaches include the use of hydrophilic CDs to enhance bioavailability of water-insoluble drug, hydrophobic CDs for sustained-release formulations of water-soluble drugs to prolong therapeutic effect, enteric-type CDs such as *O*-carboxymethyl-*O*-ethyl-*β*-CD for delayed-release formulation, and branched CD for polypeptides and proteins to prevent molecular aggregation or adsorption to the hydrophobic surface of the container. It is likely that new approaches will emerge in current and future studies, which may include further modification of the CD molecules for improved drug formulation and delivery.

IV. Drug–Protein Binding

Drug Binding to Human Serum Albumin

After drug absorption, the majority of drugs are bound reversibly to albumin that circulates in the plasma. Human serum albumin (HSA) is the most abundant protein in plasma and plays a fundamental role in the transport of drugs, their metabolites, and endogenous molecules. Protein-bound drug is held in an inactive pool in the plasma. Binding to HSA thus controls the free (active) concentration of the drug, provides a reservoir for a long duration of action, and ultimately affects the drug's absorption, metabolism, distribution, and excretion (ADME). Because many drugs bind to HSA at the same site, the free concentration of a drug can be affected by coadministered drugs or by pathological conditions that modify the binding properties of the protein, resulting in clinically significant drug interactions, particularly for drugs having a relatively narrow therapeutic index.

HSA and Its Drug Binding Sites

Unlike other plasma proteins, which tend to exert a single specific function, albumin is a multifunctional protein. It contributes strongly to the osmotic pressure in the bloodstream and provides most of the acid/base buffering action of plasma proteins. As its main function, albumin serves as a serum carrier for a variety of endogenous molecules including fatty acids, tryptophan, hormones, ions, drugs, and their metabolites.[57] Due to its high affinity for long-chain fatty acids, albumin is the primary protein for the transport of fatty acids and plays an indirect role in fatty acid metabolism. In drug binding, HSA, together with α_1-glycoprotein, accounts for the majority of drug binding in serum. As a general rule, acid drug binds mainly to albumin, whereas basic drugs usually show high affinity toward α_1-glycoprotein.

Human serum albumin consists of a single polypeptide chain containing about 585 amino acids without prosthetic carbohydrate groups and a molecular weight of 67,000 Da. The plasma concentration of albumin is about 0.04 g/mL. Albumin contains some 35 cysteine residues, of which all but one form the disulfite linkages that contribute to the stability of the protein. HSA also has a high content of ionic amino acids including glutamic acid and lysine; it is negatively charged at physiological pH (pI = 4.9). In terms of its secondary structure, albumin is highly helical, with an α-helix content of about 67%. The tertiary structure assumes a triangular shape, about 80 Å across the base and 30 Å in average thickness, with a molecular volume of about 88,000 $Å^3$.[58] The globular protein shows three domains (I, II, and III); each is divided into subdomains A and B, which contain 6 and 4 α-helices, respectively. The fatty acid binding sites are distributed throughout the protein involving all six subdomains. Drug binding to albumin is more specific, and two of the binding sites for anionic hydrophobic drugs have been located in domains IIA and IIIA, which contain pockets formed mostly of the hydrophobic and positively charged residues. These two high-affinity binding sites have been characterized and defined as the *warfarin–azapropazone binding site* (site I), which is the highest-affinity binding site for, among others, warfarin and nonsteroidal anti-inflammatory drugs such as phenylbutazone, and the *tryptophan–benzodiazepine binding site* (site II), where a number of profens (ibuprofen, fenoprofen, and ketoprofen) are known to interact.[59] Crystallographic studies[60] of the warfarin binding site in subdomain IIA have shown that the binding of warfarin involves, among others, Phe (211), Try (214), Leu (219), Leu (238), Arg (218), and His (242) residues that form a hydrophobic pocket, and Arg (222), His (242), and a water molecule for electrostatic interactions. The binding is dominated by hydrophobic contacts, and modification of the Try (214) and Arg (218) reduces the protein's binding affinity. Although higher drug concentrations can lead to additional binding to albumin at other sites, the preformed high-affinity sites account for the binding of most drugs at therapeutic concentrations.

Binding of anionic drugs to albumin may involve cationic amino acid residues such as lysine and arginine, but many studies have shown that albumin can bind molecules that are non-ionic through hydrophobic interactions. Even for anionic drugs, such as the penicillins and sulfonamides, the protein binding affinity varies with varying hydrophobicity of their side chains.[61] The classical demonstration of the hydrophobic interaction between drug and albumin was the use of 1-anilinonaphthalene-8-sulfonate (ANS) as a fluorescence probe.[61, 62] ANS is only weakly fluorescent in water (emission wavelength: 520 nm) when the molecule is excited with uv light at wavelength of 375 nm but becomes intensely fluorescent, with the emission wavelength shifted to 475 nm, in nonpolar solvents of increasing hydrophobicity, or when bound to serum albumin. Interaction of this anionic probe with the cationic amino acid residue at the binding site contributes to increased hydrophobicity of the binding site. The fluorescence change in ANS binding to albumin may be attributed to energy transfer at the excited state from the tryptophan residue, which fluoresces at about 350 nm, to the bound ANS. This phenomenon allows the determination of the average distance between the bound drug to the tryptophan residues,[63, 64] thus providing information on the location of the binding site. ANS has been used as a probe for drug–albumin binding studies based on the fact that anionic and neutral drugs compete with ANS for the binding site.

The albumin molecule, as evidenced by structural analysis and binding studies, is quite flexible and undergoes changes in tertiary structure upon binding with small molecules. Hydrophobic groups, such as the fatty acids, may penetrate into the interior of the globular albumin molecule and cause a separation of the helices of the protein. Thus, the binding properties of albumin can be significantly affected by intra- and interindividual variability related to disease states, pathological conditions, and genetics. A change in plasma level of albumin or endogenous ligands can influence drug binding and call for close monitoring of dosages.

The Binding Equilibrium

Single-Site Binding

For a protein P that has a single binding site for a drug D, the binding equilibrium can be expressed as

$$\mathrm{D} + \mathrm{P} \rightleftarrows \mathrm{PD}$$

At equilibrium,

$$K = [\mathrm{PD}]/[\mathrm{D}][\mathrm{P}]$$

where K is the binding constant, [D] is the free drug concentration (D_f), [PD] is the concentration of the drug–protein complex, i.e., the bound drug concentration, D_b, and [P] is the concentration of the unbound protein. If the total concentration of the protein is P_t, then $[\mathrm{P}] = P_t - D_b$. Hence,

$$K = \frac{D_b}{D_f(P_t - D_b)} \tag{5-13}$$

and it follows that

$$KD_fP_t - KD_fD_b = D_b \quad \text{or} \quad D_b = KD_fP_t/(1 + KD_f) \tag{5-14}$$

For the determination of the binding constant, it is useful to introduce the term v, defined as the ratio of bound drug to total protein concentration: $v = D_b/P_t$. In solutions containing a given concentration of the protein and varying concentrations of the drug, as the drug concentration increases, v will increase and approach the value of 1 as the binding approaches saturation. With this definition, Equation (5-14) can be rewritten as

$$v = \frac{D_b}{P_t} = \frac{KD_f}{1 + KD_f}$$

The above equation can be further rearranged to give

$$\frac{v}{D_f} = K - rK \tag{5-15}$$

With experimentally determined values of v and D_f, the binding constant can be easily determined by a plot of v/D_f versus v, which yields a straight line with the slope equal to $-K$. It should be mentioned that Equation (5-15) is for proteins that have a single binding site for the drug.

Drug Binding to Protein at Multiple Sites

Per the previous discussion, mathematical treatment of binding data based on chemical equilibrium involving multiple binding steps and constants can be very complicated. A protein may have several major binding sites as well as some low-affinity binding sites for a drug. But unlike small molecule interactions, such as the complexation of Co^{3+} with ammonia where the formation of the complex of a higher ligand order depends on the formation of complexes of lower ligand orders, the binding sites on a protein may be considered to be independent of one another. Scatchard[65] and others have reasoned that if these binding sites exhibit a similar intrinsic binding constant, then the equilibrium may be expressed as a 1 : 1 interaction, as shown in Equation (5-13), with the modification that the total concentration of the protein available for binding is P_t *times its number of binding sites n*. With this approach, it can be seen that

$$K = \frac{D_b}{D_f(nP_t - D_b)} \qquad (5\text{-}16)$$

$$v = \frac{D_b}{P_t} = \frac{nKD_f}{1 + KD_f}$$

and

$$\frac{v}{D_f} = nK - vK \qquad (5\text{-}17)$$

Equation (5-17), although not without shortcomings, has been the most used equation for drug–protein binding studies. The determination of the binding constant and the number of binding sites is achieved via the linear plot of v/D_f versus v, which is known as the *Scatchard plot*. Interestingly, this equation seems to take the form of a Langmuir plot that describes the adsorption isotherm of a gas onto an adsorbent. The chemisorption process, however, does not describe binding sites and is pictured as leading ultimately to a molecular film over the surface of the adsorbent.

The major question concerning the Scatchard plot is that the plot of r/D_f versus r for drug–protein interactions often does not yield a convincing straight line, but shows a downward curve. This curvature phenomenon has been addressed by many researchers. Ma et al.[62] have used the log Q approach described in previous sections to treat the data of ANS binding to human and bovine serum albumins, based on the concept that the intrinsic constants of the binding sites are not equal. The most popular approach in explaining the curvature, however, is to consider the protein as having several classes of binding sites, and within each class, all binding sites have the same intrinsic binding constant. This approach is illustrated in Equation (5-18):

$$v = \frac{n_1K_1D_f}{1 + K_1D_f} + \frac{n_2K_2D_f}{1 + K_2D_f} + \frac{n_3K_3D_f}{1 + K_3D_f} + \cdots \qquad (5\text{-}18)$$

For a protein having *three* classes of binding sites, for example, n_1, n_2, and n_3 are the number of binding sites in each class, and K_1, K_2, and K_3 are the corresponding binding constants. Equation (5-18) may be used to determine the binding parameters involving multiple classes of binding sites by regression analyses. From the chemical point of view, it can be said that the major binding sites, represented by n_1 in Equation (5-18), show considerably greater structural specificity toward drugs than those low-affinity sites, and the low-affinity sites will appear at high drug concentrations, which may not be saturable.

Fraction of Free or Bound Drug in Plasma

One of the important applications of the drug–protein binding results is to determine the fraction of bound or free drug in plasma for pharmacokinetic considerations, as it has been well demonstrated that only the free fraction of the drug is biologically active and that the displacement of bound drug by other agents from the protein can result in altered drug distribution in the body. Thus, it is desirable to calculate the fraction of bound drug based on determined binding parameters (n and K) and the protein and drug levels in the plasma. The fraction of bound drug f_b is defined as $f_b = D_b/D_t$, where D_b and D_t are the bound and total drug concentrations, respectively. From Equation (5-16), it is seen that

$$K = \frac{D_b}{(D_t - D_b)(nP_t - D_b)} \quad (5\text{-}19)$$

To solve D_b, the above equation can be rearranged to give

$$D_b^2 - (nP_t + D_t + 1/K)D_b + nP_tD_t = 0$$

By letting $B = (nP_t + D_t + 1/K)$ and $C = nP_tD_t$, the solution for D_b is

$$D_b = [B - (B^2 - 4C)^{1/2}] / 2$$

The fraction of bound drug can then be calculated as

$$f_b = D_b/D_t = [B - (B^2 - 4C)^{1/2}] / 2D_t \quad (5\text{-}20)$$

The calculation of f_b can be simplified if the protein concentration is significantly greater than the bound drug concentration, that is, $nP_t >> D_b$. In this case, $nP_t - D_b \approx nPt$, and Equation (5-19) can be rewritten as

$$K = \frac{D_b}{(D_t - D_b)(nP_t)}$$

The above equation can be derived to yield Equation (5-21) for the calculation of D_b and Equation (5-22) for the determination of the fraction of bound drug.

$$D_b = \frac{nP_tD_tK}{1 + nP_tK} \quad (5\text{-}21)$$

and

$$f_b = \frac{D_b}{D_t} = \frac{nP_tK}{1 + nP_tK} \quad (5\text{-}22)$$

Equation (5-22) is quite valid for drugs that have moderate and low plasma concentrations. With a plasma level of about 40 g/L, the molar concentration of human serum albumin (mol wt = 67,000) is 5.97×10^{-4} M. The plasma levels for most drugs are in the microgram per milliliter range. Assuming a molecular weight range of 150–600 for small drug molecules, their molar concentrations are usually at the 10^{-6} M level. This indicates that $nP_t >> D_b$. It is important to point out that the fraction of bound drug for a given system varies with varying drug concentrations if the protein and drug concentrations are in the same range. However, when the protein concentration is relatively high compared to the drug concentration range, the fraction of bound drug does not change with changing total drug level, as shown by Equation (5-22).

Methods in Drug–Protein Binding Studies

The determination of binding constants and the number of binding sites for a drug–protein interaction requires the determination of the bound and free drug concentrations. The data can then be treated according to Equation (5-17). A wide variety of biochemical techniques have been applied to protein binding studies. In general, these methods include techniques that separate the free drug from the bound drug, or spectrophotometric methods that measure the change in molecular properties as a result of protein binding. Equilibrium dialysis, ultrafiltration, and ultracentrifugation are the most commonly used separation techniques to determine drug–protein binding as well as competitive binding displacement by drugs sharing the same binding sites. These techniques are based on the separation of the free drug from the bound one after equilibrium is reached. In equilibrium dialysis, a protein-free drug solution and a protein solution are separated by a membrane in a dialysis cell that allows only the drug but not the protein to pass through. The permeation of the drug through the membrane establishes an equilibrium between the free drug concentrations in the two solutions, from which the free and bound drug concentrations in the protein solution can be determined.[66] The *ultrafiltration* methods, similar to equilibrium dialysis, are based on separation of protein and protein-bound drug from free drug molecules. They are, however, faster and more convenient than equilibrium dialysis in that the separation is forced by hydraulic pressure or centrifugation, allowing the medium and small molecules (unbound drug) to pass through the membrane while preventing the passage of protein and protein-bound drug. The free drug concentration is then determined from the ultrafiltrate. Because these methods depend on the determination of the free drug concentration, there may be sensitivity issues related to drug analysis if the drug is highly protein-bound. Potential errors may also result from binding of the drug to the membrane, suggesting that control experiments in protein-free solutions should be carried out to define the equilibrium of free drug concentrations with respect to the membrane. Among other separation methods, drug–albumin binding has been determined using immobilized albumin via high-performance affinity chromatography.[67]

Drug–protein interactions have been studied most conveniently using absorption (uv) and emission (fluorescence) spectrophotometric methods. The fluorescence methods are more advantageous than the absorption spectroscopy due to the high sensitivity of the former in measuring changes in molecular properties. Most proteins are fluorescent (excitation, 280 nm; emission, 350 nm), and this fluorescence is due primarily to the presence of tryptophan residues, which are among the most hydrophobic amino acids. Drug may exhibit uv absorptions but not necessarily fluorescence. Upon binding to a protein, if the drug has an absorption spectrum that overlaps the emission (fluorescence) spectrum of the protein (around 350 nm), the bound drug may become fluorescent due to energy transfer from the tryptophan residue to the drug provided that the distance between the tryptophan residue and the drug is sufficiently close to allow this energy transfer to occur. The probability of fluorescence by the drug also increases if the binding site environment is hydrophobic, which prevents the loss of energy due to interaction with the aqueous solvent. Thus, it is well established that the changes in fluorescence are due to drug–protein interactions.

Because not all drugs are capable of fluorescence, many fluorescent compounds were tested for their applicability as a binding probe in drug–protein binding studies. One of the most used fluorescent probes is 1-anilinonaphthalene-8-sulfonate (ANS). This compound shows a strong binding with human or bovine serum albumin. As can be seen in **Figure 5-9**, binding of ANS to bovine serum albumin (BSA) results in a blue shift (toward shorter wavelength) of the emission (fluorescent) wavelength (from 520 to 475 nm) and a strong increase in fluorescence intensity due to energy transfer from the tryptophan residues. The addition of a drug, such as phenylbutazone, that competes for the protein binding sites lowers the fluorescence due to binding displacement that leads to a reduction of the fluorescent, bound probe. Applying the fluorescence energy transfer theory, Togashi and Ryder[64] have shown that the high-affinity ANS binding sites on BSA are located in close distance (18–27 Å) to at least one of the two tryptophan residues.

The use of the fluorescent probe for drug binding studies involves first the determination of the binding of the probe to the protein. This can be achieved by successive titration of a protein solution of a desired concentration with a stock solution of the fluorescent probe. After each titration, the enhanced fluorescence at the wavelength of the bound probe is measured as a function of the probe concentration. Separate titrations in the same probe concentration range should be made in protein-free solution for baseline calibration, and in solution containing a predetermined high protein concentration where the probe exists only in the bound form. This is indicated by a linear increase in fluorescent intensity as a function of the probe concentration. From the fluorescence data, the bound and free probe concentrations at each titration point can be calculated and used for the determination of binding parameters according to Equation (5-17). This method is illustrated in **Table 5-7**.

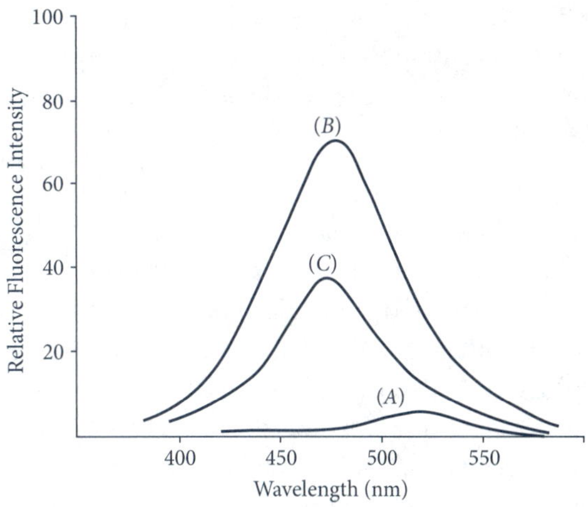

Figure 5-9 Fluorescence spectra of 5×10^{-6} *M* ANS (excitation: 375 nm) in (*A*) pH 7.4 buffer alone, (*B*) buffer + 1.38×10^{-6} *M* BSA, and (*C*) buffer + BSA + 1×10^{-4} *M* phenylbutazone.

For the study of competitive drug binding using the fluorescent probe, titrations of the protein solution with the probe can be carried out in the absence and presence of the drug at a given concentration. Binding of the drug to the protein will compete with the probe for the protein binding sites and result in a decrease of the fluorescence intensity of the protein-bound probe (see Figure 5-9). Titration curves of fluorescence intensity as a function of probe concentration in the absence and presence of protein and drug can thus be obtained at the wavelength of maximum fluorescence to determine free and bound concentrations of the probe (and drug). The binding parameters for the probe in the presence of drug can be determined using the *Scatchard equation*, and the binding constant for the drug sharing the same binding sites is calculated using the Klotz equation.[68, 69] The Klotz equation is

$$K_{\text{drug}} = K\frac{D_f}{D_b}\frac{nP_tKD_f - KD_fD_b - D_b}{C_tKD_f - P_tKD_fD_b + D_b} \qquad (5\text{-}23)$$

Table 5-7 Determination of Free and Bound ANS in BSA Solution and Binding Parameters by Fluorescence Titration†

D_t, 10^{-6} *M*	$F - F_o$ A	$F - F_o$ B	D_b, 10^{-6} *M*	D_f, 10^{-6} *M*	v	v/D_f, 10^6 M^{-1}
1	25	34	0.735	0.265	0.53	2.011
2	45	67	1.343	0.657	1.00	1.514
3	64	101	1.882	1.118	1.36	1.220
4	76	133	2.286	1.714	1.66	0.966
5	88	169	2.604	2.496	1.89	0.756
6	94	200	2.820	3.180	2.04	0.643
7	98	234	2.932	4.068	2.12	0.521
8	101	266	3.038	4.962	2.20	0.443
9	102	296	3.101	5.899	2.25	0.381

†$F - F_o$: Fluorescence intensity (arbitrary unit) after correction for baseline fluorescence, measured at excitation of 375 nm and emission of 475 nm.

Titration A: Solution contains 1.38×10^{-6} *M* BSA and varying concentrations of ANS as indicated by D_t.

Titration B: Solution contains 1.38×10^{-5} *M* BSA and varying concentrations of ANS as indicated by D_t.

Calculations: $D_b = D_t\,(F - F_o)_A \,/\, (F - F_o)_B$ $\quad D_f = D_t - D_b$ $\quad v = D_b/1.38 \times 10^{-6}$

The Scatchard plot of v/D_f versus v yields $n = 2.7$ and $K = 0.92 \times 10^6$ M^{-1}.

where K_{drug} and C_t are the binding constant and total concentration of the drug, respectively; all other symbols are previously defined parameters referring to the fluorescent probe.

The use of ANS as a fluorescence probe for drug–albumin binding studies was reported by Luzzi and coworkers for a series of drugs including warfarin, phenylbutazone, penicillins, sulfonamides, and sulfonylureas.[61–63, 70, 71] Binding of ANS to the warfarin binding site in bovine serum albumin (BSA) was tested via competitive displacement of ANS by warfarin and phenylbutazone.[70] The Scatchard plots for the binding of ANS in the absence and presence of drug to BSA are given in **Figure 5-10**. As can be seen, there is a good fit between the binding data of ANS to BSA and the Scatchard equation, which yields a binding constant of $0.92 \times 10^6\ M^{-1}$ and a value of 2.7 for the number of binding sites. The binding of ANS to the albumin is significantly diminished in the presence of warfarin or phenylbutazone, indicating that the binding of ANS involves interaction at the warfarin binding site. The calculated binding constants for warfarin and phenylbutazone using the Klotz equation are 3.1×10^4 and $9.0 \times 10^4\ M^{-1}$, respectively. These values are similar to those reported for the binding of the corresponding drug to human serum albumin.

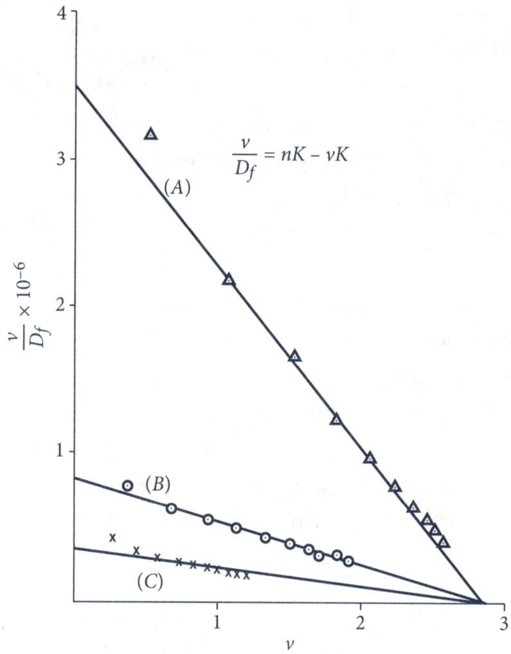

Figure 5-10 The Scatchard plots for the binding of ANS to bovine serum albumin in (*A*) the absence of drug, (*B*) the presence of $1 \times 10^{-4}\ M$ warfarin, or (*C*) the presence of $1 \times 10^{-4}\ M$ phenylbutazone in pH 7.4 buffer. Reproduced from: Jun HW, Luzzi LA, and Hsu PL. Phenylbutazone-sodium warfarin binding using a fluorescent probe technique. *J Pharm Sci.*, 1972;61:1835–1837.

The determination of binding parameters depends largely on the experimental methods used. The results from spectrophotometric techniques may differ from those of the separation-based methods in that only the high-affinity binding sites are detected by the change of molecular property, whereas separation-based methods such as equilibrium dialysis often show larger numbers of binding sites.

Role of Protein Binding in Drug Efficacy, Distribution, and Interactions

Pharmacokinetic Considerations

It is well recognized that the in vivo efficacy of drugs is determined by the free drug concentration surrounding the therapeutic target. Hence it is desirable to establish pharmacokinetic parameters based on the free drug concentration. For drugs that are extensively bound to proteins in plasma, there is the potential that the bound drug may be displaced from the proteins by coadministered drugs and/or endogenous ligands, resulting in an increase in free drug concentration in plasma. Note that the binding displacement alters the free fraction of the drug but not the total drug concentration in the plasma. One can look at this effect via pharmacokinetic modeling to delineate potential changes in drug distribution. The volume of distribution of a drug may be determined based on the unbound drug or total drug concentrations. Using diazepam, which exhibits extensive plasma protein binding and tissue distribution, as a model drug, Stepensky[72] showed that the distribution pattern and the time course of the unbound drug correlated with the unbound volume of distribution but not with the total volume of distribution. This indicates that binding displacement induces a faster elimination of the drug from the body.

The interpretation of drug levels at the steady state may be influenced by the extent of drug binding to plasma proteins. An increase in free fraction, due to binding displacement or altered protein concentration and structure in disease state, decreases the therapeutic and toxic ranges established through total drug concentration. Conversely a reduction in free fraction increases these ranges. Because drug monitoring is usually done by laboratory measurement of total rather than unbound drug concentrations, clinicians must use caution in interpreting the total drug levels in clinical situations where the binding of extensively bound drugs may be altered. Free drug concentrations are inherently more reliable than the total concentrations for indexing the intensity of drug action and may ultimately be utilized for therapeutic monitoring of drugs that are highly protein-bound. Because the plasma concentration of drugs is, in general, substantially lower than that of the drug-binding proteins, the free drug fraction can be assumed constant independent of drug concentration (see Equation (5-22)). It is thus of value that the free drug concentrations be monitored or calculated in clinical practice.

Drug Efficacy at Specific Sites

Ample studies have shown that only the unbound drug is pharmacologically active, and that only the unbound drug is capable of penetrating across the pores of the capillary membrane. Hence, one observes that the antibacterial activity of 100 μg/mL oxacillin (94% albumin-bound) in serum is equivalent only to that of 10 μg/mL of the drug in water, and that dicloxacillin (95% albumin-bound) is absorbed through intramuscular delivery at a much slower rate than that of ampicillin (18% albumin-bound). Indeed, the antibiotic drugs, in their free form, can enter muscles, bones, and synovial and interstitial fluids from intravascular sites via aqueous pores that exist in the capillaries. Significant protein binding can prevent the penetration of many antibiotics into these tissue sites, including the eye and inflamed brain tissue. One such example is sulfanilamide, which was shown to enter the cerebrospinal fluid (CSF) faster and to a larger extent than sulfamethoxypyridazine (83% albumin bound) because of the extensive binding by the latter to plasma albumin. This is despite the fact that their relative lipophilicity would predict an opposite order of action from the one observed.

The effect of protein binding on drug efficacy can be described by an equilibrium that occurs at the blood–tissue barrier between the free drug concentrations in the tissue fluid and in serum according to Equation (5-24)

$$C_t = C_s f_s / f_t \tag{5-24}$$

Here, C_t is drug concentration in the tissue fluid, C_s is the serum drug concentration, and f_s and f_t are the free fractions of the drug in serum and tissue fluid, respectively. The total concentration of a drug in tissue fluids at the therapeutic target thus depends on the serum concentration, plasma-protein binding, and drug binding to proteins in the tissue fluids. Equation (5-24) also shows that if the serum and the tissue fluid are identical in content, or if some proteins are present in both fluids, the tissue fluid concentration will be the same as that in blood serum. This is true for both high- and low-protein-containing extravascular fluids.

Drug Interactions

The most significant drug interaction involving plasma protein binding occurs where a highly bound (> 90%) drug is partially displaced by another drug or endogenous molecules. A large increase in the free drug concentration will occur, which may result in increased therapeutic or toxic effect. For example, for a drug that is 95% bound, a decrease in binding to 90% will result in a doubling of the free drug concentration. The pharmacokinetic consequences of such changes will depend on the size of the volume of distribution as well as the magnitude of the hepatic extraction and other parameters. The extent of binding displacement depends on the concentration of the competitive binding molecule. Even with a lower binding constant, significant displacement of the drug by a competitor will occur if the concentration of the competitive molecule is sufficiently high.

The most studied drug interaction through protein binding is the competitive binding between warfarin and nonsteroidal anti-inflammatory drugs such as phenylbutazone and azapropazone. Warfarin is extensively bound to human serum albumin at the subdomain IIA binding site. Studies by Diana et al.[73] showed that both phenylbutazone and azapropazone markedly inhibited warfarin binding to albumin, with an 18- and 32-fold reduction of the binding constant, respectively. Interestingly, drug binding to albumin can also be enhanced through protein conformational changes induced by the binding of the competing molecule at a different site, such as the effect of tolmetin on warfarin binding reported in the above study.[73] Such conformational change has been well studied with respect to the effect of fatty acids on warfarin binding. Fatty acids are known to enhance the binding affinity of the protein for warfarin and other site I ligands. The presence of up to 3 mol of long-chain fatty acids per mole of HSA can increase wafarin binding by a factor of about 3. As shown by Petitpas et al.,[60] the fatty acid binding induces a substantial conformational change in the protein involving rotations of domains I and III relative to domain II. One of the principal driving forces for the rotations is the binding of a fatty acid molecule to the binding site at the interface between subdomains IA and IIA in close proximity to the warfarin binding site. The hydrogen bonding interaction of the fatty acid with a tyrosine (150) residue, a helix linker, results in a rotation of the helices, through which the warfarin binding site is changed by a switch of the tyrosine residue with an arginine (257) residue in the drug pocket. This results in a more hydrophic environment for the warfarin binding site. At concentrations higher than 3 mol of fatty acid per mole of protein, fatty acids lower warfarin binding by displacement of the drug from the warfarin binding site.

V. Chapter Summary

Molecular interaction is a broad subject that applies to all aspects of drug development, drug action, and pharmacological and toxicological effects. As a general outcome, understanding the molecular forces involved in interactions and the identification of such forces based on the chemical properties and structural characteristics of both inorganic and organic compounds should be an important learning objective. This chapter also includes discussion of basic theories and quantitative methods in three key areas of molecular interactions, namely, metal ion complexation, inclusion complexation, and protein binding. Each subject has a unique position in the pharmaceutical sciences that either aids in the development of pharmaceutical products or describes the action of a drug in the biological system. The homework problems are designed to provide readers with practice for reinforced learning of the theories and methods discussed in this chapter.

VI. References

1. Easson LH and Steadman E. *Biochem J.* 27:1257, 1933.
2. Malmberg A, Nordvall G, Johansson AM, Mohell N, and Hacksell U. *Mol Pharmacol.* 46:299–312, 1994.
3. Marcus A. *Drug Cosmet Ind.* 79:456, 1956.

4. Couvreur P, Kante B, Grislain L, Roland M, and Speiser P. *J Pharm Sci.* 71:790–792, 1982.
5. Manocha B and Margaritis A. *Biotechnol Prog.* 26:734–742, 2010.
6. Janes KA, Fresneau MP, Marazuela A, Fabra A, and Alonso MJ. *J Controlled Release.* 73:255–267, 2001.
7. Rudzinski WE and Aminabhavi TM. *Int J Pharm.* 399:1–11, 2010.
8. Aziz EF, Ottosson N, Faubel M, Hertel IV, and Winter B. *Nature.* 455:89–91, 2008.
9. Alberet A. *Selective Toxcity*, New York, Wiley, 1968, p 262.
10. Grey MJ, Tang Y, Alexov E, McKnight CJ, Raleigh DP, and Palmer AG III. *J Mol Biol.* 355:1078–1094, 2006.
11. Garcia-Mayoral MF, del Pozo AM, Campos-Olivas R, Gavilanes JG, Santoro J, Rico M, Laurents DV, and Bruix M. *Biochemistry.* 45:13705–13718, 2006.
12. Pedersen S, Nesgaard L, Baptista RP, Melo EP, Kristensen SR, and Otzen DE. *Biopolymers.* 83:619–629, 2006.
13. Olson LJ, Hindsgaul O, Dahms NM, and Kim JJ. *J Biol Chem.* 283:10124–10134, 2008.
14. Kono K, Kimura S, and Imanishi Y. *Biochemistry.* 29:3631–3637, 1990.
15. Chan P, Lovric J, and Warwicker J. *Proteomics.* 6:3494–3501, 2006.
16. Chan P and Warwicker J. *BMC Biol.* 7:69, 2009.
17. Talley K and Alexov E. *Proteins.* 78:2699–2706, 2010.
18. Wang X, Lu J, Xu M, and Xing B. *Environ Sci Technol.* 42:7267–7272, 2008.
19. Li SC, Chu LN, Gong XQ, and Diebold U. *Science.* 328(5980):882–884, 2010.
20. Halliwell B and Gutteridge JMC. *Biochem J.* 219:1–14, 1984.
21. Blake DR, Hall ND, Bacon PA, Dieppe PA, Halliwell B, and Gutteridge JMC. *Lancet.* 2:1142–1144, 1981.
22. Blake DR, Hall ND, Bacon PA, Dieppe PA, Halliwell B, and Gutteridge JMC. *Ann Rheum Dis.* 42:414–419, 1983.
23. Brown CE. *J Theor Biol.* 88:245–256, 1981.
24. Faller P. *Chembiochem.* 10:2837–2845, 2009.
25. Gaggelli E, Kozlowski H, Valensin D, and Valensin G. *Mol Biosyst.* 1:79–84, 2005.
26. Badrick AC and Jones CE. *Curr Top Med Chem.* 11:543–552, 2011.
27. Oze K, Varnagy K, Suli-Vargha H, Csampay A, Sana D, Micera G, and Sovago I. *J Inorg Biochem.* 98:24–32, 2004.
28. Liu NM, Lo LSL, Askay SH, Goforth J, Viva E, Tsai MT, and Linder MC. *J Nutr Biochem.* 18:597–608, 2007.
29. Lau S and Sarkar B. *J Biol Chem.* 246:5938–5943, 1971.
30. Nagane R, Chakira M, Oumi M, Shindo N, and Antholine W. *J Inorg Biochem.* 78:243–249, 2000.
31. Tamba M and Torreggiani A. *Free Radic Res.* 32:199–211, 2000.
32. LoPachin RM, Gavin T, Geohagen BC, et al. *J Neurochem.* 116:132–143, 2011.
33. DeFord DP and Hume DN. *J Am Chem Soc.* 73:5321, 1951.
34. Li NC, Chu TL, Fujii CT, and White JM. *J Am Chem Soc.* 77:859, 1955.
35. Martin RB, Chamberli M, and Edsall JT. *J Am Chem Soc.* 82:495, 1960.
36. Conley HL and Martin RB. *J Phys Chem.* 69:2914, 1965.
37. Ma JKH and McConnell L. Unpublished data, 1980.
38. Day ST, Crouthanel WG, Martinelli LC, and Ma JKH. *J Pharm Sci.* 67:1518–1523, 1978.
39. Brown JF Jr. *Sci Am.* 207:82, 1962.
40. Biwer A, Antranikian G, and Heinzle E. *Appl Microbiol Biotechnol.* 59:609–617, 2002.
41. Abi-Mosleh L, Infante RE, Radhakrishnan A, Goldstein JL, and Brown MS. *Proc Natl Acad Sci USA.* 106:19316–19321, 2009.
42. Loftsson T, Brewster ME, and Masson M. *Am. J Drug Deliv.* 2:261–275, 2004.

43. Szejtli J. *Cyclodextrin Technology*. New York, Springer, 1988, vol 1.
44. Pendersen M, Bjerregaard S, Jacobseb J, Rommel-Mayer Larsen A, and Mehlsen Sorensen A. *Int J Pharm*. 165:57–68, 1998.
45. Higuchi T and Connors KA. *Adv Anal Chem Intr*. 4:117–212, 1965.
46. Chen Z, Lu D, and Weber SG. *J Pharm Sci*. 98:229–238, 2009.
47. Beckers O. *Int J Pharm*. 52:240–247, 1989.
48. Bakensfield T, Müller BW, Wiese M, and Seyde JK. *Pharm Res*. 7:484–490, 1990.
49. Loftsson T, Olafsdottir BJ, Fridriksdottir H, and Jonsdottir S. *Eur J Pharm Sci*. 1:95, 1993.
50. Majer V, Degrange S, and Sedlbauer J. *J Fluid Phase Equilib*. 158:419, 1999.
51. Fukahori T, Kondo M, and Nishikawa S. *J Phys Chem*. B110:4487–4491, 2006.
52. Amdidouche D, Darrouzet H, Duchene D, and Poelman MC. *Int J Pharm*. 54:175, 1989.
53. Hassan MA, Suleiman MS, and Najib NM. *Int J Pharm*. 58:19, 1990.
54. Faucci MT and Mura P. *Drug Dev Ind Pharm*. 27:909–917, 2001.
55. Beckers O, Beijnen JH, Bramel EHG, Otagiri M, Bult A, and Underberg WJM. *Int J Pharm*. 52:239, 1989.
56. Castro-Puyana M, Crego AL, Marina ML, and Gacia-Ruiz C. *Electrophoresis*. 28:2667–2674, 2007.
57. Peters T Jr. *All about Albumin, Biochemistry, Genetics and Medical Applications*. New York, Academic Press, 1996.
58. He XM and Carter DC. *Nature*. 358:209–215, 1992.
59. Sudlow G, Birkett DJ, and Wade DN. *Mol Pharmacol*. 11:824–832, 1975.
60. Petitpas I, Bhattacharya AA, Twine S, East M, and Curryl S. *J Biol Chem*. 276:22804–22809, 2001.
61. Hsu PL, Ma JKH, Jun HW, and Luzzi LA. *J Pharm Sci*. 63:27–31, 1974.
62. Ma JKH, Jun HW, and Luzzi LA. *J Pharm Sci*. 62:2038, 1973.
63. Ma JKH, Fu, PP, and Luzzi LA. *J Pharm Sci*. 66:209, 1977.
64. Togashi DM and Ryder AG. *J Fluoresc*. 18:519–526, 2008.
65. Scatchard G. *Ann NY Acad Sci*. 51:660, 1949.
66. Klotz IM, Walker FM, and Puvan RB. *J Am Chem Soc*. 68:1486, 1946.
67. Ascoli G, Bertucci C, and Salvadori P. *Biomed Chromat*. 12:248–254, 1998.
68. Klotz IM, Triwuish H, and Walker FM. *J Am Chem Soc*. 70:2935, 1948.
69. Brand L, Gohlke JR, and Rao S. *J Biochem*. 6:3510, 1967.
70. Jun HW, Luzzi LA, and Hsu PL. *J Pharm Sci*. 61:1835–1837, 1972.
71. Hsu PL, Ma JK, and Luzzi LA. *J Pharm Sci*. 63:570–573, 1974.
72. Stepensky D. *Eur. J Pharm Sci*. 42:91–98, 2011.
73. Diana FJ, Veronich K, and Kapoor A. *J Pharm Sci*. 78:195, 1989.

VII. Homework Problems

1. What organic moieties contribute to hydrophobic interaction? Briefly summarize the importance of hydrophobic interactions by naming a few biological processes that depend on hydrophobic interactions.
2. What are the end products of the Fenton reaction? Based on your previous knowledge, give another process through which iron may induce free radical formation.
3. Studies have shown that copper chelating agents are neuroprotective against copper ion–induced oxidative stress. How do copper ions induce reactive oxygen species?
4. One of the most stable of the organic nitrogen compounds is the porphyrin derivative of copper (see **Figure 5-11**), which can be sublimed at temperature of about 400°C without changing its structure. Why is this so?

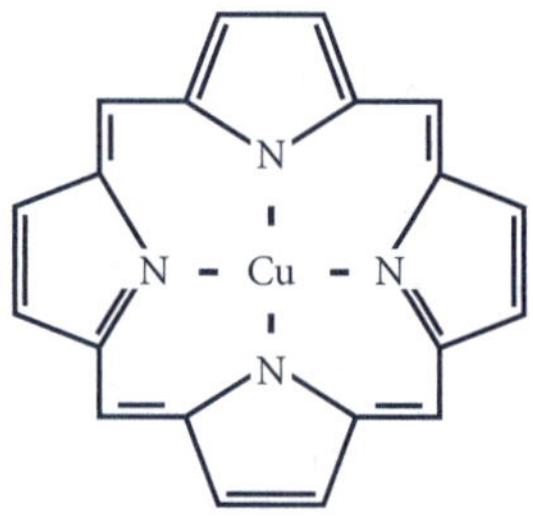

Figure 5-11 Copper porphyrin (unsubstituted).

5. Some of the compounds shown below are good chelating agents and others are not. Decide which ones are good and which ones are not, and explain your answers.
(*a*) CH_3—CH_2—C(=O)—CH_2—C(=O)—CH_3
(*b*) CH_3—C(=O)—CH_2—CH_2—C(=O)—CH_3
(*c*) CH_3—C(=O)—$C(CH_3)_2$—C(=O)—CH_3
(*d*) CH_3—C(=O)—CH=CH—C(=O)—CH_3
(*e*) CH_3—C(=O)—CH_2—C(=O)—OCH_2CH_3
(*f*) *o*-Hydroxybenzaldehyde
(*g*) 2-Formylcyclohexanol
6. Refer to Table 5-4. Determine the stability constants for the formation of $Cu(ampicillin)^+$ and $Cu(ampicillin)_2$ using the log *Q* function. (*Hint*: Plot log *Q* versus $\bar{n}$, determine the free drug concentration at $\bar{n} = 0.5$, 1, and 1.5 and the stability constants.)
7. The lack of oral liquid formulation for aspirin is due to its low solubility and its instability (through hydrolysis of the acetyl ester) in aqueous solution. Based on the chemistry of the inclusion complexes of cyclodextrins, what cyclodextrins may be the best candidates for stability and solubility testing of their applicability in forming a stable liquid aspirin formulation?
8. The binding constants for some sulfonamides to human serum albumin are shown in **Table 5-8**. Calculate the percent of bound drug in plasma, assuming the plasma albumin concentration is 5×10^{-4} *M*.
9. Using the calculated results for sulfadiazine and sulfamethoxypyridazine in Question 8, predict the free concentrations of the drugs in plasma and in tissue fluids if the total drug level in plasma is 2 μg/mL and both drugs have a tissue/blood partition coefficient of 5.
10. The reported warfarin–albumin binding constants in the absence and presence of ibuprofen, naproxen, phenylbutazone, or azapropazone are 6.1×10^5 and 3.1×10^5, 2.4×10^5, 0.33×10^5, or 0.19×10^5 M^{-1}, respectively. The number of binding sites for warfarin is 1. Estimate the free drug fractions of warfarin in plasma resulting from the drug interactions, using a plasma albumin concentration of 1×10^{-4} *M*.
11. Based on the following data (see **Table 5-9**), calculate the binding constant and the number of binding sites for the binding of 1-anilinonaphthalene-8-sulfonate (ANS) to human serum albumin using the Scatchard equation.

Table 5-8 Binding Constants for Some Sulfonamides to Human Serum Albumin

Drug	*n*	Binding Constant, M^{-1}
Sulfadiazine	2	7.8×10^2
Sulfamerazine	1.8	6.3×10^2
Sulfisomidine	1.1	5.0×10^3
Sulfamethoxypyridazine	2.0	9.8×10^3

Table 5-9 Fluorescence Titration of Solutions Containing HSA with ANS

	Fluorescence Measured at 475 nm (e.g., 375 nm)		
D_t, 10^{-6} *M*	Titration A	Titration B	Titration C
2	3.5	11.2	15.5
3	5.2	15.2	23.0
4	6.8	18.5	30.5
5	7.0	21.4	38.2

(Continues)

Table 5-9 (*Continued*)

D_t, 10^{-6} *M*	Fluorescence Measured at 475 nm (e.g., 375 nm)		
	Titration A	Titration B	Titration C
6	7.3	23.3	46.0
7	7.5	24.8	53.2
8	7.7	26.0	60.3
9	7.9	26.6	67.0
10	8.0	27.3	73.5

The concentration of HSA is (*A*) 0, (*B*) 1.45×10^{-6} *M*, and (*C*) 2.91×10^{-5} *M*.

CHAPTER 6

Chemical Kinetics: Principles and Applications

A number of kinetic processes are essential for the development of pharmaceutical products and the understanding of a drug's pharmacological effects. These processes include drug degradation, establishment of drug and product stability, enzyme kinetics, drug absorption, and pharmacokinetic evaluation of the drug in the biological system. Although all of the processes can be written in detail in separate volumes, this chapter is intended to introduce the basic kinetic principles and methods with which each of the kinetic processes can be investigated, quantitatively established, and interpreted.

CHAPTER OUTLINE

OBJECTIVES

1. Understand the definition of drug and product stability.
2. Be able to identify chemical reactions and interactions among components in a drug formulation that may lead to product instability.
3. Describe the rate equation, reaction order, and reaction mechanism.
4. Understand the role of kinetic studies in establishing reaction mechanisms.
5. Use steady-state approximation to determine the rate equations, reaction order, and kinetic equation for enzyme reactions.
6. Understand acid–base catalysis and its effect on drug stability.
7. Learn the basics of kinetic equations in first, second, and zero orders for the determination of the rate constants, half-life, and shelf life.
8. Understand the complex reactions and their application in pharmacokinetic interpretations of drug action.
9. Understand both the effect of temperature on the reaction rate and the concept of activation energy.
10. Be able to apply the Arrhenius theory for temperature-dependent modification of product shelf life and storage conditions as well as accelerated stability studies.

I. Chemical Degradation and Drug Stability

Drug and Product Stability

Both the pharmaceutical manufacturer and the pharmacist have a legal and moral obligation to ensure that their products and prescriptions maintain the therapeutic efficacy for which the drugs are intended. The legal obligation of the manufacturer, as defined by the Food, Drug, and Cosmetic Act, is to provide written evidence of product stability prior to the marketing of a new drug. Although the pharmacist does not bear this burden for each prescription, he or she must nevertheless be aware of the potential instability of the prescribed drugs. The *stability of a drug product* can be defined as the extent to which a preparation retains the same properties that it had at the time of formulation. The USP/NF[1] describes the product stability as to retain unchanged (1) physical properties, (2) chemical properties and composition, (3) microbiological sterility, and (4) therapeutic activities. This definition emphasizes that, in addition to chemical degradation of the active ingredient, changes in sterility and physical appearance have an impact on the drug therapeutic effect. Indeed, a drug product may contain several excipients, and incompatibilities may arise over time from the ingredients and result in changes of the formulation appearance and composition of the product. Hence, stability studies must be carried out based on the whole product.

Drug Degradation

The potential degradation of the active drug is obviously the most important issue to be considered in establishing a stable and safe product. Drug stability is an important issue because many drugs (e.g., fluorouracil, dioxin, carbamazepine, aspirin, and procaine) have narrow therapeutic indices, and their degradation may lead to plasma levels that are higher than the toxic level or lower than the therapeutic threshold. Chemical degradations, although not always substantial, can also produce toxic agents that, when ingested, can cause dangerous side effects. Examples, to name a few, are the conversion of tetracycline to epianhydrotetracycline, *p*-aminosalicylic acid to *m*-aminophenol, and phototoxic decomposition of chlordiazepoxide.[2, 3]

The fact that a drug is degraded via certain reactions does not preclude its use in medicine. An understanding of the degradation processes involved may, in fact, allow one to develop an acceptable product with accurately determined shelf life, expiration date, and storage conditions. Thus, it is important that pharmacists understand the types of reactions involved, the principles behind how drug stability is obtained, and how problems may be avoided to maintain drug stability. The degradation of drugs is mostly attributed to chemical and biological reactions. These reactions may be enhanced or triggered by environmental factors such as temperature, light, moisture, and oxygen, and by solution factors, such as pH, ionic strength, and the presence of metal ions that catalyze the reaction. The common degradation reactions include the following.

Photodegradation

The photons from uv light (190–400 nm), depending on the wavelength, have energy up to 150 kcal/einstein (1 einstein is the energy carried by 1 mol of light quanta of a given wavelength). This energy is more than sufficient to induce free radical formation of alkanes, alkenes, toluene, aldehydes, and ketones. Drugs that are sensitive to uv light, such as quinine sulfate and tannic acid, undergo photodegradation. The reaction is usually indicated by a change in color of the drug or solution, and it can be prevented by using light-resistant or opaque containers.

Oxidation

Air oxidation is a common degradation process for many organic molecules, including aromatic and halogenated hydrocarbons, alcohols, phenols, ethers, aldehydes, amines, and thiols. The reaction of a drug with molecular oxygen is referred to as autooxidation. Recall that oxygen may be regarded as a free radical, which forms superoxide anion and through which it induces free radical chain reactions with drugs such as morphine that contain the phenolic group. Autooxidation is catalyzed by the presence of trace amount of metal ions such as copper and iron.

Antioxidants as additives are frequently used in food and drug preparations to prevent degradation by oxidation. They are reducing agents that either undergo preferential oxidation or serve as free radical chain reaction inhibitors. A chain reaction inhibitor is a compound that can provide an electron and hydrogen (H·) in stopping the chain reaction. For example, phenols and hydroquinones are chain reaction inhibitors and are classified as strong antioxidants. The commonly used antioxidants for pharmaceutical preparations include ascorbic acid, sulfites, and bisulfate for aqueous solutions and ascorbyl palmitate, hydroquinones, and propylgallate for nonaqueous preparations. The selection of antioxidant should be based on the common factors required for all additives, i.e., stability (other than oxidation), effective pH range, effective concentration, solubility when oxidized, toxicity, and compatibility with other ingredients.

Hydrolysis and Acid–Base Catalysis

Organic acid derivatives, including esters, amides, lactams, etc., are all subject to degradation by hydrolysis to form carboxylic acid (see **Figure 6-1**). Organic esters are most susceptible to

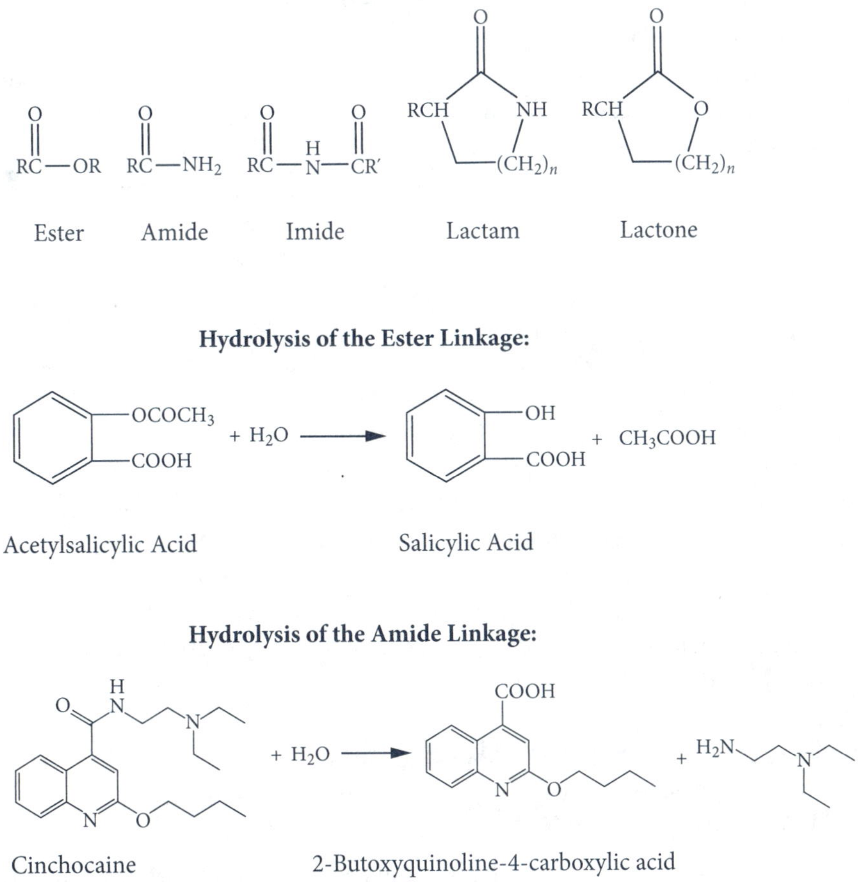

Figure 6-1 Hydrolytic degradation of acid derivatives.

hydrolysis, and many drugs, such as acetylsalicylic acid (aspirin), physostigmine, tetracaine, and procaine, exhibit an ester linkage. Amides and imides, as in cinchocaine, chloramphenicol, benzyl penicillin, and ergonovine, as well as carbonates, carbamates, and ureas also degrade through hydrolysis. The reactivity of these compounds stems from the carbonyl group (C=O), which exhibits mobile π electrons that are pulled strongly toward the electronegative oxygen atom. As a result, the carbonyl carbon is electron-deficient and thereby highly vulnerable to nucleophilic attachment by water. If acid is present, H^+ becomes attached to the carbonyl oxygen, which makes the carbonyl carbon even more electron-deficient, and catalyzes the hydrolysis reaction. Hydrolysis also occurs in alkaline solutions, and perhaps more readily than in acid solutions, due to the presence of the hydroxide ion, which, as a strong nucleophilic agent, directly attaches to the carbonyl carbon. The proton and hydroxide ion–catalyzed reactions are known as specific acid and base catalyses, where the rate of hydrolysis changes in a pH-dependent manner. Metal ions, like the proton, carry positive charges and thus are able to catalyze hydrolysis through chelation involving the carbonyl group. This process has been well demonstrated in the metal ion–promoted hydrolytic degradation of peptides.[4]

Other Degradation Processes

Aromatic compounds (phenols, polyphenols) can be easily oxidized or decomposed by microorganisms. In pharmaceutical preparations, microorganisms are undesirable regardless of whether they lead to the loss of drug potency and should be controlled using preservatives and/or aseptic techniques and sterilization. Some drug degradation processes also include decarboxylation and deamination reactions, which are catalyzed by trace metals. Still, drug molecules having a chiral carbon form optical isomers, which may exhibit different binding characteristics to proteins and receptor sites and pharmacological activity. Racemization, which leads to the formation of a racemic mixture of the enantiomers, can thus alter the drug's pharmacological effect. The commonly occurring drug stability issues also include dehydration, which changes the physical property and the chemical composition of the drug, and polymerization, such as by aldehydes that form dimers and trimers. Perhaps the most common effect of the environmental factors on drug stability is the change in solution pH. This may occur upon diluting a solution, adding another component, or even changing the packaging container during compounding, as pH may be altered by temperature, air, carbon dioxide, and possibly cationic species leaking from plastic containers.

II. Isothermal Reaction Kinetics

Our discussion of molecular properties and interactions so far has centered on chemical systems at equilibrium and the chemical nature of the compounds involved. The actual process of a chemical reaction, however, involves knowledge that describes the detailed transformation from one set of chemicals (reactants) to another (products), i.e., the *reaction mechanism*. Time, as a variable, which has been avoided in the equilibrium discussion, plays a major role in this process, and the time-dependent events that lead to the formation of the products now take the center stage. It is easy to ascertain, then, why chemical kinetics principles are also applied to other fields, such as in pharmacokinetics, where the fate of a drug in the body is traced in a time frame defined by the kinetic process.

Rate Equation and Reaction Mechanism

Introduction of Rate Equation

The experimental approach to the study of the reaction process is through the measurement of the rate at which a reaction proceeds and the dependence of this rate on (1) the concentrations of the reacting species and (2) the temperature. The results of such a study are termed the reaction kinetics, which can be summarized by a rate equation where

$$\text{Rate} = k(\text{temperature}) \times f(\text{concentrations of reactants})$$

If the function f(concentrations of reactants) correctively expresses the rate dependence on concentration, then k (temperature), which is a function only of the temperature, is called the rate constant.

It may seem presumptuous that the information on the rate of reactions would allow one to deduce how two molecules come together, how the atoms change their position, and how the electrons shift, so that one or two new molecules emerge. But the ideas arising from reaction mechanism studies have contributed to our understanding of the immense number of individual reactions that occur in organic and inorganic chemistry. In fact, it is the understanding of the reaction mechanisms, rather than that of the thermodynamics, that leads to most of the qualitative ideas as to what reactions might occur in a system of such complexity.

The information provided by one rate equation for a reaction, of course, is often not sufficient to lead to the postulation of a single mechanism while ruling out other possible mechanisms. Frequently additional experimental results are needed. For example, if a particular hydrogen atom in a compound is suspected of being involved in a reaction, it can be replaced by a deuterium atom. The analysis of the isotope content in the product molecules will aid in clarification of the proposed reaction mechanism. Likewise, the specific acid- or base-catalyzed reaction, where H^+ or OH^- is involved in the rate-limiting step, can be better understood by studying the reaction kinetics at different pH values. In addition to their usefulness in deducing reaction mechanisms, the reaction kinetics are of important practical value in establishing quantitative relationships between time and concentrations. Both the rate of the reaction and the reaction mechanism are needed to learn the details of the reaction process, and this information forms the basis of our understanding of drug stability.

Reaction Rate and Order

The rate of a reaction is usually expressed in terms of the decrease in the amount of the major reactant or the increase in the amount of the principal product in a time interval in seconds, minutes, hours, and so forth. If the volume of the reaction mixture in solution remains constant, the change in the amount of reactant or product is expressed in molar concentration. For constant volume of gaseous systems, it is generally more convenient to use the partial pressure of the reactant, which is proportional to its concentration according to the ideal gas law. The rate of a reaction is always considered to be a positive quantity. Hence, for the reaction

$$\mathrm{A} + \mathrm{B} \rightarrow \mathrm{C} + \mathrm{D}$$

the rate is written as:

$$\text{Rate} = \frac{-d[\mathrm{A}]}{dt} \quad \text{or} \quad \text{Rate} = \frac{+d[\mathrm{C}]}{dt}$$

For a general reaction that proceeds as follows

$$a\mathrm{A} + b\mathrm{B} \rightarrow c\mathrm{C} + d\mathrm{D} \tag{6-1}$$

the rate expressed with respect to A, B, C, and D (see Example 6-1) should follow this relationship:

$$-\frac{1}{a}\frac{d\mathrm{A}}{dt} = -\frac{1}{b}\frac{d\mathrm{B}}{dt} = \frac{1}{c}\frac{d\mathrm{C}}{dt} = \frac{1}{d}\frac{d\mathrm{D}}{dt} \tag{6-2}$$

Example 6-1: Consider the reaction A + 2B → products, and show the relationship between the rates expressed in A and B.

Solution: The rate may be expressed as $-d[A]/dt$ or $-d[B]/dt$, depending on whether A or B is monitored experimentally. But

$$-d[B]/dt = -2\,d[A]/dt$$

Thus, to avoid ambiguity, the rate should be expressed as in Equation (6-2); i.e., if B is monitored in this reaction, the rate should be $-d[B]/2\,dt$. If A is monitored, the rate is $-d[A]/dt$.

Most reactions have been shown to have rates that, at a given temperature, are proportional to the concentration of one, two, or possibly three of the reactants, with the concentration raised to a small integral power. If a reaction mixture contains three reactants (A, B, C), some possible rate expressions involving A would be as follows:

First Order	Second Order	Third Order
Rate = $k[A]$	$k[A]^2$	
	$k[A][B]$	$k[A]^2[B]$
		$k[A][B][C]$

Reactions that occur according to these simple rate equations are said to be reactions of the first, second, and third order. It should be immediately pointed out that although these simple rate equations do exist, many reactions have more elaborate expressions in rate equations, as dictated by their reaction mechanism. The *reaction order* is thus an experimentally verified parameter, and the correctly expressed rate equation, showing true dependency of the concentrations of the reactants, is necessary to determine the rate constant. Under this rate law, it can be seen that the reaction rate does not necessarily conform to the form of the equation for the overall reaction. The frequently used expression of the equilibrium constant, which equates the rate of the forward reaction to the rate of the reverse reaction, each written in terms of the overall equation, should not be taken as implying anything about the actual rate equation for either the forward or the reverse reaction process.

Reaction Mechanisms

First we note that *reaction mechanisms* are theoretical but the rate equation is an experimental result. We shall combine the two in a later section to show the power of the kinetic approach in understanding chemical reactions. For some reactions, the process can be accounted for by a mechanism that consists of a single step when all reactant molecules come together, rearranging atoms and electrons in the moment of impact, and fly apart as product molecules. Such a mechanism is said to involve a concerted process. In most reactions, however, such a concerted process would indicate an improbable combination of changes to get from reactants to products. It is then more satisfactory to explain the reaction as having a sequence of steps, with each step consisting of simple atomic and/or electronic moves. It has been shown that such a sequence of steps is often needed to explain the observed rate data. The idea of a stepwise reaction has led to the consideration that some *reactive intermediates* are formed, whose reactivity leads to the formation of the products. Based on the types of intermediates postulated, or demonstrated, chemical processes can be classified as free radical reactions or as ionic, or polar, reactions. Gaseous reactions appear to involve generally free radical intermediates; so do those photochemical reactions. The bulk of reactions in solution, in contrast, are characterized by ionic intermediates. Some of the charged intermediates may be familiar ions that are encountered in aqueous solutions, but most of the postulated ionic intermediates in organic reactions are never observed directly.

In organic systems, both positively and negatively charged carbon, namely, the carbonium and carbanion ions, have been recognized as reactive intermediates. These ions, being unstable intermediates, must react further to give the final products. A carbonium ion may form an alkene, react with a negative ion, alkylate an aromatic ring, form a larger carbonium ion with an alkene, and rearrange to a more stable carbonium ion. The formation of carbanion ion occurs in, among other reactions, nucleophilic aromatic substitutions. We shall see how kinetic studies contribute to the understanding of the reaction mechanism involving these species.

Relation between Rate Equation and Reaction Mechanism

To characterize a reaction process based on rate determination and theoretical consideration of the reaction mechanism, it is necessary to clarify the basis from which a rate equation can be formulated. The kinetic theory on molecular collisions shows that in a gas mixture of components A and B, the number of collisions per unit of volume per unit of time between molecules A and B is proportional to the product of their partial pressures $P_A P_B$, or, according to the ideal gas law, [A][B]. Extending this theory to solution, it seems reasonable that the rate of collision of two reacting molecules can be equated to the product of their concentrations, at least in a dilute solution. Hence, the rate equation used in the deduction of reaction mechanisms is defined as follows: The rate of a single reaction step is proportional to the product of the concentrations of the reactants in that step. The emphasis here is that the rate equation defined above applies only to a single reaction step; if a reaction involves a series of steps and if some or all of these steps control the rate, then the rate of the overall reaction will not necessarily be indicated simply by any concentration terms.

The rate equation defined above allows one to analyze the reaction mechanism expressed in a series of reaction steps. For example, if the initial step of a reaction forms the intermediate, as shown in Equation (6-3), and if this step is slow relative to all succeeding steps, then the first step is said to be rate-determining.

$$\begin{aligned} &\mathrm{A} + \mathrm{B} \rightarrow AB \\ &AB \rightarrow \text{products} \end{aligned} \tag{6-3}$$

In such cases, the intermediate *AB* formed will quickly undergo a series of transformations to give the final products, the rate of the overall reaction will depend only on the initial rate-determining step, and the mechanism will be consistent with a rate equation involving [A][B]. If, however, a single slow step followed by fast steps cannot be expected, then the relation of the mechanism to the rate equation will be more complicated. Usually, the treatment of the rate equations for stepwise reactions can lead to a simplification of the reaction kinetics by using the method of steady-state approximation, which involves the formation of an unstable intermediate. In this method, one recognizes that the concentration of the intermediate is either constant with respect to time or always very small or not detectable. Either way, $d[\text{intermediate}]/dt = 0$.

An example of using reaction kinetics to deduce the reaction mechanism can be seen from the extensively studied reaction of alkaline hydrolysis of chloroform. The overall reaction is shown in Equation (6-4):

$$2CHCl_3 + 7OH^- \rightarrow CO + HCOO^- + 6Cl^- + 4H_2O \tag{6-4}$$

The rate of the reaction was determined to follow the rate equation

$$-d\,[CHCl_3]/dt = k_{obs}[CHCl_3][OH^-]$$

where k_{obs} is the observed rate constant. To aid in the deduction of the reaction mechanism, it was also found that the rate of deuterium exchange of $CHCl_3$ in alkaline D_2O is much faster than that of the hydrolysis reaction. These results have led to a proposed mechanism that involves a first-step formation of the intermediate $:CCl_3$, subsequent formation of $:CCl_2$ by the intermediate, and the reaction of $:CCl_2$ with OH^- in a series of steps to yield the final products. The deuterium exchange data suggested that a reverse reaction of the intermediate with water to form $CHCl_3$ retards the rate of formation of the intermediate and makes the first step a slow reaction. Hence, the first two steps of this reaction mechanism are

$$CHCl_3 + OH^- \underset{k_{-1}}{\overset{k_1}{\rightleftarrows}} :CCl_3^- + H_2O$$

$$:CCl_3^- \xrightarrow{k_2} :CCl_2 + Cl^-$$

Based on this mechanism, which considers the first step to be rate-determining, it can be seen that

$$-\frac{d\,[CHCl_3]}{dt} = k_1[CHCl_3][OH^-] - k_{-1}[:CCl_3^-] \qquad (6\text{-}5)$$

The concentration of water is a constant and does not enter into the rate equation for the reverse reaction in step 1. To determine the final rate equation, one applies the method of steady state, i.e.,

$$\frac{d\,[:CCl_3^-]}{dt} = k_1[CHCl_3][OH^-] - k_{-1}[:CCl_3^-] - k_2[:CCl_3^-] = 0 \qquad (6\text{-}6)$$

Combining Equations (6-5) and (6-6) gives

$$-\frac{d\,[CHCl_3]}{dt} = \frac{k_1k_2[CHCl_3][OH^-]}{k_{-1} + k_2} \qquad (6\text{-}7)$$

Equation (6-7) is the rate equation according to the proposed mechanism, which agrees with the observed rate equation when k_{obs} is identified as $k_1k_2/(k_{-1} + k_2)$. Because the rate of deuterium exchange is much faster than hydrolysis, suggesting that k_{-1} is much greater than k_2, it follows that $k_{obs} \approx k_1k_2/k_{-1}$. Alternatively, one may also view the reaction mechanism as involving an equilibrium process for the first step, followed by a rate-determining second step. In this approach, the rate equation can be derived as

$$-\frac{d\,[CHCl_3]}{dt} = \frac{d[:CCl_2^-]}{dt} = \frac{k_1k_2[CHCl_3][OH^-]}{k_{-1}} \qquad (6\text{-}8)$$

which is the same as in Equation (6-7) when $k_{-1} >> k_2$.

The above example shows how a rate equation is deduced from a stepwise reaction (see also Example 6-2 for additional exercise). It should now be clear that the rate equation for a stepwise reaction may be—but need not be—a simple function of the reactant concentration or related to the equation for the overall reaction. It would indeed be wrong to assume that the alkaline hydrolysis of chloroform may proceed by a reaction order of $[CHCl_3]^2[OH^-]^7$, as one would if the stoichiometry of the overall reaction were followed.

Example 6-2: Consider the schematic hypothetical reaction mechanism

$$A \underset{k_{-1}}{\overset{k_1}{\rightleftarrows}} B \qquad B + A \xrightarrow{k_2} C$$

(*a*) Write the net rate of change for each species.
(*b*) If B is present in only undetectable amounts, obtain [B].

(*c*) Obtain rate equations for A and C.

(*d*) What relative values of the rate constants would result in the reaction being first order with respect to A? What values would make it second order?

Solution: (*a*) $-dA/dt = k_1[A] - k_{-1}[B] + k_2[B][A]$

$$dB/dt = k_1[A] - k_{-1}[B] - k_2[B][A]$$

$$dC/dt = k_2[B][A]$$

(*b*) Now B is the intermediate; thus,

$$dB/dt = k_1[A] - k_{-1}[B] - k_2[B][A] = 0$$

$$[B] = k_1[A]/(k_{-1} + k_2[A])$$

(*c*)

$$-dA/dt = k_1[A]\left(1 - \frac{k_{-1}}{k_{-1} + k_2[A]} + \frac{k_2[A]}{k_{-1} + k_2[A]}\right)$$

$$= 2k_1k_2[A]^2/\,(k_{-1} + k_2[A])$$

$$-dA/2\,dt = k_1k_2[A]^2/(k_{-1} + k_2[A])$$

$$dC/dt = k_2[B][A] = k_1k_2[A]^2/(k_{-1} + k_2[A])$$

(*d*) If $k_2[A] >> k_{-1}$, $dC/dt = k_1[A]$ (first step is rate-determining). first order with respect to A

If $k_1 >> k_2[A]$, $dC/dt = k_1k_2[A]^2/k_{-1}$ (second step is rate-determining) second order with respect to A

Determination of Rate Constant

First-Order Kinetics

The first-order kinetics describe a reaction in which the *rate of reaction* is proportional to the first power of the concentration of a single reacting species A. The rate equation can be written as

$$-dA/dt = k[A]$$

If the initial concentration of A, at $t = 0$, is C_A, and the concentration is reduced to [A] at a later time t, then the rate equation can be integrated as follows:

$$-\int_{C_A}^{[A]} \frac{dA}{[A]} = k\int_{o}^{t} dt$$

The resulting concentration–time relationship is $[A] = C_A e^{-kt}$, or

$$\log([A]/C_A) = -kt/2.303 \qquad \text{or} \qquad \log[A] = \log C_A - kt/2.303 \tag{6-9}$$

A reaction can be said to be first-order if a plot of $\log([A]/C_A)$ or $\log[A]$ versus t gives a straight line. If a straight line is obtained, the slope of the line relates to the rate constant k by this equation: slope $= -k/2.303$. If the initial concentration is not known, it can be determined from the y axis intercept, which yields the value of $\log C_A$ at $t = 0$.

In the treatment of kinetic data, it is customary to use not only the rate constant but also the half-life and shelf life (used to indicate product stability) of the reaction. These values are calculated using the rate constant. The half-life ($t_{1/2}$) is the time required for 50% elimination of the reactant, whereas the shelf life (t_{90}) of a pharmaceutical product is defined, in general, as the time elapsed for a 10% degradation of the initial concentration. With these definitions, from Equation (6-9)

$$t_{1/2} = 0.693/k \qquad t_{90} = 0.1054/k \tag{6-10}$$

The use of Equations (6-9) and (6-10) is shown in Example 6-3.

Example 6-3: From the following decomposition data of a drug solution, determine (*a*) the reaction order, (*b*) the rate constant, the half-life, and the shelf life, and (*c*) the initial concentration of this drug.

[A] (mg/5 mL)	Time (mo)	log [A]
200	0.25	2.301
145	0.38	2.164
100	0.50	2.000
78	0.60	1.892
50	0.76	1.699
36	0.90	1.544

Solution:

(*a*) The data are graphically represented in **Figure 6-2**. The plot of [A] versus time shows a curve, but the plot of log [A] versus time gives a straight line. This indicates a first-order kinetic process.

(*b*) From the plot of log [A] versus *t*:

$$\text{Slope} = (\log[\text{A}]_1 - \log[\text{A}]_2)/(t_1 - t_2) = -k/2.303$$

$$(2.301 - 2.000)/(0.25 - 0.50) = -k/2.303 \qquad k = 2.773\ \text{mo}^{-1}$$

$$t_{1/2} = 0.693/k = 0.25\ \text{mo} \quad \text{or} \quad 0.25 \times 30 = 7.5\ \text{days}$$

$$t_{90} = 0.1054/k = 0.038\ \text{mo} \quad \text{or} \quad 0.038 \times 30 = 1.14\ \text{days}$$

(*c*) Determine $\log C_A$ from the graph as log [A] at $t = 0$:

$$\log[\text{A}] \text{ at time } 0 = 2.602 \qquad C_A = 400\ \text{mg/5 mL}$$

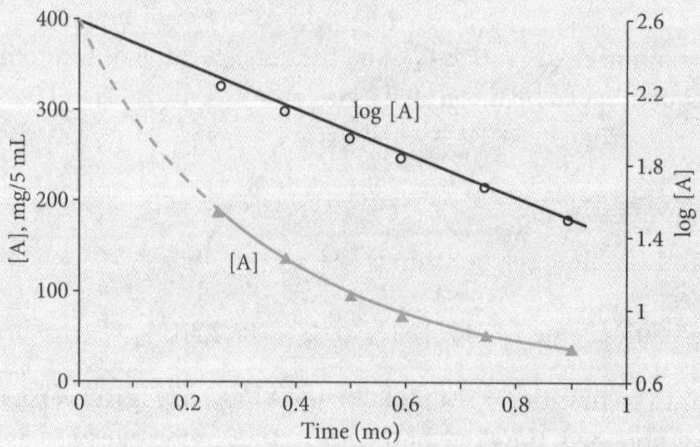

Figure 6-2 Plots of [A] or log [A] versus time for a first-order kinetic process.

It is characteristic of first-order kinetics that one can alter the rate of reaction by changing the initial concentration, but the change in the percent of the initial drug concentration as a function of time will be the same. This property of first-order kinetics leads to a characteristic rate constant, and the half-life as well, that is independent of the drug concentration. An important application of first-order kinetics is to describe the distribution of the drug in the biological systems. Imagine that if the rate constant and half-life were to change with changing doses, as in zero- or second-order reactions, it would not have been an efficient model for the pharmacokinetic evaluation of drugs.

Even though chemical reactions usually involve two reacting molecules, the first-order kinetic process, which requires relatively easy mathematical treatment, occurs readily in drug stability studies. Reaction of the drug with water, e.g., in an aqueous solution, is considered first-order, or pseudo first-order, due to the high concentration of water compared to that of the drug. The catalytic action of H^+ and OH^- can also be treated as first-order if the reaction is monitored at constant pH.

Second-Order Kinetics

The rate equation for a second-order reaction between molecules A and B may be written as

$$\mathrm{A} + \mathrm{B} \rightarrow \text{products} \qquad -d\mathrm{A}/dt = k[\mathrm{A}][\mathrm{B}]$$

It may be more convenient to develop the rate equation by introducing a term of x for the amount of reaction that has occurred at time t. The kinetic data can then be treated in terms of the following quantities:

C_A = initial concentration of A

C_B = initial concentration of B

x = decrease in A and B, or concentration of product formed, at time t

$C_A - x$ = concentration of A at time t

$C_B - x$ = concentration of B at time t

The rate equation can then be taken as

$$dx/dt = k[\mathrm{A}][\mathrm{B}] = k\,(C_A - x)(C_B - x)$$

$$\frac{dx}{(C_A - x)(C_B - x)} = k\,dt$$

or

$$\frac{1}{(C_A - C_B)} \int_o^x \left(\frac{dx}{(C_B - x)} - \frac{dx}{(C_A - x)} \right) = k \int_o^t dt$$

which, on integration, gives

$$\frac{1}{C_A - C_B} \left| \ln (C_A - x) - \ln (C_B - x) \right|_0^x = kt$$

Rearranging the above equation following insertion of the limits, one obtains

$$\frac{1}{C_A - C_B} \log \frac{C_B\,(C_A - x)}{C_A\,(C_B - x)} = \frac{kt}{2.303} \tag{6-11}$$

An example of a second-order reaction may be seen from the data shown in **Table 6-1**. In this study, the reaction of hydralazine with acetaldehyde in the formation of 3-methyl-*S*-triazolo[3,4-a] phthalazine in pH 7.4 phosphate buffer was monitored using a fluoresence technique.[5] This

Table 6-1 Kinetic Data for the Second-Order Reaction of Hydralazine ($15.27 \times 10^{-6}\,M$) with Acetaldehyde ($52.27 \times 10^{-6}\,M$) in pH 7.4 Buffer at 25°C

$$\frac{1}{C_A - C_B}\log\frac{C_B(C_A - x)}{C_A(C_B - x)} = \frac{kt}{2.303}$$

where C_A = initial concentration of acetaldehyde; C_B = initial concentration of hydralazine, x = concentration of product (3-methyl-*s*-triazolo[3,4-*a*]phthalazine)

Time, min	x, $10^{-6}\,M$	$[1/(C_A - C_B)]\log[C_B(C_A - x)/C_A(C_B - x)]$, M^{-1}
10	0.15	82.1
28	0.38	210.2
45	0.61	340.7
65	0.88	532.0
80	1.07	644.6
95	1.30	783.4
105	1.43	863.2
130	1.73	1050.9
140	1.90	1160.0
150	2.00	1224.5
170	2.25	1389.2

reaction may occur at physiological conditions and play a role in the drug's metabolism. The calculation of the second-order rate constant using Equation (6-11) is illustrated in Table 6-1, whereas the appropriate plot is shown in **Figure 6-3,** to demonstrate the linearity of the data. Either test shows that the reaction is second-order with respect to [hydralazine][acetaldehyde].

If the initial concentrations of A and B can be made equal, with a value of C_A, and the two reactants are used up at the same rate, then the kinetics may be expressed as

$$\frac{x}{C_A(C_A - x)} = kt \qquad (6\text{-}12)$$

Here the half-life can be calculated as $t_{1/2} = 1/C_A k$. As can be seen, for a second-order reaction, both the rate constant and the half-life vary with varying initial concentrations of the reactants.

Third-Order Kinetics

Very few examples of third-order reactions are known. In the gaseous phase, the reactions of nitric oxide are the only thoroughly studied reactions that involve the chemical reaction of three species. For example, the gas phase reaction of

$$2NO + Cl_2 \rightarrow 2NOCl$$

proceeds according to the rate equation

$$-d[NO]/dt = k[NO]^2[Cl_2]$$

In solution, few examples of a third-order reaction exist. It is likely that some potential

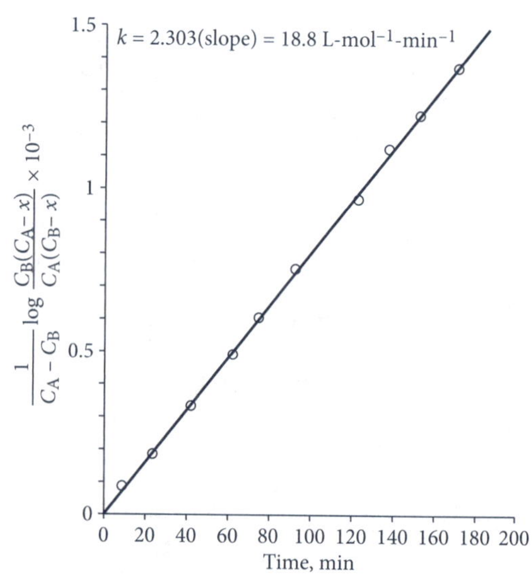

Figure 6-3 Plot of Equation (6-11) for the second-order reaction of hydralazine with acetaldehyde in pH 7.4 buffer at 25°C. The slope of the line gives k as 18.8 L/mol-min.

third-order reactions are not observed because one or two of the reactants may be solvent molecules. The displacement reaction of methyl bromide with pyridine in the formation of *N*-methylpyridinium bromide offers a good example of a third-order reaction.[6] When studied in benzene, this reaction exhibited second-order kinetics. The addition of an alcohol, however, increased the rate of reaction, even though the added alcohol does not enter into the equation of the overall reaction. The rate of the accelerated reaction was found to be not only first-order in the bromide, and first-order in pyridine, but also first-order in the alcohol. The mechanism of reaction was proposed to involve the rate-determining formation of a three-molecule intermediate in which the hydroxyl compound is hydrogen bound to the bromine, which aids in pulling the bromide from the *N*-methylpyridinium moiety.

Zero-Order Kinetics

If the rate of a reaction can be made independent of any of the reactant concentrations, the reaction will follow zero-order kinetics where the elimination of a reactant will be linear with time. The rate equation for the zero-order kinetics is

$$-dA/dt = k_0$$

where A is the reactant of interest and k_0 is the zero-order rate constant. On integration, it gives

$$[A] = C_A - k_0 t \tag{6-13}$$

where C_A is the concentration of A at time 0. The half-life and shelf life can be determined by using the rate constant, in that

$$t_{1/2} = 0.5C_A/k_0 \qquad t_{90} = 0.1C_A/k_0 \tag{6-14}$$

The zero-order kinetic feature serves as a perfect reminder that the reaction order is dependent upon the reaction conditions. Consider a drug undergoing hydrolytic degradation; the reaction will likely be second-order when carried out in a nonaqueous medium but first-order if the solvent is water and zero-order if the aqueous concentration of the drug can be maintained at saturation. From the drug formulation point of view, the zero-order kinetics offer some formulation advantage in that dry powders for suspensions may be used to maintain drug concentration at saturation, and the shelf life of the formulation may be adjusted based on C_A. This is illustrated in calculations shown in Example 6-4.

Example 6-4: (*a*) If the rate of degradation of a drug in a suspension formulation (C_A = 10 mg/mL) is 1.2 mg/mL-mo, calculate t_{90}. (*b*) If the drug solubility *S* is 0.1 mg/mL, what are the first-order rate constant and t_{90} for the drug in solution?

Solution: (*a*) The rate of degradation in zero-order kinetics is equal to k_0; hence,

$$t_{90} = 0.1\,C_A/k_0 = 0.1 \times 10/1.2 = 0.833 \text{ mo or 25 days}$$

(*b*) The zero-order rate constant is related to the first-order rate constant k_1 by the equation $k_0 = k_1(S)$. Thus,

$$k_1 = k_0/S = 1.2\,/\,0.1 = 12\,\text{mo}^{-1}$$

$$t_{90} = 0.1054/k_1 = 0.1054/12 = 0.00878 \text{ mo or } 6.3\,\text{h}$$

Table 6-2 Reaction Kinetics of Concerted Processes

	Rate	Concentration vs. Time	Unit of k	Half-life	Shelf Life
Zero-order	k	$[A] = C_A - kt$	Conc./unit time	$0.5C_A/k$	$0.1C_A/\mathrm{k}$
First-order	$k[A]$	$\log [A]/C_A = -kt \neq 2.303$	1/unit time	$0.693/k$	$0.1054/k$
Second-order	$k[A]^2$ or $k[A][B]$†	$(C_A - [A])/C_A[A] = kt$	1/conc.-unit time	$1/C_Ak$	$1/9C_Ak$
Second-order	$k[A][B]$	$\frac{1}{C_A - C_B}\log\frac{C_B[A]}{C_A[B]} = \frac{kt}{2.303}$			

†$k[A][B]$ becomes $k[A]^2$ if the initial concentrations of A and B are equal, that is, $C_A = C_B$, and at any time t, $[A] = [B]$.

The reaction kinetics based on reaction orders are summarized in **Table 6-2**. In learning kinetics, frequently one is asked to decide what reaction order should be followed to determine the kinetic parameters of a given set of data. The first answer is to look at the unit of the rate constant. The first-order rate constant has a unit of 1/unit time, but no concentration term. In contrast, both zero-order and second-order rate constants have concentration expression in their units. One can see from the half-life equations that an increase in the initial concentration will increase the half-life of a zero-order reaction, decrease the half-life of a second-order reaction, but will not change the half-life of a first-order reaction. The plot of the data according to the integrated equations (concentration versus time) will ultimately determine the reaction order. In some kinetic studies, rather than measure concentrations, some physicochemical property, such as spectroscopic measurements or drug potency, is monitored as a percentage of the initial condition. In this case, it is likely that the measurement indicates first-order kinetics.

III. Catalysis

A catalyst is a material that increases the rate of chemical reaction without itself being used up, and usually, a small amount of catalyst can result in remarkable acceleration of reactions. A catalyst may be anything from a solid metal used in heterogeneous systems to solutes in solutions or enzymes of complicated structures and reaction mechanisms. It will be shown in this section that the analysis of the catalytic phenomena using rate equations has provided the basis for the establishment of drug product stability and alternative approaches for kinetic studies.

Acid–Base Catalyses

One of the most frequently encountered type of catalysis in solution is the acceleration of reaction rate by the presence of an acid or base. It is well established that the acid–base catalysis consists of general acid–base catalysis, where the catalytic action derives from the whole and part of the acid or base molecule, and specific acid–base catalysis, where the catalytic action is attributed specifically to H^+ or OH^-. It may be upsetting to some that in specific base catalysis, the OH^- is actually used up in the reaction; but as a strong nucleophilic agent, the effect of OH^- on reaction rates is well worth noting.

General Acid–Base Catalysis

The catalytic action of an acid or base can be easily understood in terms of the reaction intermediate. For *general acid catalysis* involving a weak acid HX, to alter the reaction rate, the catalyst must enter into the rate-determining step. Consider the following reaction in an aqueous solution:

$$A \xrightarrow{k} C$$

The rate of the noncatalyzed reaction is $d[C]/dt = k[A]$. The weak acid may catalyze the reaction through either the H^+ or the conjugated base X^-. If the acid catalysis is due to the formation of the intermediate HA^+, the following reaction steps can be written to account for all the acid-catalyzed reactions:

$$A + HX \xrightarrow{k_1} HA^+ + X^- \qquad \text{rate-determining}$$

$$A + H_3O^+ \xrightarrow{k_1'} HA^+ + H_2O \qquad \text{rate-determining}$$

$$HA^+ \xrightarrow{k_2} C + H^+$$

In this case, the reaction is catalyzed by HX and by H_3O^+, and the overall rate equation is

$$d[C]/dt = k[A] + k_1[A][HX] + k_1'[A][H_3O^+] \qquad (6\text{-}15a)$$

The first, second, and third terms indicate noncatalyzed, HX-catalyzed, and H^+-catalyzed reactions, respectively. Equation (6-15*a*) illustrates that proton transfer by the acid is rate-limiting (or rate-determining).

In cases where the catalytic action comes from the X^-, the rate-determining step involves the abstraction of proton from HA^+ by the bases X^- and H_2O, as shown in the following equations:

$$A + HX \underset{k_{-1}}{\overset{k_1}{\rightleftharpoons}} HA^+ + X^-$$

$$HA^+ + X^- \xrightarrow{k_2} C + HX \qquad \text{rate-determining}$$

$$HA^+ + H_2O \xrightarrow{k_2'} C + H_3O^+ \qquad \text{rate-determining}$$

The overall rate equation can thus be obtained:

$$d[C]/dt = k[A] + k_2[HA^+][X^-] + k_2'[HA^+] \qquad (6\text{-}15b)$$

where the first term represents the uncatalyzed process, the second term is for the X^--catalyzed reaction, and the third term involves water acting as a base. Because the water concentration is always in excess, it is considered a constant and is incorporated into the rate constant in Equation (6-15*b*).

Is Equation (6-15*b*) different from Equation (6-15*a*)? The answer is no. By letting

$$K = k_1/k_{-1} = [HA^+][X^-]/[A][HX] \qquad \text{(from the first reaction step)}$$

and

$$K_a = [H_3O^+][X^-]/[HX] \qquad \text{(the acidity constant of HX)}$$

Equation (6-15*b*) can be rewritten as

$$d[C]/dt = k[A] + Kk_2[A][HX] + Kk_2'[A][H_3O^+]/K_a$$

Notice that the above equation is not differentiable from that of Equation (6-15*a*). This shows that the measured kinetics will not differentiate the mechanism of acid catalysis mediated by either H^+ or X^-, and that the catalysis by the conjugated base X^- in an acidic solution is often obscured by its low concentration and the acid (proton)-catalyzed reaction.

Analogous to the acid catalysis, the *general base catalysis* requires proton abstraction by the bases as the rate-determining steps. Consider the catalytic action of the base NaX. Both the general base X^- and OH^- will be involved in this process. Hence, the rate-limiting steps and the overall rate equation can be written as

$$A + X^- \xrightarrow{k_X} A^- + HX \qquad \text{rate-determining}$$

$$A + OH^- \xrightarrow{k_{OH}} A^- + H_2O \qquad \text{rate-determining}$$

$$d[C]/dt = k[A] + k_X[A][X^-] + k_{OH}[A][OH^-] \tag{6-16}$$

The mechanism of the general acid–base catalysis described above may be seen from the reaction of acetone with chlorine, which showed that the rate of chlorination at moderate pH values was enhanced by both acids and bases through the formation of the enol intermediate as the rate-determining step, but was independent of the concentration of chlorine. This shows that the first step is rate-determining.

$$CH_3COCH_3 \xrightarrow[\text{rate-determining}]{HX} CH_3C(OH){=}CH_2 \xrightarrow{Cl_2} CH_3COCH_2Cl$$

Pharmaceutical solutions usually contain various buffer systems, such as the phosphate, bicarbonate, citrate, borate, and acetate. The phosphate, as a general base, has been shown to catalyze the hydrolysis of streptozotocin,[7] whereas the acetate system has been shown to catalyze the degradation of thiamine,[8] both in alkaline pH. Studies have also shown that the monocyclic β-lactam antibiotics aztreonam and nocardicin A undergo general acid and base catalyses but are weak in their reaction with the hydronium ion.[9] In comparison to other β-lactam antibiotics, which are subjected to specific acid–base catalysis,[10] these compounds are much more stable in acidic and neutral aqueous solution.

Specific Acid–Base Hydrolysis

In general acid–base catalysis, the rate-determining step is the proton transfer to the reactant or proton abstraction by the base. But if the rate-determining step occurs after the proton transfer or before proton abstraction, it is known as the *specific acid* or *base catalysis*. The mechanism of the specific acid catalysis in the presence of a weak acid HX may be written as

$$A + HX \underset{k_{-1}}{\overset{k_1}{\rightleftharpoons}} HA^+ + X^-$$

$$HA^+ \xrightarrow{k_2} HC^+ \qquad \text{rate-determining}$$

where A is the reactant and C is the product. Applying steady-state approximation, it can be shown that the rate of the catalyzed reaction is

$$\frac{d[C]}{dt} = \frac{k_1k_2[A][HX]}{k_{-1}[X^-]} = \frac{k_1k_2[A][H_3O^+]}{k_{-1}K_a}$$

where K_a is the acidity constant of HX. The use of H_3O^+ directly rather than HX for the proton source yields the same equation. But the purpose here is to show that at constant pH, the rate of the reaction will remain the same even if one raises the concentration of HX while maintaining the same pH (i.e., by using both HX and NaX) because the ratio of $[HX]/[X^-]$ will not change at a given pH. Analogously, one can develop an equation for the specific base catalysis where the rate is dependent on only the hydroxide ion concentration in the aqueous solution. Hence, a general equation for the specific acid–base catalysis takes the following form:

$$-d[A]/dt = k_H[A][H_3O^+] + k[A] + k_{OH}[A][OH^-] \quad (6\text{-}17)$$

provided that reactant A as a starting material is in the same form throughout the pH range. Here, k_H, k, and k_{OH} are the rate constants for the H^+-catalyzed, noncatalyzed, and OH^--catalyzed reactions, respectively.

The pH–Rate Profile

If one determines the rate constant in a very acidic region of a specific acid-catalyzed reaction as a function of pH, then k_{obs} is likely to involve only the first term of Equation (6-17). In this case, $k_{obs} = k_H[H_3O^+]$, and

$$\log k_{obs} = \log k_H - \text{pH}$$

A plot of $\log k_{obs}$ versus pH should yield a straight line with the slope equal to −1. If the experiments are carried out in the high-pH region, where acid catalysis is diminished and the noncatalyzed reaction is obscured, it can be shown that

$$\log k_{obs} = \log k_{OH} - pK_w + \text{pH}$$

The plot of $\log k_{obs}$ versus pH now shows a straight line with a slope equal to +1. If a drug undergoes both specific acid and base catalyses, the display of the $\log k_{obs}$ on the pH scale may show a V- or U-shaped curve,[10] with the minimum indicating the pH region of noncatalyzed reaction. This is known as the *pH–rate profile*, which is very useful for understanding pH-dependent drug stability problems. But many drugs exhibit complicated degradation patterns that deviate significantly from what can be explained by the specific acid and base catalysis.

One of the best examples of the specific acid- and base-catalyzed reaction processes is the degradation of aspirin (acetylsalicylic acid) in water.[11, 12] Aspirin undergoes hydrolysis to yield salicylic acid (see Figure 6-1). The pH–rate profile shows a descending curve of $\log k_{obs}$ in the pH region below 2.5, an increase in $\log k_{obs}$ in the pH region of 2.5–5, a somewhat plateau region between pH 5 and 8, and a sharp increase in $\log k_{obs}$ above pH 9 (see **Figure 6-4**). This pH dependency of the rate constant has been shown to involve the specific acid and base catalyses in the very low and very high pH regions, respectively, and an

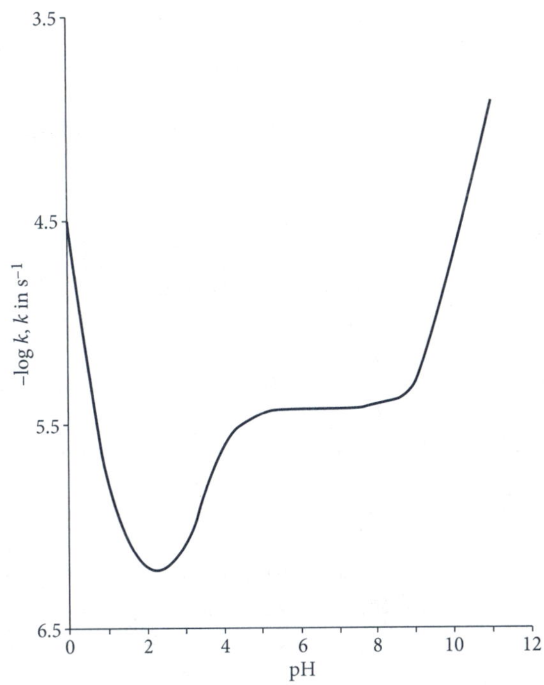

Figure 6-4 The pH–rate profile for aspirin degradation at 25°C. Reprinted from: Garrett Edward, R. The kinetics of solvolysis of acyl esters of salicylic acid. *J Am Chem Soc.*, 1957, 79(13), pp 3401–3408. Copyright 1957 American Chemical Society.

acid dissociation–controlled middle region where the rate profile can be explained as the combination of two uncatalyzed reactions involving the protonated acid, HA, and the dissociated base, A^-:[12]

$$\mathrm{HA} \xrightarrow{k_1} \text{salicylic acid}$$

$$\mathrm{A^-} \xrightarrow{k_2} \text{salicylate}$$

The overall rate equation for the noncatalyzed reactions is

$$-d[C_{\text{aspirin}}]/dt = k_1[\mathrm{HA}] + k_2[\mathrm{A^-}]$$

where $k_{\text{obs}} = k_1 + K_a k_2/[\mathrm{H_3O^+}]$. Because the negative charge on A^- enhances the departure of the CH_3COO group, $k_2 > k_1$. The pK_a for aspirin is 3.49, which corresponds to about the midpoint of the pH region where the $\log k_{\text{obs}}$ increases from the minimum to the plateau level. As can be seen from the above equation, an increase in pH will increase k_{obs} due to the increase in $[A^-]$.

Enzyme Kinetics

The enzyme-catalyzed reaction kinetics were first described by Michaelis and Menten[13] using the method of steady-state approximation. This approach has provided a convenient alternative to the use of integrated equations to monitor the elimination of a drug or the formation of the product in enzyme-catalyzed reactions. Michaelis and Menten showed that the conversion of a substrate S to the product P by enzyme E can be described by the following mechanism:

$$\mathrm{E} + \mathrm{S} \underset{k_2}{\overset{k_1}{\rightleftarrows}} ES$$

$$ES \xrightarrow{k_3} \mathrm{P} + \mathrm{E} \qquad \text{rate-determining}$$

where the rate-determining step is the conversion of the enzyme–substrate complex to the product. It follows that

$$d[\mathrm{P}]/dt = k_3[ES]$$

The steady-state condition is such that $d[ES]/dt = 0$ (see illustration in **Figure 6-5**), with which it can be shown that

$$[ES] = \frac{k_1[\mathrm{E}][\mathrm{S}]}{k_2 + k_3}$$

and

$$\frac{d[\mathrm{P}]}{dt} = \frac{k_1 k_3[\mathrm{E}][\mathrm{S}]}{k_2 + k_3} \qquad (6\text{-}18)$$

If one defines the quantity of $(k_2 + k_3)/k_1$ to be K_m (the *Michaelis–Menten constant*) and the total enzyme concentration is E_t, that is, $[\mathrm{E}] = E_t - [ES]$, the following equation is obtained and is recognized as the Michaelis–Menten equation:

$$\frac{d[\mathrm{P}]}{dt} = k_3 E_t[\mathrm{S}]/(K_m + [\mathrm{S}]) \qquad (6\text{-}19)$$

It should be mentioned that as k_3 is involved in the slow rate-determining step, k_2 is likely greater than k_3, and the Michaelis–Menten constant is then regarded as the dissociation constant of the substrate–enzyme complex, with a larger value of K_m indicating a lesser enzymatic reaction.

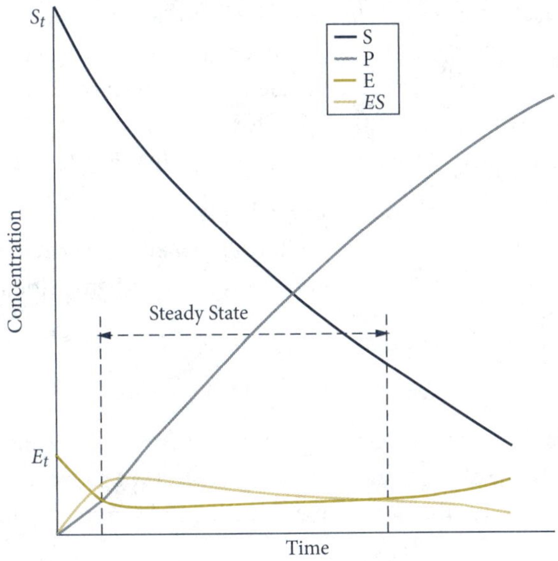

Figure 6-5 Concentration–time curves for E + S = *ES* → P + E.

For practical use of Equation (6-19), the rate of the reaction measured at steady-state conditions may be defined as the velocity V; the value of k_3E_t is thus the maximum velocity V_m obtainable by the system. A rearrangement of Equation (6-19) using the velocity terms gives

$$V = \frac{V_m[\mathrm{S}]}{K_m + [\mathrm{S}]}$$

or

$$\frac{1}{V} = \frac{1}{V_m} + \frac{K_m}{V_m}\frac{1}{[\mathrm{S}]} \tag{6-20}$$

Equation (6-20) is known as the Lineweaver–Burk equation. As can be seen, the plot of $1/V$ versus $1/[\mathrm{S}]$will give a straight line, with the intercept on the y axis equal to $1/V_m$. The slope of the plot is equal to K_m/V_m. The equation also indicates that the straight line intercepts the x axis at a value of $-1/K_m$.

Now let us consider the effect of an inhibitor I, which competes with the substrate for the binding to the enzyme in such way that the inhibitor-bound enzyme loses its catalytic action. The dissociation constant K_i, for the inhibitor binding to the enzyme, and the total enzyme concentration E_t can be written as

$$K_i = [\mathrm{I}][\mathrm{E}]/[\mathrm{EI}]$$

$$E_t = [\mathrm{E}] + [ES] + [\mathrm{EI}]$$

With these relationships, Equation (6-18) can be modified and converted to the Lineweaver–Burk form as follows:

$$\frac{d[\mathrm{P}]}{dt} = \frac{k_1k_3(E_t - [ES] - [\mathrm{EI}])\,[\mathrm{S}]}{k_2 + k_3}$$

$$V = \frac{V_m[\mathrm{S}]}{K_m + [\mathrm{S}] + K_m[\mathrm{I}]/K_i}$$

and

$$\frac{1}{V} = \frac{1}{V_m} + \frac{K_m}{V_m}\left(1 + \frac{[\mathrm{I}]}{K_i}\right)\frac{1}{[\mathrm{S}]} \tag{6-21}$$

Equation (6-21) is very useful for *competitive inhibition* studies. The plot of $1/V$ versus $1/[S]$ in the presence of the inhibitor gives a straight line that passes through the y axis at the same point as that of the noninhibited enzyme kinetics, but the slope of the plot is now $(K_m/V_m)(1 + [I]/K_i)$, from which the dissociation constant for the inhibitor–enzyme complex (K_i) can be calculated. An illustration of the Lineweaver–Burk plot is shown in Example 6-5.

The enzyme inhibition phenomena can be exceedingly complex. They can be classified as competitive, uncompetitive, and noncompetitive inhibitions; each is governed by a different reaction mechanism and thus requires individual considerations in kinetic treatment. Readers are referred to texts of biochemistry for details.

Example 6-5: The metabolite formed following a 2-h incubation of a drug with liver microsomal enzymes at 37°C in the absence and presence of 40 μM of an inhibitor was determined as follows. Calculate K_m and V_m for the drug and K_i for the inhibitor, using the Lineweaver–Burk equation.

C (Total Substrate), μM	[P] (without I), μM	[P] (with I), μM
5	2.30	1.80
7.5	3.10	2.50
10	3.85	3.15
20	5.50	4.56
40	7.25	6.02

Solution: Velocity V can be calculated as $[P]/2$ μM/h; $[S] = C - [P]$. Thus,

In the absence of I:

$1/V$ (h/μM)	0.87	0.65	0.52	0.36	0.28
$1/[S]$ (μM^{-1})	0.37	0.23	0.16	0.07	0.03

In the presence of I:

$1/V$ (h/μM)	1.11	0.80	0.64	0.44	0.33
$1/[S]$ (μM^{-1})	0.31	0.20	0.15	0.07	0.03

The plot of $1/V$ versus $1/[S]$ is given in **Figure 6-6**, which shows competitive inhibition of drug metabolism by the inhibitor.

Calculation of V_m and K_m from plot A:

From y axis intercept: $1/V_m = 0.24$ $\quad V_m = 4.05$ μM/h

From slope: $K_m/V_m = 1.7$ $\quad K_m = 6.90$ μM

From x axis intercept: $1/K_m = 0.145$ $\quad K_m = 6.90$ μM

Calculation of K_i using both plots A and B (see Equations (6-20) and (6-21)):

$1 + [I]/K_i =$ slope B/slope $A = 2.76/1.7 = 1.62$

$[I] = 40$ μM $\quad K_i$ is calculated to be 64.5 μM

The quantity $1 + [I]/K_i$ can also be obtained as the ratio of intercept A/intercept B on the x axis, which gives the same answer.

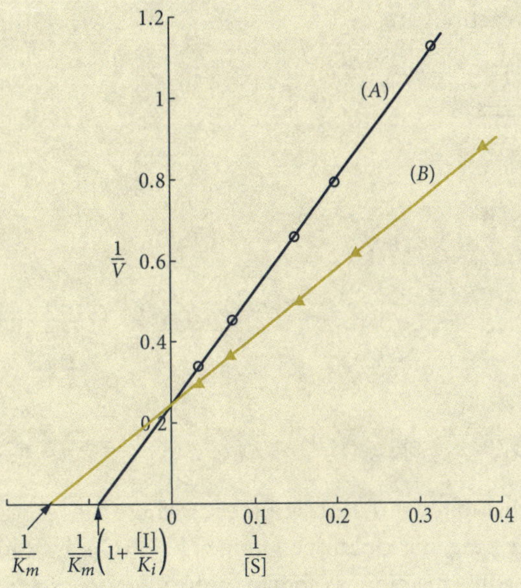

Figure 6-6 The Lineweaver–Burk plots in the absence (*A*) and presence (*B*) of competitive inhibition using data in Example 6-5.

IV. Complex Reactions

Reaction Types and Their Kinetic Processes

Complex Reactions

Many chemical reactions involve more than one step in their reaction schemes, and for each step, the product formed is measurable. They are called *complex reactions* because they are not a concerted process nor can they be treated by the steady-state approximation. Depending on the nature of the reaction or the kinetic process, complex reactions may include reversible, parallel, consecutive, autocatalytic, induced, and chain reactions. Aside from the chain reactions, which have been previously mentioned to cause drug degradation, autocatalytic and induced reactions may play a role in determining drug stability in solutions. *Autocatalysis* occurs in reactions that start slow but become much faster when the reaction generates sufficient catalyst such as H^+ to accelerate the reaction rate. The hydrolysis of esters, e.g., is autocatalytic because of the formation of a carboxylic acid. Certain reactions normally do not occur but are observed in the presence of another agent. An example of this induced reaction is the autooxidation of sodium arsenite in water, which does not occur alone. When sodium sulfite is added, however, the arsenite is oxidized. The mechanism may involve generation of oxygen radicals by the sulfite in its own oxidation by oxygen.

The kinetic processes of complex reactions include reversible reactions, in which the reaction ceases to occur when a finite concentration ratio of the reactant and product is reached; parallel reactions, in which the reactant is degraded or eliminated via two or more reaction schemes; and consecutive reactions, in which the product of a reaction undergoes further reaction to form other products. We describe these reaction processes in first-order kinetics because, as will be made clear later, these kinetic processes are very useful in describing not only a chemical reaction but also the kinetic behavior of a drug in the biological system. The first-order kinetic models for the reversible, parallel, and consecutive reactions are

Reversible reaction: $A \underset{k_{-1}}{\overset{k_1}{\rightleftarrows}} B$

Parallel reactions: $A \overset{k_1}{\longrightarrow} B$, $A \overset{k_2}{\downarrow} C$

Consecutive reaction: $A \overset{k_1}{\longrightarrow} B \overset{k_2}{\longrightarrow} C$

Reversible Reaction

Recall that for a reaction that follows first-order kinetics where the reactant essentially reaches zero concentration at some time, the kinetic equation is $[A] = C_A e^{-kt}$, or $\log [A]/C_A = -kt/2.303$ (Equation (6-9)). In a reversible reaction, as shown in the following scheme, however,

$$A \underset{k_{-1}}{\overset{k_1}{\rightleftarrows}} B$$

the kinetic process will stop when the reaction reaches an equilibrium, where the equilibrium concentrations A_{eq} and B_{eq} will no longer change and are related to the initial concentration of A by the following relationship:

$$C_A = A_{eq} + B_{eq}$$

The rate equation for this reversible reaction is

$$-d[A]/dt = k_1[A] - k_{-1}[B]$$

It should be apparent that at any time t, $[B] = C_A - [A]$, and that at equilibrium,

$$k_1 A_{eq} = k_{-1} B_{eq} \tag{6-22}$$

With these relationships, it can be seen that

$$-d[A]/dt = (k_1 + k_{-1})([A] - A_{eq}) \tag{6-23}$$

Integration of Equation (6-23) from C_A to [A], as t goes from 0 to t, gives

$$\log \frac{[A] - A_{eq}}{C_A - A_{eq}} = -\frac{k_1 + k_{-1}}{2.303} t \tag{6-24}$$

Equation (6-24) shows the kinetics of a reversible reaction. The use of this equation requires determination of the equilibrium concentration. This equation is similar to Equation (6-9), but indicates that the elimination kinetics stop as [A] becomes A_{eq} rather than at zero concentration. The rate constant thus measured is equal to $k_1 + k_{-1}$. The individual rate constants can be calculated by further determining the ratio of k_1/k_{-1} according to Equation (6-22). If the reaction is studied by monitoring the formation of product B, Equation (6-24) can be rewritten as

$$\log \frac{B_{eq}}{B_{eq} - [B]} = \frac{k_1 + k_{-1}}{2.303} t \tag{6-25}$$

Parallel Reaction

In a parallel kinetic process, reactant A is eliminated by more than one reaction or process. But even so, the mathematical treatment of the kinetic data is rather simple because the rate equation can be written as

$$-d[\mathrm{A}]/dt = (k_1 + k_2 + k_3 + \cdots)[\mathrm{A}]$$

Integration of the above equation gives

$$\log \frac{[\mathrm{A}]}{C_\mathrm{A}} = -\frac{(k_1 + k_2 + k_3 + \cdots)\,t}{2.303} \qquad (6\text{-}26)$$

It is clear that Equation (6-26) can be used to determine only the sum of the rate constants of all parallel reactions. The individual constants can be determined if the products of the parallel reactions are simultaneously monitored, because the product formation is directly proportional to the rate constant. (See Example 6-6 for calculation.)

Example 6-6: A reaction of chlorobenzene with Cl_2 was carried out in CS_2 using 0.05 *M* chlorobenzene and an excess amount of chlorine. At 35 min, 0.03 *M* of chlorobenzene was found chlorinated at either the *ortho* or *para* position, with an *ortho/para* molar ratio of 3:5. Calculate the rate constants for these two parallel reactions.

Solution: The pseudo first-order rate constant is

$$\log 0.02/0.05 = -(k_1 + k_2) \times 35/2.303$$

$$k_1 + k_2 = 0.0262\ \mathrm{min}^{-1}$$

As $k_1/k_2 = 3/5$,

$k_1 = 0.0262 \times 3/8 = 0.0098\ \mathrm{min}^{-1}$ (*ortho* chlorination)

$k_2 = 0.0262 \times 5/8 = 0.0164\ \mathrm{min}^{-1}$ (*para* chlorination)

Consecutive Reactions

In many instances the products of one reaction are themselves capable of undergoing further reaction, so that the bridge between the initial reactants and the ultimate products consists of a series of consecutive, independent steps. The simplest process involves two reaction steps, which can be shown as follows:

$$\mathrm{A} \xrightarrow{k_1} \mathrm{B} \xrightarrow{k_2} \mathrm{C}$$

Assuming first-order kinetics for both reactions, the rate equations for the first and second steps are

$$-d[\mathrm{A}]/dt = k_1[\mathrm{A}]$$

and

$$d[\mathrm{B}]/dt = k_1[\mathrm{A}] - k_2[\mathrm{B}]$$

Integration of the first rate equation gives

$$[\mathrm{A}] = C_\mathrm{A} e^{-k_1 t}$$

The expression of [B] as a function of time is the key to understanding this type of kinetics. It is thus worth the effort to derive this equation, so that one can have a greater appreciation of the reaction kinetics. The rate equation can be rewritten as

$$d[\mathrm{B}]/dt + k_2[\mathrm{B}] = k_1[\mathrm{A}] = k_1 C_\mathrm{A} e^{-k_1 t}$$

This expression is used because the right-hand quantity of the equation is known and the left-hand side of the equation needs to be transformed so that it can be integrated. This can be done by multiplying both sides of the equation by $e^{k_2 t}$. Thus,

$$e^{k_2 t}\, d[\mathrm{B}]/dt + k_2 e^{k_2 t}[\mathrm{B}] = k_1 e^{k_2 t} C_\mathrm{A} e^{-k_1 t}$$

Now, the above equation can be written as

$$d\,(e^{k_2 t}[\mathrm{B}])/dt = k_1 C_\mathrm{A} e^{(k_2 - k_1)t}$$

It follows that

$$\int d(e^{k_2 t}[\mathrm{B}]) = \int k_1 C_\mathrm{A} e^{(k_2 - k_1)t}\, dt$$

and

$$e^{k_2 t}[\mathrm{B}] = \frac{k_1 C_\mathrm{A}}{k_2 - k_1} e^{(k_2 - k_1)t} + E$$

where E is the integration constant. When $t = 0$, $[\mathrm{B}] = 0$, hence $E = -k_1 C_\mathrm{A}/(k_2 - k_1)$. Substituting $-k_1 C_\mathrm{A}/(k_2 - k_1)$ for E, the above equation can be rearranged to give

$$[\mathrm{B}] = \frac{k_1 C_\mathrm{A}}{k_2 - k_1} e^{-k_1 t} - \frac{k_1 C_\mathrm{A}}{k_2 - k_1} e^{-k_2 t} \qquad (6\text{-}27)$$

Equation (6-27) shows the concentration–time relationship for B in a consecutive first-order reaction. Because both [A] and [B] are now expressed as a function of time, the formation of the product C can be determined as $[\mathrm{C}] = C_\mathrm{A} - [\mathrm{A}] - [\mathrm{B}]$.

Equation (6-27) exhibits a maximum at $d[\mathrm{B}]/dt = 0$. From that it can be shown that

$$k_1 e^{-k_1 t} = k_2 e^{-k_2 t}$$

and

$$t_{\max} = \frac{2.303 \log (k_2/k_1)}{k_2 - k_1} \qquad (6\text{-}28)$$

Here, $t_{\max}$ is the time when B reaches its maximum concentration, $[\mathrm{B}]_{\max}$, which can be determined as

$$[\mathrm{B}]_{\max} = C_\mathrm{A}(k_1/k_2)^r \qquad \text{where } r = k_2/(k_2 - k_1) \qquad (6\text{-}29)$$

The use of Equations (6-27), (6-28), and (6-29) can be found in Example 6-7.

Example 6-7: For a first-order consecutive reaction A → B → C, if the initial concentration is 1 m*M*, $k_1 = 0.01\ \mathrm{min}^{-1}$, and $k_2 = 0.02\ \mathrm{min}^{-1}$, calculate and plot the time curves for [A], [B], and [C]. Calculate $t_{\max}$ and $[\mathrm{B}]_{\max}$.

Solution: From Equations (6-9) and (6-27),

$$[\mathrm{A}] = C_\mathrm{A} e^{-0.01t} = e^{-0.01t}$$

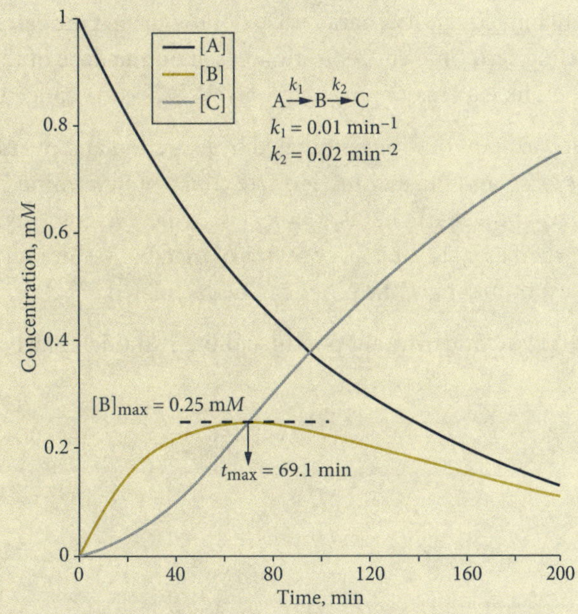

Figure 6-7 The concentration–time curves of a consecutive reaction with $k_1 = 0.01\ min^{-1}$, $k_2 = 0.02\ min^{-1}$, and an initial concentration of 1 m*M*.

$[B] = 0.01C_A(e^{-0.01t} - e^{-0.02t}) / (0.02–0.01) = e^{-0.01t} - e^{-0.02t}$

$[C] = 1 - e^{-0.01t} - e^{-0.01t} + e^{-0.02t} = 1 - 2e^{-0.01t} + e^{-0.02t}$

$= (1 - e^{-0.01t})^2$

The plot of concentrations as a function of time is shown in **Figure 6-7.** It is found that

$t_{max} = (2.303 \log 2) / 0.01 = 69.1\ min$

$[B]_{max} = C_A\ (k_1/k_2)^r = (0.01/0.02)^{0.02/0.01} = 0.25\ mM$

Complex Kinetics and Pharmacokinetics

Equation (6-27) is directly applicable for the interpretation of drug kinetics in the body following a one-compartment model via extravascular absorption of the drug. The absorption is usually assumed to be a first-order process. If the absorbed drug is rapidly distributed in the body, the plasma concentration–time curve will show an elimination phase following the absorption, and this kinetic process is described by Equation (6-27). By letting $k_1 = k_a$, the absorption rate constant; $k_2 = k_e$, the elimination rate constant; $[B] = C_P$, the plasma concentration; and $C_A = D_o/V_d$, the dose per volume of distribution; Equation (6-27) becomes

$$C_P = \frac{k_a D_o}{V_d(k_e - k_a)} e^{-k_a t} - \frac{k_a D_o}{V_d(k_e - k_a)} e^{-k_e t}$$

or

$$C_P = \frac{k_a D_o}{V_d(k_a - k_e)} (e^{-k_e t} - e^{-k_a t}) \qquad (6\text{-}30)$$

Equation (6-30) is written by taking into consideration that usually $k_a > k_e$. It should be mentioned that the initial concentration, which is critical in calculating reaction kinetic parameters, is not a known quantity and must be determined by the kinetic data. Because the dose of a drug is expressed in weight expressions, this gives the concept of volume of distribution, which is not the volume of the blood compartment but a quantity characteristic of the drug. One calculates the volume of distribution by extrapolating zero time concentration based on the dose of the drug that was given. A large volume of distribution, e.g., may indicate low levels of plasma concentration.

Drug in the blood compartment may be eliminated by excretion and by metabolism. Hence, parallel kinetic processes exist, and the elimination rate constant determined using plasma data usually is the sum of the two processes, that is, $k_e = k_u + k_m$, where k_u is the excretion rate constant measured in urine data, whereas k_m is the rate constant of metabolic elimination. If one of these processes is determined experimentally, the other can be calculated.

A commonly employed two-compartment pharmacokinetic model may be represented by the following diagram:

$$\text{IV} \rightarrow C_P \underset{k_{21}}{\overset{k_{12}}{\rightleftarrows}} C_T$$

$$C_P \xrightarrow{k_e} \text{Elimination}$$

This model involves transfer of the drug (1) from the blood (central) compartment to the peripheral tissue compartment at a rate of $k_{12}C_P$; (2) from the tissue to the blood compartment at a rate of $k_{21}C_T$; and (3) from the central compartment to outside the body at a rate of k_eC_P. The plasma concentration–time curve is characterized by a fast distribution phase (or α phase), which may occur within a few minutes or hours, followed by a postdistribution β elimination phase. When the distribution of the drug reaches equilibrium, such as when $k_{12}C_P = k_{21}C_T$ per the reversible reaction mechanism, the plasma and tissue levels will have a finite ratio, and elimination of the drug from the plasma and the tissue compartments will proceed with the same rate constant. The pharmacokinetic data allow the measurement of the rate constants of α and β for the distribution and elimination phases, respectively, according to the following equations:

$$C_T = \frac{D_o k_{12}}{V_t\,(\beta - \alpha)}\,(e^{-\alpha t} - e^{-\beta t}) \qquad (6\text{-}31)$$

$$C_P = \frac{D_o}{V_p\,(\beta - \alpha)}\,[(k_{21} - \alpha)\,e^{-\alpha t} - (k_{21} - \beta)\,e^{-\beta t}] \qquad (6\text{-}32)$$

where D_o is the dose given intravenously, and V_t and V_p are volumes of distribution in the tissue and central compartments, respectively. The rate constants α and β depend solely on k_{12}, k_{21}, and k_e in that $\alpha + \beta = k_{12} + k_{21} + k_e$ and $\alpha\beta = k_{21}k_e$.

Example 6-8: A drug that follows a one-compartment open model was eliminated from the plasma by the following pathways:

Metabolism	$k_m = 0.18\,\text{h}^{-1}$
Excretion by the kidney	$k_e = 0.15\,\text{h}^{-1}$
Excretion through the bile	$k_e = 0.50\,\text{h}^{-1}$

Calculate the half-life of the drug, and predict the half-life if (*a*) the metabolism were completely blocked, (*b*) the metabolism were doubled, and (*c*) the patient suffered from liver disease such that biliary flow was completely blocked.

Solution: The overall elimination constant is $0.18 + 0.15 + 0.5 = 0.83\,h^{-1}$.

$t_{1/2} = 0.693/0.82 = 0.83\,h$

(*a*) $\beta = 0.15 + 0.50 = 0.65\,h^{-1}$ $t_{1/2} = 0.693/0.65 = 1.07\,h$

(*b*) $\beta = 0.36 + 0.15 + 0.50 = 1.01\,h^{-1}$ $t_{1/2} = 0.693/1.01 = 0.69\,h$

(*c*) $\beta = 0.18 + 0.15 = 0.33\,h^{-1}$ $t_{1/2} = 0.693/0.33 = 2.10\,h$

Example 6-9: A drug was given by IV infusion, and the following rate constants were determined: $k_{12} = 0.75\,h^{-1}$, $k_{21} = 0.55\,h^{-1}$, and $\beta = 0.15\,h^{-1}$. Calculate the half-life and the tissue/plasma concentration ratio at steady state.

Solution: $t_{1/2} = 0.693/\beta = 0.693/0.15 = 4.6\,h$

$C_T/C_P = k_{12}/k_{21} = 0.75/0.55 = 1.36^{\dagger}$

†In a two-compartment model, if the drug is given by rapid injection, $C_T/C_P = k_{12}/(k_{21} + \beta)$.

The above discussion shows that complex reaction mechanisms are useful in understanding both chemical and nonchemical processes. Our knowledge of drug disposition in the body, in particular, has been generated by scientists who applied these kinetic principles to pharmacokinetic drug research.

V. Temperature Dependency of the Rate Constant

Theories of the Rate Constant

Temperature Effect on Reaction Rate

In 1889, *Arrhenius* showed that while the dependence of the reaction rate on concentration remains unchanged, there exists a linear relationship between $\log k$ and $1/T$; that is, the rate constant increases in an exponential manner with the temperature:

$$k \propto e^{\text{constant}/T}$$

In later deductions, this empirical relation becomes

$$k = Ae^{-E_a/RT} \qquad (6\text{-}33)$$

where A is called the preexponential factor and E_a is the activation energy. With this notation, one writes the logarithmic form as

$$\log k = -E_a/2.303RT + \log A$$

The constants E_a and A can thus be deduced from the slope and intercept of the plot of $\log k$ versus $1/T$. For reactions that proceed with a half-life in minutes or hours, the E_a value is about 20 kcal/mol. The chemist's rule of thumb is that reactions go 2 or 3 times as fast when the temperature increases by 10°C.

It is perhaps best to recognize that Arrhenius could have found this rate constant–temperature relationship by an entirely empirical procedure. Numerous experiments have been done since to verify its validity, and as we shall see, more refined theories have been developed in attempt to explain both the preexponential term A and the exponential term E_a. For a first look, the Arrhenius equation appears to be consistent with the temperature dependency of the equilibrium constant. The thermodynamic equation of the change in equilibrium constant K as a function of temperature is

$$d(\ln K)/dT = \Delta H/RT^2$$

or $$K = Ae^{-\Delta H/RT}$$

If the Arrhenius equation is interpreted as an equilibrium between the forward (k_1, A_1) and reverse (k_{-1}, A_{-1}) reactions, then the following equation can be written, which would be in agreement with the Arrhenius equation (Equation (6-33)):

$$K = k_1/k_{-1} = (A_1/A_{-1})\, e^{-(E_{a1} - E_{a-1})RT}$$

The Arrhenius Theory

Arrhenius himself had provided a qualitative theory for the molecular behavior that leads to the empirical Equation (6-33). His theory is centered on the concept that any and all reaction processes involve the formation of some high-energy species, now known as the activated complex, which can break down into the products. This concept may be illustrated using the second-order gas-phase reaction of hydrogen and iodine in the formation of hydrogen iodide. The reaction is reversible and proceeds by a single-step four-center process as shown below. It is easily recognizable that the four-center complex allows atoms and electrons to be rearranged to go in either reaction direction.

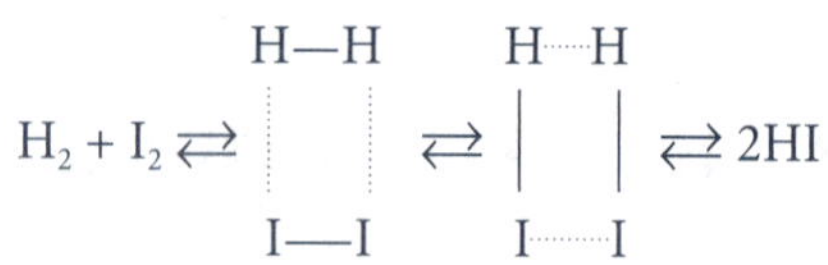

Arrhenius' original ideas were elaborated later into quantitative expressions. If the activated complex is assumed to have an energy E_a greater than the reactants, the number of activated complexes compared to the number of reactant molecules can be written in terms of the Boltzmann distribution as

No. of activated complexes/no. of reactant molecules $= e^{-E_a/RT}$

The theory of Arrhenius now says that the rate of a reaction is proportional to the number or concentration of the activated complex. The idea of a high-energy activated complex is illustrated in **Figure 6-8**, which gives a qualitative description of the extent of the transformation from reactants to products. Although the Arrhenius theory improved our understanding of the reaction process, it does not show how the preexponential factor A depends on the molecular properties of the reaction system; nor does it attempt to predict the value of E_a. Two later theories made progress in the interpretation of the factor A, but the energy of the activated complex remains too subtle a quantity for evaluation.

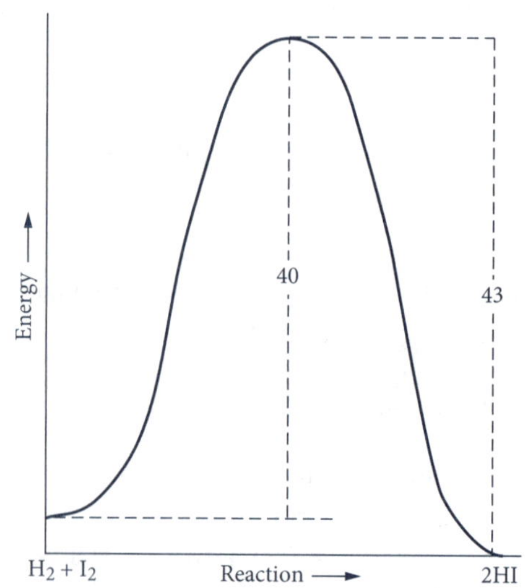

Figure 6-8 Activation energy of the reaction of $H_2 + I_2 \rightleftarrows 2HI$.

Collision Theory

The collision theory stems from the idea that reactions occur only when reactant molecules are coming together, and the rate of reaction should be proportional to the number of collisions per unit time between reactant molecules. The idea of activation energy also enters because only molecules that have enough energy will undergo the necessary rearrangement of atoms and electrons in the moment of impact and fly away as product molecules. However, because the number of collisions can be calculated only for gases, the collision theory is therefore restricted to the interpretation of gaseous reactions.

Consider the reaction A + B → products. The total number of collisions of gaseous molecules in this mixture includes collisions between A and B and between like molecules. Clearly, for a reaction to occur, collisions must come from those between molecule A and molecule B, and only a fraction of these collisions result from molecules that have enough energy to permit the reaction to occur. With these stipulations, the number of collisions between A and B per cubic centimeter, with the average speed derived from the Maxwell–Boltzmann distribution, can be obtained as

$$Z_{AB} = (\sigma_A + \sigma_B)^2(\pi RT/2\mu_m)^{1/2}N_A N_B$$

Here, σ_A and σ_B are the diameters of A and B molecules, respectively; μ_m is the molar reduced mass, which is related to the molecular weights of A and B by the relation $\mu_m = M_A M_B/(M_A + M_B)$; and N_A and N_B are the numbers of A and B molecules per cubic centimeter. The above equation can be modified by a factor of $\theta/10^3$, where θ is the Avogadro number, so that A and B can be expressed in molar concentrations as in normal kinetic treatment. This modification yields

$$Z_{AB} = (\sigma_A + \sigma_B)^2(\theta/10^3)(\pi RT/2\mu_m)^{1/2}[A][B]$$

The basic relation for sorting out the number of molecules that have various speeds or energy is Boltzmann's distribution. In terms of molar expressions (based on Avogadro's number of molecules), it can be shown, without going into detail, that the fraction of the molecular collisions between A and B that has more energy than E_a is

$$\text{Fraction of effective collisions} = \Delta N/N = e^{-E_a/RT}$$

The rate of a reaction ($-d[A]/dt$ or $-d[B]/dt$), according to the collision theory, is therefore

$$\begin{aligned}\text{Rate} &= (\text{no. of collisions/s})(\text{fraction of effective collisions})\\ &= Z_{AB}\, e^{-E_a/RT} \qquad (6\text{-}34)\end{aligned}$$

From Equation (6-34) and the molar expression of Z_{AB}, it is seen that

$$-d[A]/dt = (\sigma_A + \sigma_B)^2(\theta/10^3)(\pi RT/2\mu_m)^{1/2}e^{-E_a/RT}[A][B]$$

$$k = (\sigma_A + \sigma_B)^2(\theta/10^3)(\pi RT/2\mu_m)^{1/2}e^{-E_a/RT}$$

and

$$A = (\sigma_A + \sigma_B)^2(\theta/10^3)(\pi RT/2\mu_m)^{1/2} \qquad (6\text{-}35)$$

The principal accomplishment of collision theory is that the preexponential term A is seen as a constant that depends on the molecular diameters and molecular weights of the reactants. If A and B exhibit similar σ and molecular weights, the calculated A value will be the same for different reactions. Assuming that A and B have the same molecular weight of 50 and a σ of 3.5 Å, A is

Table 6-3 The Arrhenius Constants of Some Second-Order Gaseous Reactions

Reaction	A, M^{-1} s^{-1}	E_a, cal/mol
$H_2 + I_2 \rightarrow 2HI$	$2.0 \times 10^9\ T^{1/2}$	42,500
$2HI \rightarrow H_2 + I_2$	$3.3 \times 10^9\ T^{1/2}$	38,900
$2NO_2 \rightarrow 2NO + O_2$	$2.6 \times 10^8\ T^{1/2}$	26,600
$2NOCl \rightarrow 2NO + Cl_2$	$3.3 \times 10^9\ T^{1/2}$	25,800
$CH_3I + HI \rightarrow CH_4 + I_2$	$5.2 \times 10^{10}\ T^{1/2}$	33,100

calculated to be $6.6 \times 10^9\ T^{1/2}$. **Table 6-3** shows the Arrhenius constants for a number of second-order gaseous reactions. It can be seen that whereas some of the *A* values are in line with the theory, others showed quite appreciable disagreement. Part of the reason for this disagreement is that collision theory is rather rigid and does not account for the fact that the reaction may also depend on a suitable orientation of the reactant molecules when the collision takes place.

Transition State Theory

The major point of the transition state theory is that the activated complex, now known as the *transition state*, is treated as a molecule and thus a thermodynamic entity, in spite of its transitory existence. This theory is attributed mainly to the work of Henry Eyring. Consider the reaction

$$A + B \rightleftarrows (AB)^{\ddagger} \rightarrow \text{products}$$

The equilibrium of the transition state can be written as

$$K^{\ddagger} = (AB)^{\ddagger}/[A][B]$$

Because the transition state is quite unstable, a suitable vibration with sufficient amplitude can break up the complex, resulting in flying apart of the product molecules. The energy required for this action is small and corresponds to the classical energy of kT, where k is the Boltzmann constant (we shall use k_r later to represent the rate constant). Using Planck's expression $\Delta\varepsilon = h\upsilon$, the average frequency of such vibration is $\nu_{av} = kT/h$. With this notation, the rate of the reaction can be written as

$$-d[A]/dt = K^{\ddagger}(kT/h)[A][B]$$

and

$$k_r = K^{\ddagger}(kT/h)$$

Now if we consider the equilibrium constant $K^{\ddagger}$ a thermodynamic entity, the rate of the reaction will depend on the free energy of activation in that

$$(\Delta G^{\circ})^{\ddagger} = -RT \ln K^{\ddagger}$$

or

$$K^{\ddagger} = e^{-(\Delta G^{\circ})^{\ddagger}/RT}$$

Because at a given temperature $\Delta G = \Delta H - T(\Delta S)$, it follows that

$$K^{\ddagger} = e^{+(\Delta S)^{\ddagger}/R}e^{-(\Delta H)^{\ddagger}/RT}$$

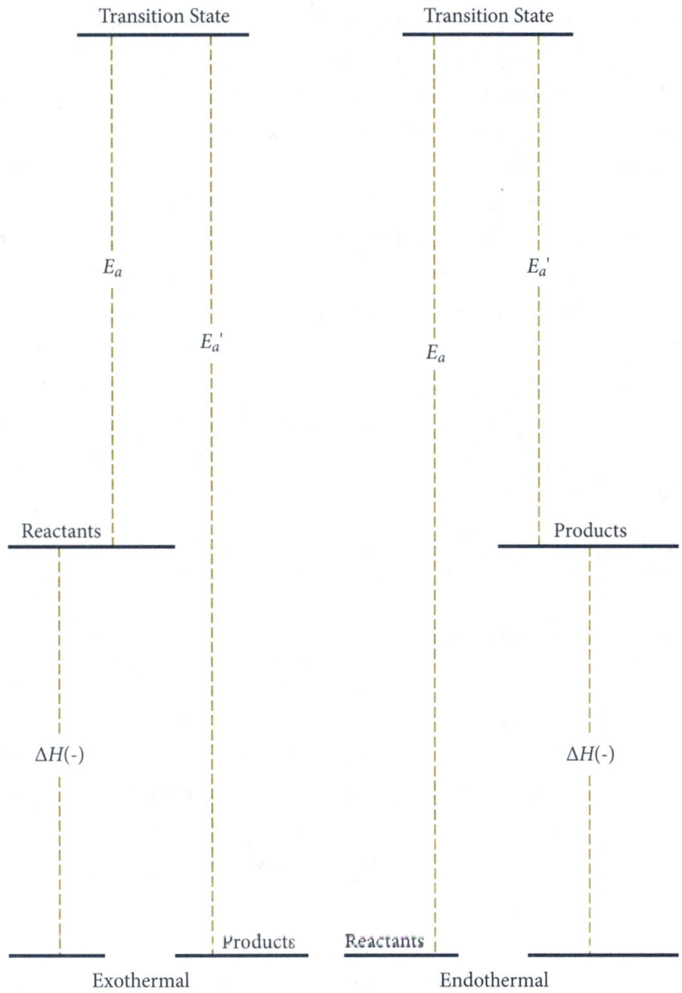

Figure 6-9 Relation between activation energy and heat of reaction.

and

$$k_r = (kT/h)e^{+(\Delta S)^{\ddagger}/R}e^{-(\Delta H)^{\ddagger}/RT} \tag{6-36}$$

Compared to the Arrhenius expression, it is seen that the exponential temperature dependence now involves enthalpy rather than the energy of activation. This perhaps offers a better explanation of the energy change in the reaction process in that $\Delta H^{\ddagger}$ is the energy needed in addition to the heat of reaction to reach the energy level of the transition state. If the reaction is exothermal, the activation energy will be less than that of the reverse reaction. This concept is shown in **Figure 6-9**.

The transition state theory is specially noted for its theoretical interpretation of the preexponential factor A of the Arrhenius equation. As shown in Equation (6-36), the factor A is now entropy-dependent:

$$A = (kT/h)e^{+(\Delta S)^{\ddagger}/R}$$

The entropy of activation represents the tendency through which the reactant molecules rearrange to form the activated complex, which depends largely on the molecular structure of the reactants as well as that of the complex. Because the reaction does not occur naturally, $\Delta S^{\ddagger}$ is usually negative. Structurally, formation of the activated complex appears to bring rigidity to the molecules. For example, when hydrogen and iodine come together to form the transition state, the number of translational and rotational degrees of freedom decreases from those of the two molecules to that of the complex. The energy levels of the complex will be more widely spaced, and the entropy of the complex will be less than that of the two reactant molecules. If, however, the rigidity imposed by the complex is quite small or the reactant molecules act as rigid spherical particles themselves, then the entropy of activation will be less negative. In this case, the *A* value of the transition state theory will approach the collision numbers as predicted by collision theory. The entropy-based interpretation of factor *A* has also provided insight into some reactions in solutions. When oppositely charged ions, e.g., react to form a neutral molecule, the extent of solvation is greatly reduced. The activated complex, in which the opposite charges will be close together, should also exhibit a decrease in solvation and thus positive entropy of activation. This is indeed the case in the reaction of $Cr(OH_2)_6^{3+}$ with CNS^- to form $[Cr(OH_2)CNS]^{2+}$ ($\Delta S^\ddagger = +29$ cal/deg-mol). In contrast, the formation of a charged transition state complex from neutral reactants should lead to a large negative $\Delta S^\ddagger$ because of the added loss of freedom of motion by the solvating molecules, as has been seen in the reaction of aniline with bromomethyl phenyl ketone ($\Delta S^\ddagger = -50$ cal/deg-mol).

Accelerated Stability Testing

Use of the Arrhenius Equation

The Arrhenius theory shows that chemical degradation of drug is predictably more rapid at higher temperatures than at room temperature, the normal storage condition. With the linear relationship of $\log k$ versus $1/T$, the kinetic results obtained by studies at higher temperatures can be used to determine the rate constant and shelf life of the drug at room or other storage temperatures (see Example 6-10). These "accelerated stability studies," through which much information on drug degradation can be gained in a relatively short time, are both practical and necessary in drug product development.

Example 6-10: The rate constants for the decomposition of a drug in an aqueous solution were determined to be 0.00011 and 0.00062 h^{-1} at 40 and 60°C, respectively. Determine (*a*) the activation energy and (*b*) the rate constant at 25°C for this decomposition reaction.

Solution: (*a*) Equation (6-33) shows that

$$\log k = -E_a/2.303RT + \log A$$

If we designate k_1 and k_2 as the rate constants at 40 and 60°C, Equation (6-33) becomes

$$\log(k_2/k_1) = E_a(T_2 - T_1)/2.303RT_1T_2$$

$$E_a = 2.303 \times 1.987 \times 313 \times 333 \log(0.00062/0.00011)/(333 - 313)$$

$$= 17{,}910 \text{ cal/mol}$$

(*b*) Let $T_2 = 333$ K, $T_1 = 298$ K, $k_2 = 0.00062\ h^{-1}$, and $k_1 = k_{25}$.

$$\log(k_2/k_{25}) = E_a(T_2 - T_1)/2.303RT_1T_2$$

$$= 17{,}910\ (333 - 298)/2.303 \times 1.987 \times 333 \times 298 = 1.3804$$

$$k_2/k_{25} = 24.01$$

$$k_{25} = 0.00062/24.01 = 2.58 \times 10^{-5}\ h^{-1}$$

Stability studies, as required by current good manufacturing practices (cGMP) established by the FDA, include testing of those attributes of the drug or drug product that are susceptible to change during storage and are likely to influence quality, safety, and/or efficacy. Drug products must bear an expiration date determined by appropriate stability testing methods. As part of the formal studies, the accelerated stability data can be used to aid in the assessment of long-term chemical effects at normal storage conditions, to evaluate the effect of shorter excursions outside the label storage conditions, and in certain cases to support tentative expiration dates in the event that full shelf life studies are not available. It should be apparent that the accelerated stability testing applies only to chemical or thermal processes, where the linear relationship of $\log k$ versus $1/T$ can be verified. It is suggested that the Arrhenius equation is valid if E_a is in the range of about 10–30 kcal/mol. Many of the physical stability issues in solution and in polyphasic systems such as precipitation, coagulation, and contamination are not described by the Arrhenius theory. In such cases, accelerated stability studies based on temperature changes would have little value. Should some of these phenomena occur at higher temperature in a solution, they can certainly affect the reaction kinetics of the drug, thus causing complexity to the stability study. The main purpose of the accelerated stability studies is to establish a quantitative relationship between rate and temperature. The mechanism of the reaction has presumably been studied or known. It should be pointed out, however, that the reaction at higher temperature may be complicated by changes in reaction order and/or potential parallel reactions. For example, induced reaction by acid formation (autocatalysis) in ester hydrolysis would be more pronounced at higher temperature due to increased degradation of the drug at the higher temperature.

Temperature-Dependent Methods

Accelerated drug stability studies have been carried out using traditional isothermal conditions where drug degradation is measured as a function of time at a constant temperature and nonisothermal conditions where the temperature changes continuously with time. The isothermal studies require that the kinetic process be carried out at various temperatures, normally ranging from 30 to 70°C. For each experiment, the rate constant is determined. The kinetic data can be treated in various fashions. A plot of concentration or the percent of drug remaining (in log scale) versus time gives a straight line and can provide a visual identification of t_{90} at different temperatures. The plot of $\log k$ values determined at different temperatures versus $1/T$ also yields a straight line, from which the value of $\log k$ corresponding to a desired temperature, such as at 25°C, can be easily determined. Still, a plot of t_{90} (in log scale), which is inversely proportional to the rate constant, versus $1/T$ in both Kelvin and Celsius scales can be made for easy identification of the shelf life at room temperature.[14] The isothermal kinetic studies, although somewhat time-consuming, are very reliable in their accuracy.

The method of *nonisothermal kinetics* of drug degradation was developed to reduce the experimental effort. This is achieved by a study design in which the temperature of the system is programmed to change as a function of time according to some algorithm[15–18] that permits the measurement of kinetic parameters, such as reaction order, activation energy, and rate constants, from a single set of drug concentration versus time data. Studies by Zoglio et al.[15] and by Edel and Baltzer[16] have shown that, using consecutive equal-stepped temperature increases, the degradation of drug can be described by a series of isothermal stages in between temperature changes. With this approach, they reasoned that the arithmetic mean of the rate constants for these stages may be taken as the ratio of the total degradation of the drug to the duration of the experiment. Thus, for a first-order kinetic process with n stages, it can be shown that

$$\ln C - \ln C_0 = t(k_1 + k_2 + k_3 + \cdots + k_n)/n$$

where C and C_0 are the concentrations of the drug at time t and time 0, respectively. Here, $\ln C - \ln C_0$ and t/n are determined experimentally, from which the rate constants and the activation energy can be determined with computer-assisted calculations. Using this method, Edel and Baltzer showed that the activation energy determined by both isothermal and nonisothermal kinetics for the degradation of benzazepine in pH 5.0 buffer–ethanol solution is approximately the same.

The complexity of a nonisothermal study is primarily related to the temperature program and the associated data treatment method.[17, 18] But there has been advancement on both fronts. Recent studies by Oliva et al.[19] showed that a linear heating model allows the temperature of the system to be controlled as

$$T_i = T_0 + vt$$

where v is the heating rate constant and T_0 and T_i are the temperature at time 0 and at time t, respectively. For nonisothermal analysis of a first-order kinetic process, the combination of the first-order and Arrhenius equations gives

$$C = C_0 \exp\left\{-A \int_0^t \exp\left[\frac{-E_a}{RT(t)}\right] dt\right\}$$

Direct evaluation of the integrated expression on the right side of the equation can be made with the nonlinear Fit function from the Mathematica program,[20] which allows a direct nonlinear estimation of the activation energy, the factor A, and the initial drug concentration C_0 that enables the percentage expressions of drug degradation. With this approach, Oliva et al.[19] studied the thermal degradation of cholecystokinin peptide and found that the activation energies determined by both isothermal and nonisothermal kinetics are quite similar, but there is a significant difference in shelf life determined by the two methods. It appears that the methods of the nonisothermal kinetics will create a high demand for sophisticated equipment as well as experimental accuracy.

Estimation of Shelf Life

The shelf life and expiration date of a drug product are always referred to the specific temperature condition. If a product is stored under a nonstandard temperature condition for a significant time, modification of the shelf life or expiration date must be made by the pharmacist to ensure product quality. In the normal sequence of determining a shelf life at a new temperature, one would have to know the activation energy, calculate the rate constant for that new temperature based on the activation energy, and then calculate the shelf life using the newly calculated rate constant. Chances are that none of the required information may be available at the time of need. Connors et al.[21] provided a very user-friendly approach to allow estimation of the new shelf life with respect to changes in temperature by using the function Q_{10}, originally defined by Simonelli and Dresback.[22] Function Q_{10} is the ratio of two rate constants measured at temperatures separated by 10 degrees. Because the rate constant is inversely proportional to the shelf life ($k = 0.1054/t_{90}$), knowledge about the Q_{10} value will be useful for computing the shelf life due to change in temperature or rate constant. Using the Arrhenius equation, it can be shown that when the temperature change is 10 degrees, say, from 20 to 30°C, the ratio of the two rate constants, or Q_{10}, is 2, 3, or 4, with E_a equal to 12.2, 19.4, or 24.5 kcal/mol, respectively. Reactions with reasonable rates (with the half-life in hours) have E_a values close to 20 kcal/mol; thus, it is reasonable to assume that Q_{10} will fall in the range of 2–4. With this notation, one can calculate the change in shelf life using the following equation:

$$t_{90,T_2} = t_{90,T_1}/(Q_{10})^{\Delta T/10} \quad (6\text{-}37)$$

where T_1 and T_2 are the two temperatures under consideration, and $\Delta T = T_2 - T_1$. This equation is used by letting Q_{10} equal 2, 3, or 4. The pharmacist can then make a reasonable judgment of the estimated shelf life based on the intended use of the drug product (see Example 6-11).

Example 6-11: A newly reconstituted product is labeled to be stable for 24 h in a refrigerator. What would be the shelf life of this product at room temperature?

Solution: Now

$$\Delta T = T_2 - T_1 = 25°C - 5°C = 20°C$$

Hence,

$$t_{90,\,25} = t_{90,\,5} / Q_{10}^{20/10}$$

At $Q_{10} = 2$, $t_{90,\,25} = 24/4 = 6.0\,h$

At $Q_{10} = 3$, $t_{90,\,25} = 24/9 = 2.7\,h$

At $Q_{10} = 4$, $t_{90,\,25} = 24/16 = 1.5\,h$

Some considerations:

1. For a drug having a narrow therapeutic index, a conservative estimation of the shelf life as 1.5 h is advised. The average value of Q_{10} is 3, which makes the shelf life of 2.7 h reasonable for most drugs.
2. The shelf lives in Equation (6-37) can also be considered as the equivalent storage times at two temperatures. For example, if the product is left at 25°C for 1.2 h and then returned to the refrigerator, what will be the new shelf life, assuming $Q_{10} = 3$?

Answer: Let

$t_{25} = t_5 / Q_{10}^{\,2}$ $\quad t_5 = 1.2 \times 9 = 10.8\,h$

New shelf life at 5°C: $t_{90} = 24 - 10.8 = 13.2\,h$

VI. Chapter Summary

From the discussion of this chapter, it is seen that the principles of chemical kinetics provide the basic tools to study both the chemical degradation and nonchemical kinetic processes that govern the development and use of pharmaceutical products. Kinetic studies are used to elucidate reaction mechanisms and to determine the extent to which a drug is degraded under solution and temperature conditions. It is quite apparent that the first-order kinetic process occurs readily in many reactions of pharmaceutical concern and in biological systems with which drug absorption, distribution, and elimination can be studied. Thus, it is especially important that the first-order kinetic equations and their properties be thoroughly understood. The temperature effect on the reaction rate provides an important tool in drug product development. For a factor of such importance, readers may appreciate the fact that the Arrhenius equation is an empirical expression, numerous studies over the past 120 years have been carried out to verify its validity, and among the most important works are the theories of the rate constant, which greatly improve our understanding of the temperature-dependent rate process.

VII. References

1. Stability considerations in dispensing practice, in *USP 31/NF 26, United States Pharmacopeia, National Formulary.* Rockville, MD, United States Pharmacopeial Convention Inc., 2008, vol 1, chap 1191, pp 656–659.

2. Dearborn EH in Windheuser JJ, and Blackstein WL: *The Dating of Pharmaceuticals.* Madison, WI, University Extension, University of Wisconsin, 1970, p 29.
3. Cornelissen PJG, Beijersbergen van Hensgouven GMJ, and Gerritsma KW. *Int J Pharm.* 1:173, 1978.
4. Koltun WL, Roth BH, and Gurd RN. *J Biol Chem.* 238:124–131, 1963.
5. O'Donnell JP, Proveaux WJ, and Ma JKH. *J Pharm Sci.* 68:1256–1258, 1979.
6. Swain CG. *J Am Chem Soc.* 70:2989, 1948.
7. Garrett ER. *J Pharm Sci.* 49:767, 1960.
8. Windheuser JJ and Higuchi T. *J Pharm Sci.* 51:354, 1962.
9. Mendez R, Alemany T, and Martin-Villacorta J *Chem Pharm Bull. (Tokyo)* 40:3222–3227, 1992.
10. Tsuji A, Nakashima E, Hamano S, and Yamana T. *J Pharm Sci.* 67:1059–1066, 1978.
11. Edward IJ. *Trans Farady Soc.* 46:723, 1950.
12. Garrett ER. *J Am Chem Soc.* 79:3401, 1957.
13. Michaelis L and Menten ML. *Biochem. Z.* 49:333, 1913.
14. Amirjahed AK. *J Pharm Sci.* 66:785, 1977.
15. Zoglio MA, Windheuser JJ, Vatti R, et al. *J Pharm Sci.* 57:2080, 1968.
16. Edel B and Baltzer MO. *J Pharm Sci.* 69:287–290, 1980.
17. Zhan X, Yin G, and Ma B. *J Pharm Sci.* 86:1099–1104, 1997.
18. Zhan X, Yin G, Wang L, and Ma B. *J Pharm Sci.* 86:709–715, 1997.
19. Oliva A, Hidalgo M, Alvarez C, Llabres M, and Farina JB. *Drug Dev Ind Pharm.* 32:947–953, 2006.
20. Wolfram S. *Mathematica: A System for Doing Mathematics by Computer.* Redwood City, CA, Addison-Wesley, 1988.
21. Connors KA, Amidon GL, and Kennon L. *Chemical Stability of Pharmaceuticals.* New York, Wiley, 1979, pp 28–32.
22. Simonelli AP and Dresback DS, in Francke DE and Whitney HAK (eds), *Perspectives in Clinical Pharmacy*, Hamilton, IL, Drug Intelligence Publications, chap 19, 1972.

Recommended Readings

Guidance for Industry Q1A(R2) Stability Testing of New Drug Substances and Products. http://www.fda.gov/cber/gdlns/ichstab.pdf. Published November 2003. Accessed October 24, 2008.

Britlain HG (ed). *Analytical Profiles of Drug Substances and Excipients*, San Diego, CA, Academic Press, 2000, vol 27.

Connors KA, Amidon GL, and Stella VJ. *Chemical Stability of Pharmaceuticals: A Handbook for Pharmacists.* New York, Wiley, 1986, 2nd ed.

Yoshioka S and Stella VJ. *Stability of Drugs and Dosage Forms.* Boston, Kluwer Academic Publisher, 2002.

VIII. Homework Problems

1. Consider the hydrolysis of ethyl ester of acetic acid in the following equation:

$$CH_3CO\text{—}OCH_2CH_3 + H_2O \rightarrow CH_3COOH + HOCH_2CH_3$$

(*a*) Describe the point of attack by H^+ and OH^- and the reaction mechanism of this reaction.

(*b*) If a radiolabeled hydroxide, that is, $O^{18}H^-$, is used for the specific base catalysis, where is the radioisotope ending up, in CH_3COO^- or CH_3CH_2OH?

2. Plot the following data and determine (*a*) the reaction order and (*b*) the rate constant, half-life, and the shelf life of the drug product.

% Potency	Time (mo)
100.0	0
94.4	1
89.0	2
84.0	3
70.6	6
49.9	12
35.2	18

3. A suspension shows zero-order kinetics with a rate constant of 1.0 mg/mL-mo. (*a*) If the suspension has a concentration of 10 mg/mL, calculate the shelf life. (*b*) If the drug solubility is 0.1 mg/mL, what are the first-order rate constant and the shelf life for the drug in solution?

4. Consider the *bromoform reaction* of acetone with bromine. The overall reaction is

$$CH_3COCH_3 + 3Br_2 + 4OH^- \rightarrow CH_3COO^- + HCBr_3 + 3Br^- + 3H_2O$$

Kinetic studies showed that the rate of this reaction is second-order:

$$-d[\text{acetone}]/dt = k[\text{acetone}][OH^-]$$

If the first, second, and third steps of this reaction are

$$CH_3COCH_3 + OH^- \underset{k_{-1}}{\overset{k_1}{\rightleftharpoons}} CH_3COCH_2^- + H_2O$$

$$CH_3COCH_2^- + Br_2 \xrightarrow{k_{-2}} CH_3COCH_2Br + Br$$

$$CH_3COCH_2Br + OH^- \rightarrow CH_3COCHBr^- + H_2O$$

what is the reaction mechanism? Derive a rate equation to explain the observed reaction kinetics.

5. The decomposition of a colorant in a multisulfa preparation shows the following temperature dependence:

t (°C)	k (day^{-1})
40	0.00011
50	0.00028
60	0.00062
70	0.00156

What is the activation energy for this reaction?

6. The half-life of a drug that decomposes by first-order kinetics is 55 days. What are the rate constant and the shelf life?

7. The rate constant for procaine at 40°C is 0.011 s^{-1}. The activation energy is 13,800 cal/mol. Calculate k and the half-life at 0°C.

8. Atropine base decomposes with a rate constant of 0.016 s^{-1} at 40°C. The energy of activation is 7.7 kcal/mol. Calculate k and the half-life at 10°C.

9. A product you currently possess has an expiration date of 20 mo from the current date when stored in a refrigerator (5°C). It is inadvertently left at room temperature (25°C) for 1 mo. Calculate a new estimate of the expiration date.

10. A product has a t_{90} of 48 h in a refrigerator. What would t_{90} be at 20°C?

11. If a suspension that has a 14-day shelf life at 5°C is left at room temperature for 1 day, by how much might the expiration date be reduced?
12. Calculate Q_{10} for the temperature interval of 15 to 25°C at E_a values of 10, 15, and 20 kcal/mol.
13. A pharmacist found a 5-year-old bottle of tablets in his supply, and from the drug monograph she learned that the decomposition rate constant at room temperature is 4.46×10^{-2} yr^{-1}. What is the calculated potency of the tablets?
14. Consider the following reaction:

$$A + B + H^+ \xrightarrow{k_{obs}} \text{products} + H^+$$

If the condition is such that (1) the initial concentration of A is much greater than that of B and (2) the reaction was carried out at constant pH, what are the rate equation and k_{obs}?
15. An acid (H^+) catalyzed reaction of A and B was found to follow this mechanism:

$$A + H^+ \underset{k_2}{\overset{k_1}{\rightleftarrows}} X$$

$$X + B \xrightarrow{k_3} P + H^+$$

Here X represents the formation of an intermediate, and P represents the products.
(*a*) What is the rate of change for X (dX/dt)?
(*b*) What is the overall rate of product formation (dP/dt)?
(*c*) In what condition does the reaction rate follow pseudo first-order kinetics?
16. If the initial concentrations of A and B in a second-order reaction are the same, the kinetic expression can be written as follows:

$$(C_A - [A])/[A] = C_A k_t$$

Here C_A is the initial concentration of A (or B), and [A] is the concentration of A (or B) at time t. If the initial concentration C_A is 0.01 M, and the rate constant is 6.364 M^{-1} min^{-1}, what is the half-life (t_{50}) of this reaction? What would be the half-life if the reaction were started with an initial concentration of 0.005 M?
17. The rate constants of a reaction at 45 and 25°C were found to be 0.045 and 0.006 min^{-1}, respectively. What is the activation energy E_a for this reaction?
18. If the shelf life of a drug product is calculated based on a minimum potency of 95% of the initial preparation, what is the relationship of this shelf life with the rate constant, assuming that the degradation follows first-order kinetics?
19. Calculate the shelf life of a suspension formulation containing 325 mg of aspirin per 5 mL of solution buffered at pH 6.0. The first-order rate constant for aspirin at 25°C is 3.7×10^{-6} s^{-1}, and the solubility of aspirin in water is 1 g per 100 mL.
20. The rate constant for the degradation of a drug following zero-order kinetics was determined to be 0.02 mg/mL-day. If the initial concentration of the drug was 500 mg/mL in a 20-mL package, determine the shelf life.
21. A single oral dose (100 mg) of an antibiotic was given to an adult male. The equation that best fits the plasma–time curve of this drug for this patient is

$$C_p = 450(e^{-0.175t} - e^{-1.5t})$$

Calculate (*a*) t_{max}, (*b*) C_{max}, and (*c*) $t_{1/2}$ for the drug in this patient. Here C_p is in micrograms per milliliter and the rate constants are in hour^{-1}.

PART

II

PHARMACEUTICAL DEVELOPMENT I: SOLID DOSAGE FORMS

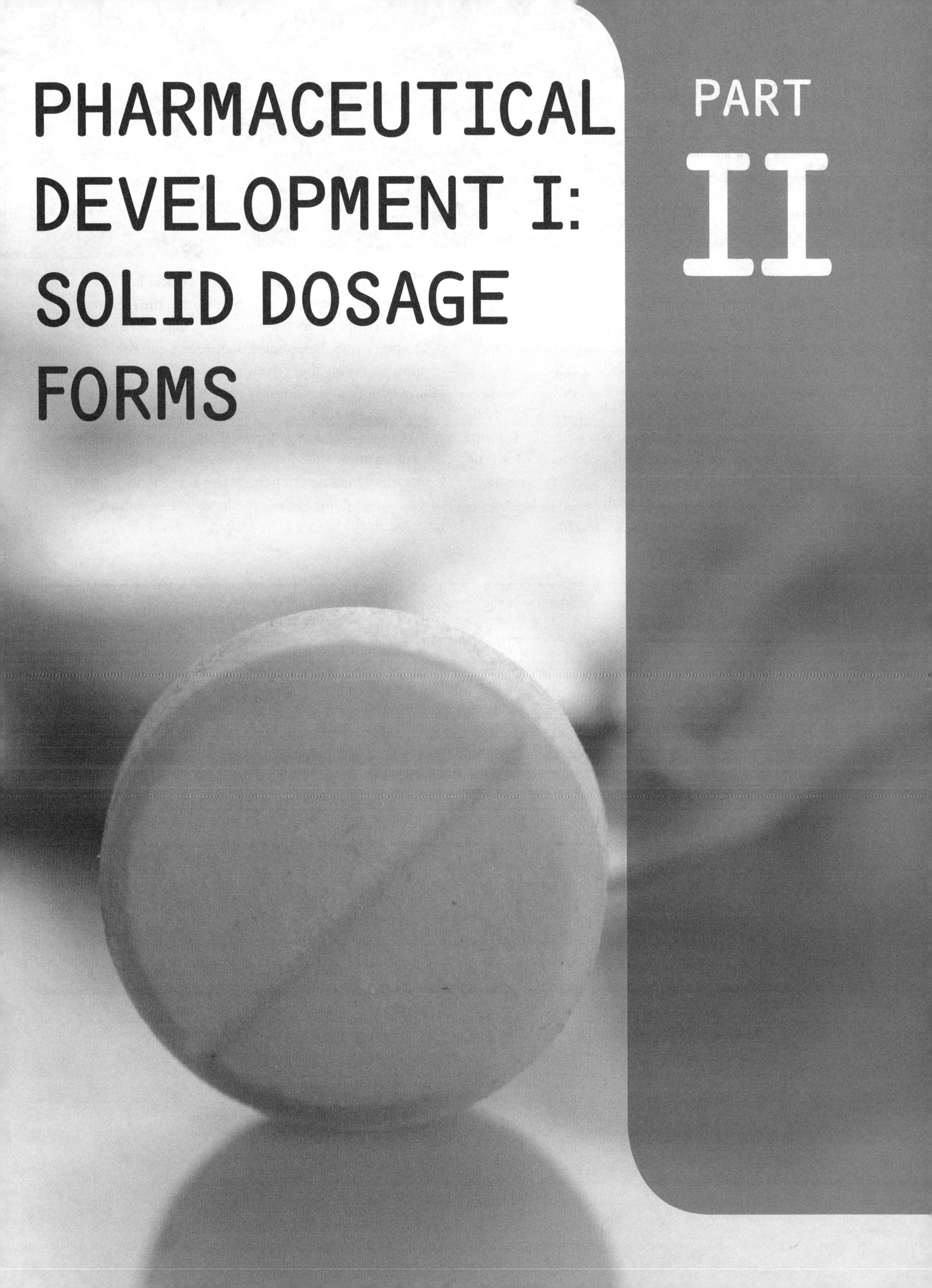

Drug Absorption, Bioavailability, and Dosage Forms: A Regulatory Perspective

CHAPTER 7

Hae-Young Ahn

When a drug product is administered to a person, it is absorbed, distributed to different tissues and organs, metabolized, and excreted via urine and feces. A drug's therapeutic effects depend on how much drug is available at the effect site, and the concentrations of drug at the effect site are dependent on how much of and how fast a drug is absorbed. If you suffered from headache, you would want to take a drug product that is both fast and effective. If you were afflicted with a chronic disease such as cancer, it would be important for drug concentrations to be above the minimal effective concentrations for a certain period of time (amount of absorption), and the rate of absorption may not be as much a concern.

The study of drug absorption is of critical importance in developing new drugs and establishing the therapeutic equivalence of new formulations or generic versions of existing drugs. Different dosage forms and routes of administration affect the drug's absorption and bioavailability, and ultimately its therapeutic effects. Because most drugs are administered orally, the discussion here will focus on oral dosage forms. This chapter will review drug absorption and bioavailability related to their dosage forms from a regulatory perspective as regulatory agencies, through their guidance and the drug review process, get involved in guiding drug development in this area.

CHAPTER OUTLINE

OBJECTIVES

1. Understand the process of drug absorption.
2. Learn the factors affecting drug absorption and regulatory tools to assess their effects on drug absorption.
3. Describe different dosage forms and their clinical significance.
4. Understand bioavailability and bioequivalence, how bioavailability and bioequivalence are assessed, and the criteria for biowaiver.

I. Drug Absorption

Absorption is the process of movement of a drug from the site of administration into the extracellular compartment of the body. Normally, after a drug is administered, a drug is absorbed, distributed to different tissues, metabolized by enzymes, and excreted in urine and feces, with the exception being the case of intravenous administration. When a drug is administered intravenously, absorption does not take place, as the drug is injected into the blood directly and goes directly into the distribution phase. Understanding drug absorption is of critical importance in developing new drugs, as a drug product's efficacy and safety depend on the amount of drug that is absorbed from its formulation (extent of absorption) and how rapidly the absorption process takes place (rate of absorption).

Drugs are most commonly administered orally, and therefore the gastrointestinal (GI) tract plays an important role in determining the rate and extent of drug absorption. The biologic factors such as surface area for absorption, blood flow to the site of absorption, gastrointestinal pH, GI emptying, and GI motility influence drug absorption. Drug absorption also depends upon solubility, particle size, chemical form, and other physicochemical characteristics of the drug itself. Additionally, the rate and extent of drug absorption can be affected by biopharmaceutical factors related to the dosage form (e.g., tablet, capsule, solution, suspension, emulsion, and gel). These biopharmaceutical factors (i.e., formulation characteristics) influence the rate of drug disintegration and dissolution as well.

From the physiologic standpoint, passive non-ionic diffusion is the mechanism by which most drugs are absorbed. Absorption by passive diffusion is largely governed by the molecular size and shape, degree of ionization, and lipid solubility of a drug. Classical explanations of the rate and extent of drug absorption have been based on the pH-partition theory. Based on this theory, one would predict that weakly acidic drugs are largely un-ionized and lipid-soluble in acid medium, and hence would be better absorbed from the stomach (pH 1–2) than from the upper intestine (pH 3–6). Conversely, weakly basic drugs should be absorbed primarily from the more alkaline contents of the small intestine. In reality, the stomach, however, does not appear to be a major site for the absorption of even acidic drugs. The epithelium of the stomach is lined with a thick mucous layer, and its surface area is small; by contrast, the villi of the upper intestine provide an extremely large surface area (approximately 200 m^2). Accordingly, the rate of absorption of a drug from the intestine is greater than that from the stomach even if the drug is predominantly ionized in the intestine and largely non-ionized in the stomach. Because absorption from the stomach is poor, the rate of gastric emptying becomes an important determinant of the rate of drug absorption. Any factors that accelerate gastric emptying will be likely to increase the rate of drug absorption, whereas any factor that delays gastric emptying is expected to have the opposite effect, regardless of the characteristics of the drug. Slow gastric emptying not only may retard drug absorption but also, in some cases, may lead to less complete drug absorption.

Once the drug is systemically absorbed, normal physiologic processes for distribution and elimination occur, which usually are not influenced by the specific formulation of the drug. The rate of drug release from the product and the rate and extent of drug absorption are important in determining the onset, intensity, and duration of drug action.

II. Factors Affecting Oral Drug Absorption

The rate and extent of drug absorption from the GI tract are affected by many factors. These include physicochemical factors (pK_a, solubility, lipophilicity, polar–nonpolar surface area, presence of hydrogen bonding functionalities, particle size, and crystal form) and physiological factors (GI pH, GI blood flow, gastric emptying, small intestinal transit time, and absorption mechanism).

These are in addition to and affected by specific factors related to the dosage form (e.g., tablet, capsule, solution, suspension, emulsion, and gel). In this section, factors related to the solid oral dosage forms will be discussed from a regulatory perspective.

Disintegration

For solid oral dosage forms, a drug product must first disintegrate into small particles that allow for release of the drug. To monitor uniform tablet disintegration, the United States Pharmacopeia (USP) has established an official disintegration test. It should be borne in mind that disintegration does not imply complete solution of the drug unit or drug substance. The USP defines complete disintegration as "that state in which any residue of the unit, except fragments of insoluble coating or capsule shell, remaining on the screen of the test apparatus is a soft mass having no palpably firm core." The official apparatus for the disintegration test and procedure is described in USP 23.[1] Solid drug products exempted from disintegration tests include troches, tablets that are intended to be chewed, and drug products intended for sustained release or prolonged or repeat action.

Dissolution and Solubility

Dissolution is the process by which a solid drug substance becomes dissolved in a solvent. It is the next step following disintegration in the release of drug product from a solid formulation. Solubility is defined as the mass of solute that dissolves in a specific mass or volume of solvent at a given temperature. Solubility is affected by many factors. One of the most important factors is pH. Other factors that affect the solubility of the drug include temperature, hydrophobicity of the drug, solid form of the drug, and the presence of complexation agents in solution. For pharmaceutical development, the solubility of a drug is determined by dissolving the highest unit dose of the drug in 250 mL of buffer adjusted between pH 1.0 and 8.0. In biologic systems, drug dissolution in an aqueous medium is an important prior condition for systemic absorption. The rate at which drugs with poor aqueous solubility dissolve from an intact or disintegrated solid dosage form in the gastrointestinal tract often controls the rate of systemic absorption of the drug. Thus, a dissolution test can be used to characterize the quality and (in certain specific cases) the performance of the drug product. A dissolution test and release specification is required for all U.S. Food and Drug Administration (FDA)-approved solid oral drug products. The following dissolution testing conditions are recommended by the U.S. FDA through its *Guidance for Industry—Dissolution Testing of Immediate Release Solid Oral Dosage Forms*.[2]

Apparatus

The most commonly employed dissolution methods are the basket method, using *Apparatus 1*, and the paddle method, using *Apparatus 2*, as described in USP 23.[3] The basket and paddle methods are simple, robust, and well standardized and are used worldwide. These methods are flexible enough to allow dissolution testing for a variety of drug products. The in vitro dissolution procedures, such as the reciprocating cylinder (*Apparatus 3*) and a flow-through cell system (*Apparatus 4*) described in the USP,[4] may be considered if needed.

Dissolution Medium

Dissolution testing should be carried out under conditions that mimic physiological conditions, if possible. This allows interpretation of dissolution data with regard to in vivo performance of the product. The testing conditions should be based on physicochemical characteristics of the drug substance and the environmental conditions the dosage form might be exposed to after oral administration. The volume of the dissolution medium is generally 500, 900, or 1000 mL.

An aqueous medium with pH range of 1.2 to 6.8 should be used. Use of water as a dissolution medium is discouraged because test conditions such as pH and surface tension can vary depending on the source of water and may change during the dissolution test itself, due to the influence of the active and inactive ingredients. The use of surfactants to enhance solubility is generally discouraged. All dissolution tests should be conducted at 37 ± 0.5°C.

Agitation

In general, mild agitation conditions should be maintained during dissolution testing to allow maximum discriminating power and to detect products with poor in vivo performance. With the basket method, the common agitation is 50–100 rpm, and with the paddle method it is 50–75 rpm.

Permeability

Permeability indirectly measures the extent of absorption of a drug substance in humans and directly measures the rate of mass transfer across human intestinal membrane. The determination of drug permeability can be carried out in both human and nonhuman systems (e.g., in vitro epithelial cell culture methods) capable of predicting the extent of drug absorption in humans. The permeability of a drug substance in human subjects can be determined using mass balance, absolute bioavailability, or intestinal perfusion approaches. Recommended methods not involving human subjects include in vivo or in situ intestinal perfusion in a suitable animal model (e.g., rats), and/or in vitro permeability methods using excised intestinal tissues, or monolayers of suitable epithelial cells. These methods are described by the FDA via its guidance for industry on dissolution testing and waiver of in vivo bioavailability and bioequivalence studies for immediate-release solid oral dosage forms based on the biopharmaceutics classification system.[2]

Rate-Limiting Steps in Drug Absorption

Systemic drug absorption from a drug product consists of a succession of rate processes. For solid oral, immediate-release drug products, the rate processes include (1) disintegration of the drug product and subsequent release of the drug, (2) dissolution of the drug in an aqueous environment, and (3) absorption across cell membranes into the systemic circulation. In the process of drug disintegration, dissolution, and absorption, the rate at which the drug reaches the circulatory system is determined by the slowest step in the sequence. The slowest step in a series of kinetic processes is called the rate-limiting step. In general, disintegration of a solid oral immediate-release drug product is usually more rapid than drug dissolution and drug absorption. For drugs that have very poor aqueous solubility, the dissolution rate is often the slowest step and therefore exerts a rate-limiting effect on drug bioavailability. For a drug that has a high aqueous solubility, however, the dissolution rate is rapid, and the rate at which the drug crosses or permeates cell membranes is the slowest or rate-limiting step.

III. Dosage Forms

Drugs are not generally given as pure chemical drug substances but are formulated into finished dosage forms (drug products) with various excipients. *Excipients* are defined as substances other than the pharmacologically active drug or product, but are included in the manufacturing process or are contained in a finished pharmaceutical product dosage form. These include binders to form a tablet, aggregates to keep the tablet together, disintegrants to aid dissolution once the drug is administered, and coloring or flavoring agents. Excipients help keep the drug in the desired form until administration, aid in delivering the drug, control the release rate of the drug, or make the product more appealing in some way to the patient.

Drug products are designed to deliver drug for local or systemic effects. Therefore, dosage forms must be viewed as a drug delivery "system." As such, its selection could be important to the clinical outcome of a given course of therapy, as a drug product may exhibit several fold difference in the rate or extent of gastrointestinal drug absorption when compared to other products for the same drug, depending on the dosage form or the formulation thereof. As a general principle, the bioavailability of a drug would decrease in the following order: solution > suspension > capsule > tablet. Although this ranking is not universal, it nevertheless provides a useful guideline. This section discusses some of the potential effects on absorption that may be observed with conventional dosage forms.

Solutions

With rare exception, drugs are absorbed more rapidly when administered as an aqueous solution than in any other oral dosage forms. In most instances, the rate-limiting step in the absorption of a drug from a solution dosage form is likely to be gastric emptying. Many drugs, unless converted to a soluble salt, are poorly soluble in water. Aqueous solutions can be prepared by adding cosolvents such as alcohol or propylene glycol, complexing agents that form water-soluble complexes with the drug, or surfactants.

Suspensions

In general, the aqueous suspension is second in the rate of absorption to a solution dosage form. Unlike solution dosage form, however, suspensions require a dissolution step for a drug to be absorbed. Among critical factors to consider in formulating suspension dosage forms for maximal absorption are particle size of the suspended particle, inclusion of wetting agents, formation of insoluble complexes, crystal form, and viscosity. The higher the viscosity of a suspension, the slower is the dissolution rate as the time to achieve dispersion of the suspension would be increased.

Capsules

The capsule dosage form is generally an efficient drug delivery system. The hard gelatin shell encapsulating the formulation should disrupt quickly and expose the contents to the gastrointestinal fluids. Upon disruption of the shell, the drug content, being a loose powder, should disperse rapidly, exposing a large surface area to the fluids in the GI tract. Factors that may influence drug absorption from capsule dosage forms include the particle size, crystal form of the drug, and selection of diluents and fillers.

Tablets

After ingestion, the tablet breaks down first to granules and then to drug particles. The disintegration and dissolution processes take place in the gastrointestinal fluids after oral administration of a tablet. A tablet that fails to disintegrate or disintegrates slowly may cause incomplete absorption or an undue delay in the onset of clinical response at best and a blunting or failure to achieve efficacious levels at worst. However, tablet disintegration, although important, is unlikely to be the rate-limiting step in the absorption of drugs administered as conventional tablets. In most instances, granule disintegration and drug dissolution occur at a slower rate than tablet disintegration.

Many factors related to the formulation or manufacture of tablets may affect drug dissolution and absorption. Most formulations require the incorporation of hydrophobic lubricants such as magnesium stearate to produce an acceptable tablet. In general, lubricants, being generally hydrophobic, reduce the rate of drug dissolution from a formulation: the larger the quantity of lubricant, the slower the dissolution rate. Compression force may also be an important factor in drug availability from compressed tablets. The in vitro disintegration time of tablets has been shown to be directly proportional to compression force and tablet hardness. High compression forces may also increase the strength of the internal structure of the granules and retard dissolution of drug from the granules and disintegration of the granules.

Controlled-Release Preparations

The rate of absorption of a drug administered as a tablet or other solid oral dosage form is partly dependent on its rate of dissolution in GI fluids. This is the basis for controlled-release preparations that are designed to produce slow, uniform absorption of the drug. Potential advantages of such preparations include the reduction in the frequency of administration of the drug as compared with conventional dosage forms (possibly with improved compliance by the patient), maintenance of a therapeutic effect for longer periods, and decreased incidence and/or intensity of both undesired effects (by reduction of the peaks in drug concentration) and subtherapeutic blood levels of the drug (by increase of troughs in concentration) that often occur after administration of immediate-release dosage forms (see **Figure 7-1** for illustration). The controlled-release dosage forms are most appropriate for drugs with short half-lives (< 4 h).

There are, however, some drawbacks related to the controlled-release formulation. Generally, interindividual variability in terms of the systemic concentration of the drug achieved by controlled-release dosage form is greater than that of the immediate-release dosage form. During repeated drug administration, trough drug concentrations resulting from controlled-release dosage forms may not be markedly different from those achieved with immediate-release preparations, although the time interval between trough concentrations is greater for a well-designed controlled-release product than for the conventional dosage form. It is also possible that the dosage form may fail, and "dose dumping" may occur and result in serious toxicity, as the total dose of drug ingested at one time via the controlled-release preparation may be several times the amount contained in the conventional preparation. Factors that may contribute to dose dumping for certain controlled-release preparations include stomach pH and administration along with a high-fat meal.

IV. Bioavailability and Bioequivalence

Bioavailability

Although the formulation concern of a solid dosage form places its emphasis on the absorption of drug following its dissolution, the clinician is concerned primarily with the drug's bioavailability rather than absorption per se. *Bioavailability* is a term used to indicate the fractional extent to which a dose of drug reaches its site of action or a biological fluid from which the drug has access to its site of action. For orally administered products, it depends on the formulation-specific dissolution process and resulting absorption, but also on the interaction of the drug with the systemic system. For example, a drug given orally must be absorbed first from the stomach and intestine, but this may be limited by the characteristics of the dosage form and the drug's physicochemical properties.

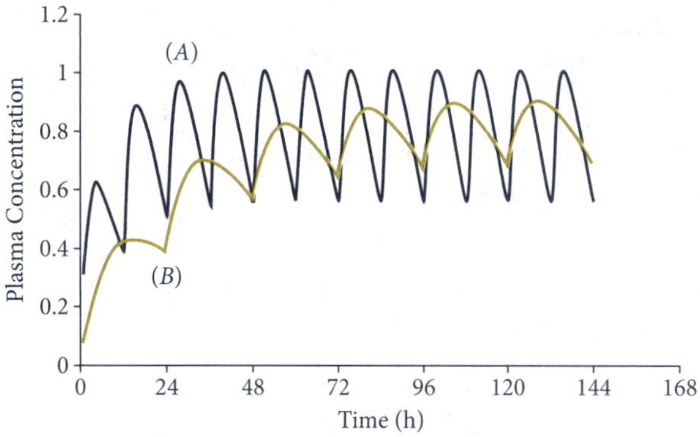

Figure 7-1 Comparison of plasma concentration–time curves of immediate-release (*A*) and controlled-release (*B*) dosage forms.

A drug then passes through the liver, where metabolism and biliary excretion may occur before the drug enters the systemic circulation. If the metabolic or excretory capacity of the liver for the drug is large, bioavailability will be reduced substantially.

The stability of the drug in the gastrointestinal tract is another factor that alters the bioavailability of the drug. Some drugs, such as penicillin G, are unstable in the acidic medium of the stomach. The addition of buffering in the formulation or the use of an enteric coating on the dosage form will protect the drug from degradation at a low pH by retarding the disintegration and dissolution processes until the dosage form reaches a more favorable pH environment in the upper intestine. Some drugs have poor bioavailability because of first-pass effects (presystemic elimination). If the oral drug bioavailability is poor due to metabolism by enzymes in the gastrointestinal tract or in the liver, then a higher dose may be needed, as in the case of propranolol, or an alternative route of drug administration, as in the case of insulin. Drugs that are only partially absorbed after oral administration usually leave residual drug in the gastrointestinal tract, which may cause local bowel irritation or alter the normal gastrointestinal flora. If the drug is not absorbed after the oral route or causes toxicity at the required high doses to achieve bioavailability, then the drug might be given by an alternative route of administration, and a different dosage form, e.g., a parenteral drug product, might be needed.

Bioavailability (BA) is best defined as the rate and extent to which the active ingredient or active moiety is absorbed from a drug product and becomes available at the site of action. This definition focuses on the processes by which the active ingredients or moieties are released from an oral dosage form and move to the site of action. Bioavailability is the term most often used to characterize drug absorption. For orally administered drug products, BA can be documented by developing a systemic exposure profile that monitors the concentration of active ingredients and/or active moieties over time in samples collected from the systemic circulation. As shown in **Figure 7-2**, three *indices of drug bioavailability* usually are estimated: the maximum drug concentration in plasma (C_{max}), the time needed to reach this maximum (t_{max}), and the area under the plasma concentration–time curve (AUC). The C_{max} and AUC measured after administration of a drug dose are related to the rate and extent of drug absorption, respectively. The clinical significance of variations in the bioavailability of drug products has been the subject of intense debate, and one regulatory objective of a BA study is to assess the performance of the formulations used in the clinical trials that provide evidence of safety and efficacy.

Bioequivalence

The term *bioequivalence* (BE) is usually used to assess the bioavailability of a drug in two formulations. Bioequivalence is defined as the absence of a significant difference in the rate and extent to which the active ingredient or active moiety from the two pharmaceutical equivalents becomes available at the site of action when administered at the same molar dose under similar conditions. In other words, the two drug products having the same active moiety and at the same molar dose are considered bioequivalent if their rate and extent of absorption are similar enough to ensure comparable in vivo performance. Bioequivalence must be demonstrated between a pharmaceutically

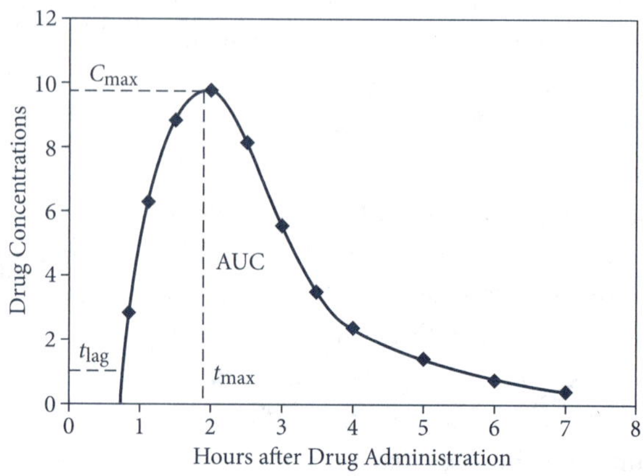

Figure 7-2 Determination of the bioavailability of a drug dose through oral administration.

equivalent generic drug product and the corresponding referenced drug product. In addition, bioequivalence must be established between pre- and postchange products if significant changes in the manufacturing site and process occur.

The extent and rate of absorption constitute the basis of bioequivalence testing. Assessment of BE is generally achieved by performing in vivo human pharmacokinetic studies that intend to prove the similarity between two products. However, there are situations in which BE studies can be substituted with in vitro data. The term *biowaivers* refers to these exceptions to the requirement to perform clinical studies. A common type of biowaiver adopted by the regulatory authorities includes the application of the Biopharmaceutics Classification System (BCS).

V. Biopharmaceutics Classification System

As discussed earlier, the rate and extent of drug absorption from the gastrointestinal drug product are affected by many factors including physicochemical factors (pK_a, solubility, stability, lipophilicity, and particle size), physiological factors (GI pH, GI blood flow, and gastric emptying), and dosage form–related factors. Despite this complexity, recent research has revealed that the fundamental events controlling oral drug absorption are the permeability of the drug through the GI membrane and the solubility of the drug in the GI milieu.[5,6] These key parameters are characterized in the *Biopharmaceutics Classification System* (BCS). Based on the BCS, drug substances are classified as follows:

Class I: high solubility—high permeability

Class II: low solubility—high permeability

Class III: high solubility—low permeability

Class IV: low solubility—low permeability

When combined with the dissolution of the drug product, the BCS provides a framework to consider three major factors that govern the rate and extent of drug absorption from immediate-release (IR) solid oral dosage forms: dissolution, solubility, and intestinal permeability. Within this framework, when certain criteria, as defined by the solubility, permeability, and dissolution of the drug, are met, the BCS can be used as a drug development tool by drug sponsors in justifying requests for biowaivers.

Solubility Consideration

Drug solubility can be measured in vitro and related to the volume of fluid required to dissolve the drug dose completely. The solubility classification of a given drug is based on the highest dose strength in an IR product. According to the FDA guidance on waiver of in vivo bioavailability and bioequivalence studies for immediate-release solid oral dosage forms,[2] a drug substance is considered highly soluble if the highest strength is soluble in 250 mL or less of aqueous media throughout the pH range of 1.2–6.8. Otherwise, the drug substance is considered poorly soluble.

Permeability Consideration

A drug substance is considered highly permeable if the extent of intestinal absorption is determined to be 90% or higher. Otherwise, the drug substance is considered poorly permeable. The permeability classification is based either directly on the extent of intestinal absorption of a drug substance in humans determined by mass balance or in comparison to an intravenous reference dose, or indirectly on the measurements of the rate of mass transfer across the human intestinal membrane. Alternatively, animal or in vitro models that predict human intestinal absorption, e.g., intestinal rat perfusion models or epithelial cell culture models, can be used.

Dissolution

In vitro dissolution tests have been standardized and are widely used for manufacturing quality control and in the evaluation of new formulations and generic products. An IR product is characterized as rapidly dissolved if not less than 85% of the labeled drug amount is dissolved within 30 min using USP *Apparatus 1* at 100 rpm or USP *Apparatus 2* at 50 rpm in a volume of 900 mL or less of each of the following media: (1) acidic media, such as USP-simulated gastric fluid without enzymes; (2) pH 4.5 buffer; and (3) pH 6.8 buffer or USP-simulated intestinal fluid without enzymes. Otherwise, the drug product is considered to be slow-dissolving.

Biowaiver

The BCS of drugs is now adopted by many regulatory authorities including the FDA, the European Medicines Agency (EMA), and the World Health Organization (WHO) for setting bioavailability and bioequivalence (BA and BE) standards for immediate-release oral drug product approval. It is used as a regulatory tool to allow biowaivers of in vivo BA and BE requirements for immediate-release drug products. A drug product belonging to BCS class I can be granted a biowaiver if it dissolves very rapidly (namely, more than 85% dissolution in less than 30 min) in media with pH 1.2, 4.5, and 6.8. In general, the role of excipients is very critical for a BCS-based biowaiver, as excipients may modify gastrointestinal and/or absorption kinetics. Initially, waivers of in vivo BE were accepted only for Scale-Up and Post Approval Changes (SUPAC), but later the biowaiver principle was extended to the approval of new generic drug products, thus avoiding unnecessary human experiments and reducing both the cost and the time of developing generic IR oral drug products.

VI. Chapter Summary

This chapter is written to provide a basic understanding of drug product development from the clinical and regulatory perspectives of oral dosage forms and their effects on drug absorption. The physical pharmacy of dosage form development is discussed in later chapters. The prime considerations in the design of a drug product and dosage form are safety and efficacy. The drug product must effectively deliver the active drug at an appropriate rate and amount to the target site so that the intended therapeutic effect is achieved. Drug absorption varies depending on dosage forms, and therefore it is important to understand the factors that govern the drug absorption and to apply biopharmaceutic knowledge in designing the drug products. Most importantly, the finished drug product should meet the therapeutic objective by delivering the drug with maximum bioavailability and minimum adverse effects.

VII. References

1. USP 23/NF 18. General Chapters on General Tests and Assays, Section ‹701›, *Disintegration*, Rockville, MD, U.S. Pharmacopeial Convention, Inc., 1995, pp 1790–1791.
2. FDA, Center for Drug Evaluation and Research, *Guidance for Industry: Immediate Release Solid Oral Dosage Forms. Scale-up and Post-Approval Changes: Chemistry, Manufacturing and Controls, In Vitro Dissolution Testing, and In Vivo Bioequivalence Documentation* [SUPAC-IR], November 1995. Accessed at http://www.fda.gov/cder/guidance.htm.
3. USP 23/NF 18. General Chapters on General Tests and Assays, Section ‹711›, *Dissolution*, Rockville, MD, U.S. Pharmacopeial Convention, Inc., 1995, pp 1791–1793.

4. USP 23/NF 18. General Chapters on General Tests and Assays, Section ‹724›, *Drug release*, Rockville, MD, 1995, The United States Pharmacopeial Convention, Inc., pp 1793–1795.
5. Amidon GL, Lennernas H, Shah VP, and Crison JR. A Theoretical Basis For a Biopharmaceutic Drug Classification: The Correlation of In Vitro Drug Product Dissolution and In Vivo Bioavailability. *Pharm Res.* 12:413–420, 1995.
6. Skelly JP, Amidon GL, Barr WH, Benet LZ, Carter JE, Robinson JR, Shah VP, and Yacobi A. In Vitro and In Vivo Testing and Correlation for Oral Controlled/Modified-Release Dosage Forms. *Pharm Res.* 7:975–982, 1990.

CHAPTER 8

Diffusion, Dissolution, and Permeability

The core idea of the FDA's Biopharmaceutics Classification System (BCS) is to rationalize the use of in vitro models to predict oral drug absorption by centrally embracing a drug's solubility and permeability as the crucial parameters. Solubility and solution pH are deciding factors for the dissolution of drugs from solid dosage forms. Thus, dissolution and permeability are the key processes for the determination of oral drug absorption. The physicochemical principle that describes these processes is the diffusion law, which when certain conditions are met becomes a product of solubility and permeability. This chapter examines the diffusion principles, the processes and methods from which drug substances are transported from solid dosage forms to solution and from solution to solution through a membrane barrier, and the use of in vitro experiments to predict in vivo oral drug absorption. The diffusion process also plays an important role in controlling drug release from special dosage forms. However, we postpone this discussion to a later chapter when advanced drug delivery strategies are being discussed.

CHAPTER OUTLINE

OBJECTIVES

1. Be able to define the process of diffusion through Fick's first law, the diffusion coefficient, and molecular properties relating to the diffusion coefficient.
2. Understand the concept of diffusion layer and thickness.
3. Understand the nature of Fick's second law of diffusion and sink conditions.
4. Be able to describe the time–diffusion layer thickness relationship.
5. Define permeability and its relationship with the diffusion coefficient.
6. Describe the dissolution process based on Fick's law of diffusion involving a constant surface area and a change in particle size.
7. Be able to discuss conditions in dissolution testing experiments and the use of biorelevant simulated intestinal fluids.
8. Understand the concept of unstirred water layer (UWL) and drug permeability through UWL.
9. Understand the role of solubility in determining the dissolution and oral absorption of drugs that are poorly soluble in water.

I. The Diffusion Phenomena

Fick's Law of Diffusion

Fick's First Law of Diffusion

The hydrodynamic nature of a solution is such that the molecules of a dissolved solute will move from a region of higher concentration to a region of lower concentration until the system reaches a homogeneous concentration. This process is termed *diffusion*, and it occurs naturally because the process is accompanied by a decrease in chemical potential or partial free energy change. In a carefully defined liquid boundary into pure solvent, one can show that the rate of diffusion is proportional to (1) the concentration gradient dc/dx, across the boundary, where c is the concentration of the solute in grams per milliliter of solution, and (2) the cross-sectional area A. If the diffusion rate is written as dW/dt, the number of grams of solute transferred across the boundary per second is then

$$dW/dt = -DA\, dc/dx \qquad (8\text{-}1)$$

Here, the proportional constant D is called the diffusion coefficient, and the negative sign is introduced so that D will have a positive value. Equation (8-1) is known as *Fick's first law of diffusion*. The diffusion coefficient can be recognized as the amount of solute that diffuses across a 1 cm^2 area in 1 s under the influence of a concentration gradient of 1 g/mL-cm. The diffusion coefficient (in units of square centimeters per second) is, therefore, characteristic of the diffusing tendency of the solute for a given solvent and temperature. If the amount of solute is measured in grams per second per unit area, that is, $dw = dW/A$, then Equation (8-1) can also be written as

$$J = dw/dt = -D\, dc/dx \qquad (8\text{-}1a)$$

where dw/dt is known as the *flux* (J).

Molecular View of Diffusion Coefficient

The diffusing tendency of a solute can be analyzed based on the driving forces and counterforces in the diffusion process. This can be best appreciated by considering the solute to be a macromolecule of high molecular weight. Because diffusion is spontaneous, the driving force for diffusion is the partial free energy change of the solute. If diffusion occurs in a distance interval of dx over which the concentration changes from c to $c - dc$, then the free energy change (work done in the transfer of one molecule across a distance of dx) will be

$$dG = (RT/N)\ln[(c - dc)/c] = (RT/N)\ln(1 - dc/c) = -(RT/N)\, dc/c$$

where N is Avogadro's number, and the relation $\ln(1 - y) = -y$ for small y is used. The driving force is then dG/dx, or

$$dG/dx = -(RT/N)\, dc/c\, dx \qquad (8\text{-}2)$$

It should be pointed out that $c\, dx$ is essentially dW/A (or dw), as both terms indicate the amount of solute diffusing across the boundary per area A of the cross section by traveling a distance of dx in a time of dt.

The counterforce to diffusion that allows the system to reach homogeneity is the frictional force exerted by the solution viscosity η. According to *Stokes' law*, for a macromolecule with a radius r,

$$\text{Frictional force} = 6\pi r\eta\, dx/dt \qquad (8\text{-}3)$$

By combining Equations (8-2) and (8-3), it can be seen that

$$6\pi r\eta\, dx/dt = -(RT/N)\, dc/cdx$$

or $$c\, dx/dt = -(RT/6\pi r\eta N)\, dc/dx$$

Substituting dW/A for $c\,dx$, one obtains

$$dW/dt = -(RT/6\pi r\eta N)(A)\, dc/dx$$

Comparing the above expression with Equation (8-1) yields

$$D = RT/6\pi r\eta N \tag{8-4}$$

Equation (8-4) shows that the diffusion coefficient is a function of temperature/viscosity (T/η) and is related to the radius of the solute molecule. For macromolecules, it is perhaps easy to see that the diffusion coefficient will decrease with a large increase in molecular weight. It may be possible to determine the radius of a macromolecule using Equation (8-4). But such a procedure may not be satisfactory because both the viscosity and the effective radius are subject to change with respect to the solvent type, concentration, and temperature. As we shall see, Equation (8-4) may be refined with further experiments.

Sedimentation and Ultracentrifugation

The above section shows the natural tendency for a molecule to diffuse across a concentration gradient. If the solute molecules have a density higher than that of the solvent, they can be made to alter their distribution in space by added forces. The simplest phenomenon is sedimentation, which can be obtained by letting the solution stand so that the force of gravity acts. A greater effect, however, can be produced by means of an ultracentrifuge in which the solution rotates at a very high speed (10,000 to 80,000 g). One can start with a well-defined boundary, or layer of solution, near the center of rotation and follow the movement of this layer toward the outside of the cell as a function of time (a sedimentation velocity experiment). The centrifugal force that moves the solute to the outside of the cell is given by

$$f_{\text{centrifugal}} = m'r'w^2$$

where m' is the effective mass of the solute, r' is the distance to the center of rotation, and w is the angular velocity. Because the centrifugal force is effective only when the density of the solute is greater than the density of the solvent, the effective mass can be calculated as

$$m' = m(1 - v\rho)$$

where m is the actual mass, v is the volume of 1 g of solute, and ρ is the density of the solvent. The term $v\rho$ gives the weight of solvent at the same volume of the solute. Hence, $1 - v\rho$ is the weight difference between solute and solvent at the specific volume (mL/g) of the solute. When the centrifugal force is balanced by the frictional force ($= 6\pi r\eta\, dr/dt$) given by Stokes' law (Equation (8-3)), it can be seen that

$$dr/(r'w^2)\, dt = S = m(1 - v\rho)/6\pi r\eta \tag{8-5}$$

The term on the left-hand side of the equation, $dr/(r'w^2)\, dt$, is a characteristic value of a macromolecule, known as the *sedimentation coefficient* S. It is defined as the velocity (dr/dt) with which a macromolecule moves per unit centrifugal field $r'w^2$. Rearrangement of Equation (8-5), followed by converting the mass into molecular weight using Avogadro's number N, gives

$$M = 6\pi r\eta NS/(1 - v\rho) \tag{8-6}$$

Table 8-1 Diffusion and Sedimentation Coefficients of Some Proteins

Protein	Sp. Volume (mL/g)	Diffusion Coeff. (cm^2/s)	Sedimentation Coeff. (s)	Mol Wt
Insulin	0.75	8.2×10^{-7}	3.5×10^{-13}	41,000
Hemoglobin	0.73	6.3×10^{-7}	4.4×10^{-13}	67,000
Catalase	0.73	4.1×10^{-7}	11.3×10^{-13}	250,000

When Equation (8-6) is combined with Equation (8-4), the following equation is obtained:

$$M = RTS/D(1 - v\rho) \tag{8-7}$$

It can now be seen that the diffusion (D) and sedimentation (S) coefficients are both dependent on the well-defined quantities of the molecular weight of the solute and the densities of the solute and solvent, rather than the terms of viscosity and radius. With experimental determination of S and D, the molecular weights of macromolecules can be calculated. The use of Equation (8-7) to obtain information for a number of proteins is illustrated in **Table 8-1**.

Fick's Second Law of Diffusion

The diffusion process in a given direction x is manifested by mass transport through a cross section and changes in concentration along the direction of diffusion. This process can be simply illustrated in **Figure 8-1**. Consider the diffusion of the solute from x to $x + dx$ in a time dt, and the concentration changes from c to $c - dc$. According to Fick's first law of diffusion, the amount of solute diffusing across the plane at point x is dW, in that

$$dW/dt = -DA\, dc/dx \tag{8-1}$$

Now if we consider the cross section at $x + dx$, where the concentration is $c - dc$, the mass transfer of the solute dW'/dt at this point can be similarly written as

$$dW'/dt = -DA\frac{\partial}{\partial x}\left[c - \left(\frac{\partial c}{\partial x}\right)dx\right] = -DA\frac{\partial c}{\partial x} + DA\left(\frac{\partial^2 c}{\partial x^2}\right)dx \tag{8-8}$$

In Equation (8-1), dc/dx can be rewritten as $\partial c/\partial x$. Thus, from Equations (8-1) and (8-8), one obtains

$$\frac{dW - dW'}{dt} = -DA\left(\frac{\partial^2 c}{\partial x^2}\right)dx$$

or

$$\frac{dW - dW'}{A\,dx\,dt} = D\frac{\partial^2 c}{\partial x^2}$$

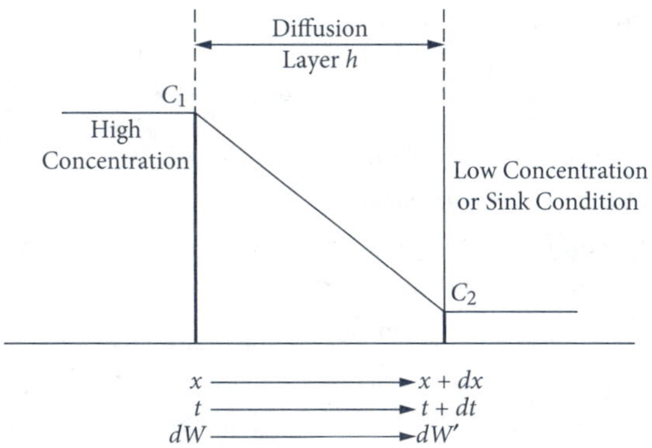

Figure 8-1 Fick's first and second laws of diffusion.

Because $A\,dx$ is the volume between the cross section x and cross section $x + dx$, the left-hand side of the above equation is essentially the change in concentration as a function of time dc/dt, thus,

$$\frac{dc}{dt} = -\frac{dW - dW'}{A\,dx\,dt} = D\frac{\partial^2 c}{\partial x^2} \qquad (8\text{-}9)$$

Equation (8-9) shows that the concentration change per time in the diffusion distance is directly proportional to changes in the difference between concentrations at x and $x + dx$. In other words, if the concentrations are C_1 and C_2 at x and $x + dx$, respectively, then $C_1 - C_2$ is the concentration gradient, and $dc/dt \propto (C_1 - C_2)$. This is known as Fick's second law of diffusion.

Interpretation of Fick's Law of Diffusion

As shown in Figure 8-1, Fick's first law describes the rate of diffusion (dW/dt) through a unit area at plane x under the existence of a concentration gradient in the direction of x. The second law describes the concentration change (dc/dt) at $x + dx$, which is proportional to the concentration gradient ($C_1 - C_2$). The diffusion slows down when the concentration gradient decreases and stops when $C_1 = C_2$, so that the second law is generally referred to as a non-steady-state flow. But the concentration gradient can be made constant through experimental conditions, such as by keeping C_1 at saturation and removing C_2 constantly to create a sink condition. In such a case, $dc/dt = D\partial^2 c/\partial x^2 = 0$. When the second derivative is zero, dc/dx is taken to be a constant, meaning that in the diffusion layer, the concentration changes linearly with changing distance. Thus, the flux can be written as

$$J = -D\,dc/dx = -D\,\Delta C/\Delta x$$

The change in concentration in the diffusion layer (ΔC) is $C_2 - C_1$. If the diffusion layer thickness is h, that is, $h = \Delta x$,

$$J = D(C_1 - C_2)/h \qquad (8\text{-}10)$$

The above discussion shows that the second law defines the necessity of having a concentration gradient, whereas the first law describes the mass transport according to this concentration gradient. It is apparent that a sink condition will ensure the diffusion flow.

Time–Distance Relationship

So far the discussion on diffusion has centered on the relationship of concentration or flux with the diffusion distance. The relation between time and the diffusion distance is also of interest because it can be used to determine the diffusion coefficient. The time–distance relation can be easily understood using Einstein's *random walk* theory. Consider two connected boxes containing a solute. The average concentrations within a distance of x for the two boxes are C_1 and C_2, respectively, where $C_1 > C_2$ (see **Figure 8-2**). Diffusion occurs because of the concentration gradient. Assuming that at time t the diffusion is complete, meaning that one-half of the concentration in box 1 flows to box 2 and one-half of the concentration in box 2 flows to box 1, the net flow (flux) is thus

$$J = C_1x/2t - C_2x/2t$$

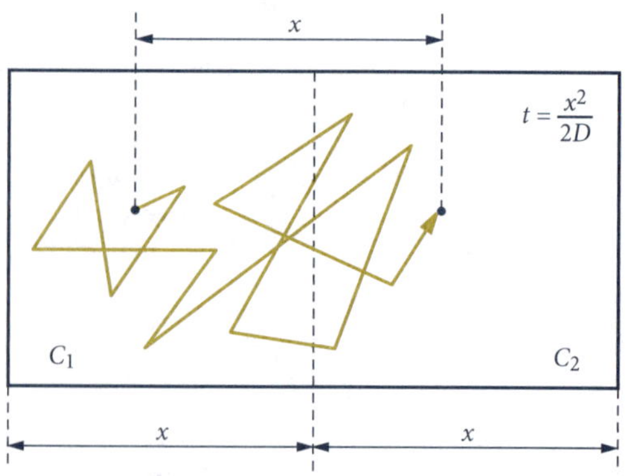

Figure 8-2 Time–distance relationship of diffusion by random walk.

Because $C_2 - C_1 = x\,dC/dx$, where dC/dx is the concentration gradient, it gives

$$J = (1/2t)\,[C_1x - x(C_1 + x\,dC/dx)] = -(x^2/2t)\,dC/dx$$

Substituting for J while using the relation that $J = -D\,dC/dx$, one obtains

$$D = x^2/2t \qquad \text{or} \qquad x = (2Dt)^{1/2} \qquad \text{or} \qquad t = x^2/2D \tag{8-11}$$

Equation (8-11) shows that as a result of random walk (kinetic molecular theory), the time required for a molecule to travel a distance x is $x^2/2D$. If we now consider a diffusion layer with a thickness of h, the time required to reach the outer boundary is thus $h^2/2D$, which may be considered to be the lag time for a natural diffusion system. Using the more complicated diffusion law, one can obtain the same relationship as indicated by the Einstein Equation of (8-11).

Membrane Diffusion and Permeability

The determination of diffusion coefficient of a solute is most commonly done using a system where two solution chambers are separated by a porous membrane that allows the diffusion of the solute. The system should be calibrated with a compound of known diffusion coefficient, from which the area/thickness (A/h) of the membrane can be determined. The diffusion coefficient of the solute can then be determined based on measured flux using the calibrated value of A/h. The diffusion coefficients for compounds in liquid are about $10^{-5}\,\text{cm}^2/\text{s}$ or less, and they can be theoretically calculated using Equation (8-7). As we shall see, a more useful term known as permeability (cm/s) can be determined using the membrane diffusion system.

Passive Diffusion

The passage of molecules through a barrier (a membrane or a drug device) is frequently studied to gain information on the mass transport processes as they relate to drug absorption or drug release from a dosage form design. One of the important processes is passive diffusion, where the mass transfer of molecules is driven by a concentration gradient. The diffusion studies can be carried out using a diffusion cell such as the one shown in **Figure 8-3**.[1] In such a device, the donor and receptor chambers are separated by a natural or synthetic polymeric membrane permeable by the solute, and they contain a drug solution in the donor chamber and the solvent in the receptor chamber. Diffusion of drug from the donor to the receptor compartments is monitored as a function of time under constant temperature and stirring by sampling drug concentrations in the donor and receptor chambers at appropriate time intervals. According to Fick's law, diffusion occurs as long as a diffusion layer exists, which in this case is the thickness of the membrane (see **Figure 8-3B**). Here, the concentration

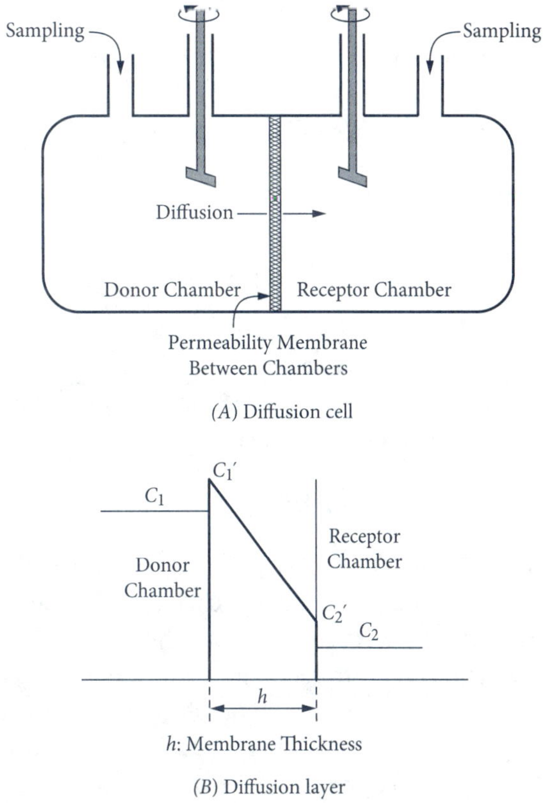

Figure 8-3 (*A*) Diffusion cell and (*B*) concentration gradient in diffusion layer.

gradient is indicated by concentrations C_1' and C_2' inside the membrane boundary, whereas C_1 and C_2 are the concentrations in the donor and receptor chambers, respectively. The C' is related to C by a partition coefficient. Because C_1 decreases while C_2 increases with time, the rate of diffusion will decrease with time and becomes zero when $C_1 = C_2$. In this experiment, C_1 and C_2 are measured experimentally. The concentrations inside the membrane can be determined by the partition equilibrium (K), in that

$$K = C_1'/C_1 = C_2'/C_2$$

The above relationship assumes that the partition coefficient is the same on both sides of the membrane. If the membrane thickness is h, the diffusion phenomenon according to Fick's first law can be written as $dW/A\,dt = D(C_1' - C_2')/h$ or

$$dW/dt = DAK(C_1 - C_2)/h = PA(C_1 - C_2) \qquad P = DK/h \tag{8-12}$$

Here, P is defined as the permeability *or* permeability coefficient, which has units of centimeters per second.

Sink Conditions and Kinetics

Alternative to the above experiment, the studies can be carried out in a manner in which the drug in the receptor chamber is constantly removed, such as by replacing the sample volume collected for drug analysis with the solvent system. In this case, the concentration of the drug in the receptor chamber can be kept very low ($C_2 \approx 0$). Depending on the rate of removal of drug from the receptor chamber, a steady-state (or quasi-stationary) condition may be reached with time where the concentration gradient may become a constant. This is known as the *sink condition* under which the rate of diffusion becomes

$$dW/dt = DAKC_1/h = PAC_1 \qquad (C_2 \approx 0) \tag{8-13}$$

In actual determination of the permeability for a particular membrane system at the sink condition, the diffusion kinetics depends largely on the concentration of C_1. If C_1 is constant, Equation (8-13) can be integrated to give

$$W = PAC_1t \tag{8-14}$$

The diffusion kinetics are zero-order, and the permeability can be determined from the slope of the linear plot of W versus t, and the surface area of the membrane. If C_1 changes appreciably with time, however, Equation (8-13) shows a first-order kinetic model, where C_1 is related to the permeability by the following equation:

$$\log C_1 = \log C_0 - PAt/2.303V_1 \tag{8-15}$$

where C_0 and C_1 are the concentrations in the donor chamber at $t = 0$ and $t = t$, respectively, and V_1 is the volume of the donor chamber. The above discussion shows that the diffusion kinetics through a barrier depend on the drug concentration on both sides of the barrier, as both concentrations affect the concentration gradient across the barrier. The kinetics will be zero-order if excess amount of drug is at the absorption site or in a drug release device and the diffused drug is quickly removed. But the kinetics will be first-order if drug concentration depletes appreciably from the absorption site or the drug-releasing device with time. Indeed, Baker and Lonsdale have shown that a zero-order release of steroids from a zero-order release drug device was achieved only by saturated solution with excess solid drug.[2]

II. Dissolution

Dissolution is a kinetic process by which a solid of moderate solubility enters into solution. Because most commonly the oral drug absorption process begins with the intake of a drug in the solid dosage form, the in vivo dissolution process is of vital importance in determining the bioavailability of the drug. In this light, in vitro drug dissolution tests, which can be used to gain knowledge of the in vivo process, are of equal importance. Indeed, mandatory drug dissolution testing for several drug formulations began in the late 1960s, and it has remained today as one of the most important quality-control tests for many pharmaceutical preparations.

Theory of Dissolution

Diffusion-Based Dissolution Model

Consider a drug particle in a solution under constant mixing. The drug molecules at the particle surface will dissolve, where the concentration will reach the solubility of the drug (C_s) and move to the bulk of the solution by diffusion, because the bulk solution will have an initial concentration of zero and a concentration at time *t* of C_t, which is lower than C_s. Under sufficient mixing, if the bulk concentration can be detected at a distance *h* to the particle surface, then a concentration gradient is established, which can be used to determine the diffusion of dissolved drug from the particle surface by Fick's law:

$$dw/dt = D(C_s - C_t)/h$$

If the particle has a surface area *A* and the solution volume is *V*, then

$$dC/dt = (dw/dt)(A/V) = DA(C_s - C_t)/Vh \quad (8\text{-}16)$$

If the amount of solid particles is sufficiently large, *A* is a constant. Because *D, A, V,* and *h* are all constants, the above equation can be written as

$$dC/dt = k_s(C_s - C_t)$$

where $k_s = DA/Vh$, which is termed the solubilization coefficient. Equation (8-15) shows a first-order kinetic process. But under sink conditions, that is, $C_s >> C_t$,

$$dC/dt = DA(C_s)/Vh$$

The dissolution will show a linear increase in dissolved drug with time according to zero-order kinetics.

The above diffusion-controlled dissolution model was first described by Noyes and Whitney[3] and later modified by Nernst[4] and Brunner.[5] They postulated that a static (unstirred) diffusion layer, with a thickness of *h*, is first formed around the particle surface. This rapid equilibrium process is followed by a slow step in which the dissolved drug diffuses across the boundary layer into the bulk solution. The Nernst–Brunner equation is written as

$$\frac{dW_s}{dt} = -\frac{DA}{h}\left(C_s - \frac{W_d}{V}\right) \quad (8\text{-}17)$$

where W_s is the amount of drug remaining in solid form, W_d is the total amount of drug dissolved at time *t*, *V* is the volume of the solution, and C_s is the solubility of the drug in the bulk solution. Equation (8-17) is essentially the same as Equation (8-16). The diffusion model based on Equation (8-17) is effective in describing the general trend of the dissolution process, but at the same time falls short in explaining the solubility- and particle size–dependent dissolution processes. It can be seen that the dissolution process will have a rapid initial rate, where the slope of the curve is DAC_s/h, followed by gradually slowed rates as W_d/V increases to the value of C_s. This indicates that the solubility at the particle surface determines the initial rate of dissolution, whereas the solubility of the drug in the bulk solution determines the plateau concentration in the bulk solution (see **Figure 8-4** for illustration). Both the initial dissolution rate and the plateau concentration are critical to the drug absorption process. Equation (8-17) considers the solubility of the drug at the particle surface and in the bulk to be the same. But in reality, this is not true for drugs that undergo acid–base dissociation and for dissolution media, such as the biological or biorelevant simulated fluids, which contain bile salts that can alter the solubility of the drug. Greater discussion of the Nernst–Brunner equation is given in later sections.

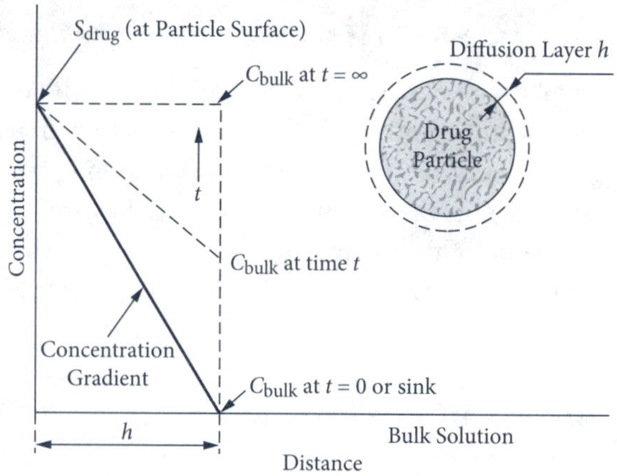

Figure 8-4 Dissolution of solid drug particle.

The Hixson–Crowell Cube Root Dissolution

The Nernst–Brunner equation assumes that the surface area of the solid particles remains constant during the dissolution process. But it is possible to show that, for spherical particles, the solubilization of surface molecules will lead to a reduction in the particle radius r, surface area A, and volume V in that

$$dW = \rho\, dV = \rho 4N\pi r^2\, dr \qquad \text{and} \qquad A = 4N\pi r^2$$

where W is the solid mass, ρ is the density of the solid, and N is the number of particles. Using this approach, it can be shown that the Nernst–Brunner equation at sink condition ($dW/dt = -DAC_s/h$) can be rewritten as

$$\rho\, dr = -(D/h)C_s\, dt$$

Integration from r_0 to r and t from 0 to t gives

$$r = r_0 - (D/h\rho)C_s t \qquad \text{or} \qquad r/r_0 = 1 - DC_s t/\rho h r_0$$

The above equation expresses the dissolution process as a change in the radius of the particles as a function of time. The values of r and r_0 can be changed to mass by the relationship $W = N\rho(\pi/6)(2r)^3$ (mass = density × volume × number of particles). With this substitution, one obtains

$$(W_s/W_0)^{1/3} = 1 - DC_s t/\rho h r_0 \qquad (8\text{-}18)$$

where W_0 and W_s are the weights of the undissolved particles at 0 and time t, respectively. Equation (8-18) is one of the expressions of the *Hixson–Crowell cube root law*,[6] which can be used in dissolution testing assuming the surface area is described by one size (r_0).

Wetting and Drug Release from Dosage Form

The release of drug from a solid dosage form consists of the following steps:

- Wetting of the solid dosage form
- Penetration of the solvent into the formulation
- The swelling process
- Disintegration and disaggregation
- Dissolution

If the adhesive force between a solid and liquid is strong, a liquid film will form around the solid particles, known as wetting. Under moderate adhesive forces, however, where the liquid cannot displace completely other adsorbed molecules on the particle surface, such as air, there will be a contact angle between the solid and liquid phases varying from 0° (complete wetting) to 180° (no wetting). This phenomenon can be described by surface free energy changes expressed in *surface tension* (γ), which can be defined as the energy per unit area or work required to form a unit area of surface. The surface free energy change due to wetting (going from nonwetting to wetting states) involves the change of surface area from solid and liquid surfaces to a solid–liquid interface. Thus the surface free energy change (erg/cm^2) is $\gamma_{SL} - (\gamma_S + \gamma_L)$, where γ_{SL} is the interfacial tension and γ_S and γ_L are the surface tensions of the solid and liquid, respectively. When the free energy change is negative, the process is spontaneous. Thus, the thermodynamic requirement for wetting is $\gamma_{SL} - (\gamma_S + \gamma_L) < 0$, which can be brought about by a surfactant (wetting agent) incorporated in the dosage form that lowers the interfacial tension. The penetration characteristics of the fluid, indicated by $\gamma_S + \gamma_L$, also play an important role in each of the processes mentioned above. The presence of hydrophobic additives in tablets and capsules will reduce the rate of penetration and thus slow down the disaggregation process. Extensive studies have shown that the disintegration process is a poor indicator of bioavailability because of the turbulent and fast agitation used in the test, and this process is generally not affected by factors such as solubility, particle size, and crystallinity of the drug, which are known to be deciding factors for drug dissolution. Nevertheless, all processes shown above affect the rate of drug dissolution and hence the absorption process.

Dissolution Testing

Dissolution Methods

Dissolution testing experiments are carried out by simulating the in vivo sink condition in such a way that the dissolution medium is replaced constantly with fresh solvent so that the solute concentration does not reach more than 10% to 15% of its maximum solubility. Under such conditions, the dissolution process is considered to be under sink conditions; i.e., the initial rate is not affected by the concentration gradient. Several methods are used for dissolution assessment and are accepted as valid procedures. Among these are the rotating filter/stationary basket method, rotating bottle method for sustained-release formulations, open flow-through dissolution system, and several others.

The dissolution tests are described in the USP in individual monographs of solid dosage forms (tablets or capsules), and appropriate apparatuses are specified. All instruments allow the dissolution testing to be carried out at constant temperature of 37 ± 0.5°C. A speed-regulating device allows the rotation speed to be selected and maintained at the rate specified for each monograph. The dissolution medium is usually either water or a buffered solution with pH adjusted to within 0.05 unit of the desired pH as described in the individual monograph.

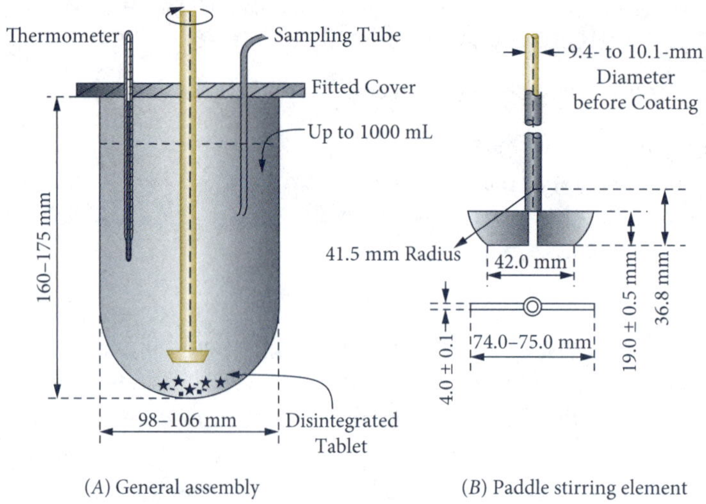

Figure 8-5 USP paddle dissolution apparatus.

Note that the diffusion-based dissolution model assumes the surface area A of the solid and the diffusion layer thickness h to be constants. One can readily see that the surface area is obviously not a constant as the powder, granule, or tablet dissolves, and the diffusion layer thickness is likely changed due to the force of agitation at the surface of the dissolving tablet or granules. These considerations have led to the design of different dissolution apparatuses as well as alternative theories on drug dissolution.[7,8] Detailed descriptions of the various apparatuses and methods are available in the literature.[9] The USP/NF has designated the rotating basket apparatus and paddle apparatus the USP dissolution *Apparatuses 1* and *2*, respectively, and has described the dissolution testing instruments and methods for formulations in the form of uncoated, coated, and enteric-coated tablets. These guidelines are important for pharmaceutical manufacturers and pharmacists to provide tests for drug release and product quality control. **Figure 8-5** shows *Apparatus 2* with the paddle stirring element of standard dimensions. The assembly consists of a covered vessel made of glass or other inert transparent material, a motor, and a metallic rotating paddle. The vessel is partially immersed in a suitable water bath that permits holding the temperature inside the vessel at 37 ± 0.5°C during the test and keeping the bath fluid in constant smooth motion. The vessel is cylindrical, with a hemispherical bottom and a capacity of 1000 mL. A paddle formed from a blade and a shaft is used as the stirring element. The shaft is positioned so that its axis is not more than 2 mm at any point from the vertical axis of the vessel, and it rotates smoothly without significant wobble. In dissolution testing, the distance between the blade and the inside bottom of the vessel, where the tablet was allowed to rest, is maintained at 25 ± 2 mm.

Simulated Intestinal Fluids

The primary objective of dissolution rate studies is to assess oral drug absorption. Hence, it is necessary to keep in mind the physiological conditions with which the dissolution assessment is applied. The volume of GI fluids available for dissolution depends on the volume of coadministered fluids and the secretion of water flux across the gut wall. It has been suggested that the actual volume of the intestinal fluid is around 600 mL.[10] The biopharmaceutics classification system uses 250 mL as the fluid volume when a drug is administered with a cup of water. The major factors that influence the rate of drug dissolution in the gastrointestinal tract are the pH, buffer capacity, and surfactant concentrations of the intestinal fluid. The physiological conditions of the human GI system have been reported in a number of studies.[11–14] In the fasting state, the pH in the stomach after the administration of 250 mL of water varies from 1.2 to 7.4 (median 1.7), and the pH in duodenum and jejunum are 6.2–7.0 and 6.8, respectively. In the fed state, the pH of the stomach is

Table 8-2 Simulated Intestinal Fluids (FaSSIF and FeSSIF)

	Fasting State	Fed State
pH	6.5	6.0
Buffer capacity (M/ΔpH)	0.012	0.076
Taurocholic acid (mM)	3.0	15
Egg lecithin (mM)	0.75	3.75
Osmolarity (mosmol/kg)	270	635

about 6.4.[11] The main buffer species in the intestine is the bicarbonate system, with a reported concentration of about 6.7 mM in the fasting state.[11] The average bile salt concentration in the jejunum is about 3 mM in the fasting state and 5–15 mM in the fed state with a bile salt/phospholipids ratio of about 4 : 1.[11, 15] Because these substances can aggregate into micelles, the solubility of lipophilic drugs can be significantly increased through incorporation into the micelles. This action can result in changes in not only the solubility but also the diffusion coefficient of the drug, as micelle-incorporated drug will diffuse more slowly than free drug in the dissolution process. It is noteworthy that the aggregation state of bile salts varies with varying concentrations.[16, 17] Smaller micelles (< 10 nm) are formed at high concentration, comparing to vesicles (60–70 nm) found in low bile salt/lipid concentration, and upon dilution, the diameter of the aggregates increases to 50 nm.[14] Various simulated biorelevant gastrointestinal fluids have been developed. The most widely studied ones are the fasting state simulated intestinal fluid (FaSSIF) and the fed state simulated intestinal fluid (FeSSIF) (see **Table 8-2**), which contain taurocholic acid and egg lecithin (phosphatidylcholine) in a 4 : 1 molar ratio.[18]

Factors Influencing Dissolution Rate

Diffusion Layer Thickness and Agitation

The dissolution testing usually involves rotational agitation, which is important for the dissolution of coarse particles or disintegration of formulations and granules. The effect of agitation on a dissolution system, such as the paddle apparatus seen in Figure 8-5, can be readily visualized. At low rpm the flow is passive, and the dissolution rate depends on the way solid particles are scattered over the bottom of the vessel. Neither the solid nor the solution may move to the top of the system, which may result in layers of solutions with different concentrations. At very high rpm, the flow is turbulent and the centrifugal force of the rotating solution will force the particles upward and outward. It is thus likely that the force of agitation will change the thickness of the static diffusion layer. Indeed, studies have shown that an increase in agitation strength (in rpm) results in an increase in the dissolution rate constant, and there is an inverse relationship between agitation strength and the diffusion layer thickness.

It is possible to determine the apparent diffusion layer thickness through hydrodynamic theories.[19] For spherical particles with a radius r, the diffusion layer thickness h can be expressed as

$$\begin{aligned} h &= 2r/\mathrm{Sh} \\ \mathrm{Sh} &= 2 + 0.6\mathrm{Re}^{1/2}\mathrm{Sc}^{1/3} \end{aligned} \qquad (8\text{-}19)$$

where Sh is the Sherwood number, Re is the Reynolds number, and Sc is the Schmit number. Equation (8-19) is a semi-empirical equation known as the Ranz–Marshall correction. For large particles, the estimated diffusion layer thickness under low agitation is about 30 μm.[19] For small particles (< 30 μm), where the Reynolds number is negligible, Sh is 2 and $h = r$. This suggests that with low agitation, the agitation strength does not affect the dissolution rate of small particles, as has been confirmed by studies,[20] because there is no further reduction of h. It is worth noting that during dissolution, there is time-dependent reduction of particle size or radius. The diffusion layer thickness is reduced with time, thus resulting in an increase of the intrinsic dissolution rate by first-order kinetics. Can the USP paddle method be used to represent in vivo hydrodynamics? Studies have shown that the agitation strength in the human intestine corresponds to 10–30 rpm in the 900-mL scale paddle method.[21]

Solubility and the Dissolution of Weak Electrolytes and Salts

The solubility term in the Nernst–Brunner equation refers to the solubility of the drug in the bulk solution. For a weak acid or a weak base, the solubility in the bulk is the sum of the intrinsic solubility S_o and the concentration of the dissociated species. For a weak acid HA, for example, $S_{bulk} = S_t = S_o + [A^-]$. Consider the dissolution of a free acid (HA) into a medium where $pH \geq pK_a$. It is apparent that the pH at the particle surface will be lower than that of the bulk solution due to the self-buffering effect of the dissolved drug, and the solubility will be less than the solubility of the bulk.[22–24] The same is true for the dissolution of a weak base into a medium where $pH \leq pK_a$. Because the initial dissolution rate is dependent upon the solubility of the drug at the particle surface, the use of S_{bulk} in the Nernst–Brunner equation will overestimate the dissolution rate. This effect is shown in **Figure 8-6**, where the dissolution of a weak acid in an acidic medium based on a solubility of S_o (curve *A*) is compared to the rate of dissolution at a higher pH, with a solubility of S_t (curve *B*), using the Nernst–Brunner equation. Curve *C* indicates a dissolution rate based on the correct solubility at the surface, which is lower than that of the bulk solution. The pH at the particle surface can be calculated based on the diffusion coefficients and concentrations of the ionic species involved in the diffusion process[24] (see the next section for the calculation of surface pH and solubility). This, in turn, allows the calculation of the solubility of the drug at the particle surface. Sugano et al.[25] have demonstrated that the higher the intrinsic solubility of the drug, the greater is the difference between the bulk and particle surface pH; and they suggested that, in predicting the dissolution rate, a factor *Z*, which is the ratio of drug solubility at the particle surface to that in bulk solution, can be used to modify the constant of the Nernst–Brunner equation.

The dissolution of a salt, such as the sodium salt of the weak acid, is also mediated by the pH of the dissolution medium. The solubility of a salt depends on the combined effect of pH and its K_{sp}. In a medium where the pH determines the salt concentration, the dissolved salt may precipitate in solution and at the solid surface. It is recalled that the precipitation process may result in the formation of very fine particles and supersaturated solution.[26] This would lead to an increase in dissolution rate that is not predicted by the Nernst–Brunner equation. This effect is also illustrated in Figure 8-6, where the predicted rate curve has a plateau concentration of S_t, whereas the supersaturation phenomenon may lead to a higher concentration plateau of S_t' (curve *D*). If the supersaturated state can be maintained for longer than the transition time for absorption, it may be used as the bulk solubility. If not, precipitation will occur, as shown in curve *E* of

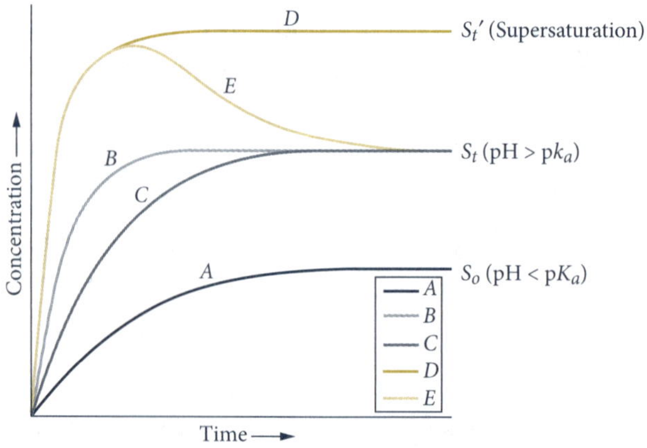

Figure 8-6 The pH-dependent dissolution behavior by a weak acid–base drug (curves *A*, *B*, and *C*) and its salt (curves *D* and *E*).
Courtesy of: The Japanese Society for the Study of Xerobiotics (JSSX).

Figure 8-6. It has been shown that the rate of dissolution of sodium tolbutamide is greater in the simulated gastric fluid than in the simulated intestinal fluid,[27] suggesting that supersaturation is associated with the dissolution of salts.

Determination of Surface pH

A detailed model describing the surface pH and the dissolution of weak electrolytes was given by Ozturk et al.[24] In an abbreviated view, one can consider the dissolution of a weak acid (HA) into a nonbuffered medium as involving concentration gradients of the positive (H^+) and negative (OH^- and A^-) ions in the diffusion boundary layer. Applying the electroneutrality rule, the dynamic presences of these ions can be written as

$$D_H([H^+]_s - [H^+]_b) = D_{OH}([OH^-]_s - [OH^-]_b) + D_A([A^-]_s - [A^-]_b)$$

where D is the diffusion coefficient, the subscripts H, OH, and A represent H^+, OH^-, and A^-, and the subscripts s and b indicate particle *s*urface and *b*ulk solution, respectively. The equilibrium expressions for the weak acid, $K_a = [H^+][A^-]/[HA]$, and for water, $K_w = [H^+][OH^-]$, apply both at the particle surface and in the bulk solution. In addition, $[A^-]_b$ is considered to be zero at the sink condition. With this notation, it can be seen that

$$D_H[H^+]_s - D_{OH}[OH^-]_s - D_A[A^-]_s = D_H[H^+]_b - D_{OH}[OH^-]_b$$

$$[H^+]_s - \frac{D_{OH}K_w}{D_H[H^+]_s} - \frac{D_AK_a[HA]_s}{D_H[H^+]_s} = \frac{D_H[H^+]_b}{D_H} - \frac{D_{OH}[OH^-]_b}{D_H} \qquad (8\text{-}20)$$

or

$$[H^+]_s^2 - \frac{D_{OH}K_w}{D_H} - \frac{D_AK_a[HA]_s}{D_H} = [H^+]_s\left(\frac{D_H[H^+]_b}{D_H} - \frac{D_{OH}[OH^-]_b}{D_H}\right)$$

It is known that $D_H = D_{OH}$ (= 2.7×10^{-5} cm²/s).[22] $[HA]_s$ is the intrinsic solubility of the drug S_o. All other quantities, except $[H^+]_s$, in the above equation are known or measurable. Hence, a simple rearrangement of the above equation as follows allows for the calculation of $[H^+]_s$ and the surface pH.

$$[H^+]_s^2 - ([H^+]_b - [OH^-]_b)[H^+]_s - (K_w + D_AK_aS_0/D_H) = 0$$

$$[H^+]_s = [b + (b^2 + 4c)^{1/2}]/2 \qquad (8\text{-}21)$$

where $b = [H^+]_b - [OH^-]_b$ and $c = K_w + D_AK_aS_0/D_H$. It should be noted that for an alkaline bulk solution, b is a negative value.

In the presence of a buffer agent, HB, the relation of the ionic species at the particle surface and bulk solution, includes, in addition to those shown in Equation (8-20), $[B^-]_s$ and $[B^-]_b$. Hence, one can rewrite Equation (8-20) for the buffer system as

$$D_H[H^+]_s - D_{OH}[OH^-]_s - D_A[A^-]_s - D_B[B^-]_s = D_H[H^+]_b - D_{OH}[OH^-]_b - D_B[B^-]_b \qquad (8\text{-}22)$$

If the dynamic total buffer concentration $(D_B[B^-]/D_{HB}) + [HB]$ at the particle surface is the same as that of the bulk solution, the concentration of $[B^-]_s$ can be written as

$$[B^-]_s = \frac{D_{HB}K_a'C_b}{D_BK_a' + D_{HB}[H^+]_s}$$

where K_a' is the acidity constant of the buffer system and C_b is the total buffer concentration. Because D_B and D_{HB} are essentially the same, the above equation may be rewritten as

$$[B^-]_s = K_a'C_b/(K_a' + [H^+]_s)$$

Similarly, one obtains

$$[B^-]_b = K_a'C_b/(K_a' + [H^+]_b)$$

With these relationships, the equation of $[H^+]_s$ for the buffered medium can now be written as

$$[H^+]_s^2 - \frac{D_{OH}K_w}{D_H} - \frac{D_A K_a [HA]_s}{D_H} - \frac{D_B K_a' C_b}{D_H(K_a'/[H^+]_s + 1)}$$

$$= [H^+]_s \left(\frac{D_H[H^+]_b}{D_H} - \frac{D_{OH}[OH^-]_b}{D_H} - \frac{D_B K_a' C_b}{D_H(K_a' + [H^+]_b)} \right)$$

The above equation is solvable using the quadratic expression if the pK_a of the buffer system is 2 or more pH units higher than the particle surface pH (that is, $1 + K_a'/[H^+]_s \approx 1$). With such a condition,

$$[H^+]_s^2 - \{[H^+]_b - [OH^-]_b - D_B K_a' C_b / D_H(K_a' + [H^+]_b)\}[H^+]_s$$
$$- (K_w + D_A K_a S_o / D_H + D_B K_a' C_b / D_H) = 0 \quad (8\text{-}23)$$

where $b = [H^+]_b - [OH^-]_b - D_B K_a' C_b / D_H(K_a' + [H^+]_b)$

$c = K_w + D_A K_a S_o / D_H + D_B K_a' C_b / D_H$

$[H^+]_s = [b + (b^2 + 4c)^{1/2}]/2$

The use of equations (8-21) and (8-23) is illustrated in Example 8-1.

Example 8-1: Calculate the pH and the dynamic total concentration of 2-naphthoic acid at the particle surface in (*a*) a nonbuffered dissolution medium and (*b*) a buffered dissolution medium at pH 9.0, based on the following data[24]:

2-Naphthoic acid: $K_a = 9.55 \times 10^{-5}$ $S_o = [HA]_o = 1.3 \times 10^{-4}\ M$

$D_A = D_{HA} = 9.6 \times 10^{-6}\ cm^2/s$

$D_H = D_{OH} = 2.7 \times 10^{-5}\ cm^2/s$

Buffer (imidazole): $K_a' = 6.76 \times 10^{-8}$ Buffer concentration: $C_b = 0.01\ M$

$D_B = D_{HB} = 8.20 \times 10^{-6}\ cm^2/s$

Solution:

(*a*) In a nonbuffered medium, pH = 9.0:

$[H^+]_s^2 + ([H^+]_b - [OH^-]_b)[H^+]_s - (K_w + D_A K_a S_o / D_H) = 0$

$b = [H^+]_b - [OH^-]_b = 10^{-9} - 10^{-5} = -10^{-5}\ M$

$c = K_w + D_A K_a S_o / D_H = 10^{-14} + 9.6 \times 10^{-6} \times 9.55 \times 10^{-5} \times 1.3 \times 10^{-4} / 2.7 \times 10^{-5}$

$= 44.1422 \times 10^{-10}$

$[H^+]_s = [b + (b^2 + 4c)^{1/2}]/2 = [-10^{-5} + (10^{-10} + 4 \times 44.1422 \times 10^{-10})^{1/2}]/2$

$= 6.1627 \times 10^{-5}\ M$ $(pH_s = 4.21)$

$[A^-]_s = K_a S_o / [H^+]_s = 9.55 \times 10^{-5} \times 1.3 \times 10^{-4} / 6.1627 \times 10^{-5}$

$= 2.015 \times 10^{-4}\ M$

Total conc. at particle surface $= S_o + [A^-]_s$

$= 1.3 \times 10^{-4} + 2.015 \times 10^{-4} = 3.315 \times 10^{-4}\ M$

Answer: $pH_{surface} = 4.21$; surface conc. = 3.315×10^{-4} *M*. Note that the pH at the surface is much lower than that of the bulk solution, indicating that the weak acid buffers the solution layer adjacent to the solid surface.

(*b*) In the buffered medium, pH = 9.0:

$$b = [H^+]_b - [OH^-]_b - D_B K_a' C_b / D_H (K_a' + [H^+]_b)$$

$$= 10^{-9} - 10^{-5} - \frac{8.2 \times 10^{-6} \times 6.76 \times 10^{-8} \times 0.01}{2.7 \times 10^{-5}\,(6.76 \times 10^{-8} + 10^{-9})} = -3.0027 \times 10^{-3}\ M$$

$$c = K_w + D_A K_a S_o / D_H + D_B K_a' C_b / D_H \approx D_A K_a S_o / D_H + D_B K_a' C_b / D_H$$

$$= \frac{9.6 \times 10^{-6} \times 9.55 \times 10^{-5} \times 1.3 \times 10^{-4}}{2.7 \times 10^{-5}} + \frac{8.2 \times 10^{-6} \times 6.76 \times 10^{-8} \times 0.01}{2.7 \times 10^{-5}}$$

$$= 44.1422 \times 10^{-10} + 0.2053 \times 10^{-9} = 4.6195 \times 10^{-9}$$

$$[H^+]_s = \{b + (b^2 + 4c)^{1/2}\}/2$$

$$= \{-3.0027 \times 10^{-3} + [(3.0027 \times 10^{-3})^2 + 4 \times 4.6195 \times 10^{-9}]^{1/2}\}/2$$

$$= 1.537 \times 10^{-6}\ M \qquad (pH_s = 5.81)$$

Total concentration of drug at particle surface:

$$S_{t,surface} = 1.3 \times 10^{-4} + 9.55 \times 10^{-5} \times 1.3 \times 10^{-4} / 1.537 \times 10^{-6}$$

$$= 8.21 \times 10^{-3}\ M$$

Answer: $pH_s = 5.81$; surface concentration: 8.21×10^{-3} *M*. Comparing parts (*a*) and (*b*), notice that the presence of a buffer system reduces the difference in pH between the particle surface and the bulk solution. In fact, this pH difference decreases with increasing buffer concentration.

Effects of Excipients and Bile Salts on Dissolution

Among the various excipients used in the formulation of solid dosage forms, some modified cyclodextrins have been shown to enhance the dissolution of hydrophobic drugs. This is due to the fact that cyclodextrins enhance the aqueous solubility of the drugs. Studies have also shown that polymeric compounds in some cases can increase, but in other cases can decrease the dissolution of hydrophobic drugs depending on the nature of the interactions. The use of lactose and starch may increase the dissolution of hydrophobic drugs in solid formulations, whereas lubricating agents such as stearic acid and magnesium stearate can decrease dissolution of the drugs by forming a hydrophobic layer that prevents the interfacial interaction with water. In addition to solubility considerations, drugs that form complexes with additive or biorelevant materials, such as the bile salts (bile acids and phospholipids), may exist in various states, and each state is characterized by its own diffusion coefficient. In the case of micelle formation, it is shown that the drug can exist as monomeric molecules but also as aggregates associated with micelles. Although the solubility of lipophilic drugs in the bile media is enhanced, diffusion of the aggregates is much slower than that of monomer drugs.[28–31] The diffusion coefficient measured in a bile medium is a function of those of the different aggregates. The overall effect of micelle formation on the dissolution of lipophilic drugs, however, is the product of D and C_s. The data of Takano et al.[31] on 12 such drugs showed that the value of DC_s is consistently higher in FeSSIF than in simulated intestinal

Table 8-3 Particle Size and Surface Area

Spherical Particle Size	Number of Particles	Total Surface Area (Arbitrary Unit)
r	1	1
$0.1r$	10^3	10
$0.01r$	10^6	100
$0.001r$	10^9	1000

fluid without the bile salts, indicating that the bile material increases the dissolution rate of poorly water-soluble drugs.

Particle Size and Surface Area

Equation (8-17) shows a direct relationship between the surface area of the drug particles and the dissolution rate, although it has been noted that the particle surface area does not remain constant during the dissolution process. Still, for the characterization of the initial dissolution rate under the sink condition, the particle size of the drug plays a very important role in drug dissolution. According to the Nernst–Brunner equation, the greater the surface area, the greater the dissolution. By reducing particle size, one increases the surface area, as can be seen from **Table 8-3**.

Hence, even for sparingly soluble drugs such as griseofulvin, chloramphenicol, and phenacetin, micronization of the particles increases significantly their rate of dissolution and oral absorption.

It should be mentioned that the total surface area is calculated based on particle size distribution. For spherical particles,

$$A = \sum_j A_j = N_j 4\pi r_j^2$$

where N_j is the number of particles in the size group of j, with a radius of r_j. The number of particles N can be calculated based on the weight (W), density (ρ), and volume (V) of the drug, in that

$$N = W/\rho V = W/\rho(4\pi r^3/3)$$

As has been mentioned previously, the surface area does not remain constant during dissolution, but decreases as a function time through reduction of particle sizes. The time-dependent decrease in radius of the spherical particles may be calculated from

$$r_{j,t} = r_{j,0}\,(W_{j,t}/W_{j,0})^{1/3}$$

where the ratio of the radius of group j particles at time t to time 0 is the cube root of the weight ratio at time t and time 0. Hence, the surface area of a drug sample may be expressed as

$$A = \sum_j A_{j,t} = N_j 4\pi r_{j,t}^2 = N_j 4\pi (r_{j,0})^2\,(W_{j,t}/W_{j,0})^{2/3} \tag{8-24}$$

Equation (8-24) provides a more accurate calculation of the surface area for better analysis of the dissolution rate, but it does not change the fact that the surface area is not a constant in dissolution. In the actual dissolution process, the decrease in particle radius reduces the total surface area (by second order) but may increase the intrinsic dissolution rate if the radius becomes equal to or smaller than the diffusion layer thickness.

Other Factors

Solid-state properties including polymorphism, hydration, and amorphous and crystalline characteristics all affect the rate of dissolution. For example, the amorphous form of novobiocin has a higher solubility and dissolution rate than the crystalline form and shows greater bioavailability than the crystalline form. The salts of weak acid and base drugs are more water-soluble than the drugs themselves and can thus be used to enhance dissolution and absorption. The presence of counterions in the medium may influence the rate of dissolution, if the solubility is K_{sp}-dependent, in which case lower ionic strength corresponds to a faster rate of dissolution. It is important to point out, however, that not all acids and bases can form a dosage form developable salt. Studies have shown that to make a stable salt for development, the difference in pK_a between the drug and the counterion must be larger than 2–3 pH units,[32] and in the case of very weak acids (p$K_a > 7$) or bases (p$K_a < 5$), it is difficult to find a successful salt form product.

III. Permeability and Oral Drug Absorption

Permeability Involving the Unstirred Water Layer

Multilayer Diffusion

The membrane barrier for diffusion may involve multiple diffusion layers. Even with an artificial membrane such as siloxane, *unstirred water layers* may exist on both sides of the membrane. The thickness of the static water layer of some in vitro planer membranes could reach 1500–2000 μm without stirring.[33] In the GI system, there exists an unstirred water layer adjacent to the intestinal membrane that has been measured to be about 30–100 μm. Although the membrane itself can be the major diffusion barrier, the existence of the unstirred water layer has been shown to play a very important role in determining the absorption of some drugs across a biological membrane, and to offer valuable insight into the structure-dependent behavior of drugs in the absorption process. As most membrane diffusion involves multiple diffusion layers, the overall permeability measured from such a system (see Equation (8-12)) is designated as the apparent permeability (P_{app}). With this notation, Equation (8-12) can be rewritten as

$$dW/dt = DAKC_1/h = P_{app}AC_1 \qquad P_{app} = DK/h \tag{8-25}$$

Now, consider a multilayer diffusion involving P_1, P_2, P_3, etc. The intrinsic effect of each diffusion layer on flux is $(1/P)(dW/dt)$, so that the overall diffusion process can be written as

$$\frac{1}{P_{app}}\frac{dW}{dt} = \frac{1}{P_1}\frac{dW}{dt} + \frac{1}{P_2}\frac{dW}{dt} + \frac{1}{P_3}\frac{dW}{dt} + \cdots = AC_1$$

The term $1/P$ has been described as the resistance to passage for each diffusion layer. If we consider a diffusion system with an artificial membrane having an unstirred water layer on both sides of the membrane, where the two water layers have equal layer thickness, the diffusion process is then

$$\frac{1}{P_{app}}\frac{dW}{dt} = \frac{2}{P_w}\frac{dW}{dt} + \frac{1}{P_m}\frac{dW}{dt} = AC_1$$

or

$$\frac{dW}{dt} = P_{app}AC_1 = \frac{P_w P_m}{P_w + 2P_m}AC_1$$

or

$$J = \frac{dW}{A\,dt} = P_{app}C_1 = \frac{P_w P_m}{P_w + 2P_m}C_1 \tag{8-26}$$

Here, the subscripts w and m denote the unstirred water layer and membrane, respectively. It is seen from Equation (8-26) that $P_{app} = P_w P_m/(P_w + 2P_m)$. Substituting DK/h for P (for the water layer, where $K = 1$), the above equation yields

$$J = \frac{D_w D_m K_m}{D_w h_m + 2h_w D_m K_m} C_1 \tag{8-27}$$

The significance of Equation (8-27) is twofold. First, the maximum flux from this diffusion process is set by the solubility of the drug in the donor medium; i.e., when $C_1 = C_s$, J is maximum. Second, a drug may cross the membrane via two different mechanisms. If the drug is highly soluble in the medium, diffusion across the unstirred water layer will be fast and the rate-limiting step will be its membrane permeability. In this case, $D_w h_m >> 2h_w D_m K_m$ (10-fold difference or more), Equation (8-27) is reduced to

$$J = \frac{D_m K_m}{h_m} C_1$$

The permeability is *membrane-controlled*. If, in contrast, the drug has only limited solubility in the medium, then the permeability will be *solubility-controlled*, in which the diffusion of the drug through the unstirred water layers (UWLs) will be the limiting step, and Equation (8-27) may be written as

$$J = \frac{D_w}{2h_w} C_1$$

As can be seen, the measured flux will depend on the diffusion coefficient in the medium and the water layer thickness. Note that in some in vitro studies, the unstirred water layer at the receptor side of the membrane can prevent the drug from reaching the bulk of the receptor solution and can result in high retention of drug in the membrane. This would underestimate the permeability of the drug compared to in vivo experiments in which the absorbed drug will be quickly washed away by the blood.[34]

The solubility-controlled permeability can also be explained using the lag time concept. The lag time for a membrane system is the time required for the drug to establish a uniform concentration gradient within the membrane boundary. For multilayer diffusion, studies[35, 36] have shown that the lag time for the membrane-controlled permeability is $t_1 = h_m^2/6D_m$, but for the solubility-controlled process described above, $t_1 = h_m h_w K/2D_w$. This equation contains the partition coefficient as a deciding factor for the lag time. Because the membrane partition coefficient for water-insoluble drugs is usually very large, the lag time increases with increasing drug lipophilicity. The membrane- and solubility-controlled permeability can be seen from the study of Flynn and Yalkowsky.[36] Using a well-characterized siloxane membrane of known thickness and the alkyl esters of *p*-aminobenzoate, they showed that the steady-state flux of the transferred drug increased with increasing carbon chain length of the esters from zero to three carbons, but decreased with increasing chain length from four to seven carbons. The latter was also accompanied by a linear increase in lag time. These results showed that for the smaller derivatives, the concentration gradient resided almost entirely inside the siloxane membrane, making the permeability membrane-controlled. There was, however, a shift to the solubility- or UWL-controlled permeability when the partition coefficient (of the longer-chain-length derivatives) became sufficiently large.

Caco-2 Cell Monolayers

The Caco-2 cell line is a continuous line of heterogeneous human epithelial colorectal adenocarcinoma cells, developed by the Sloan-Kettering Institute for Cancer Research. Although derived from a colon carcinoma, when cultured under specific conditions, the cells differentiate into a phenotype that morphologically and functionally resembles the enterocytes lining the small intestine. Caco-2 cells express tight junctions, microvilli, and a number of enzyme and transporters such as P-glycoprotein and uptake transporters for amino acids and bile acids, which are characteristic of the enterocytes. They formed continuous monolayers when grown on permeable filters of polycarbonate. The transmembrane resistance of the Caco-2 monolayer is about 260 Ω-cm^2,[37] which is typical of the intestinal mucosa.[38] Hence, the Caco-2 monolayer has been widely used across the pharmaceutical field as an in vitro model of the human intestinal mucosa for oral drug absorption studies. Since the initiation of this model, drug development failures in the pharmaceutical industry due to unrecognized poor absorption and pharmacokinetic properties have been markedly reduced. It is now well characterized that the permeability of lipophilic drugs through Caco-2 monolayers increases with increasing drug lipophilicity and is linearly correlated with the in vivo permeation process. In fact, Caco-2 monolayers are more applicable to prediction of oral drug absorption than isolated intestinal membranes, which have been found to interact with lipophilic drugs in a manner different from the in vivo intestinal absorption process.[39] The reliability of the Caco-2 model has led to the development of a quantitative biopharmaceutics classification system using the apparent permeability (P_{app}) across the Caco-2 monolayer as a standard.[40] In this approach, high permeability is defined by $P_{app} > 10^{-5}$ cm/s, and low permeability is defined as $P_{app} < 2 \times 10^{-6}$ cm/s.

Several types of in vitro systems have been reported[41, 42] in which the dissolution and permeability studies are concurrently carried out. Kataoka et al.[42] showed a dissolution/permeation (D/P) system using the Caco-2 cell monolayer for the prediction of oral absorption of drugs that are poorly soluble in water. The D/P system consists of two side-by-side chambers separated by the Caco-2 monolayer. The apical side contains simulated intestinal fluid, such as the isotonic FaSSIF, whereas the basal side contains a pH 7.4 buffer with or without serum albumin. For a given experiment, drug is applied to the apical side as powder, suspension, or solution, and both sides are under constant mixing with magnetic stirring. The concentrations of drug in both chambers are then monitored as a function of time. With this approach, Kataoka et al. showed that there is positive correlation between the permeated amount in the D/P system and the in vivo absorption of some 13 poorly water-soluble drugs.

Solubility, Dissolution, Permeability, and Drug Absorption

Intestinal Permeability

The effective intestinal surface area for the oral absorption is about 800 cm^2.[10] Because of the expansion of surface area by villous structure in the intestine, the intestinal permeability, commonly referred to as the *effective permeability* P_{eff}, is usually magnitude 10^{-4} cm/s. In comparison, the permeability from in vitro experiments using the Caco-2 cell monolayer and other parallel artificial membrane permeability assay (PAMPA) are in the range 10^{-5}–10^{-6} cm/s. There is a static or unstirred water layer (30–100 µm) adjacent to the intestinal membrane unaffected by luminal agitation, which plays an important role in drug absorption and limits the maximum P_{eff} value to about 5–10 × 10^{-4} cm/s. As mentioned earlier, in vitro membrane can have extensive retention of drugs that leads to underestimation of permeability. In vivo, the blood flow washes away drug from the intestinal membrane. In the intestinal fluid, drugs can exist in various states, including pH-mediated acid–base forms, micelle incorporated aggregates, and as complexes with polymeric substances. Because of the presence of the unstirred water layer, these aggregated or acid–base drug forms are expected to be in equilibrium with the free drug in the unstirred water layer. Previously, it was thought that only the free monomer state of the drug was effective for membrane permeation. It has since been determined that the free fraction theory applies to membrane-controlled permeability, but is largely nonapplicable to solubility- or UWL-limited permeation.

For drugs of high membrane permeability, e.g., their absorption is UWL-limited and the apparent permeation should not be affected by pH because the diffusion coefficients of both the aggregated and monomer species are similar. Once they pass through the UWL, the drug can be released as free monomers and quickly can penetrate the intestinal membrane. The free fraction theory also suggests that for poorly water-soluble drugs, even if the bile increases its solubility, oral absorption may not be increased due to the formation of micelle aggregates. But studies have shown that the oral absorption of poorly soluble drug is often increased in the fed state compared to the fasting state,[43] where the bile concentration is largely increased in the latter. In addition, the use of biorelevant media, such as the FeSSIF and FaSSIF, tends to give a more accurate prediction of oral absorption than the use of a simple buffer.[31, 44] Compounds with poor solubility tend to have high membrane permeability, and as shown in the previous section, the effective permeability is limited by the unstirred water layer. Using an artificial membrane, Amidon et al.[45] showed that when the membrane permeability is limited by UWL, not only free drug but also micelle-incorporated drug are effective in crossing the rate-limiting layer and membrane, because the micelles can diffuse the UWL. In effect, micelles can act as a carrier of solute across the UWL to the membrane surface, where the drug can be released from the micelles and can quickly penetrate the epithelial membrane. It should be mentioned, however, that the UWL superimposes the mucus layer on the intestinal membrane, which may add to the membrane resistance to permeability by micelle-incorporated drug.

Oral Absorption Profiles

In the Biopharmaceutics Classification System (BCS), drug candidates are classified into high solubility–high permeability, low solubility–high permeability, high solubility–low permeability, and low solubility–low permeability categories. This is largely based on the fact that the product of solubility and permeability is a determining factor for drug dissolution and absorption. Justifications for waiver of in vivo bioavailability and bioequivalent studies by the FDA may be granted for substances that are classified as having high solubility and high permeability (class I) in the development of immediate-release products. More significantly, three of the four BCS groups indicate a poor oral absorption profile for compounds so classified based on the balance among the solubility, dissolution rate, and permeability of the drug. These considerations indicate that the dissolution and permeability studies are both important tools in drug development work, especially for drug candidates that are in the poor oral absorption categories. The following is a brief discussion of the challenges involved in the drug development process.

Class II (low solubility–high permeability): The absorption is dissolution-limited. Because the rate of permeation is greater than the rate of dissolution, the intestinal concentration will remain low as the dissolved drug quickly disappears. The percentage of drug dose absorbed can be increased by increasing the dose and reduction of particle size.

Class III (high solubility–low permeability): The absorption is permeability-limited. The dissolution rate is fast. Because the solubility of the drug is high, the administered dose may be completely dissolved, while the intestinal concentration remains lower than the drug solubility in the intestinal fluid. Thus, an increase in dose will increase the percentage of drug dose absorbed. Particle size reduction would not affect the absorption.

Class IV (low solubility–low permeability): The absorption is solubility-limited. If the intestinal concentration reaches drug solubility, solid drug can no longer dissolve. An increase in dose may increase the absorbed amount, if the dissolution rate is slow, but the increase is limited to the intestinal solubility of the drug. The low permeability indicates a UWL-controlled permeation, which again indicates an upper limit of absorption set by the solubility. Similarly, the particle size reduction can increase the dissolution rate, but may not increase the absorbed amount because of the solubility limit.

Simulation of Oral Absorption

The use of in vitro data to simulate in vivo drug absorption can be a valuable tool for drug development research. Such results can be used to guide the product design, screening for lead compounds, selection of drug candidates, and optimization of drug formulation. Oral drug absorption from a solid dosage form is determined by the dissolution rate, solubility, and intestinal membrane permeability. A number of computer models of dissolution and permeation processes in the GI tract have been developed to simulate oral absorption.[31, 46, 47] The following is an example through which the intestinal absorption of drugs with low solubility but high permeability (BCS class II) can be predicted with significantly high correlation with clinical results.[31]

Studies of Takano et al.[31] showed that the model accounting for the dissolution and passive permeation of a BCS class II drug in the small intestine can be expressed as follows:

$$\frac{dW_d}{dt} = zX_0\left(\frac{W_s}{W_0}\right)^{2/3}\left(C_s - \frac{W_d}{V}\right) - P_{\mathrm{UWL}}A\left(\frac{W_d}{V}\right) \quad (8\text{-}28)$$

where W_d and W_s are the masses of the dissolved and solid drug at time t, respectively, W_0 is the initial mass, C_s is the solubility of the drug, V and A are the fluid volume and absorption surface area of the small intestine, respectively, z is a dissolution factor that will be described later, and P_{UWL} is the drug's UWL permeability. On the right-hand side of the equation, the first term describes the dissolution process, and the second term describes the absorption process. The rate of drug absorption can be written as

$$dW_a/dt = P_{\mathrm{UWL}}AW_d/V$$

where W_a is the mass of absorbed drug at time t. This model assumes that (1) drug dissolution and drug absorption occur in the small intestine only, (2) the membrane permeability of the drug is high, so that the permeation is UWL-limited, and (3) the dissolution follows the Hixson–Crowell cube root law for spherical particles, in which the radius or total surface area decreases with time.

The z factor is a combined parameter that includes the diffusion coefficient (D), initial particle radius (r_0), and the density (ρ) of the drug and the diffusion layer thickness (h) in that

$$z = 3D/\rho h r_0$$

This parameter along with the solubility of the drug in a biorelevant solvent (such as FaSSIF) is determined by in vitro experiments. Takano et al. have also shown that the P_{UWL} values of drugs can be estimated using existing information on the UWL of the human intestine and theoretical considerations. The UWL permeability is the diffusion coefficient divided by the diffusion layer thickness. Combining this relationship with Equation (8-4), one obtains

$$P_{\mathrm{UWL}} = D/h = (kT/6\pi\eta h)(1/r)$$

where k is the Boltzmann constant, T is the absolute temperature, η is the viscosity of the solution, and r is the radius of the compound. It has been shown that the effective permeability of glucose in humans, which is rate-limited by the UWL, is 10×10^{-4} cm/s.[48] The radius of glucose is calculated to be 3.6 Å.[49] Using glucose (mol wt. = 180) as a reference, it can be shown that the P_{UWL} of a drug is related to either the drug's radius or its molecular weight as follows:

$$P_{\mathrm{UWL}} = 10 \times 10^{-4}\,(3.6/r)$$

or

$$P_{\text{UWL}} = 10 \times 10^{-4}\,(180/\text{mol wt})^{1/3} \tag{8-29}$$

Because oral absorption is a kinetic process, the transit time through the GI tract is an important factor that determines the absorbed amount of a drug. In humans, in fasting state, the average transit time in the stomach and the small intestine is 12 min and 3–4 h, respectively. The available surface area for absorption and the fluid volume in the small intestine are 800 cm^2 and about 600 mL, respectively. With these data, Equation (8-28) can be used for computer simulation of absorption with the input of the z value, solubility, P_{UWL}, and dose, from which the mass absorbed W_a, the total mass dissolved $W_{d,\text{total}}$, and the concentration ratio C_{ratio} of the intestinal concentration versus solubility as a function of time can be determined. The total mass dissolved $W_{d,\text{total}}$ is given by the difference between dose X_o and solid mass W_s remaining at any time t. The concentration ratio C_{ratio}, as shown below, is an important indicator of the dissolution process.

$$C_{\text{ratio}}\,(\%) = (W_d/V) \times 100/C_s$$

If the C_{ratio} is small, $C_s >> W_d/V$, the dissolution is in sink conditions. If C_{ratio} increases with time, drug dissolution decreases due to a decrease of the concentration gradient. The fraction of dose absorbed F_a can be calculated as the ratio between W_a at time of 4 h (transit time) and the initial dose.

$$F_a\,(\%) = W_{a,4\text{h}} \times 100/W_0$$

The study of Takano et al. yielded several characteristics regarding the oral absorption process. A partial list of the compounds studied is given in **Table 8-4**. These compounds exhibit a P_{app}, measured across the Caco-2 cell monolayer, in the range of 3–10 × 10^{-5} cm^2/s, which classifies them as compounds of high permeability. First, there appears to be a general trend in that a larger value of the dissolution parameter z tends to lead to a greater percentage of the absorbed drug dose. This becomes more apparent if the predicted F_a is compared to zC_s, which represents, practically, the first-order rate constant of the dissolution based on particle size change. Second, for quantitative prediction of oral drug absorption, in vitro data obtained from biorelevant media are more appropriate. When compared to clinical data, the predicted F_a (%) using parameters generated from FaSSIF (pH 6.5) showed a significant correlation with the in vivo data on absorption ($r^2 = 0.82$; $p < 0.001$). This correlation became much lower ($r^2 = 0.59$), however, when the in vitro parameters used for in vivo prediction were generated from simulated intestinal fluid (SIF) without the bile salts. This indicates that interactions of drugs with taurocholic acid and phospholipids in the micelle formation are part of the in vivo process.

Third, the effect of the bile material on drug dissolution and permeability is such that it increases drug solubility but decreases the drug's diffusivity. The overall effect, however, leads to increased dissolution of poorly water-soluble drugs. Although the zC_s value measured in FaSSIF is generally greater than that of the SIF, the increased solubility also plays a key role in determining the concentration gradient. It has been reported that the oral absorption of BCS class II drugs is dissolution-limited if the dose/solubility ratio is low.[10] This can be explained by the solubility factor. For a drug used in low dose, the amount of drug dissolved versus solubility will be low. An increase in solubility by the bile can make this ratio much lower, thus creating a sink condition for the in vivo dissolution. If the dose is high, the dissolution is not in a sink condition. Solid drug will no longer dissolve if the fluid concentration already reaches the solubility value. Hence, an increase in solubility by the bile material will greatly increase the amount of drug dissolved. For example, the data of Takano et al. showed that ivermectin dissolves under sink condition whereas efavirenz

Table 8-4 The Dissolution Parameter, Solubility, and Predicted Oral Absorption of Drugs with High Permeability and Low Solubility[†]

Drug	Molecular Weight	z (mL/mg-min)[‡]	C_s (mg/mL)[‡]	P_{UWL} (10^{-4} cm/s)[§]	zC_s (min^{-1})	F_a (%)[¶]	Dose (mg)
Ketoconazole	531.4	0.022 ± 0.006	0.021 ± 0.001	6.97	0.00046	9 ± 2	200
Griseofulvin	352.8	0.183 ± 0.033	0.019	7.99	0.00348	23 ± 1	500
Danazol	337.5	0.269 ± 0.023	0.012 ± 0.001	8.11	0.00323	40 ± 2	100
Ivermectin	875.1	0.026 + 0.006	0.120 ± 0.01	5.90	0.00312	53 ±10	12
Gefitinib	446.9	0.315 + 0.028	0.034 ± 0.006	7.39	0.01071	69 ± 2	250
Efavirenz	315.7	0.053 ± 0.004	0.194 ± 0.007	8.29	0.01028	76 ± 2	1200
Exemestane	296.4	0.411 ± 0.074	0.061 ± 0.002	8.47	0.02507	100	25
Phenytoin	252.3	1.142 ± 0.172	0.043 ± 0.002	8.94	0.04911	100	300
Spironolactone	416.6	1.427 ± 0.163	0.042 ± 0.002	7.56	0.05993	100	200

[†]All data are taken from Takano et al., *Pharm. Res.* 23:1144–1156, 2006.
[‡]Determined in FaSSIF.
[§]Calculated based on molecular weight of drug.
[¶]Predicted by computer simulation using Equation (8-28).

Table 8-5 Effect of Solubility on F_a (%) in Simulated Oral Absorption of Ivermectin and Efavirenz

	SIF		FaSSIF	
Drug	C_s (mg/mL)	F_a (%)	C_s (mg/mL)	F_a (%)
Ivermectin	0.0007 ± 0	5 ± 0	0.120 ± 0.01	53 ± 10
Efavirenz	0.01 ± 0.001	8 ± 0	0.194 ± 0.007	76 ± 2

Data from: Takano et al., *Pharm. Res.* 23:1144–1156, 2006.

dissolves under nonsink conditions according to the simulated oral absorption experiments. The time curves of dissolved (W_d) and absorbed (W_a) drug showed that, for both drugs, the dissolved amount is almost completely absorbed as a function of time, so that the absorption is dissolution rate limited. The total absorption, however, is significantly limited by solubility, which sets an upper limit on the dissolved amount. This effect can be seen for the data shown in **Table 8-5**, where a marked increase of the solubility of the drugs by the bile material leads to a large increase in the percentage of dose absorbed.

Under sink conditions, the dissolution of the drugs based on radius change can be calculated using Equation (8-18). Some calculations that demonstrate the potential effect of dose and particle size on the dissolution and absorption of poorly water-soluble drug are given in Example 8-2.

Example 8-2: Assuming sink condition for the dissolution of ivermectin in the small intestine, predict the absorption of this drug if the dose is 10 mg, using the data given in Table 8-4. The simulated results showed a percent ratio of 1% between the intestinal drug concentration and solubility at the end of 4 h.

Solution: The following information is given:

Dose (W_0) = 10 mg $z = 0.026$ mL/mg-min

$C_s = 0.12$ mg/mL $C_{\text{ratio,4h}} = 0.01$ $V = 600$ mL

The calculation of the amount of drug remaining in solid state when particles change their radius as a function of time is based on the Hixson–Crowell cube root equation (Equation (8-18)), that is,

$$(W_s/W_0)^{1/3} = 1 - zC_st/3 = 1 - 0.026 \times 0.12 \times 240/3 = 0.7504$$

$$W_s = (0.7504)^3 W_0 = 4.226\text{ mg}$$

Total drug dissolved in 4 h:

$$W_{d,\text{total}} = W_0 - W_s = 10 - 4.226 = 5.774\text{ mg}$$

Drug concentration at $t = 240$ min:

$$W_{d,\,4\text{h}} = C_{\text{ratio}} \times C_s \times V = 0.01 \times 0.12 \times 600 = 0.72\text{ mg}$$

Thus, the amount absorbed is

$$W_{a,\,4\text{h}} = 5.774 - 0.72 = 5.054\text{ mg}$$

$$F_a(\%) = 5.054 \times 100/10 = 50.5\%$$

Answer: $F_a = 50.5\%$. If one calculates F_a using a z value of 0.052, which corresponds to a reduction of the particle radius to one-half of its value, $F_a = 80\%$. For BCS class II drugs, dose increase and particle size reduction may increase drug absorption.

IV. Chapter Summary

The majority of the most needed pharmaceutical products are for oral administration. The dominating role of this route in drug therapy stems from it being safe, efficient, and easily accessible with minimal discomfort to the patient compared to other routes of administration. Oral drug absorption is thus an important subject for pharmacy practitioners who either participate in the making of the products or dispense such products for patient use. This chapter shows that the in vivo oral drug absorption is readily demonstrated by the theory of diffusion and can be predicted by in vitro experiment that utilizes this theory. Note that when certain simplifying assumptions are made, the flux of Fick's law simply reduces to a product of solubility and permeability. Solubility is a deciding factor for drug dissolution, making available the drug at the absorption site. Permeability describes the passive diffusion of a drug through a membrane that impedes absorption. Both phenomena are described by Fick's first law. That the diffusion processes also apply to the intestinal absorption has been the basic rationale of the FDA's BCS initiative. It is also important to point out that the diffusion-based phenomena usually involve mass transport through phase changes, such as from solid to liquid, liquid to liquid, and from one side of the membrane to the other side. The values of some important factors such as pH and solubility will vary with varying microenvironments; hence, they must be used appropriately. This is illustrated by the fact that in the dissolution of acid and base drugs, neither the solubility nor the pH at the particle surface is the same as that of the bulk solution.

V. References

1. Karth MG, Higuchi WI, and Fox JL. *J Pharm Sci.* 74(6):612–617, 1985.
2. Baker RW and Lonsdale HK. In Tanquary AC and Lacey RE (eds), *Controlled Release of Biologically Active Agents.* New York, Plenum Press, 1974, pp 30–33.
3. Noyes AA and Whitney WR. *J Am Chem Soc.* 19(12):930–934, 1897.
4. Nernst W. *Zeit Physikal Chem.* 47:52–55, 1904.
5. Brunner E. *Zeit Physikal Chem.* 47:56–102, 1904.
6. Hixson A and Crowell J. *Ind Eng Chem.* 23:923, 1931.
7. Skelley JP, Amidon GL, Barr WH, et al. *J Pharm Sci.* 79:849, 1991.
8. Levich V. *Physicochemical Hydrodynamics.* Englewood Ciffs, NJ, Prentice-Hall, 1982.
9. McGinity J, Stavchansky S, and Martin A. Bioavailability in tablet technology, in Lieberman HA and Lachman L (eds.), *Pharmaceutical Dosage Forms: Tablets*, New York, Marcel Dekker, 1981, Vol II.
10. Yu LX. *Pharm Res.* 16:1883–1887, 1999.
11. Kalantzi L, Goumas K, Kalioras V, Abrahamsson B, Dressman JB, and Reppas C. *Pharm Res.* 23:165–176, 2006.
12. Vertzoni M, Fotaki N, Kostewicz E, et al. *J Pharm Pharmacol.* 56:453–462, 2004.
13. Sutton SC. *Adv Drug Deliv Rev.* 56:1383–1398, 2004.
14. Leng J, Egelhaaf SU, and Cates ME. *Biophys J.* 85:1624–1646, 2003.
15. Perez de la Cruz Moreno M, Oth M, Deferme S, Lammert F, Tack J, Dressman J, and Augustijns P. *J Pharm Pharmacol.* 58:1079–1089, 2006.
16. Andrieux K, Forte L, Lesieur S, Paternostre M, Ollivon M, and Grabielle-Madelmont C. *Pharm Res.* 21:1505–1516, 2004.

17. Nibbering CP, Frederik PM, van Berge-Henegouwen GP, van Veen HA, van Marle J, and van Erpecum KJ. *Biochim Biophys Acta, Mol Cell Biol Lipids*, 1583:248–255, 2002.
18. Dressman JB, Amidon GL, Reppas C, and Shah VP. *Pharm Res.* 15:11–22, 1998.
19. Harriott P. *AICHE J.* 8:93–102, 1962.
20. Scholz A, Kostewicz E, Abrahamsson B, and Dressman JB. *J Pharm Pharmacol.* 55:443–451, 2003.
21. Katori N, Aoyagi N, and Terao T. *Pharm Res.* 12:237–243, 1995.
22. Mooney KG, Mintun MA, Himmelstein KJ, and Stella VJ. *J Pharm Sci.* 70:13–22, 1981.
23. Mooney KG, Mintun MA, Himmelstein KJ, and Stella VJ. *J Pharm Sci.* 70:22–32, 1981.
24. Ozturk SS, Palsson BO, and Dressman JB. *Pharm Res.* 5:272–282, 1988.
25. Sugano K, Okazaki A, Sugimoto S, Tavornvipas S, Omura A, and Mano T. *Drug Metab Pharmacokinet*. 22:225–254, 2007.
26. Sugano K, Kato T, Suzuki K, Keiko K, Sujaku T, and Man T. *J Pharm Sci.* 95:2115–2122, 2006.
27. Banker GS and Rhodes CT. *Modern Pharmaceutics*, New York, Marcel Dekker, 1979, p 164.
28. Naylor LJ, Bakatselou V, and Dressman JB. *Pharm Res.* 10:865–870, 1993.
29. Balakrishnan A, Rege BD, Amidon GL, and Polli JE. *J Pharm Sci.* 93:2064–2075, 2004.
30. Sun W, Larive CK, and Southard MZ. *J Pharm Sci.* 92:424–435, 2003.
31. Takano R, Sugano K, Higashida A, Hayashi Y, Nachida M, Aso Y, and Yamashita S. *Pharm Res.* 23:1144–1156, 2006.
32. Morissette SL, Almarsson O, Peterson ML, et al. *Adv Drug Deliv. Rev.* 56:275–300, 2004.
33. Youdim KA, Avdeef A, and Abott NJ. *Drug Dis Today*. 8:997–1003, 2003.
34. Krishna G, Chen KJ, Lin CC, and Nomeir AA. *Int J Pharm.* 222:77–89, 2001.
35. Higuchi T. *J Soc Cosm Chem.* 11:85, 1960.
36. Flynn GL and Yalkowsky SH. *J Pharm Sci.* 61:838, 1972.
37. Artursson P. *J Pharm Sci.* 79:476–482, 1990.
38. Rojanasakul Y, Wanf L, Bhat M, Glover DD, Malanga CJ, and Ma JKH. *Pharm Res.* 9:1029–1034, 1992.
39. Yamashita S, Tanaka Y, Endoh Y, Taki Y, Sakane T, Nadai T, and Sezaki H. *Pharm Res.* 14:486–491, 1997.
40. Rinaki E, Valsami G, and Macheras P. *Pharm Res.* 20:1917–1925, 2003.
41. Ginski MJ and Polli JE. *Int J Pharm.* 177:117–125, 1999.
42. Kataoka M, Masaoka Y, Yamazaki Y, Sakane T, Sezaki H, and Yamashita S. *Pharm Res.* 20:1674–1680, 2003.
43. Singh BN. *Clin Pharmacokinet*. 37:213–255, 1999.
44. Wei H and Loebenberg R. *Eur J Pharm Sci.* 29:45–52, 2006.
45. Amidon GL, Higuchi WI, and Ho NFH. *J Pharm Sci.* 71:77–84, 1982.
46. Yu LX, Lipka E, Crison JR, and Amidon GL. *Adv Drug Deliv Rev.* 19:359–376, 1996.
47. Dressman JB and Reppa C. *J Pharm Sci.* 11:S73–S80, 2000.
48. Lennernas H. *J Pharm Sci.* 87:403–410, 1998.
49. McGowan JC. *J Appl Chem Biotechnol.* 28:599–607, 1978.

Recommended Readings

Lee SL, Raw AS, and Yu L. Dissolution testing, in Krishna R and Yu L (eds), *Biopharmaceutics Applications in Drug Development.* New York, Springer, 2007; pp 47–74.

Sugano K, Okazaki A, Sugimoto S, Tavornvipas S, Omura A, and Mano T. Solubility and dissolution profile assessment in drug discovery. *Drug Metab Pharmacokinet.* 22(4):225–254, 2007.

VI. Homework Problems

1. From the diffusion coefficient of Table 8-1, estimate the radius of insulin using Equation (8-4), calculate its molecular weight [based on the formula mol wt = $\rho(4\pi r^3/3)N$], and compare this value with the one determined by Equation (8-7). Avogadro's number is N, ρ can be found in Table 8-1, and the viscosity of water at 25°C is 0.894 cp.
2. For a diffusion layer thickness of 100 μm, what is the time required for a molecule to clear the diffusion boundary by random walk, if the diffusion coefficient is 1×10^{-6} cm²/s?
3. Predict the dissolved amount of 10 mg of a drug in 1 h using the Nernst–Brunner equation, Equation (8-17), under sink conditions. The diffusion coefficient of the drug is 1×10^{-5} cm²/s, the particle size of the drug is 100 μm, the density of the drug is 1.2 g/mL, the diffusion layer thickness is 30 mm, and the solubility of the drug is 0.1 mg/mL. What is the dissolved amount if the dissolution is based on particle size reduction using Equation (8-18)?
4. What is the estimated time for complete dissolution of the above drug if the particle size is 25 mm? *Hint:* For particles that are equal to or smaller than the diffusion layer thickness, the equation $r = r_0 - (D/h\rho)\,C_s t$ may be written as

   $$r^2 = r_0^2 - (D/\rho)C_s t$$

   For r to be zero for complete dissolution, $r_0^2 = DC_s t/\rho$.
5. Calculate the pH and the solubility of benzoic acid at the particle surface for the dissolution of benzoic acid in (*a*) a nonbuffered medium of pH 7.0 and (*b*) a buffered medium of pH 7.0, where the total buffer concentration is 0.02 *M*. Physical constants are as follows: for benzoic acid, $K_a = 9.33 \times 10^{-5}$ ($pK_a = 4.03$), $S_o = 0.0216\,M$, $D_{\mathrm{HA}} = D_{\mathrm{A^-}} = 9.6 \times 10^{-6}$ cm²/s,[24] $D_{\mathrm{H}} = D_{\mathrm{OH}} = 2.7 \times 10^{-5}\,M$; for buffer, $K_a = 4.31 \times 10^{-7}$; $D_{\mathrm{HB}} = D_{\mathrm{B}} = 5 \times 10^{-6}$ cm²/s.
6. The intestinal permeability of exemestane (mol wt = 296.4), a BCS class II drug, is UWL rate-limited. (*a*) Calculate P_{UWL} in the small intestine. (*b*) The solubility of this drug in FaSSIF is 0.061 mg/mL.[31] If this solubility is the same as that in the intestinal fluid, calculate the maximum absorbable amount in 2 h. (*c*) For any given intestinal concentration, how long does it take for 99% absorption of that concentration?
7. Assuming sink conditions for the dissolution of ketoconazole, calculate the percentage of dose dissolved at the end of 4 h, using data given in Table 8-4. How could the absorption rate be improved?

CHAPTER 9

Micromeritics and Pharmaceutical Powders

Our discussion of physicochemical activities of drugs has been confined to molecular behaviors. As we begin to examine the pharmaceutical dosage forms, it is apparent that the starting point of a pharmaceutical preparation begins almost always with the powdered material. Earlier we learned that the dissolution process of drugs, through which their pharmacological activities are realized, depends primarily on the properties of the solid particles. It will be made clear with discussion in this chapter that the making of the pharmaceutical systems also depends on the properties of small particles. The science and technology of small particles is termed *micromeritics.* These properties, on one hand, demonstrate how particles interact with the surrounding environment (interfacial phenomenon) and, on the other hand, form the basis from which solid dosage forms are developed, thus serving as a bridge between the making of the therapeutic product and its therapeutic effect.

CHAPTER OUTLINE

OBJECTIVES

1. Understand the definitions of mean diameters used for particle size expressions.
2. Perform calculations to determine the mean diameter and particle size distributions.
3. Understand the U.S. sieving standard and the determination of particle size based on sieving and the interfacial phenomenon known as sedimentation.
4. Understand the effect of particle size reduction on particle surface activity and perform calculations of the surface area of small particles.
5. Understand the surface area and pore size measurements based on interfacial gas adsorption principles.
6. Understand the effects of porosity on the surface activity, density, and flow properties of pharmaceutical powders.
7. Know the density expressions in pharmaceutical powders.
8. Understand and perform basic pharmaceutical techniques in comminution and blending of powders.
9. Know the type and use of various medicated powders.

I. Micromeritics

Solid particles consist of molecules arranged in crystalline forms, which are fundamental in determining the property of a solid and how the surface molecules interact with the environment. Particles also vary in size. As particle size reduces, different particle activities may arise compared to those of particles of a larger size scale, due primarily to the increase in surface/volume ratio and the exposure of surface molecules. In the nanosize range, even the quantum effects may be observed due to the large increase in exposed surface electrons. The involvement of particles in pharmaceutical use, as given in **Table 9-1**, shows a clear particle size–dependent application and thus the importance of controlling particle size and range in pharmaceutical preparations. Besides, particulates are inherently associated with human activities and our environment. Many diseases including pulmonary inflammation, gastric ulceration, and asthma are caused by various particulates. Hence, for health and disease, there are good reasons for the properties of small particles to be closely examined.

Most pharmaceutical ingredients exist in the solid state as amorphous powders or as crystals of different morphological structures. The word powder refers to a solid compound or a solid formulation with or without added ingredients to the active drug(s), known as a medicated or compounded powder. Powders are characterized by a number of properties including particle shape, size, and distribution; active surface area; porosity; density and packing; solubility; and flow characteristics. These properties are determined early in the pharmaceutical process and used for decision making in the development of a product and for quality control to ensure batch-to-batch uniformity in the production procedure. The science and technology of small particles is given the name, by J. M. Dalla Valle,[1] micromeritics.

Particle Size and Distribution

Particle Size

The particle size of a drug plays a key role in determining the rate of drug dissolution. There are, in fact, specific requirements of particle size and distribution for many therapeutic applications and formulation processes. For inhalation use, powders are required to have a specific size range (1–5 μm) in order for the particles to reach the alveoli of the deep lungs; and for formulation of ophthalmic suspensions and ointments and dermal ointments and creams, the particle size and shape of the powder are known to play an important role in formulation stability, drug absorption, and side effects. In solid dosage forms, particle size and distribution influence powder mixing, compression, wettability, and the mechanical flow of the powder during dosage form fabrication.

Table 9-1 Size and Size Range of Particles in Pharmaceutical Preparations

Type	Particle Size (μm)	Use
Granulation	1000–3360	Tablet preparation
Coarse powder	150–1000	Drug powders
Fine powder	50–100	Drug powders
Emulsions and suspensions	10–50	Coarse emulsions and flocculated suspensions
Dry powder	1–5	Inhalation
Emulsions and suspensions	0.5–10	
Nanoemulsion	0.01–0.5	Colloids
Nanoparticles	0.001–0.1	Novel drug delivery systems

Often, a narrow particle size distribution is desirable, for if the size distribution is wide, the powder can segregate according to different particle sizes, and this can result in inaccurate dosing, inconsistent performance, and deformation of solid dosage forms with time.[2]

If all fine particles were spheres, their size would be defined explicitly by their diameter or radius; or if they were all cubical, the length along one edge would be characteristic. The great majority of particles from any batch of powder, however, are quite irregular in shape and size. It appears that a practical definition of size is needed, short of detailed examination of each particle, where the particle size so defined permits a great number of particles to be examined so as it represents the characteristics of the powder sample. In this light, it is both convenient and practical to use an equivalent spherical diameter to express the particle size. The diameter (d) thus implies that the particle has a surface area equivalent to πd^2 and a volume equivalent to $\pi d^3/6$. The presence of different particle sizes necessitates the derivation of an average particle size and size distribution expression so that the variation of particle size of the powder from batch to batch can be evaluated. Edmundson[3] has shown that different mean diameters (d_{mean}) as an average particle size can be obtained for specific applications according to Equation (9-1)

$$d_{\text{mean}} = \left(\frac{\sum nd^{(p+f)}}{\sum nd^{f}}\right)^{1/p} \tag{9-1}$$

where n is number of particles in a given size group with an arithmetic mean of d. The terms p and f are indexes, which, in combination, determine whether the weighted average is based on total length, surface area, or volume (or weight), with $p = 1, 2,$ or 3 and $f = 0, 1, 2,$ or 3. Based on the f value, the frequency term nd^f indicates a weighted total of particle number ($f = 0$), length ($f = 1$), surface area ($f = 2$), or volume ($f = 3$). For example, if $p = 1$ and $f = 0$, d_{mean} ($= \sum nd/\sum n$) is a weighted average of the measured particle diameter, which may be designated as $d_{length/number}$ or $d_{l/n}$. This expression is generally used if the size range is narrow and the distribution is normal. If $p = 1$ and $f = 2$, d_{mean} is calculated based on the total volume divided by the *total surface area*, that is, $\sum nd^3/\sum nd^2$, and it may be designated as $d_{v/s}$. This expression is of value if the intended use of this powder involves surface area considerations. The calculation of the mean particle diameter of a sample analysis is given in **Table 9-2**.

Table 9-2 Calculation of Mean Diameters Based on the Following Particle Size

Size Group (µm)	Arithmetic Mean (µm)	n	nd, 10^2	nd^2, 10^3	nd^3, 10^6
20–40	30	2	0.6	1.8	0.054
40–60	50	14	7.0	35.0	1.750
60–80	70	59	41.3	289.1	20.237
80–100	90	96	86.4	777.6	69.984
100–120	110	95	104.5	1149.5	126.445
120–140	130	75	97.5	1267.5	164.775
140–160	150	50	75.0	1125.0	168.750
160–180	170	30	51.0	867.0	147.390
180–200	190	17	32.3	613.7	116.603
200–220	210	5	10.5	220.5	46.305
	Total	443	506.1	6346.7	862.293

d_{mean}: $d_{v/s} = \sum nd^3/\sum nd^2 = 862.293 \times 10^6/6346.7 \times 10^3 = 135.9\ \mu\text{m}$

$d_{l/n} = \sum nd/\sum n = 506.1 \times 10^2/443 = 114.2\ \mu\text{m}$

Distribution

A complete understanding of the particle size effect requires also knowledge of the particle size distribution. The deciding factors of a distribution are the frequency (f), mean (m), and standard deviation (σ). The distribution curve can be readily obtained by plotting the frequency (n) as a function of the arithmetic mean of the particle size groups such as the data given in Table 9-2. For a normal distribution, the curve is symmetrical to the mean, and the mean, where the maximum frequency occurs, is identical with the median (50% size). The standard deviation of the normal distribution can be determined based on basic statistical calculations or the cumulative frequency of the distribution (described later). The equation for a normal distribution is

$$f(x) = \frac{1}{\sigma\,(2\pi)^{1/2}} \exp\{-[(x-\mu)/\sigma]^2/2\} \qquad (9\text{-}2)$$

where $f(x)$ is the probability density or frequency as a function of x on the x axis (abscissa). This equation shows that the maximum frequency (f_{max}) occurs at $x = \mu$ and is equal to $1/\sigma(2\pi)^{1/2}$, or $0.3989/\sigma$. At the point x where $x - \mu = \sigma$, $f = 0.6056\, f_{max}$. For a normal particle size distribution, when n is the frequency, 68, 95.5, or 99.7% of total particles will have particle sizes within 1, 2, or 3 standard deviations, respectively, from the mean.

Pharmaceutical powders, however, often do not show normal distribution in particle sizes, such as the one shown in **Figure 9-1** based on data given in Table 9-2. In this figure, the distribution is positively skewed where the mean ($d_{l/n}$ = 114.2 mm) is larger than the median and mode. Statistical methods have shown that many nonsymmetrical continuous distributions may be logarithm normal or *lognormal*, in that if the variable x exhibits a lognormal distribution, then the function $\log x$ will assume a normal distribution. The reverse is also true. One can thus transform the unsymmetrical distribution of $f(x)$ into a normal distribution by substituting $\log x$ for x on a linear abscissa scale. The frequency for the distribution of $\log x$ is

$$f(\log x) = \frac{1}{\sigma_{\log x}\,(2\pi)^{1/2}} \exp\{-[(\log x - \mu_{\log x})/\sigma_{\log x}]^2/2\} \qquad (9\text{-}3)$$

where $\mu_{\log x}$ is the mean, representing the median (in log scale) of the distribution, and $\sigma_{\log x}$ is the corresponding standard deviation in log scale. For particle size distribution, the median value for a lognormal distribution is known as the *geometric diameter d_g*, which indicates that 50% of the particles will be either under or over this size. The logarithmic transformation is useful in that it allows the determination of the median (d_g), the corresponding geometric standard deviation (σ_g), and the mean diameter ($d_{l/n}$), based on the normal distribution with respect to $\log x$. As an example, the data in Table 9-2 are recalculated in logarithms and are presented in **Table 9-3.**

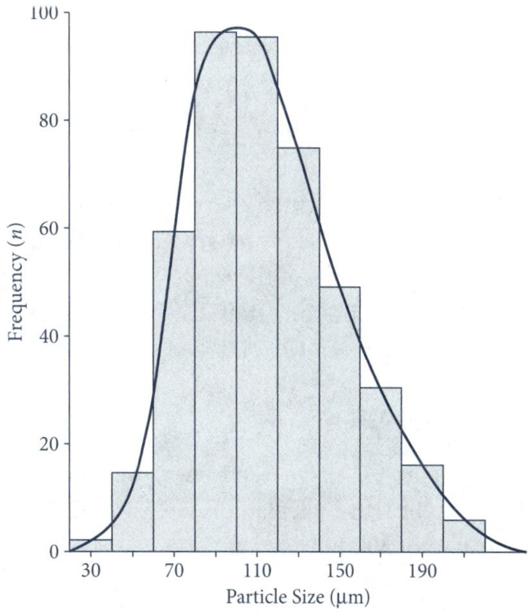

Figure 9-1 Plot of frequency (n) as a function of the measured arithmetic mean diameter shown in Table 9-2.

Here, from **Figure 9-2**, we see that the plot of %n (or n) versus $\log x$ gives a normal distribution, with the mean at maximum frequency being the median of the particle sizes. Figure 9-2 also shows that the plot of the cumulative %n (f) versus $\log x$ yields a sigmoid curve. Thus, the median can be determined by plotting $\log [f/(100 - f)]$

Table 9-3 Distribution of Particle Sizes According to the Logarithm of the Arithmetic Mean of Particle Size Groups

Arithmetic Mean x (μm)	$\log x$	n	$\%n$	f ($\%n$ cumulative)	$\log[f/100-f)]$
30	1.477	2	0.45	0.45	−2.345
50	1.699	14	3.16	3.61	−1.427
70	1.845	59	13.32	16.93	−0.691
90	1.954	96	21.67	38.60	−0.202
110	2.041	95	21.44	60.04	0.177
130	2.114	75	16.93	76.97	0.524
150	2.176	50	11.29	88.26	0.876
170	2.230	30	6.77	95.03	1.282
190	2.279	17	3.84	98.87	1.941
210	2.322	5	1.13	100.00	—

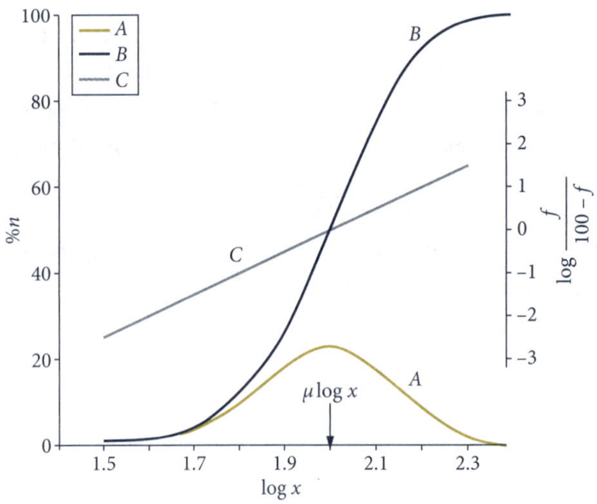

Figure 9-2 Particle size distribution as a function of the log arithmetic mean (log x) for data given in Table 9-3: (*A*) plot of $\%n$ versus log x, (*B*) plot of cumulative $\%n$ versus log x, (*C*) plot of log $[f/(100-f)]$ versus log x.

versus log x, from which a straight line (curve *C*) will be obtained. When $\log[f/(100-f)] = 0$, $\log x = \mu_{\log x}$. Because for a normal distribution about 68% of the population is within 1 standard deviation of the mean, the range of 1 standard deviation is from 16% to 84% of the cumulative $\%n$ of the distribution. Thus, the particle size corresponding to the 16% size is 1 standard deviation from the mean ($\mu_{\log x}$), or

$$\mu_{\log x} - \log x_{16\%} = \sigma_{\log x} \tag{9-4}$$

From Figure 9-2 curve *C*, it is determined that $\mu_{\log x} = 2.00$ and $\log x_{16\%} = 1.84$; hence, $\sigma_{\log x} = 2.00 - 1.84 = 0.16$. These calculations yield a median particle size (d_g) of 100 μm and a geometric standard deviation of 30.8 μm.

From the above discussion, we see that for any normal distribution, the mean is the median and the standard deviation can be determined by the cumulative frequency as the difference between the 50% and 16% sizes.

The mean diameter of the particle size distribution of Table 9-2 can also be calculated based on the Hatch–Choate equations[4] using the logarithmic transformation. For $d_{l/n}$, it is shown that

$$\log d_{l/n} = \mu_{\log x} + (2.303/2)\sigma^2_{\log x} \qquad (9\text{-}5)$$

Using the results given above, $d_{l/n}$ is calculated to be 107.0 μm. Notice that this value is smaller than the value given in Table 9-2 because the latter is positively skewed with more data on larger particle sizes.

Determination of Particle Size

The science on the measurement of particle size and distribution is diverse. For nanoparticles (1–100 nm), electron microscopy (EM) including scanning and transmission EM and scanning probe microscopy is generally necessary. Light scattering techniques with a laser particle sizer, through which the particle size is deduced from quantified Brownian diffusion of the particles, also allows the determination of particle size and distribution in the colloidal size range (1–500 nm). In addition, there are electric migration techniques such as mass spectrometry and differential mobility analysis that can be used to measure the ultrafine particles. A number of techniques exist for the determination of particle size in the size range above 1 μm. These methods include optical microscopy (size range of 0.2–100 μm), through which particles are sized using a calibrated grid background; sieving (37–9500 μm), in which particles are sized by passing through a series of sieves of known and successively smaller sizes under mechanical shaking; coulter counter (size range of 1–500 μm), an automated apparatus for sizing and counting particles or cells based on changes in electrical conductance of the conductive channel as the particles pass through; and sedimentation method (size range of 1–200 μm), through which the particle size is determined by measuring the terminal settling velocity of particles in a liquid medium under gravitational or centrifugal force. In the following sections, the sieving and sedimentation methods are discussed.

Sieving

Standardized woven-wire sieves defined by the National Bureau of Standards for particle size analysis are given a sieve number that indicates the number of openings in the mesh screen per inch. For example, a #40 sieve has 40 openings per inch in the screen mesh. Particles that can sieve through that mesh are said to be "40 mesh" size, which is equivalent to about 420 μm. The correlation of mesh size with micrometer length is given in **Table 9-4**. The finest mesh readily available is 400 mesh, with openings of 38 μm.

The sieving method uses a set of standard sieves arranged in a column such that the mesh openings become smaller as one descends through the column. At the bottom is a pan that catches particles small enough to pass through all the sieves. A weighted sample of powder is placed in the uppermost sieve and covered with a lid. The joints between sieves are taped to keep particles from working through the joints during shaking; the sieve column is then placed on an automatic shaker. For fine, insoluble particles, wet sieving is appropriate. Here the top sieve is washed with a water stream to move the particle to its appropriate level. With this technique, the sieves must be dried before the particles can be weighed. The size or weight of the sample used is the most important factor that affects the consistency of the particle size analysis. In general, the sample should be sufficiently large that the first sieve retains enough particles to be representative. However, clearly the smaller the sample, the more consistent will be the results, as every particle must present itself to the screen openings for rejection or passing through to the next-finer sieve. If there are six or seven sieves in the nest, a fine-mesh particle must repeat this operation six or seven times. If the sieves are overloaded, the fine-mesh particle may never get a chance to get to its proper sieve. To prevent overloading of the sieves, samples of different weights may be tested in a short time.

Table 9-4 Mesh Opening Sizes in U.S. Standard Sieves

Sieve Number	Millimeters (mm)	Micrometers (μm)
2	9.52	9520
4	4.76	4760
8	2.38	2380
10	2.00	2000
20	0.84	840
30	0.59	590
40	0.42	420
50	0.297	297
60	0.250	250
70	0.210	210
80	0.177	177
100	0.149	149
120	0.125	125
200	0.074	74

A comparison of these results should be sufficient to point out the correct sample size. In general, if the particle size range is very wide, such as in a crushed sample, a large sample (500 to 1000 g) may be required. For finely ground powder, a sample of 25 to 100 g should be used. Completion of sieving usually takes from a few minutes to one-half hour.

After completion of sieving, the entire nest of sieves is brought to the weighing station. Weighing is done in grams with a sensitivity of 0.1 g. The total weight of the material retained on the various sieves and in the pan should be very close to the weight of the original sample. The weight of the material retained on each sieve is never used directly but is expressed as a percentage, for the particle size group, of the total sample. The frequency of the size distribution is thus expressed as a mass distribution, which indicates the fraction of total mass found for particles in a certain size range. **Table 9-5** is an example of particle size analysis based on sieving.

The mean diameter calculated from mass distribution corresponds to the Edmundson expression of $(\Sigma nd^3/\Sigma n)^{1/3}$, that is, $d_{v/n}$, which refers to particles having a finite relationship of volume, weight, and number of particles per weight. Consider spherical particles with a diameter of $d_{v/n}$.

Table 9-5 Determination of Particle Size by Sieving Method

Sieve No.	Arithmetic Mean (d_a; μm)	Weight (wt) Retained (g)	% wt	% wt Cumulative	(% wt) (d_a)
50/60	274	3.5	3.51	3.51	961.9
60/70	230	15.8	15.85	19.36	3,644.9
70/80	194	24.3	24.37	43.73	4,728.4
80/100	163	37.3	37.41	81.14	6,098.2
100/120	137	14.6	14.64	95.78	2,006.2
120/200	100	4.2	4.21	100	421.0
					17,860.6
$d_{mean} = \Sigma$ (%wt)(d_a)/100 = 17,860.6/100 = 178.6 μm					

The volume of a single particle is $\pi d_{v/n}^3/6$, and the mass is the volume times the density (ρ) of the particle. Assuming that the number of particles per gram of powder is N, then

$$N = 6/\pi d_{v/n}^3/6 \qquad (9\text{-}6)$$

Equation (9-6) is an important expression in particle technology. The woven-wire sieves are effective for the analysis of coarse particles with diameters larger than 50 to 100 µm. Smaller particles, which can easily stick to screen surfaces, may bring difficulty to proper sieving.

Sedimentation

It is possible to measure the size of a particle by the speed with which it moves through a liquid medium under the influence of some force, such as gravity. A particle of mass m, in such a case, experiences a downward pull of mg, opposed in solution by the buoyancy of the medium. In effect, the particle displaces a volume of m/ρ_2, or $\pi d^3/6$, corresponding to a mass of medium equal to $(m/\rho_2)\rho_1$, where ρ_1 and ρ_2 are the densities of the medium and particle, respectively. The net force due to gravity is then

$$mg\,(1 - \rho_1/\rho_2) = \pi d^3 g\,(\rho_2 - \rho_1)/6$$

The particle will fall through the medium if $\rho_2 > \rho_1$, but as it accelerates, a viscous drag develops that is proportional to the velocity (v), or equal to fv, where f is the friction coefficient. A *terminal settling velocity* is reached when the force due to gravity and that of the viscous drag have become equal, i.e., when

$$v = \pi d^3 g\,(\rho_2 - \rho_1)/6f$$

According to Stokes, the friction coefficient depends, in a complicated way, on the shape of the particle and the viscosity (η) of the solvent. The effect of irregular shapes is mathematically unattainable. But for a spherical particle, $f = 6\pi\eta r$ *or* $3\pi\eta d$, where r is the radius and d is the diameter of the particle. This is known as Stokes' law. Thus,

$$v = \pi d^3 g\,(\rho_2 - \rho_1)/6(3\pi\eta d) = d^2 g\,(\rho_2 - \rho_1)\,/18\eta \qquad (9\text{-}7)$$

One can determine the terminal settling velocity and thus the *Stokes* (*spherical equivalent*) *diameter* (d_{St}) of the particles by using Equation (9-7).

A number of methods have been developed for the measurement of particle sizes based on the sedimentation phenomenon. Among these the *Andreasen pipette* method has been extensively used in various fields of study. The apparatus for the Andreasen pipette consists of a special graduated cylinder (500 mL) with a ground tapered neck for particle suspension and special stopper with a pipette immersed at a depth h below the surface of the suspension. Samples (10 mL) of the suspension at depth h can be withdrawn using the pipette for analysis. The system is secured in a constant-temperature bath during operation. Note that temperature, which strongly affects the viscosity of the solution, will have a significant effect on the particle sedimentation rate. The procedure is straightforward. A powder sample is dispersed by vigorous agitation into a liquid with a suitable deflocculating agent in an initial concentration C_0 of 0.5–1%, and it is allowed to settle beginning at time 0. At desired time intervals, samples of the fluid are pipetted from the depth h below the surface. These samples are evaporated to dryness and weighed to yield the concentration C_t at various time intervals. Based on the sedimentation theory, at any time t, the particles from the withdrawn sample will have a terminal settling velocity equal to or less than h/t, and the larger particles will have already settled below the pipette tip. Hence, the ratio of C_t/C_0 gives the weight fraction of particles that have a terminal velocity equal to or less than h/t, where the Stokes diameter is

$$d_{St} \leq [(h/t)(18\eta)/g(\rho_2 - \rho_1)]^{1/2} \quad (9\text{-}8)$$

The use of Equation (9-8) for particle size determination can be seen from Example 9-1. Although there are some drawbacks related to poor dispersion, possible thermal gradients, and accelerated sedimentation due to sampling, the pipette method for particle size measurement is considered to be accurate and economical in terms of equipment in the size range of 2–50 μm.

Example 9-1: An air pollution dust sample was analyzed using the Andreasen pipette method for particle sizes. The dust sample has a density of 2.92 g/cm³. When it was suspended in an aqueous medium (η = 0.01 P or g/cm-s, ρ_1 = 1.01 g/cm³) at 25°C, the following sedimentation rate data were obtained:

Particle group	1	2	3	4
d_{St} (μm)	?	?	?	≤ 4
h (cm)	10	10	10	5
t (s)	100	400	1610	?

(*a*) Calculate the Stokes diameters of the particle groups.

(*b*) Calculate the time needed for sedimentation of particles with size equal to or less than 4 μm.

Solution: $d_{St} \leq [(h/t)(18\eta)/g(\rho_2 - \rho_1)]^{1/2} = (h/t)^{1/2}\,[18 \times 0.01/(2.92 - 1.01) \times 981]^{1/2}$

$$= 0.0098(h/t)^{1/2} \quad \text{cm}$$

(*a*) Group 1: $d_{St} \leq 0.0098 \times (10/100)^{1/2} = 0.0031$ cm or 31.0 μm

Group 2: $d_{St} \leq 0.0098 \times (10/400)^{1/2} = 0.00155$ cm or 15.5 μm

Group 3: $d_{St} \leq 0.0098 \times (10/1610)^{1/2} = 0.00077$ cm or 7.7 μm

(*b*) Group 4: h = 5 cm $\quad d_{St} \leq 0.0004$ cm

$t = 5/(0.0004/0.0098)^2 = 3001$ s or 50.02 min†

†The Andreasen pipette method is a time-consuming process.

Particle Shape and Surface Area

There is an inverse relationship between particle size and surface area. A cube 1 cm on an edge has a surface area of 6 cm². If the cube were fragmented into smaller cubes having edges of 0.1 cm, there would be 1000 smaller cubes and the total surface area would become 60 cm². This ideal relationship is unlikely to ever be encountered because particles break into smaller particles with a range of sizes and shapes. Actual particles of whatever size, if examined on a molecular scale, may display planar regions, but also lattice distortions, dislocations, and cracks. This means that the actual surface area of the resulting smaller particles will be greater, sometimes very much greater, than would be calculated by assuming any one geometric shape. Particle shape may also affect the particle surface activity, as has been shown in the catalytic properties of metallic nanoparticles, where different crystal facets result in different selectivity.[5]

Particle Shape

Shape reflects the history of the formation of the particles. From crystallization, particles may exist as single crystals that assume various crystalline structures such as plates, needles, and cubes, or as amorphous aggregate if formed by rapid precipitation from solution. The characteristics of the existence of multiple forms in shape and structure are called polymorphism and potentially can be found in any crystalline material. Polymorphs have different stabilities and may spontaneously convert from a metastable form to a stable shape or structure at a particular temperature. Polymorphism is very important in the development of active pharmaceutical ingredients, as it can affect, via changes in particle surface area and solubility, drug absorption and bioavailability. The metastable forms usually exhibit higher solubility and dissolution rates than the stable form, but for many drugs, regulatory approval is given only to the stable crystalline structure.

For small particles in the colloidal size range (1–500 nm), particle shape can have a direct effect on the performance of small particles, when used for drug delivery purposes, in the biological system. As revealed by electron microscopy, colloidal and nanoparticles can be generally classified as spherical or ellipsoid, disc- or plate-like, or rod- and needle-shaped particles. It is obvious that the particle surface area will be different depending upon the shape. Computer simulation studies have shown that the translocation of nanoparticles across the lipid bilayer depends on the orientation of particles at the membrane and the contact surface area,[6] both of which are shape-dependent. The penetrating capability of a nanoparticle across a lipid bilayer is determined by the contact area between the particle and the lipid bilayer, and the local curvature of the particle at the contact point. Cell culture studies on the uptake of colloidal gold nanoparticles of different sizes and shapes have also shown that spherical particles were taken up 500% more than rod-shaped particles of similar size by Hela cells,[7] which was explained by the greater membrane wrapping time required for the elongated particles. An understanding of how nanoparticles with different shapes interact with the cell membrane is important in drug delivery. Greater discussion of this subject will be given later.

Surface Area

The surface area of a powder sample is expressed in terms of *specific surface area*, defined as the surface area per unit volume (S_v) or per unit weight (S_w). The term surface area/volume ratio refers to S_v. These two expressions are related in that $S_v = \rho S_w$, where ρ is the density of the particle. With known particle size and distribution, the total or specific surface area of a powder sample can be calculated using the equivalent spherical diameter and the relationships that the volume of sphere = $\pi d^3/6$ and surface area = πd^2. The weight of a particle group with a single particle size is the weight of the particle times the number of particles (N); the weight of a particle is the volume of the particle times its density; and the total surface area is the surface area of the single particle times N. Hence,

$$w \text{ (weight of particle group)} = N(\pi d^3/6)\rho$$

$$S \text{ (total surface area)} = N\pi d^2$$

It follows that

$$S = 6w/\rho d \tag{9-9}$$

and

$$\begin{aligned} S_w &= 6/\rho d \\ S_v &= 6/d \end{aligned} \tag{9-10}$$

Table 9-6 Calculation of Surface Area of Individual Particle Size Groups and Specific Surface Area (S_w) from the Particle Size Distribution

Sieve No.	Arithmetic Mean (d_a; μm)	Weight (w) Retained (g)	%w	(%w)(d_a)	S ($6w/\rho d_a$)† cm², 10²
50/60	274	3.5	3.51	961.9	5.11
60/70	230	15.8	15.85	3,644.9	27.48
70/80	194	24.3	24.37	4,728.4	50.10
80/100	163	37.3	37.41	6,098.2	91.53
100/120	137	14.6	14.64	2,006.2	42.63
120/200	100	4.2	4.21	421.0	16.80
		99.7		17,860.6	233.65
$S_w = 233.65 \times 10^2/99.7 = 2.34 \times 10^2$ cm²/g					

†$\rho = 1.5$ g/cm³

Consider the data given in Table 9-5, where the mean diameter of the powder sample was determined to be 178.6 μm and the total weight of the sample was 99.7 g. If the density of the particle is 1.5 g/cm³, the total surface area according to Equation (9-9) will be 2.23×10^4 cm², and the specific surface area per weight (S_w) according to Equation (9-10) will be 2.24×10^2 cm²/g. Alternatively, one can calculate the surface area for each particle size group and take the weighted mean as S_w as shown in **Table 9-6**.

Surface Activity

The surface activity of small particles derives from the surface area, surface characteristics, and the energy storage capacity of the particles. Particle size reduction in pharmaceutical formulations has a significant impact on product performance. A large increase in particle surface areas affects not only drug adsorption but also interparticle interactions that can alter the overall properties of the drug delivery system, such as suspensions and emulsions. In addition, there is a concomitant increase in surface energy as the material is finely divided. It is worth noting that the increase in surface energy from 1 cm to 10 nm is about 10 million J, indicating that nanoparticles have a great capacity in the storage and charge and discharge of energy through a huge increase in surface area. As the particle size is reduced, the internal area of the particle also becomes exposed, and with it there is a potential change in the number and type of surface chemical sites and groups. In a particle of 1 cm³, the surface molecules are only a few compared to millions of nonexposed molecules. When divided into 10 nm, more molecules or atoms become surface moieties and the ratio rises to nearly 1:4; and at 1 nm, 80% of molecules are at the surface.[8] The most noted effect of such changes is that, in the colloidal size range, electrical effects that are normally negligible for particles of the macro scale become dominant in the description of colloidal properties. Studies have also shown that nanoparticles exhibit novel optical, magnetic, and electronic properties, and that the surface area may be a defining metric that controls the properties of a nanoparticle system, be it physiochemical, toxicological, or therapeutic.[8, 9]

Surface Area Measurement

Adsorption

Whereas it is possible to calculate the surface area based on the spherical assumption, this condition is clearly not met by most real-world powder samples. Different particle shapes, surface irregularities, and porosity will inevitably lead to an estimation that is significantly less than the

Table 9-7 Comparison of the Physicochemical Features Involved in Physical Adsorption and Chemisorption

	Physical Adsorption	Chemisorption
Forces	van der Waals forces	Valence electron interactions
Heat of adsorption	< 10 kcal/mol	> 20 kcal/mol
Temperature	Below boiling point of adsorbate	Occurs at high temperature
Pressure (P)	Adsorption increases with P	Adsorption decreases with P
Dependency	More on adsorbate than adsorbent	Characteristics to both
Activation energy	No	May be involved
Multilayer adsorption	Yes	At most, a monolayer
Reversibility	Reversible	Irreversible

true value. Hence, it is essential that the surface area be measured directly. Indeed, all the fine attributes to the significance of surface activities could not have been achieved without precise measuring means. With well-defined theories, such measurement can yield information on not only the surface area but also the nature of the particle surface and surface activity. Surface area has been, and still is, determined using the classical *adsorption theory*, except that the instrumentation has been much improved to allow accurate determination with computer-assisted calculations of experimental results.[10] The basic theory is that under appropriate conditions, gas molecules will be adsorbed onto the particle surface, and if the gas layer is one molecule deep, then the area covered by gas can be calculated from the area occupied by one molecule and the total number of gas molecules in the monolayer.

Adsorption of gases or solutes from a solution, as in suspensions, is a fundamental property of small particles. Hence, much can be gained from a basic review of this important phenomenon. It is convenient to recognize that most adsorptions can be placed in one of two categories. These categories are differentiated by surface interactions involving essentially physical forces in one and chemical bonding at the solid surface in the other, from which arise the terms physical adsorption and chemical adsorption. The latter is more commonly known as chemisorption. **Table 9-7** outlines the experimental features that allow a process to be so categorized.

These features show that physical adsorption of gases such as N_2 and H_2 occurs at very low temperature, where the incremental increase in the amount adsorbed increases with each incremental increase in the pressure of the gas. This suggests a condensation process. The heat of adsorption is relatively low and is in the range of the heat of vaporization. Hence, in surface area measurement, the particles are routinely degassed to provide a clean or free surface. In chemisorption, however, the gases may exist in atomic state through interaction with surface electrons and penetrate into the interior of the particles. As a result, the heat of adsorption is in the range of the heat of reactions (20–100 kcal/mol), and such adsorption is nonreversible.

Langmuir Isotherm

Most adsorption studies involve the measurement of the amount of gas adsorbed (in volume) by a given amount of the adsorbent (particles) and the pressure of the adsorbate (gas). Such measurement is usually made at constant temperature, and the results are presented graphically as an *adsorption isotherm*. A great variety of adsorption isotherm shapes exist. We discuss two theoretical treatments of the adsorption isotherm for the purposes of determining the surface area. A simple model of the adsorption process was given by Langmuir in 1916 based on the formation of a gas monolayer over the surface of the adsorbent. This type of adsorption

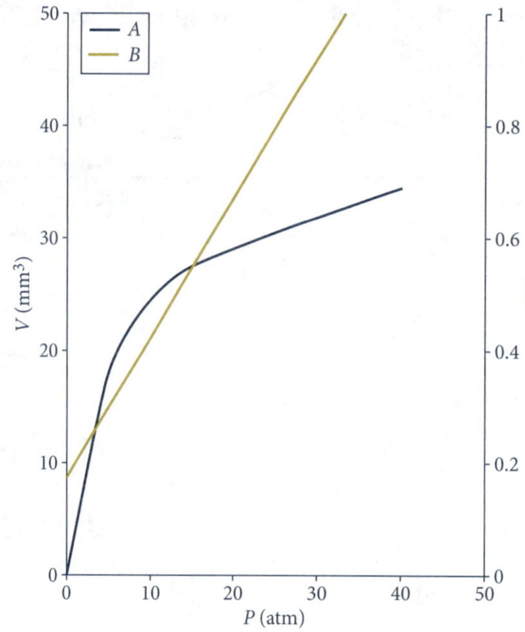

Figure 9-3 The Langmuir adsorption isotherm for N_2 on mica at 90 K: (*A*) Plot of *V* versus *P*; (*B*) plot of *P*/*V* versus *P*.[11]

typically shows an initial steeply rising curve that gradually flattens out (**Figure 9-3**). The initial rise is taken as the strong tendency of the surface to bind the gas molecules, and the leveling off can be attributed to the saturation of such binding forces or the active sites on the surface. Langmuir suggested that the rate of evaporation is proportional to the fraction of the surface covered with gas (θ), whereas the rate of condensation is proportional to the amount of gas (as indicated by pressure *P*) and the fraction of the surface not covered by adsorbed gas ($1 - \theta$). Thus, at equilibrium, where the rate of evaporation is the same as the rate of condensation, one can write

$$\text{Rate of evaporation} = k\theta = \text{rate of condensation} = k'P(1 - \theta)$$

where *k* and *k'* are the proportionality constants. Rearrangement and introduction of $K = k/k'$ give

$$\theta = k'P/(k + k'P) = P/(K + P)$$

If the saturated volume of the gas that can be adsorbed (to form a monolayer) is V_m, whereas the volume of adsorbed gas at any pressure *P* is *V*, then $V/V_m = \theta$. With this relation, the above equation can be rewritten as

$$\frac{P}{V} = \frac{K}{V_m} + \frac{P}{V_m} \qquad (9\text{-}11)$$

Equation (9-11) is known as the *Langmuir isotherm*. A plot of *P*/*V* versus *P* will yield a straight line with a slope equal to $1/V_m$ and an intercept of K/V_m, if the experimental data are in accord with the Langmuir theory (see Example 9-2 and Figure 9-3 for the use of the above equation).

BET Isotherm

The Langmuir theory is based on the formation of a monolayer film of gas molecules. The application of this approach is limited mostly to chemisorptions. Other theories have been developed to explain the more complete adsorption process that involves multilayer formation

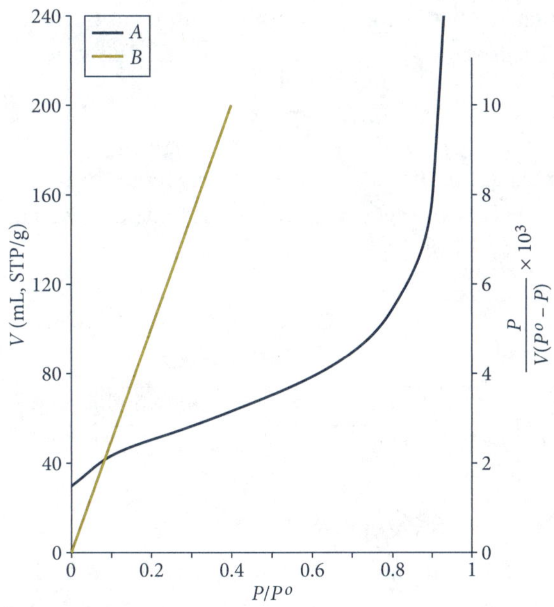

Figure 9-4 The BET adsorption isotherm of N_2 on silica gel[12]: (*A*) Plot of *V* versus P/P^o; (*B*) plot of $P/V(P^o - P)$ versus P/P^o.

and S-shaped adsorption curve (see **Figure 9-4**). One such treatment, developed by Brunauer, Emmet, and Teller, is known as the *BET isotherm.* It should be pointed out that whether more than a monolayer is being formed is not directly observable. But one can consider the multilayer adsorption (of gas on gas) above the first layer as a condensation process having the same heat of condensation for each layer. If the basic assumption of the Langmuir approach holds, i.e., if the particle surface contains a finite number of sites for the gas molecules to occupy, then the saturation of gas or liquid at the particle surface will lead to the saturated vapor pressure of the liquefied gas as the adsorbed amount reaches infinity. In this approach, the isotherm can be written as

$$\frac{P}{V(P^o - P)} = \frac{1}{cV_m} + \frac{c-1}{V_m c}\frac{P}{P^o} \qquad (9\text{-}12)$$

where P^o is the saturation vapor pressure of the liquefied gas and c is a constant expressing the difference between heat of condensation (E_{cond}) and heat of adsorption (E_{ad}), $c = \exp - (E_{cond} - E_{ad})$. The heat of condensation is the energy change from the surface to the outer layer, whereas the heat of adsorption is the energy change for the first layer adsorption. The volumes V and V_m are as previously defined, which are calculated at standard temperature and pressure (STP) conditions. To use Equation (9-12), a plot of $P/V(P^o - P)$ versus P/P^o should yield a straight line with a slope of $(c - 1)/V_m c$ and an intercept of $1/V_m c$, from which both V_m and c can be determined. Studies have shown that for S-shaped isotherm, the plot indeed gives a straight line in the P/P^o range of 0.05–0.35 (see Example 9-3 and Figure 9-4). The BET theory has been the basis for surface area determinations.

Determination of Surface Area

Once V_m is obtained, it can be converted to the number of molecules required for the formation of a monolayer. For example, if 1 g of particles is covered by an amount of gas that occupies a volume of 1.5 mL at STP, then the number of gas molecules is $(1.5/22{,}400) \times 6.02 \times 10^{23} = 4.03 \times 10^{19}$ molecules. Next, one estimates the area covered by one molecule. A crude estimate of the effective area per molecule is $(V_{liq}/N)^{2/3}$, where V_{liq} is the volume of 1 mol of liquid gas and N is Avogadro's number. Emmet and Brunauer[13] have shown that for common gases, the close-packed area (A) covered by one gas molecule is

$$A = 4(0.866)\,[M/4(2)^{1/2}N\rho]^{2/3} = 1.53(M/\rho)^{2/3} \quad \text{Å}^2 \tag{9-13}$$

where M is the molecular weight of the gas and ρ is the density of the gas at its boiling point. The following examples will show how the specific surface area is determined using the adsorption data.

Example 9-2: The data of Langmuir for the adsorption of N_2 on mica at 90 K give[11]

P (atm)	2.8	3.4	4.0	4.9	6.0	7.3	9.4	12.8	17.1	23.5	33.5
V (mm^3)†	12.0	13.4	15.1	17.0	19.0	21.6	23.9	25.5	28.2	30.8	33.0

†Amount adsorbed (at 20°C, 1 atm).

(*a*) Show that these data fit a Langmuir isotherm expression and evaluate the constants.
(*b*) Calculate the area covered by a single nitrogen molecule; the density of liquid nitrogen is 0.812 g/cm^3.
(*c*) Estimate the surface area of the mica sample.

Solution:

(*a*) The Langmuir expression can be tested by plotting V as a function of P or P/V versus P. The latter gives a straight line. The results are shown in Figure 9-3. From the linear plot,

Slope = 0.0255

$V_m = 39.2\ \text{mm}^3/\text{g}$ adsorbent or 39.2×10^{-6} L/g

$n = PV/RT = 1 \times 39.2 \times 10^{-6}/0.082 \times 293 = 1.63 \times 10^{-6}$ mol

Monolayer of N_2 over mica:

$N = 1.63 \times 10^{-6} \times 6.02 \times 10^{23} = 9.81 \times 10^{17}$ molecules

y-intercept $= K/V_m = 0.165 \qquad K = 6.47$ atm

(*b*) $A = 1.53(M/\rho)^{2/3} = 1.53(28.01/0.812)^{2/3} = 1.53 \times 10.61 = 16.2$ Å^2

(*c*) $S_w = NA = 16.2 \times 10^{-16} \times 9.81 \times 10^{17} = 15.89 \times 10^2\ \text{cm}^2/\text{g}$

Example 9-3: The adsorption of N_2 up to the vapor pressure of nitrogen on a silica gel at 90 K is shown in Figure 9-4. In the $P/P°$ region of 0.05 to 0.35, the parameters are as follows:

V (mL STP/g)	39	41	44	48	50	53	58	61
$P/P°$	0.05	0.07	0.10	0.16	0.20	0.25	0.30	0.35

Calculate the specific surface area of the silica gel according to the BET isotherm.

Solution: The parameter $P/V(P° - P)$ can be calculated as $1/V(P°/P - 1)$ to give the following:

$P/P°$	0.05	0.07	0.10	0.16	0.20	0.25	0.30	0.35
$P/V(P° - P) \times 10^3$	1.35	1.74	2.53	3.97	4.72	6.29	7.45	8.83

Using Equation (9-12), a plot of $P/V(P^o - P)$ versus P/P^o yields a straight line (see Figure 9-4), where

Slope = $(c - 1)/V_m c = 24 \times 10^{-3}$ cm^{-3}

Intercept = $1/V_m c = 0.2 \times 10^{-3}$ cm^{-3}

Calculation of c:

$c - 1$ = slope/intercept = 24/0.2 = 120

$c = e^{-\Delta E/RT} = 121 \qquad \Delta E = 858$ cal/mol

Calculation of surface area:

$V_m = 1/0.2 \times 10^{-3} \times 121 = 41.3$ mL STP/g

Molecules in monolayer:

$N = (41.3/22{,}400) \times 6.02 \times 10^{23} = 1.11 \times 10^{21}$ molecules

Area occupied by single nitrogen molecule = 16.2 Å^2 (see Example 9-2)

Thus,

$S_w = NA = 1.11 \times 10^{21} \times 16.2 \times 10^{-16} = 17.98 \times 10^5$ cm^2/g

Particle Porosity and Density

Porosity, either as a function or independent of the particle size, is also an important physical characteristic of particles. Solid particles from grinding, milling, and leaching processes often exhibit cracks, cavities, and holes (collectively called *pores*) within the structure. Particles produced by condensation or crystallization may contain or acquire, after a period of time, cracks along grain boundaries and at positions where impurities are occluded. Fine particles also tend to adhere to one another to form aggregates or larger secondary particles, giving rise to another level of pore size. Then there are organized porous structures in which polished particles such as silicon[14] are converted, by electrochemical etching methods, to tailored pore sizes and volumes that are controllable for the scale of micrometers to nanometers. Pore size is expressed either in terms of the diameter, assuming it is cylindrical, or simply as the width of the pore opening. Pores of widths less than 2 nm (20 Å) are referred to as micropores, those from 2 to 50 nm are called *mesopores*, and those of larger widths are referred to as macropores. The volume of all cracks, fissures, holes, and channels within the body of particles is the total pore volume.

Measurement of Pore Size

The evaluation of pore size and porous structures may be achieved by gas adsorption, as in surface area measurement, and by the mercury intrusion method. We confine the discussion to gas sorption in order to gain greater insight into how the porous structure is studied. The surface area determinations involve creating the conditions required to adsorb an average monolayer of gas molecules onto a sample. By extending this process so that gas is allowed to condense in the pores, the sample's pore structure can also be evaluated. Experimentally, adsorption is carried out by admitting the gas to the particles in controlled increments. After each increment, the pressure is allowed to equilibrate, and the quantity of gas adsorbed is determined. As pressure increases, the gas condenses first in the pores with the smallest dimensions. The pressure is increased until saturation is reached, at which time all pores are filled with liquid. The adsorptive

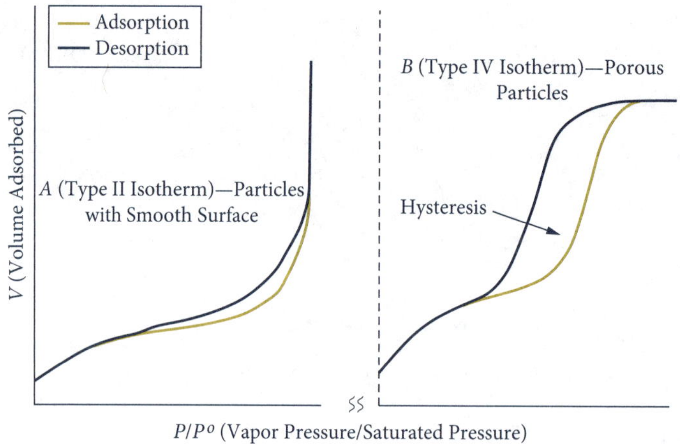

Figure 9-5 (*A*) Type II adsorption isotherm and (*B*) adsorption isotherm with a closed hysteresis of a porous material.

gas pressure then is reduced incrementally to evaporate the condensed gas from the system. The characteristics of a porous structure can be seen from **Figure 9-5**, which shows the plot of absorbed gas as a function of its vapor pressure over saturated vapor pressure (P/P^o). For particles of smooth surface, the desorption curve is nearly identical with the adsorption curve. For porous particles, however, the gas volume and pressure diagram exhibits hysteresis, in which the desorption curve is above the adsorption curve, indicating that the absorbed gas volume is larger than that of the adsorption curve at the same P/P^o ratio due to, in the most likely case, trapped or condensed gas in the pores. The trapped gas effectively reduces the radius or diameter of the pore size, suggesting that in desorption, only at a lower value of P/P^o will the absorbed amount of gas be the same as that of the adsorption process. The relation of pore size to gas pressure can be deduced using the *Kelvin equation*, which is one of the principal equations in surface chemistry, along with the *Laplace equation*, the Gibbs adsorption equation, and the equation of Young and Dupre.[15]

The Kelvin equation relates the surface free energy change to the pressure-induced change in the size (radius) of a spherical bubble. One recalls that the surface free energy change, $RT \ln(P_2/P_1)$, from P_1 to P_2 can be expressed as

$$\Delta G = RT \ln(P_2/P_1) = V\,\Delta P \qquad (9\text{-}14)$$

where V is the molar volume and ΔP is the applied pressure. This can be numerically illustrated as follows. Water has a molar volume of 18 cm^3/mol. If a 100 atm mechanical pressure is applied, assuming the volume of water is not compressed, $V\,\Delta P = 18 \times 100 = 1800$ cm^2-atm. At 25°C, $RT = 82.06 \times 298.2 = 24{,}470$ cm^2-atm. Thus, $\log (P_2/P_1) = 1800/24{,}470 \times 2.303 = 0.0319$, and $P_2/P_1 = 1.076$. This indicates that the vapor pressure is increased 7.6% by the application of 100 atm pressure. Now consider a bubble of radius r, where the total surface free energy is $4\pi r^2 \gamma$ and γ is the surface tension. If the radius were to decrease by dr, which must be brought about by a pressure change of ΔP on the bubble film, then the change in surface tension is $8\pi r\gamma\, dr$, and the work against this pressure change is $(\Delta P)4\pi r^2\, dr$. Thus, we have

$$\Delta P\, 4\pi r^2\, dr = 8\pi r\gamma\, dr$$

or

$$\Delta P = 2\gamma/r \qquad (9\text{-}15)$$

Equation (9-15) is the Laplace equation for a spherical shape, which shows that the larger the ΔP, the smaller the bubble will become. When Equations (9-14) and (9-15) are combined, one obtains the Kelvin equation, which describes the effect of mechanical pressure on the vapor pressure of a liquid:

$$RT\ln(P_2/P_1) = 2\gamma V/r$$

If we substitute the ratio of molecular weight to density (M/ρ) for V, and P and P^o for P_1 and P_2, respectively, then the above equation can be written, for gas adsorption studies, as

$$RT\ln(P/P^o) = -2\gamma M/r\rho \qquad (9\text{-}16)$$

Here, P is the incremental pressure in gas adsorption measurement and P^o is the saturated vapor pressure. Notice that the pressure ratio is written as P/P^o for pore size measurement, and the right-hand side of the equation is now negative, because $P^o > P$. In pore size determination, the trapped gas in pores during desorption makes the pore radius smaller; consequently, P/P^o is smaller, and the desorption curve is shifted to the left of the adsorption curve.

Evaluation of the adsorption and desorption branches of the isotherms and the hysteresis between them reveals information about the pore size, pore volume, pore area, and pore shape. The Kelvin model allows the determination of pore radius at various P/P^o points, which represent pore size equal to or smaller than the radius calculated (see Example 9-4 for application of the Kelvin equation). This method applies to only the mesopores and macropores. Micropore size and distribution may also be determined based on experimental isotherm using different models.[10]

Example 9-4: The data on water adsorption and desorption on a clay sample at 20°C are partially given in the following table:

P/P^o	V_1 (adsorption), mL/g	V_2 (desorption), mL/g
0.35	0.129	0.150
0.56	0.150	0.188
0.89	0.182	0.209

Calculate the pore size at each relative pressure point.

Solution:

The surface tension of water at 20°C is 72.8 erg/cm^2, the gas constant is 8.3143 erg/deg-mol, and the molecular volume (V_w) of water is 18.02 cm^3/mol. Based on the Kelvin equation

$$r = -2\gamma V_w/RT\ln(P/P^o) = -(2)(72.8)(18.02)/(8.3143\times 10^7)(293.16)[\ln(P/P^o)]$$

$$= -1.077\times 10^{-7}/\ln P/P^o \quad \text{cm}$$

Thus,

P/P^o	0.35	0.56	0.89
r (Å)	≤10.25	≤18.57	≤92.39

The adsorption of water vapor by pharmaceutical powders will have an important consequence on the formulation, manufacturing, and performance of pharmaceutical products. Studies have shown that many pharmaceutical agents such as methylcellulose and povidone show water vapor sorption characterized by hysteresis in their adsorption isotherms.[16] Povidone was shown to exhibit increased water adsorption when treated with acetone, which increases the pore size and the number of adsorption sites.

Porosity and Density of Particles

Porosity is the measure of the void volume in a powder material, and it is expressed as a fraction or a percentage of the total volume. The total volume of the material, which can be measured with a graduated cylinder, is usually known as the bulk volume, whereas the void volume is the difference between the bulk volume and the true volume that must be measured with specialized methods. In association with the volume is the particle density, which, as in all density expressions, is defined as the weight per unit volume. There are three density expressions associated with powders: (1) the *true density* (or absolute density), which excludes the volume of pores and interparticle spaces; (2) envelope density (also called the apparent density), which includes the pore volume but excludes interparticle spaces; and (3) the *bulk density*, which includes both pore volume and the interparticle spaces. For a powder, the bulk density changes with vibration and applied forces due to changes in volume. The true and envelope densities of a nonporous powder are identical, but the two will differ significantly if the material is of irregular shape with cracks, internal pores, and capillary spaces.

True Density

Because most particle samples are porous, the determination of the true density is best carried out using a helium densitometer. A sample of the material is placed in a sealed chamber of known volume and is exposed to a series of elevated and then released helium gas pressures. The release of the pressure is directed to a connected chamber of known volume. The pressures in both chambers are determined before and after the expansion of the gas, from which the volume of the sample excluding pore volume is calculated as the true volume, and the density determined from the weight and volume as the true density. For inorganic salts of sodium, potassium, magnesium, and calcium, the true densities are in the range of about 1.5–4.0 g/cm^3, whereas for organic drugs, the average density is about 1.3 g/cm^3.

Envelope Density

The envelope density can be determined by the principle based on liquid displacement. For a powder that is insoluble and heavier than a suitably selected liquid, the difference in total weight between the liquid alone and a particle suspension of known particle weight at the same volume is the amount of liquid displaced by the powder sample. This permits the calculation of the volume and thus the density of the sample. This determination requires the liquid to penetrate and fill the intraparticle pore structures. The envelope density of a solid, when compared to its true density, allows one to evaluate the solid's porosity and specific pore volume.

Bulk Density

A standard method for the determination of bulk density may be followed.[17] A sample of about 50 mL of powder, which has been passed through a U.S. #20 sieve, is introduced into a 100-mL graduated cylinder. The cylinder, held 1 inch above a hardwood surface, is dropped three times onto the surface at 2-second intervals. The bulk density is then obtained as the ratio of the sample weight in grams to the measured volume in cubic centimeters by the graduated cylinder. Bulk density is the parameter that defines how granular, fibrous, and powdery materials pack or consolidate under a variety of conditions. Powder materials compressed under a force of 100,000 lb/in^2 have been shown to yield true densities of the materials.[18]

Relation of Porosity to Density

As mentioned earlier, the porosity (Φ) is defined as the fraction of the void volume over the total volume of the powder sample. Because the volume is inversely proportional to density, it follows that

$$\Phi_{total} = (V_{bulk} - V_{true})/V_{bulk} = 1 - V_{true}/V_{bulk} = 1 - \rho_{bulk}/\rho_{true} \quad (9\text{-}17)$$

The above definition is termed *total porosity*, because it includes interparticle void spaces as well as pore volumes of the particles. Similarly, one can define the intraparticle and interparticle porosities as

$$\Phi_{intraparticle} = 1 - \rho_{envelope}/\rho_{true} \quad (9\text{-}18)$$

$$\Phi_{interparticle} = 1 - \rho_{bulk}/\rho_{envelope} \quad (9\text{-}19)$$

The use of these equations is illustrated in Example 9-5.

Example 9-5: (*a*) A powder mixture has a true density of 2.054 g/mL. When 50 g of this mixture was placed in a graduated cylinder, the bulk volume was determined to be 41 mL. Calculate the porosity of this powder mixture. (*b*) If the volume of the sample were measured to be 35 mL using a tapped density tester, by repeated tapping of the graduated cylinder until the change in volume is within 2% of the total volume, how would you calculate the porosity? (*c*) Calculate the Hausner ratio,† defined as $\rho_{tapped} = \rho_{bulk}$.

Solution:

(*a*) The bulk density:

$\rho_{bulk} = 50/41 = 1.220$ g/mL

$\Phi_{total} = 1 - \rho_{bulk}/\rho_{true} = 1 - 1.220/2.054 = 40.6\%$

(*b*) The tapped density:

$\rho_{tapped} = 50/35 = 1.429$ g/mL

$\Phi_{total} = 1 - \rho_{tapped}/\rho_{true} = 1 - 1.429/2.054 = 30.4\%$

(*c*) $H = \rho_{tapped}/\rho_{bulk} = 1.429/1.220 = 1.17$†

†This parameter is related to the flowability of the powder, and a value greater than 1.25 is considered to indicate poor flowability.

Flow Property

The flow property of powders and the constancy of flow are of great importance for the manufacture of solid dosage forms. In making tablets, e.g., a powder die must be filled with the same amount of powder each and every time. *Powder flowability* is defined as the ease with which a powder will flow under a set of conditions. Some of the conditions include the pressure on the powder, the humidity of the air around the powder, and the equipment the powder is flowing through or from. A number of factors have been used to describe the flow characteristics. These factors include cohesive strength, which measures the potential arching (bridging) and rat-holing tendencies; internal and wall frictions that affect the hopper angles to achieve mass flow; compressibility related to bulk density; and angle of repose, *tapped density*, and chute angle required to maintain flow after impact. Although particle size, shape, and distribution, surface area and porosity, and moisture content all play a role in determining the flow characteristics, there is no direct correlation that would allow these variables to be used to calculate or infer the powder material's flow properties.

Qualitatively, it is known that particle shape and particle size influence how powders flow. Spherical particles flow better than needle-shaped particles, and fine particles do not flow as well as large particles. There is a general correlation between particle size and flowability. Particles in the size range of 250–2000 μm with suitable shape flow freely. Those in the size range of 75–250 μm may or may not flow freely depending on the shape and other factors of the particles. When the particle size is less than 100 mm, flow rate is a problem for most powder substances. Particle size distribution also affects the flow properties of powders. In a test of the flowability of ibuprofen powders, Liu et al.[19] showed that the bulk powder does not flow as well as the separated fractions, and for powders of narrow size distributions, the flowability increases with increasing particle size.

The angle of repose measures the angle of pile of material at rest and gives some recognition of a powder's ability to flow. To determine the angle, the powder flows through a funnel and falls freely onto a surface. As the powder is added to the pile, it slides down the sides until the mutual friction of the particles is in equilibrium with the gravitational force. The height (h) and radius (r) of the resulting cone are measured, and the angle is calculated as

$$\tan \alpha = h/r \tag{9-20}$$

This parameter gives some recognition of a powder's ability to flow. There is a correlation of smaller particle sizes, which flow poorly, to larger angle of repose.[20] Surface roughness also plays a role in a powder's bulk density and flowability.[21] For particles having a rough and irregular surface, the angle of repose will be high and the flow of powder is generally poor.

The tapped density (ρ_{tapped}) is measured using a tapped density tester by repeated tapping (over 1000 times) until a consistent tapped volume (less than 2% change) is achieved. This value has been used to calculate the Hausner ratio H as a parameter to indicate the flowability of powders.[22]

$$H = \rho_{tapped}/\rho_{bulk} \tag{9-21}$$

A ratio of 1.25 or above is considered an indication of poor flowability. Although it gives only an empirical relationship, Dahlinder et al.[23] have shown that the Hausner ratio and the angle of repose correlate well with each other and are applicable even to fairly cohesive tablet granulations. All the studies appear to indicate that porosity is necessary to enhance the flow properties of powders. In manufacturing procedures, compounds such as magnesium stearate, starch, and talc are frequently added as glidants, which enhance powder flow at relatively low concentrations ($\leq 1\%$), possibly by decreasing the repose angle and by reducing the internal friction angle.[19]

II. Pharmaceutical Powders

Pharmaceutical Techniques of Powder Formulation

Methods of Comminution

Comminution is the process of reducing the particle size or aggregates of powder materials. This is mainly performed on active ingredients, as the reduction of particle size can be used to enhance drug dissolution and absorption and to achieve content uniformity. A variety of methods can be used to reduce particle sizes, depending on the purpose, the desired particle size range, and the chemical properties of the powder. Large-scale comminution mills used in industrial settings may be classified into three types: coarse crushers, intermediate grinders, and fine grinding mills. The coarse crushers are used when the diameter of the powder material is 1.5 to 60 in, but as most powders are not in this size range, they are not often used in the pharmaceutical setting. Intermediate grinders provide powders that are between 20 and 200 mesh, and fine grinding mills yield particles that are smaller than 200 mesh.

Mills (or grinders) reduce particle size by attrition, rolling, and impact. Attrition involves rubbing the particles between two surfaces. Most mills use two stones or revolving steel grinding plates to provide the grinding action. Hammer mills result in particles in the range of 20–50 μm.

When particle size reduction is desired on a small scale (e.g., in extemporaneous compounding), there are three methods of comminution:

- Trituration
- Pulverization by intervention
- Levigation

Trituration is the continuous rubbing or grinding of the powder in a mortar with the aid of a pestle, and it is used in working with hard powders. Pulverization by intervention is used for hard crystalline powders that do not crush or triturate easily or for gummy-type substances. In this method, one uses an "intervening" solvent (alcohol or acetone) to dissolve the compound, and then the dissolved powder is mixed in a mortar or spread on an ointment slab to allow evaporation of the solvent. As the solvent evaporates, the powder recrystallizes or precipitates out of solution as fine particles. Levigation reduces the particle size by triturating it in a mortar or spatulating it on an ointment slab with a small amount of a liquid in which the solid is not dissolved. The solvent should be somewhat viscous; compounds such as mineral oil or glycerin are often used for this purpose. This method is of special use for the reduction of particle size of insoluble materials when compounding ointments and suspensions.

Blending

Medicated powders require that the mixed ingredients be blended into a homogeneous mixture, so that consistent doses can be obtained from the powder formulation. As is true with the comminution, there are large- and small-scale blending methods. Large-scale methods involve equipment designed to mix large portions of the powder sample. There are different types of industrial blenders. Some are double-coned or twin-shelled blenders that rotate about an off-center axis; others consist of a vertical impeller mixer, which is cone shaped with a screw-type impeller along the interior wall. In terms of the blending process, there are paddle blenders, fluidized air mixers, and motionless mixers, which rely on a series of flow-twisting or flow-splitting components. The blending processes are routinely monitored, by sampling and analyzing mixed powder at different parts of the powder bed, to ensure that the blender produces a powder bed that is uniformly mixed.

Small-scale methods involve spatulation and geometric dilution. Spatulation mixes powders using a spatula. The mixing can be done in a mortar, on an ointment slab, or in a plastic bag. Because this method does not reduce particle size, the powders must be of fine particle size and uniform before the blending begins. There is also no pressure applied to the mixture as it is already blended and the resulting blend is light and "fluffy." This method is useful for mixing compounds that form eutectic mixtures, i.e., mixtures that have the propensity to liquefy, such as aspirin, benzocaine, camphor, lidocaine, menthol, resorcinol, salicylic acid, and thymol.

Table 9-8 Advantages and Disadvantages of Powders for Medicinal Use

Advantages	Disadvantages
Easy administration to children and geriatric patients	Possible objectionable taste and odor
	Time-consuming and costly preparation
Rapid-onset action	Possible cause of nausea
Improved stability over liquid formulation	
Multiple choices in dosage forms (tablets, capsules, dusting and inhalation powders, etc.) for drug delivery	

Trituration of mixed powders in a mortar with a pestle blends powders more strongly than spatulation. When mixing two powders of unequal quantity, a technique called *geometric dilution* is used. First, the smaller-quantity powder, usually the active ingredient, is triturated with an equal portion of the larger-quantity powder. This first "dilution" is then mixed and triturated again with an equal portion of the larger-quantity powder. This process continues, each time the diluted active ingredient being mixed with an equal portion of the diluent, until all of both powders have been mixed. The geometric dilution method is especially indicated when the active ingredient and the excipient are of the same color and a visible sign of mixing is lacking.

Medicated Powders

Medicated or compounded powders are made for either internal or external uses. Although their application in medicine is limited, there are conditions where extemporaneous compounding of powder dosage forms is necessary for specialized dosage and patients. There are a number of advantages and disadvantages regarding the use of pharmaceutical powders, as can be seen from **Table 9-8**.

Bulk Powders

Bulk powders are those that can be reasonably dosed using inaccurate measuring devices such as a teaspoon, cap, or insufflator. Bulk powders have a large surface area, which exposes them to potential degradation. For example, if a powder is hygroscopic, it will absorb moisture from the air. Some powders absorb so much moisture that they liquefy (called deliquescent powders). Bulk powders may also be volatile and can evaporate if exposed to the air. Therefore, these powders must be packaged in tightly closing, screw-capped glass containers or foil envelopes.

Oral Powders

Pharmaceutical powders intended for oral administration may be dispensed as either bulk powders or divided powders (charts). The latter represent accurately premeasured individual dosages for the dispensing of relatively more potent drugs. Orally administered bulk powders include antacids, dietary supplements, laxatives, and some analgesics. Many oral powders are fine powder mixtures to be taken by patients with a glass of water or juice. Another type of oral powder is an effervescent granulation. Granules, in general, have less surface area than the fine powder mixture because of their larger particle sizes; hence, granules are more slowly hydrated and dissolved than the fine mixtures. An effervescent granulation, however, will rapidly dissolve in water owing to the liberation of carbon dioxide, which makes water "fizz." These formulations contain sodium bicarbonate and a mixture of citric acid monohydrate and tartaric acid. The amounts of the weak acids are in a ratio of 1:2. Through neutralization, both weak acids promote the release of carbon dioxide from the bicarbonate, according to the following reactions.

$$3NaHCO_3 + \underset{\text{citric acid}}{H_3C_6H_5O_7(H_2O)} \rightarrow \underset{\text{citrate}}{C_6H_5O_7^{3-}} + 3CO_2\uparrow + 4H_2O + 3Na^+$$

$$2NaHCO_3 + \underset{\text{tartaric acid}}{H_2C_4H_4O_6} \rightarrow \underset{\text{tartrate}}{C_4H_4O_6^{2-}} + 2CO_2\uparrow + 2H_2O + 2Na^+$$

The amount of sodium bicarbonate in such a formulation is calculated based on the stoichiometry of the above reactions. For example, the molecular weights of sodium bicarbonate, citric acid monohydrate, and tartaric acid are 84, 210, and 150 g/mol, respectively. For 1 g of citric acid monohydrate and 2 g of tartaric acid, the amount of sodium bicarbonate needed is

$$Wt_{NaHCO_3} = 3 \times 84/210 + 2 \times 84 \times 2/150 = 3.44\,g$$

Granules are prepared agglomerates of small particles. A number of pharmaceutical products of small granules, which contain mostly antibiotic drugs that are unstable in aqueous solution, are prepared for constitution by the pharmacist with purified water prior to dispensing. The granules are prepared to contain the active drug as well as excipients such as colorant and flavorant, so that upon constitution, the liquid will have the desired features of a pharmaceutical solution.

Divided powders are single doses of a powder formulation individually wrapped in plastic, metallic foil, parchment paper, or white bond paper. The divided powder is a more accurate dosage form than bulk powder, with which patients are not required to make a measurement decision on dose. Such preparation may be carried out by the pharmacist in extemporaneous compounding. For example, if a pediatric patient is to receive 5-mg doses of captopril according to the prescription shown in Example 9-6, divided doses can be prepared using available tablets made at a different strength. The following is a demonstration how the prescription should be prepared.

Example 9-6: Describe how you would prepare the following prescription for a pediatric patient with 95% weighing accuracy.

Rx	Captopril	5 mg
	Lactose qs	100 mg
	#10 (powder papers)	
	Sig: powder doses	

In stock, you have 25-mg tablets, each weighing about 75 mg.

Solution:

If the sensitivity of the prescription balance is 5 mg (modern instruments should exhibit better sensitivity), the least amount weighable (LAW) is 100 mg. This quantity can be the weight of a single dose.

For 10 doses, the total weight is 1000 mg. Because a total of 50 mg of captopril is needed, two regular captopril tablets are to be used. The tablets are weighed to give the tablet weight.

The amount of diluent (lactose) needed is $wt_{lactose}$ = 1,000 – tablet weight. If the two tablets weigh 150 mg, then the lactose needed is 850 mg. These quantities are summarized as follows:

Balance sensitivity:	5 mg
LAW:	100 mg
Aliquot (weight of divided dose):	100 mg
Multiple (no. of doses):	10
Total dilution:	1,000 mg
Weight of drug (tablets):	150 mg
Weight of diluent:	850 mg

Tablets should be crushed and triturated in a mortar with a pestle via a circumferential motion and mixed with lactose, using the geometric dilution method described above. The doses are divided by weight, with each 100 mg of the total dilution containing 5 mg of captopril.

Dusting Powders

Dusting powders are fine powders intended to be dusted on the skin by means of sifter-top bottles or containers. A single medicinal agent may be used as a dusting powder, but compounds may be frequently added to protect the skin from irritation and friction. Bentonite, kaolin, magnesium carbonate, starch, and talc are used as inert bases for dusting powders. These agents, however, can absorb skin secretions, exert a drying effect, and impart a cooling sensation.

Douche Powders

Douche powders are used to prepare aqueous solutions to cleanse the vagina. Most douche powders are used for their hygienic effects, but a few contain antibiotics. Douche powders are a matter of convenience for the patient over solutions as a powder is more portable than a bulky solution. The reconstituted solution usually is acidic, with solution pH varying from 3.5 to 5.

Insufflations

Insufflations are extremely fine powders to be introduced into various parts of the body cavities. The powder is usually administered using a device called an *insufflator*. The powder is placed in the insufflator. Upon squeezing the rubber bulb, turbulence in the device is created, which forces some of the powder into the airstream and out of the device through the orifice in the tip.

Inhalation Powders

Medicated powders may be administered by inhalation in metered quantities with the aid of a dry-powder inhaler. Such products are currently used for the treatment of asthma, bronchitis, COPD, and other bronchial conditions. The particle size plays an important role in the distribution of particles in the lungs. Particle sizes in the range of 6–10 μm are respirable but are distributed mainly in the tracheal bronchial region. For deep lung penetration (the alveolar region), the size range is 1–5 μm. In addition to the active drug, the products contain inert propellants and lactose as a diluent to aid in the formulation's flow property and metering uniformity.[24]

III. Chapter Summary

Pharmaceutical powders are used either as medicated powders or for the preparation of various solid and suspension dosage forms. The uniformity and stability of these products depend on the desired particle characteristics including particle size, size distribution, porosity, surface area, and flowability. It is crucial that students have an understanding of these characteristics based on the physical and chemical principles that control these properties. There are several useful concepts that can aid in studying the properties of small particles. Calculation of basic parameters such as particle size, surface area, and density is mostly based on equivalent spherical diameters. Students will do well by knowing the spherical system in expressing volume, surface area, and other parameters based on radius or diameter. Because the use of spherical diameter is only an approximation, it should be emphasized that experimental methods in the determination of parameters such as surface area and porosity are of practical value in the preparation of pharmaceutical product. Last, but not the least, as particle size is reduced, the surface area as well as the percentage of molecules that makes the surface active increases; hence, there is likely a change in particle activity. With the advent of using nanoparticles for pharmaceutical development, there are yet new properties that may "surface" in the near future.

IV. References

1. Dalla Valle JM. *Micromeritics*, New York, Pitman, 1948, 2nd ed.
2. Fichtner F, Rasmuson A, and Alderbotn G. *Int J Pharm*. 292:211–225, 2005.
3. Edmundson IC. Particle size analysis, in Bean HS, Careless JE, and Beckett AH (eds), *Advances in Pharmaceutical Sciences*, New York, Academic Press, 1967, vol 2, pp 95–179.
4. Hatch T and Choate SP. *J Franklin Inst*. 207:369, 1929.
5. Ahmadi TS et al. *Science*. 272:1924, 1996.
6. Yang K and Ma YQ. *Nat Nanotechol*. 5:579–583, 2010.
7. Verma A and Stellacci F. *Small*. 6:12–21, 2010.
8. Oberdorster G, Oberdorster E, and Oberdorster J. *Environ Health Perspect*. 113:823–839, 2005.
9. Van Hoecke K, Schamphelaere KA, Van der Meeren P, Lucas S, and Janssen CR. *Environ Toxicol Chem*. 27:1948–1957, 2008.
10. Micromeritics Instrument Corp., Norcross, GA, United States. (A series of instruments are available for measurement of surface area and pore size, including methods of density function theory that determine the population density profile of gas sorption from zero to saturation pressure. The population density profile at equilibrium reveals how various layers of molecules have formed on or near the solid surface.)
11. Langmuir I. *J Am Chem Soc*. 40:1361, 1918.
12. Emmet P. *Catalysis*, New York, Reinhold Publishing Corp., 1954, vol 1.
13. Emmet PH and Brunauer S. *J Am Chem Soc*. 59:1553, 1937.
14. Anglin EJ, Cheng L, Freeman WR, and Sailor MJ. *Adv Drug Deliv Rev*. 60:1266–1277, 2008.
15. Adamson AW. *Physical Chemistry of Surfaces*. New York, Wiley (Interscience), 1967, 2nd ed.
16. Sadek HM and Olsen J. *Pharm Technol*. 5:40, 1981.
17. Butler AQ and Ransey JC Jr. *Drug Standards*. 20:217, 1952.
18. Strickland WA Jr, Busse LW, and Higuchi T. *J Am Pharm Assoc, Sci Ed*. 45:482, 1956.
19. Liu LX, Marziano I, Bentham AC, Litster JD, White ET, and Howes T. *Int J Pharm*. 362:109–117, 2008.
20. Nelson E. *J Am Pharm Assoc, Sci Ed*. 44:435, 1955.
21. Fonner DE Jr, Banker GS, and Swarbrick J. *J Pharm Sci*. 55:181, 1966.
22. Li Q, Rudolph V, Weigl B, and Earl A. *Int J Pharm*. 280:77–93, 2004.
23. Dahlinder LE, Johansson M, and Sjogren J. *Drug Dev Ind Pharm*. 8:455, 1982.
24. Hindle M and Byron PR. *Pharm Tech*. 16:82–86, 1992.

V. Homework Problems

1. It is said that "they exhibit anisotropic stress, elastic deformation, and yield strength; they fail along slip planes, often don't exhibit shear gradients, can slip on wall surface, and are less sensitive to strain rate; they do not really flow (as a fluid), but are measurable by shear cells." What are they?
2. Using Equation (9-2), calculate the frequency (probability density) at $x = \mu$ and at $x = \mu + \sigma$, assuming $\mu = 0$ and $\sigma = 1$. If you know, give the area under the curve from μ to $\mu + \sigma$ as a percentage of total area.
3. What is the mean diameter ($d_{l/n}$) of the following powder sample determined using Equation (9-1)?

Particle size (μm)	20	25	30	35	40	45	50	55	60	65	70
n (no. of particles)	1	9	32	40	39	33	23	15	9	4	2

4. What is a lognormal distribution? Using data given in Problem 3, plot the frequency (n) as a function of the particle size, and determine whether this is a normal distribution. Plot n versus log (particle size), and use this distribution to determine the geometric diameter (d_g) and $d_{l/n}$.
5. The liquid densities of argon (at −183°C) and carbon dixode (at −78°C) are 1.384 and 1.188 g/mL, respectively. Estimate the area covered by one molecule of these gases when adsorbed onto a particle surface.
6. A silica gel was subjected to BET isotherm measurement for surface area determination using different gases. From the data in **Table 9-9**, calculate the specific surface area per gram of particles, and compare the results obtained using different gases.

Table 9-9 Calculation of Specific Surface Area per Gram of Particles and Comparison of Results Obtained Using Different Gases

Gas	Temp., °C	Area/Gas Molecule (Å²)	V_m, cm³ STP/g
N_2	−196	16.2	127.9
O_2	−183	14.4	119.3
CO_2	−78	17.0	99.0
n-Butane	0	32.1	58.2

7. The Kelvin equation for pore size measurement using the free energy concept may be illustrated by the relation of free energy and pressure changes by working through the following problems:
(*a*) Liquid benzene has a vapor pressure of 100 mmHg at 26°C. If benzene is subjected to a 500-atm mechanical pressure, what are the vapor pressure and the increase in free energy? The molecular weight and density of benzene are 78 and 0.879 g/cm³, respectively.

$$\Delta G = RT \ln(P_2/P_1) = V\,\Delta P \qquad (9\text{-}14)$$

(*b*) Now consider a pore on a particle surface with a radius *r*. The change in vapor pressure of a condensed gas is now related to the radius *r* by the Kelvin equation

$$RT \ln(P/P^{o}) = -2\gamma M/r\rho \qquad (9\text{-}16)$$

If this pore is filled with benzene at 20°C and the vapor pressure ratio of P/P^{o} required is 0.5, what is the pore size in terms of the radius? Benzene has a surface tension of 28.88 dyn/cm (erg/cm²) at 20°C. The gas constant is 8.3143×10^7 erg/deg-mol.
8. Define mesopore, envelope density, and tapped density.
9. The true density of an organic drug is 1.30 g/mL. If the bulk and tapped volumes of 100 g of this drug are measured as 95 and 90 mL, respectively, what are the porosity and Hausner ratio for this drug?

10. Describe how you would prepare 12 divided doses of aspirin, each containing 65 mg of the drug. In stock, you have regular 325-mg aspirin tablets (assuming that they weigh 400 mg each). The prescription balance in your pharmacy has a sensitivity of 6 mg. You may use lactose as the diluents.
11. Calculate the amount of each compound needed:

Rx	Calcium carbonate	0.5 g
	Magnesium trisilicate	0.3 g
	Bismuth subcarbonate qs	1.2 g
	Dtd #42	

12. A formulation for a dusting powder is as follows:

Rx	Salicylic acid	1 part
	Benzoic acid powder	3 parts
	Starch	20 parts

How many grams of each ingredient are needed to make 12 kg of dusting powder?
13. Describe how to formulate the following prescription?

Rx	Calcium carbonate	0.6 g
	Sodium bicarbonate	1.0 g
	Lactose qs	3.0 g
	M.FI chart Dtd #12	

The prescription is written for one chart, but 12 are needed. Sodium bicarbonate and lactose are available in powdered form, but calcium carbonate is supplied by 0.5-g tablets.

CHAPTER 10

Tablets and Capsules

Aniruddha Railkar

A pharmaceutical preparation contains the drug or active pharmaceutical ingredient (API) and inactive ingredients called excipients. These components are listed on the container itself in the case of an over-the-counter (OTC) preparation or in the package insert if it is a prescription drug product. Regardless of where the components are listed, it is extremely important to understand the reason for their use as well as the processing technique used to manufacture the product. This chapter discusses drug product development as it pertains to solid oral dosage forms, tablets, and capsules.

CHAPTER OUTLINE

OBJECTIVES

1. Understand how to evaluate the active pharmaceutical ingredient (API).
2. Understand the use of various excipients in pharmaceutical dosage forms.
3. Understand various pharmaceutical processes in the development of solid dosage forms.
4. Describe the effects of the physicochemical properties of solids on the manufacturing process.
5. Understand different types of solid oral dosage forms.

I. Introduction

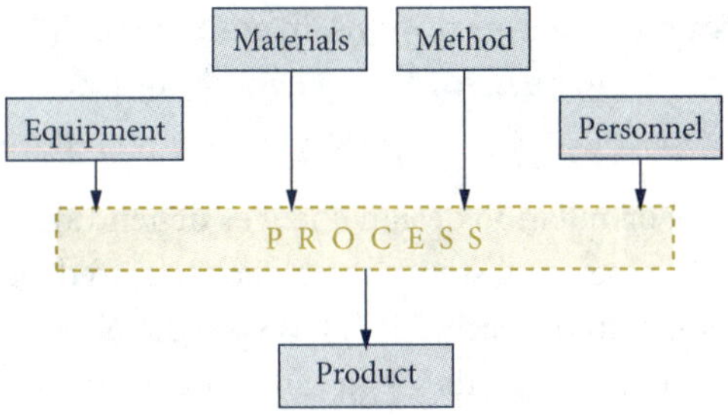

Figure 10-1 Components of a pharmaceutical product development.

The development of a pharmaceutical product requires the integration of knowledge, decision making, and appropriate methodology into a *process* to yield the product with the desired quality. The main components, upon which the process is based, are materials, method, personnel, and equipment, as illustrated in **Figure 10-1**. Each of these components, as shown in subsequent sections, will play a critical role in determining the product outcome.

Solid oral dosage forms (tablets and capsules) comprise 90% of the dosage forms administered. The oral route is the most convenient and thus a preferred route of administration. This chapter focuses mainly on the formulation design strategies, the influence of method and equipment on the product development process, and how this process affects the critical quality attributes of a solid product. Critical process parameters that need to be controlled are also discussed.

II. Formulation Design

Prior to the issuance of a report on Current Good Manufacturing Practices for the 21st Century from the Food and Drug Administration,[1] formulation design was predominantly driven by familiarity and experience with certain formulation platforms. But because of the report, formulation design is now being driven by science. Factors such as dose range (low, medium, high), stability (heat and moisture), particle size and morphology, solubility, wettability, compressibility, and flowability all influence the choice of process used. This requires that the formulation design be conducted with methods that take into account all dosage considerations, so that appropriate decisions can be made with regard to the dosage form. This science-based approach can be subdivided into two methods.

Decision Tree

A decision tree is a model of decisions and their possible consequences, including chance event outcomes and resource costs. It is often used to create a plan to reach a specific goal. The decision tree model offers a systematic method of problem solving in which one can look at the whole picture, effectively communicate one's decision, focus on the best possible scenario for success, and ultimately save time and money. In decision analysis, a decision tree can be used visually and explicitly to represent decisions and decision making. It is simple to understand and interpret. People are able to understand decision tree models after a brief explanation. It requires little data preparation, and it is possible to validate a model by using statistical tests. This model is robust and performs well with large data in a short time, and it enables stakeholders to make and/or accept decisions based on its analysis.

Design of Experiments (DOE)

Design of experiments is a method in which independent variables are manipulated and their effect on one or more dependent variables is studied. It is used to identify the critical parameters of, and their effect on, the product development process and to obtain adequate control over the critical parameters for the development of robust and reproducible processes. DOE consists of three phases. In the first or planning phase, a problem is clearly defined and the variables (factors) to be studied are identified. In the second or design phase, factors are considered such as the number of observations, magnitude of difference to be detected, sample size, and mathematical model to be used. Next a hypothesis is formulated. Finally, the third or analysis phase consists of data collection and processing, computation of test statistics, and interpretation of results.

Formulation design changes depending on the phases of development. In the preclinical phase (nonhuman testing), the objective is to develop formulations in the form of suspensions or solutions. In the early clinical phase, the objective is to develop a simple formulation so that the safety and efficacy of the drug can be determined. A simple formulation could be powder in a bottle (for reconstitution just prior to administration), or powder in a capsule, or a compressed, uncoated tablet. There is a debate among pharmaceutical companies on whether the minimalistic approach or a front-loaded approach to formulation should be used in early development. But as far as commercial development is concerned, the objective is to develop a film-coated tablet formulation.

III. Pharmaceutical Ingredients

Active Pharmaceutical Ingredient (API)

The issues with the API can be discussed under two categories: *new chemical entities* (NCEs) or new molecular entities (NMEs) and existing APIs (for generic development). A new chemical entity is the one that has never been approved before. Consequently, there is no existing clinical information on dose range and very little information about the drug's safety and efficacy. Also, at earlier stages of development, drug supply is limited. Thus, for the NCEs, preclinical development will consist of pharmacology and toxicology evaluations in different animal models, pharmacokinetic and pharmacodynamic profiling in animal models, and preformulation evaluation of the appropriate drug form (crystalline versus amorphous, salt versus neutral) and their thermal properties. In addition, studies of the physiochemical properties such as bulk and tapped density, angle of repose, wettability, solubility, and hygroscopicity as well as an excipient compatibility study could be carried out. In comparison, there is a lot of information for existing APIs, and there are also no issues with drug supply.

Excipients

According to a 1999 report of the WHO Expert Committee on Specifications for Pharmaceutical Preparations,[2] pharmaceutical excipients are defined as substances, other than the active ingredient, that have been appropriately evaluated for safety and are included in a drug delivery system to

- Aid in the processing of the drug delivery system during its manufacture
- Protect, support, or enhance stability, bioavailability, or patient acceptability
- Assist in product identification
- Enhance any other attribute of the overall safety and effectiveness of the drug during storage or use

In the context of manufacturing tablets or capsules, APIs (or actives) generally do not flow or compress well. Hence, the use of excipients is generally required. As the above definition implies, the performance of the dosage form can be influenced by the excipients, and there are potential interactions of the excipients with the active drug that could lead to toxic or allergic responses. Excipients commonly used in solid oral dosage forms fall into the categories below:

Filler/Diluent

As mentioned before, the active ingredient does not flow or compress well. These issues can be addressed to a limited extent by modifying the synthesis and crystallization parameters. But an easier approach is to use a filler. For low-dose actives that are potent, excipients may be needed to dilute the active and act as a carrier for the active. Diluents and fillers are commonly used at a concentration of 65–85% of the formulation. Sometimes more than one filler can be used. The commonly used diluents and fillers are lactose (hydrous and anhydrous), microcrystalline cellulose, dicalcium phosphate, and mannitol.

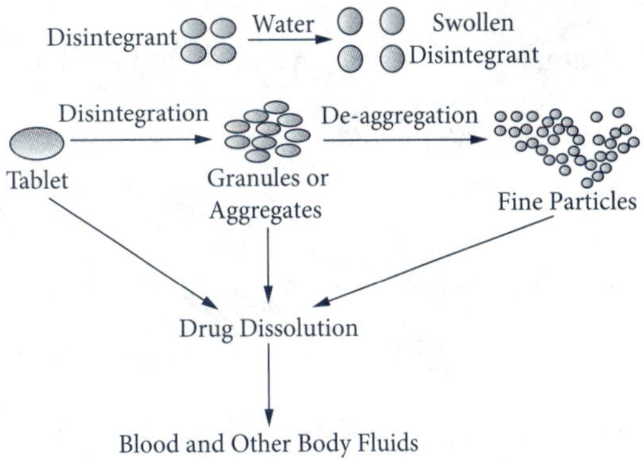

Figure 10-2 Mechanism of disintegrant action.

Binders

As the name suggests, *binders* are excipients that hold the active and inactive ingredients together like a glue. Binders can be used in their dry or powdered form. Binders that are hydrophilic can be used in a wet granulation process. A typical binder concentration is 2–5% of the formulation. Examples of commonly used binders are povidone, hypromellose (hydroxypropylmethylcellulose), and hydroxypropylcellulose.

Disintegrants

The dissolution of drug from a solid dosage form, as previously discussed, plays a central role in oral drug absorption. *Disintegrants* are excipients that are not water-soluble but have a high affinity for water. These compounds can reduce the cohesive forces holding a tablet together and induce the breakup of a tablet into smaller particles, thus increasing the surface area for drug dissolution. The primary mechanisms of action of the disintegrants are wicking or capillary action and swelling (see **Figure 10-2**). Other mechanisms such as heat of wetting, deformation, and release of gases have also been proposed.[3] Superdisintegrants exert their effect at low concentrations and have a higher swelling capacity. The concentration of disintegrants in a formulation is 2–5%. Commonly used disintegrants are croscarmellose sodium, sodium starch glycolate, and cross linked povidone.

Lubricants

Lubricants are hydrophobic waxy substances used in tablet or capsule formulations. In a tablet formulation, lubricants reduce the friction between the die wall and tablet during ejection. They also reduce wear and tear on punches and dies and prevent sticking to the punch faces. In a capsule formulation, a lubricant prevents sticking to tamping pins and dosators. The lubricant efficiency is a function of quantity and mixing time. Because lubricants are hydrophobic, use in large quantities or mixing for prolonged periods can cause a slowing of drug dissolution from the tablet and capsule dosage form. The overuse of lubricants can also result in softer tablets. Commonly used lubricants are magnesium stearate, stearic acid, and sodium stearyl fumarate, and their concentrations range from 0.25% to 5% of the formulation. Hydrophilic lubricants are available, but they generally offer poor lubrication.

Glidants

Glidants are used to enhance the flow of the powder blends by reducing interparticulate friction. Many lubricants also serve as glidants. Glidants are used in the same concentration as lubricants. A commonly used glidant is colloidal silicon dioxide.

Wetting Agents and Surfactants

If the active is hydrophobic, wetting agents or surfactants are added to improve the wettability of the dosage form and facilitate dissolution. They can also be added to binder solutions for a wet granulation process. Their concentration is 2–4% of the formulation. Commonly used wetting agents or surfactants are sodium lauryl sulfate and polysorbate 20.

Example 10-1: Develop a simple formulation for a hydrophobic active and excipients based on the discussion above.

Solution:

Active	25% w/w
Filler	65% w/w
Binder	3% w/w
Disintegrant	3% w/w
Lubricant	1% w/w
Glidant	1% w/w
Wetting agent	2% w/w
Total	100% w/w

Other Excipients

Other ingredients such as colorants, sweeteners, and flavors can also be used in pediatric formulations, but their use in adult dosage forms is largely on an as-needed basis.

Coating and Excipient Compatibility

Coating can be added to the product after it has been manufactured for aesthetic or functional reasons. Aesthetic reasons include appearance, product identification, and differentiation. Functional reasons include taste masking and delayed drug release (enteric or controlled).

Note that, by definition, excipients are inert materials. But more often than not excipients can be incompatible with the active ingredient. Thus, prior to choosing an excipient, accurate understanding of the physical and chemical properties of the active is necessary. The compatibility of excipients with the active drug should be studied under ambient and accelerated (temperature and humidity) conditions over a reasonable time (2 weeks to 3–6 months). It is recommended that the compatibility of a mixture of all excipients in the proportion they will appear in the final formulation be studied in favor of binary mixtures of the active and excipient. Sometimes an excipient is compatible by itself but is incompatible when used in combination with other excipients with the active.

IV. Processes for Solid Dosage Forms

The process of making a compressed tablet requires the drug-excipient mixture to be free-flowing from the hopper of the tablet press into the die cavities for high-speed compression of the powder mix into tablets. Granulation—a manufacturing procedure for the control of particle size, density, and internal porosity of the powder blend and prevention of demixing—provides this free-flowing quality. Many pharmaceutical excipients, including some fillers (spray-dried lactose), disintegrants (direct-compression starch), lubricants (magnesium stearate and talc), and glidants (fumed silicon dioxide) can also be used to enhance the flow of powder mix, thus allowing tablet formation through direct compression without granulation. **Figure 10-3** shows the options through which a process (direct compression, dry granulation, or wet granulation) may be selected for the manufacture of a solid dosage form. The detail and criteria for selecting these processes are discussed below.

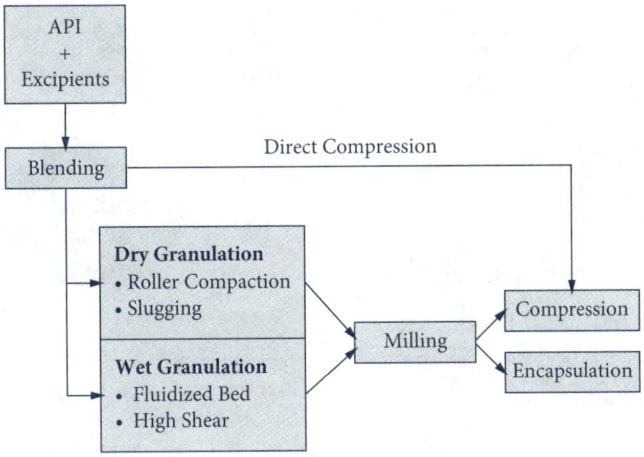

Figure 10-3 Options of pharmaceutical processes in the manufacture of solid dosage forms.

Direct Compression (DC)

Weighing and Blending

These are the initial steps that are required for all manufacturing processes. The weighing should be carried out using balances calibrated for the desired weight range, with adequate ventilation and personal protective equipment. Specified quantities of the active ingredient and excipients are then mixed, either in whole or in steps, to uniformity using a mechanical powder blender or mixer (see Section V for details). Direct compression (DC), as the name suggests, is a process in which tablets are manufactured directly from a blend of active and suitable excipients. Although wet granulation (which is discussed later) has long been the preferred process, many excipients and APIs suitable for direct compression have been developed. If the granular actives possess free-flowing and cohesive properties that enable them to be compressed directly in a tablet machine, then the selection of excipients should be made so that the physical properties such as flow and compressibility of the ingredients have not been altered by any means. For actives that do not exhibit this quality, special pharmaceutical excipients, as mentioned earlier, can be used for DC purposes. Some of the properties of an ideal DC excipient are its good flow and compressibility, low cost, compatibility with a wide range of actives, and noninterference with the drug's bioavailability and biological activity.

Direct compression is becoming the process of choice because it requires fewer processing steps and fewer parameters to control compared to other processes (**Figure 10-4**), and thus it is time- and cost-efficient. The DC process is also especially applicable to heat- and moisture-sensitive actives that could not be easily processed through wet granulation. However, several disadvantages are associated with the DC process:

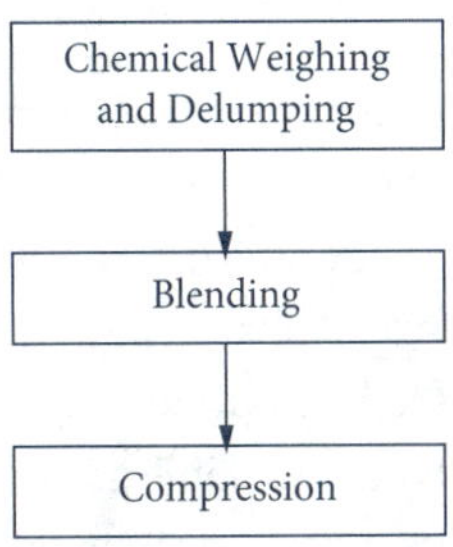

Figure 10-4 Processing steps for direct compression.

1. Actives with poor flow and compressibility cannot be processed.
2. There is nonuniformity of content for low-dose actives.
3. High-dose actives are difficult to process.
4. Segregation can occur due to differences in particle size of API and excipients.
5. Static charge can develop because of lack of moisture.

In addition, capping, splitting, or laminating of tablets is sometimes related to air entrapment during direct compression. When air is entrapped, the resulting tablets expand when the pressure of tableting is released, resulting in splits and layers in the tablets.

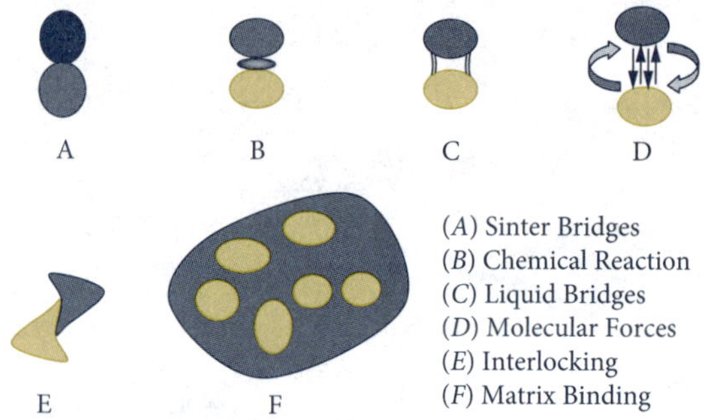

Figure 10-5 Agglomeration mechanisms. (*A*) Sinter bridges, (*B*) chemical reaction, (*C*) liquid bridges, (*D*) molecular forces, (*E*) interlocking, and (*F*) matrix binding.

Mechanisms of Agglomeration

The flow of small fine particles (10 μm or less) through an orifice is restricted because the cohesive forces of the particles are of the same order as the gravitational forces. As particle size increases, however, the gravitational force increases and flow is facilitated. There is a maximum flow rate with respect to particle size in that after reaching the maximum flow rate, the flow decreases as the particles size increases. Experience has shown that particles with a diameter of 400 to 800 μm exhibit excellent flow property, and the tablets formed using these granules show minimum weight variations. Granulation, which is used to produce optimum particle size to gain the necessary flow and compressibility of the powder blend, is thus a process of *agglomeration*, which can be defined as a process of particle size enlargement in which small particles (powders or dust) are gathered into larger masses, clusters, or pellets for use as end products or for secondary processing steps. There are six types of agglomeration mechanisms, and they are shown in **Figure 10-5**. Sinter bridges are formed when particles partially melt and then solidify as agglomerates. When a chemical bond is formed between two particles, agglomeration occurs. When a liquid is sprayed onto particles and the particles are agitated, they collide with one another, forming liquid bridges. Van der Waals, electrical, or mechanical forces also result in particle agglomeration. When irregular particles collide and lock, the mechanism is called interlocking. Finally, agglomeration occurs when particles are embedded in a binder matrix.

Dry Granulation (DG)

As the name suggests, in this process, powders are granulated in the absence of liquid. Because a liquid is not used, the agglomeration has to be carried out by compaction or densification, in which the powder mixture is compacted in large pieces and subsequently broken up and sized into granules. Dry granulation can be achieved using slugging or roller compaction methods. For slugging, a regular tablet press with large-diameter die (1 in) and punch is used. The objective is to form a large compact or slug and then mill the slug to the desired particle size. As small particles do not flow well into the die cavity, this results in large weight variation in the slugs, which in turn causes a large variation in the applied force and inconsistent mechanical strength. Slugging is used less frequently now in pharmaceutical preparations.

In a *roller compactor*, powders can be vertically fed via an auger into two counter-rotating rollers and compressed under force. The roll force is the most important parameter in this process. The result is a dense compaction in the shape of a ribbon or sheet, which can be milled to the desired granule size. Apparatuses with horizontal feed, a combination of horizontal and vertical feed, and angular feeding options are also available. The gap of the compact rolls can be fixed, or the apparatus can come with a variable gap option. In the case of a fixed roll gap, the amount of powder entering the rolls can be inconsistent, which can create problems similar to those experienced with slugging. The variable gap rolls can adjust according to the amount of powder drawn and thus apply a consistent force.

The roller compaction method is preferred over slugging because of its consistency. Binding agents such as methylcellulose or hydroxymethylcellulose have been shown to produce desired

Table 10-1 Advantages and Disadvantages of the Dry Granulation (DG) Process Compared to the Direct Compaction (DC) Process

Advantages	Disadvantages
DG can be used to densify materials.	There are more processing steps in DG than in the DC process.
DG improves flow and compressibility.	DG is less time- and cost-effective than the DC process.
Drugs susceptible to moisture can be processed by DG.	DG creates dust and fines. It cannot process drugs susceptible to high shear.

tablet hardness and friability using the roller compaction method. The major advantages and disadvantages of the DG process are listed in **Table 10-1**.

Wet Granulation (WG)

Agglomeration in the presence of liquid and binder is called *wet granulation*. Thus a binder can be added in a dry powder form or as an aqueous solution. With adequate environmental and engineering controls, organic solvent is also applicable to wet granulation, but is rarely used. The agglomeration process occurs in the presence of agitation, where liquid-coated particles come together and form liquid bridges. When the wet mass is dried, the liquid evaporates and binder particles form solid bridges. The flow chart for the WG process is shown in **Figure 10-6**. Here, after the initial blending step, binder solution is added with agitation. The next steps are continued agitation or wet massing, wet sizing, and drying. After drying, a sizing step is often necessary to reduce the granule size so that the die cavities may be completely filled by the free-flowing granulation, before lubricant blending and compression or encapsulation.

Wet granulation can be achieved by two main methods: high-shear granulation and fluid-bed granulation. Low-shear granulation using a Hobart or KitchenAid mixer is also carried out but rarely.

High-Shear Granulation (HSG)

High-shear granulation is a process in which a liquid and solid are combined by imparting force to the components. A liquid undergoes shear when one area of the liquid has higher velocity than another area. The equipment consists of a low-speed rotating impeller, which imparts higher velocity to the liquid at the tip of the impeller than at the center of the impeller, thus creating shear. The agglomeration in a high-shear process can take place by two primary mechanisms: nucleation and coalescence. In nucleation, solid and liquid particles are combined to form new particles (granules) or nuclei. Coalescence is the combination of two granules to form a larger granule. As more liquid is added, the agglomerates go through four stages depending on the amount of liquid. In the pendular stage, the particles are held together at the solid–liquid and air–liquid interphases by liquid bridges. In the funicular stage, there is a continuous liquid phase in air. In the capillary stage, granule pore spaces are completely filled with liquid. Finally in the *droplet* stage, the solid particles are surrounded by liquid. In a high-shear process, these steps occur very quickly. Regardless of the morphology of the starting material, a high-shear process tends to produce round, dense particles.

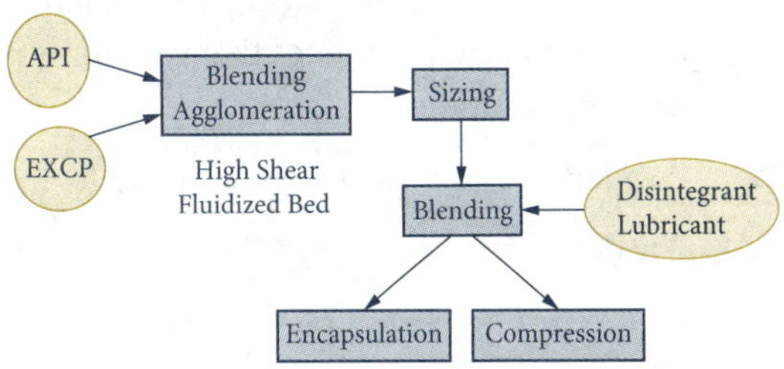

Figure 10-6 Wet granulation process flow.

The main components of a high-shear granulator, with heated upper and lower jacket, are shown in **Figure 10-7**. If the high-shear granulator does not have the heated upper and lower jacket, the granulated material is wet-sized and

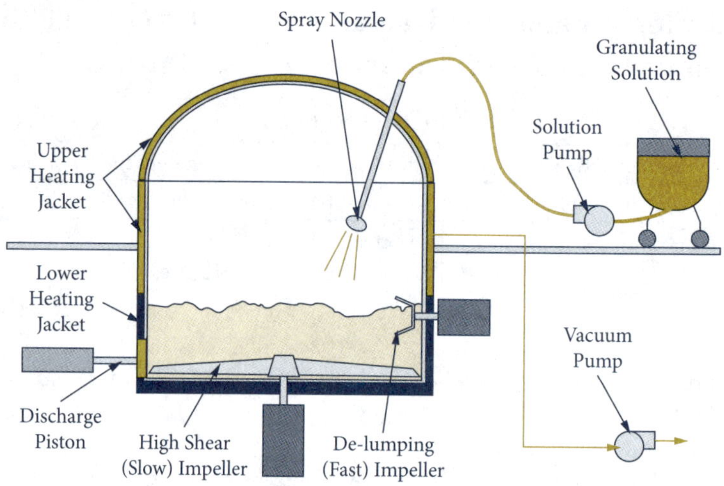

Figure 10-7 Components of a high-shear granulator.

dried in a fluidized-bed dryer. The important formulation and process parameters are the concentration of binder solution, the spray rate, and the impeller and chopper speed. Because there is a lot of shear imparted to the system, it is easy to overgranulate in a high-shear process. This makes the detection of the granulation endpoint a critical objective. Many of the processes available currently are indirect methods that do not have a direct correlation with granule properties such as density, porosity, shape, and size. However, they can be correlated to downstream properties such as bulk and tapped density, blend flow, and compressibility. These indirect methods include measurement of power consumption, impeller torque, conductivity, and capacitance and acoustic monitoring.[4] In-line methods such as focused (laser) beam reflectance measurement (FBRM) can provide real-time data about granule properties, but are evolving.[5]

Fluidized-Bed Granulation (FBG)

Fluidized-bed granulation is a process in which heated air is drawn through the unit, which suspends or "fluidizes" the particles while a binder solution is sprayed onto the fluidized particles. The wet particles collide with one another, forming granules. It is a low-shear process. It is also a "one-pot" process in which mixing, granulation, and drying are carried out in the same equipment. The fluidized-bed unit can also be used as a dryer for granulations from high-shear granulators not equipped with a heating jacket. Fluidized-bed granulation can be carried out in three different configurations through which particles are coated via a top spray (downward), bottom spray (upward), or a bottom- or side-arm spray in combination with a rotating bed known as the tangential spray.

The main components of a fluidized-bed granulator are as follows:

1. The inlet air system, which deliver the air from the bottom of the fluidized bed, consists of a coarse filter, freeze protection for colder climates, dehumidification for tropical climates, heating, and a high-efficiency particulate air (HEPA) filter. The dew point of incoming air is an important parameter that should be monitored and controlled (via humidification or dehumidification).
2. Powder charging can be done manually by scooping the materials or by a vacuum system.
3. Powder contact *areas* are subdivided as follows.
   a. Product bowl with perforated distributor plate, screen, and sample port.
   b. Expansion chamber, which can be either straight-sided, resulting in intermittent granulation, or of increasing diameter, resulting in continuous fluidization. The expansion

chamber is also equipped with windows to monitor the process as well as ports at different heights to attach a spray arm and nozzle.

4. The filter housing consists of either cloth or cylindrical stainless-steel filters. The filters are of fine-mesh size to prevent any fluidized particles from exhausting into the atmosphere. But as the process continues, accumulation of particles can clog filters. The filters are cleaned either by shaking periodically (for cloth filters) or by using a purging air pulse for stainless-steel filters.
5. *A* spray system consists of spray arm capable of delivering the binder and the air and a spray head with single or multiple nozzles. The nozzles are equipped with the ability to atomize the liquid into fine droplets, thereby increasing the surface area and resulting in a high surface/mass ratio.

In addition, the binder solution can be mixed using low- or high-shear mixers with or without heating and cooling. The solution needs to be deaerated and is delivered by means of peristaltic or gear pumps that can be controlled manually or through the control panel on the fluidized bed. Product can be discharged either manually by scooping or by using a specialized device called a *bowl inverter* coupled with a lifting device or, in larger units, through a bottom discharger.

Top Spray Granulation

In this type of process, heated air is drawn through the bottom of the unit, which suspends the particles in midair just underneath the spray nozzle. The binder is sprayed from above, and as the particles get wetted by the binder solution, they collide and form granules. A schematic of a top spray fluidized-bed granulator is shown in **Figure 10-8**. The top spray fluidized bed is commonly used in the pharmaceutical industry. The primary purpose of the top spray process is to improve the handling of the particles, i.e., make them more flowable and compressible, and so a precise film is not necessary. The motion of the particles and the distance traveled by droplets are not uniform, and this results in a porous film.

Bottom Spray Granulation

The major difference between the top and bottom spray granulators (other than how the binder is sprayed) is in the design of the equipment. Just like the top spray granulator, the bottom spray granulator also has a distributor plate and screen. However, the bottom spray granulator has a

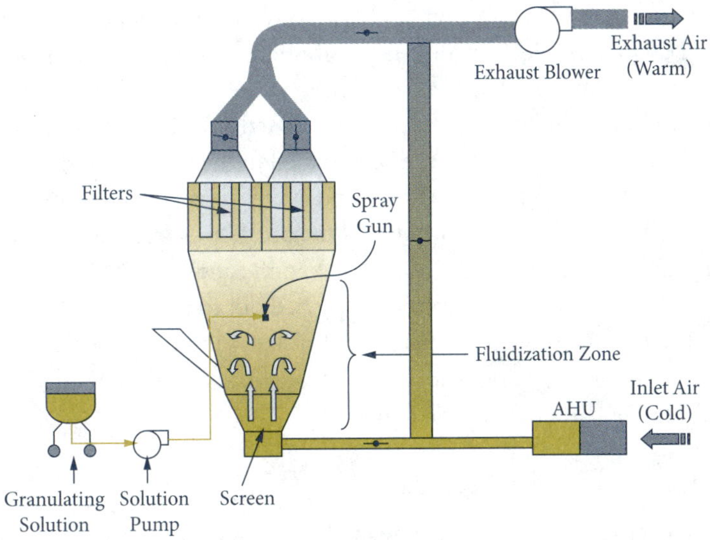

Figure 10-8 Top spray fluidized-bed granulator.

Table 10-2 Advantages and Disadvantage of the Wet Granulation Process as Compared to Direct Compaction and Dry Granulation Methods

Advantages	Disadvantages
It can densify materials (in HSG).	There are many process steps.
It improves flow and compressibility (compared to DC).	It is not time- and cost-effective.
It improves the electrostatic properties (compared to DC and DG).	Moisture- and heat-sensitive actives cannot be processed.
It improves homogeneity and content uniformity (compared to DC).	
It reduces fines (compared to DG).	
Drugs susceptible to high shear can be processed by fluidized-bed process (compared to DG).	

column through which most of the process air is drawn in creating a venturi effect. The spray nozzle is located at the base of the column. Due to the venturi effect, the velocity of the particles is low in the column, which facilitates drying of the particles, and particles that fall outside the column are drawn repeatedly into the column, resulting in a precise filming and a narrow particle size distribution.

Tangential Spray Granulation

In this type of granulation, the amount of air being drawn in is metered by a rotating disk. The binder solution is sprayed at the bottom of the unit but at an angle to the rotating plate. But due to the design of the unit, agglomeration is not possible because there is a high separation force between particles. This type of process is very useful for drug layering or pelletizing the powders.

Regardless of the configuration used, the WG process is influenced primarily by three parameters: inlet air temperature, spray rate, and air volume. Wet granulation provides enough particle size heterogeneity. This is an important quality because large particles tend to deform, but the small particles help lock these deformations, resulting in stronger interparticulate bonds. The major advantages and disadvantages of the wet granulation process are listed in **Table 10-2**.

V. Blending

Blending is a very important unit operation in pharmaceutical processing and is defined as the mixing of drug and excipients to get a uniform distribution of components. Blending involves principles of dispersion, diffusion, shear, and convection. There are two main types of blenders. In rotating-shell blenders, the container is rotated along a fixed axis. Blending is achieved by sliding or rolling the powders. Sometimes baffles can be attached to the lids to aid in the mixing process. In fixed-shell blenders, the internal parts of the blender such as paddles and impellers will rotate, thereby causing a shuffling and cutting motion and the breakup of large agglomerates. To ensure adequate blending, appropriate test methods (both scientific and validated) and in-process controls have to be established, and blend sampling is carried out to determine the uniformity of the active ingredient. The FDA has issued guidance on stratified sampling, which requires samples to be taken at various depths and at various locations throughout the blender. These samples have to meet specifications for content of the active ingredient.

Evaluation of Blend Properties

Once the active and excipients are processed by methods described above, their properties need to be evaluated prior to tableting or encapsulation.

Angle of Repose

When bulk powders are poured onto a horizontal surface, they will form a conical pile. The *angle of repose* is the angle formed between the slope of the material and the horizontal plane, as shown in **Figure 10-9**. It can be calculated as

$$\tan \alpha = H/R \quad (10\text{-}1)$$

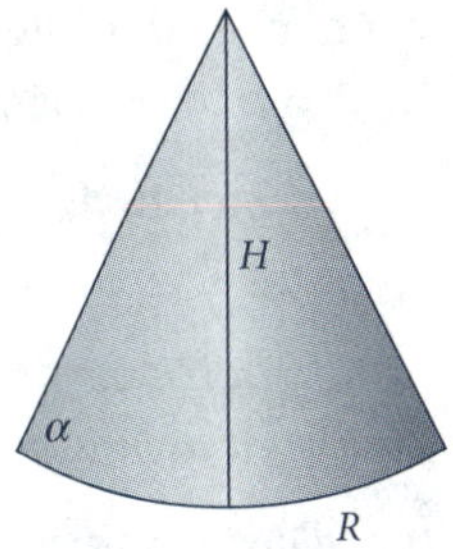

Figure 10-9 Angle of repose (α) as defined by the height of the cone (H) and the radius (R) of the base.

The angle of repose is a measure of the flowability of the blend in that the better the flow, the lower the angle of repose. As a manufacturing rule, values in the range of 20° to 40° are acceptable.

Powder flow measurement is not simple because it depends on several factors including factors related to equipment. Powder that flows well through one container may not flow well in another container. However, as an in-process quality control tool, the measurement of powder flow can be useful if the same product is made and measured in the same equipment. The *flow rate* is the weight of blend allowed to drop through a certain diameter orifice as a function of time.

Particle Size Distribution

Typically, the particle size distribution is carried out by weighing a certain amount of blend and allowing it to distribute over different sieves under vibration. The amount of blend retained on each sieve is weighed and expressed as percent retained. Other sophisticated techniques such as laser diffraction could be employed, but from a tableting or encapsulation point of view, a gross distribution is more informative.

Bulk and Tapped Density

Bulk density (ρ_b) is the density of a loosely packed powder bed, whereas the tapped density (ρ_t) is the density of a tightly packed powder bed. These two quantities can be used to determine the compressibility index (CI) or *Carr index*,[6] defined as

$$\text{CI} = [(\rho_t - \rho_b)/\rho_t] \times 100 \quad (10\text{-}2)$$

Typically, values between 15% and 25% indicate a compressible blend.

Porosity

For tableting, porosity is a measure of void spaces between particles, and typically it is calculated by forcing a nonwetting liquid such as mercury under pressure through a powder bed. This technique is called *porosimetry*. It can also be calculated from powder densities. From a performance point of view, porous particles dissolve faster than dense particles.

Blend Defects

The two major defects are flow and segregation. Powder flow depends on several material and equipment characteristics. Material properties such as electrostatic charge and the presence of fines (particles less than 10 μm in diameter) can impede flow. It is desirable to have mass flow where the powder bed moves as a unified mass. Funnel flow is observed when different regions of powder bed flow at different rates or not at all. When particles separate due to size, shape, and density, it is called segregation. Segregation can occur during transportation, due to vibration as in a hopper or while a blend is being discharged from the blender or when the blend is stationary. There are three major types of segregation:

1. *Sifting*: In this type of segregation, large particles move to the exterior of the powder bed, and small particles are in the center of the powder bed.
2. *Fluidization*: When small particles move to the top of the pile and large particles settle to the bottom, it is called fluidization segregation.
3. *Dusting*: Very fine particles separate from the bed and stick to the sides of the blender. When the bed is discharged, these fine particles stay on the surface of the blender, resulting in segregation.

Blend defects can cause variability of the content of the active ingredient in the blend, but the uniformity issues can be resolved by modifying material characteristics or equipment design or both.

VI. Tableting

Equipment and Tableting

A tablet is a compressed dosage form of any shape, size, and weight containing a pharmaceutical active and excipients. Tableting is a process in which a powder is compressed under a force to form a compact. Tablets are manufactured using a tablet press. Tablet presses come in two configurations: a single-station or multistation rotary press. All discussion will be focused on the multistation rotary press. A schematic of a multistation rotary press is shown in **Figure 10-10**.

There are three steps in tableting:

1. *Fill*: In this step the powder blend from the hopper is poured into a feeder, which in turn fills the die cavity (see **Figure 10-11**). A scraper blade attached to the feeder scrapes off excess powder.
2. *Compression*: As the powder-filled die moves forward, a precompression roll (not pictured) deaerates the powder, the upper punch starts moving into the die cavity while the lower punch is stationary, and the powder is compressed by a force applied by the main compression rolls.
3. *Ejection*: The upper punch moves up, and the lower punch travels up the die cavity to eject the tablet. A scraper blade gently moves the tablet away from the die table into the exit chute.

Note that the actual compression cycle is much more involved than the simplified explanation provided here. High-speed rotary presses have die filling times measured in milliseconds. There are two types of feed frames: a gravity feeder, where powder from the hopper flows into the die cavity

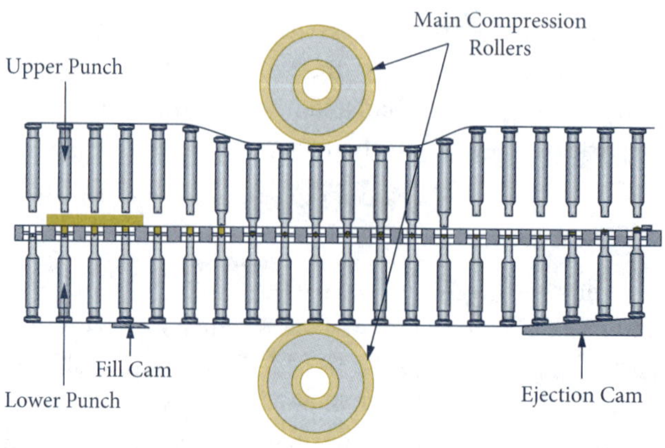

Figure 10-10 Components of a rotary tablet press.

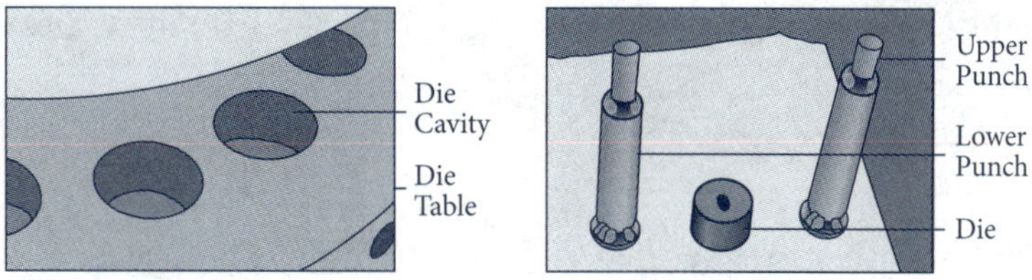

Figure 10-11 Die table, punches, and dies.

through gravity, and a force feeder, where powder from the hopper is filled into the die cavity by rotating wheels inside the feeder. After the tablets are compressed, they are passed through a metal checker and deduster.

Evaluation of Tablet Properties

In-Process and Postcompression Testing

During the compression, in-process testing of tablets is necessary to make sure that the tablet meets certain specifications determined by the operator. After compression, additional testing is carried out to ensure that the tablets meet assay and content uniformity requirements of the United States Pharmacopeia (USP). The various in-process tests are described below.

Tablet Hardness

Sometimes referred to as crushing strength or tablet-breaking force, the tablet hardness is a measure of the mechanical integrity of the tablet. Tablets that are too soft will break up during coating, packaging, or transport. Tablets that are too hard will fail to disintegrate in body fluids, resulting in inadequate absorption of the active. Hardness is measured on a hardness tester, which consists of two metal platens, one stationary and the other movable. The tablet is placed between the two platens, and the force required to break the tablet is measured. Hardness testers come in constant-speed and constant-force configurations. The constant-speed hardness testers are commonly used in the pharmaceutical industry. A related property is tablet thickness. Hardness and thickness are inversely proportional to each other.

Disintegration Testing

This test measures the amount of time required by the tablet to break into pieces under specific conditions. It does not correlate with performance *in vivo*, but is a quality control measurement. Most pharmacopeias specify that immediate-release uncoated (core) tablets should disintegrate in 15 min or less. The requirements change for modified-release tablets. The test involves putting tablets in a container with glass tubes with a 10-mesh screen at the bottom. The container is immersed in and out of a beaker containing water at 37°C. Complete disintegration is indicated when all particles fall through the mesh screen.

Friability

This is a measure of the ability of tablets to withstand mechanical shock during coating, transportation, and packaging. The equipment consists of a curved baffle inside a rotating drum, which allows the tablets to roll and drop. The difference in weight before and after testing is converted to a percentage as follows:

$$\% \text{ Friability} = 100(W_0 - W)/W_0 \qquad (10\text{-}3)$$

where W_0 is the initial weight and W is the final weight. Typically, friability values of 1% or less are considered acceptable.

Weight Variation

In this test, 10 individual tablets are weighed, and then the mean is calculated. According to USP requirements, the weights have to be between 85% and 115% of the mean, although tighter specifications are desirable.

Content Uniformity

Ten individual units are analyzed, and the results have to meet USP requirements. There are exceptions based on drug content, and they are also specified by USP.

Assay of API

A suitable number of units are combined, and then aliquots equal to the weight of the average dosage unit are analyzed for the amount of active ingredient. The results have to meet USP requirements.

Tablet Defects

Tablet defects can occur during compression. The causes can be traced to raw materials and their physicochemical properties, the formulation, or the process. Regardless of the cause of the defect, the costs can be significant, and hence it is critically important that one recognize the defects and know how to eliminate them. There are three common defects, described below.

Capping

This is a defect in which only the top of the tablet or "cap" is broken. It is primarily caused by entrapped air resulting in lack of compressibility. When the tablet is being compressed, entrapped air is pushed to the exterior of the tablet. This allows the particles to bond together. Tooling is designed such that the tip of the upper punch has a slightly smaller diameter than the tip of the lower punch, which allows air to escape as the upper punch enters the die. But as the air is escaping, fine particles also get pushed to the exterior, and these particles do not bond together, resulting in lack of compressibility. Capping can be fixed by making formulation changes (materials) or process changes. From an equipment perspective, changing the penetration depth of the upper punch, using precompression, slowing the press, or modifying the tooling design by changing the cup depth or radii can be used to solve this problem.

Lamination

This is a defect in which part of the tablet other than the top is broken. The most common cause of lamination is overcompression. Overcompression removes the irregularities in granules, making them flat, and flat surfaces cannot bond with one another. Lamination can also be caused by lack of bonding between small, lightweight particles. This defect can be eliminated, however, by making the same changes as in eliminating capping.

Picking and Sticking

Picking is indicated when the particles stick to logos or lettering on punches. Sticking is a defect in which particles are deposited on punch faces. It can be caused by particles inherently having high moisture or by inadequate drying where the outside is dry, but the inside is still moist. When compression force is applied, the particles rupture and the moist particles stick to the punch faces. Sticking can also be a result of under- or overblending. In either case, lubricant is not effective. These problems can be fixed by formulation changes, adequate lubrication, increasing compression force, or slowing down the press. Logos and lettering can also be modified.

VII. Coating

Tablet coating is a process in which tablets are covered with multiple layers of natural or synthetic materials including fillers, polymers, colors, and flavors. Coating has evolved over the years, starting with sugar coating, which was more art than science. It consisted of many steps carried out in multiple pieces of equipment including sealing and waterproofing, subcoating, grossing and smoothing, coloring, and polishing. This time-consuming and costly process sometimes took weeks to complete. The sugar coating also resulted in 30–50% weight gain, which in turn affected dissolution and bioavailability. Coating with organic solvents easily replaced sugar coating because it could be carried out in a single piece of equipment in a matter of hours. However, for environmental and safety reasons, solvent coating was less desirable, and this has led to the advances in equipment design and versatile coating materials for aqueous film coating, a method of choice for the current pharmaceutical industry.

Film Coating

Tablet coating, although it adds steps to the product development and costs, is an important operation that adds to the proprietary prestige. The purpose of tablet coating is to achieve improved appearance, improved stability, ease of swallowing, ability to modify release, taste masking, improved handling for packaging and blistering, product differentiation, and anticounterfeiting. Film coating is an operation in which a thin film of coating is applied by using a coating dispersion in the presence of heated air to facilitate solvent evaporation. There are three components of the coating operation: the substrate or core tablet, the coating equipment (coating pan, spray systems, air handling), and the coating solids, which are discussed below.

Core Tablet

If coating is anticipated for a product, some attributes should be built into the product in the design stage. Tablets need to be of a certain hardness. The friability should be less than 0.5%. Tablets come in various geometric shapes. But not all shapes tumble appropriately in a pan, which may result in inadequate coverage of the tablet surface. Sharper edges could result in chipping during the coating operation. In addition, large tablets have smaller surface areas, and smaller tablets have larger surface areas when loaded into the coating pan. An appropriate amount of coating should be sprayed based on the surface area.

Coating Equipment

A schematic diagram of the coating apparatus is shown in **Figure 10-12**. The air handling unit (AHU) draws and heats air passed through a HEPA filter. Depending upon the geographic location, humidification and dehumidification capability is also built into the AHU. The heated air is brought in through the top of the coating pan and exhausted through the tablet bed from the bottom of the pan (the side-vented pan). Prior to being exhausted, the air is filtered again to remove any dust from the tablets or coating solids. This type of AHU is currently in use in tablet coating systems.

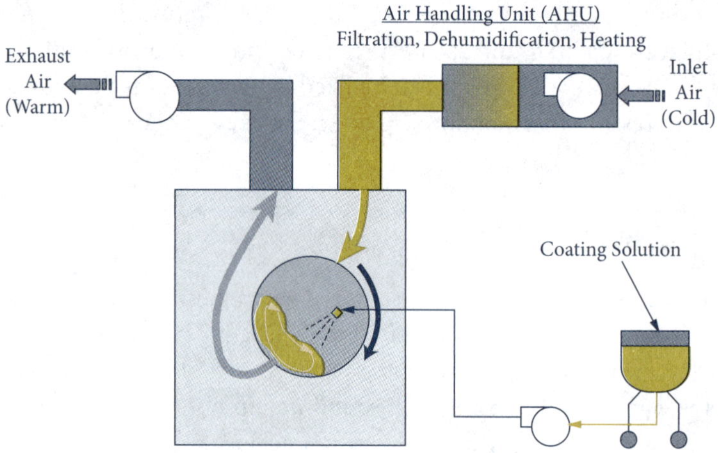

Figure 10-12 Components of a coating system.

Coating Pans

The coating pans of the older coating systems evolved from pans used in the food and candy manufacturing operations. They were hexagonal, pear-shaped, or spherical and contained two fixed ducts for inlet and exhaust air. Even with later improvement achieved by incorporating a movable inlet air duct to distribute heat to different parts of the tablet bed, the coating is generally less than desirable, due to inefficient drying of the tablets, mixing of the powder bed, and the removal of solvent vapors and dust. This led to the development of the *immersed sword system* consisting of concentric inlet and exhaust ducts attached to a perforated column embedded in the product. The pan was also closed, resulting in improved airflow and safety. Further modifications resulted in coating pans that were mounted on an angle and rotated on a horizontal axis with access in front and back. Air inlet and air exhaust were in the back. To improve the mixing of tablets, baffles were added inside the pan. This system still had the same issues with tablets drying only on the surface, but led to the development of fully or partially perforated side-vented pans that combined the advantages of rotation along a horizontal axis with superior drying efficiencies suitable for aqueous film coating. The addition of baffles, as in the earlier design, improved tablet mixing. Coating pans have different capacities starting as low as 500 g to 500 kg. Proper loading of the pan is crucial to getting a good film.

Coating Solids

Film coating basically involves the use of five types of materials including film formers, plasticizers, colorants, opacifiers, and other additives such as flavoring agent and antioxidant. The film formers are pharmaceutical polymers, which, by design, may or may not influence the release of active ingredient. Soluble polymers such as hypromellose, hydroxyethylcellulose, sodium carboxymethylcellulose, povidone, and polyvinylalcohols are commonly used polymers that do not influence the release of active ingredient. Compounds such as hypromellose phthalate, cellulose acetate phthalate, and acrylates are used for enteric coating if the drug needs to be protected from gastric fluids. Some modified acrylates and insoluble cellulose can also be used for controlled-release formulations.

Most polymers used as film formers have rigid structures that make them brittle after drying. Plasticizers are low-molecular-weight substances that have the ability to modify the physical properties of the polymers. When interspersed with polymer chains, the plasticizers reduce the polymer's glass transition temperature, making them more pliable and soft. This results in films that strongly adhere to the tablet surface. Polyols and organic esters are most commonly used plasticizers.

The colorants include both natural and synthetic dyes and lakes used to impart colors to the tablet core. Natural ingredients are not consistent and show color variation from batch to batch. Synthetic materials are preferred because the quality can be consistent from batch to batch. The opacifiers are added to mask the color of the tablet core. This reduces the amount of colorant needed to get adequate coverage on tablets. Other additives including surfactants, flavors, and antioxidants are added to film coating as needed.

Since pharmaceuticals are a very highly regulated entity, use of all ingredients described above should be carried out with proper input from regulatory experts. Many countries have restrictions on maximum amounts of ingredients that can be ingested in one day. This should also be taken into consideration, especially if the dosage form is to be administered multiple times. The three major regions—the United States, Europe, and Japan—have attempted to harmonize the specifications to some extent, but variations do exist. Other regions adopt specifications from one or more of the major regions.

Solution Preparation and Delivery

The coating solution is prepared by rapidly dispersing the solids in the presence of agitation. Once the solids have been dispersed, the agitation can be reduced, but some mixing should be done continuously. Because agitation results in air incorporation into the system, the solution needs to be deaerated prior to use. This operation also creates dust, which requires adequate protection measures. The coating solution/suspension is delivered using peristaltic pumps, piston pumps, gear pumps, or pressurized containers. Regardless of the type of pump used, calibration is very important. The solution is delivered via a manifold to spray nozzles, and calibration of flow at each nozzle is also critical. Spray nozzles are designed with inlets for coating solution, atomizing air, and pattern air. The angle and the distance of the spray nozzles to the tablet bed are also important. Ideally the spray nozzles should be spaced such that there is an overlap of the spray from each nozzle. Note that the description above is a much simplified version of a fairly intricate system.

The critical parameters in film coating that can be controlled include the inlet air temperature, inlet air volume, humidity, pan speed, spray rate, concentration of coating solids, and atomizing air pressure and volume. In addition, there are some indirect or dependent variables that need to be monitored, and they are the bed temperature, bed humidity, exhaust temperature, and exhaust humidity. These parameters can be predominantly controlled by adjusting the inlet air temperature, air volume, and spray rate.

Coating Defects

As with other unit operations, defects are observed during film coating. Some of the major defects are as follows.

Logo Bridging and Logo Filling

This problem is caused by the composition and characteristics of the core, inappropriate design or placement of the logo, or spray drying of the coating solution. The solution is to reformulate the core, deaerating the solution before spraying, adjusting the gun distance from the bed, and adjusting the inlet air temperature. The spray rate should be increased to reduce logo filling and decreased to reduce logo bridging.

Picking and Sticking

If tablets stick together and then come apart as they are tumbling, the film can peel off. Possible causes are poor mechanical strength of the coating, poor adhesion of film, or internal stress. It can be resolved by using materials with good mechanical strength, less internal stress, and better adhesion.

Twinning

When two tablets stick together and do not come apart, it is called twinning. The most probable cause is wet conditions (high spray, low temperature and air volume), low coating pan speed, or inappropriate tablet shape. It can be solved by using higher temperature and air volume, modifying the tablet shape, and increasing the pan speed.

Orange Peel

As the name indicates, the tablet surface looks like an orange peel and has a roughness to it rather than being smooth. Possible causes are overwetting, high viscosity of the coating solution (high percentage of solids content), insufficient atomization, and excessive drying. This defect can be corrected by lowering the solids content, increasing atomization, and/or lowering the spray rate and temperature.

Color Variation

This is a defect in which tablets do not have a uniform color distribution. Possible causes could be improper atomization, too high a solids content, not enough opacifier, and an insufficient number of spray guns. This can be overcome by increasing the atomization pressure, using less solids, increasing the opacifier, and using additional spray guns.

Cratering

Tablet excipients absorb water and swell, causing blisters that can break open. It can be resolved by using a seal coat or reformulating with excipients that are not water-sensitive.

Cracking

Tablets can develop cracks or defects after coating, due to differences in the thermal properties of the tablet core excipients and coating materials. Under low mechanical strength of coating for an extended time, strain relaxation of the tablet depends on the core composition and the amounts of plasticizer and pigments used. With inadequate plasticizer or excessive pigments, cracking occurs when the internal stresses in the film exceed the tensile strength of the film. This defect can be overcome by changing core composition, allowing tablets to recover from strain by waiting to coat the tablets, and adjusting plasticizer or pigment content.

Core Erosion

The possible causes for this defect are sensitivity of excipients to moisture, low friability of the cores, low spray rate, high pan speed, and inappropriate logo design or placement. This defect can be resolved by reformulating the core with excipients not sensitive to moisture, increasing the spray rate or the solids content, preheating the cores before starting the coating step, and modifying the logo design or placement.

Edge Chipping

During the coating operation, tablets are tumbling inside the pan and could get chipped at the edges. The most common causes are worn out punches, sharp edges on the tablets, low spray rate, high pan speed, and an underloaded pan. Tablet punches should be inspected, and if they are worn out, they should be replaced. Tablet shape should be modified to reduce the sharp edges. Increased spray rate, higher solids content, and low pan speed are additional means of solving the problem.

VIII. Hard and Soft Gelatin Capsules

Hard Gelatin Capsules

A common type of solid oral dosage form is a hard gelatin capsule, which consists of a locking cap and body in which a drug substance or blend containing the drug substance is enclosed. The gelatin capsule is a good alternative to tablets as it is easier to swallow, and it can be used to deliver powders, granules, beads, and even liquids encapsulated in various colors, sizes, and shapes. Most of the excipients used for tablet manufacture can be used in capsules and hence are not discussed again. Similarly, processes such as dry blending, dry granulation, and wet granulation, discussed in previous sections, can be used to obtain blends that can be either compressed into tablets or filled into capsules. There are, however, excipients that are specifically used in the manufacture of gelatin capsules, such as the ones discussed below.

Content of Gelatin Capsule

Gelatin is a protein obtained by partial hydrolysis of collagen derived from bovine or porcine skin and bones. Type A gelatin is derived from bovine or porcine skin by acid hydrolysis. The isoelectric point for this type of gelatin is pH 4.8–5.2. Type B gelatin is derived from bovine or porcine bones by alkali hydrolysis. The isoelectric point is pH 6.5–9.5. Gelatin derived from skin has plasticity, and gelatin derived from bones has firmness. Typically capsules are manufactured by using both types of gelatin. The firmness of the gel is called the *bloom strength*. For capsule manufacturing, gelatin should have a bloom strength of 150–280 g. Because of concerns about animal-derived products, especially of bovine origin, hypromellose, starch, and carrageenan capsules are available. However, manufacturers of gelatin capsules do certify that their gelatin has been derived from bovine spongiform encephalopathy (BSE)-free cattle. Gelatin capsules are still widely used. Some additives in gelatin capsules include plasticizers, preservatives, and colorants and opacifiers.

Plasticizers

Plasticizers are added to gelatin to reduce the rigidity of the polymer and make it more pliable. Common examples of plasticizers are glycerin and polyhydric alcohols. Water is also a good plasticizer and is naturally present in the gelatin.

Preservatives

Gelatin is a good substrate for bacterial and fungal growth. During capsule manufacture, gelatin is in an aqueous solution, which can further increase the possibility of bacterial and fungal growth. The most commonly used preservatives are methylparaben and propylparaben in a 4 : 1 ratio.

Colorants and Opacifiers

Natural and synthetic dyes are used to impart color to the capsules. Commonly used synthetic dyes are azo dyes and xanthene dyes. Iron oxide pigments are also used. But as with colorants used in coating, the regulatory requirements of different regions should be evaluated. The most common opacifier is titanium dioxide, and it is used to make clear gelatin opaque. Opaque capsules can protect their contents from light. As in tablet coating, flavors and sugar are occasionally added as needed.

Manufacture of Empty Hard Gelatin Capsules

The steps used in the manufacture of empty hard gelatin capsules are as follows. Stainless-steel pins are dipped into an aqueous solution of gelatin maintained at 50°C and are rotated to ensure even distribution of the gelatin without bubble formation. In these steps (dipping and spinning), the cap and body

Table 10-3 Capsule Size and Capacity

Capsule Size	Volume, cm^3	Fill-Weight,† g	
		(a)	(b)
000	1.37	0.548	1.096
00	0.95	0.380	0.760
0	0.68	0.272	0.544
1	0.50	0.200	0.400
2	0.37	0.148	0.296
3	0.30	0.120	0.240
4	0.21	0.084	0.168
5	0.13	0.052	0.104

†Based on powder bulk densities of (a) 0.4 g/cm^3 and (b) 0.8 g/cm^3.

are simultaneously formed. The drying of the capsules is carried out first in cold air and then in kilns to remove water. They are stripped from the pins and cut to desired lengths for the capsule body and cap, and the capsules are closed. Finished capsules are polished by either cloth dusting or brushing.

Storage of capsules is important. Generally capsules are stored in a controlled-temperature and controlled-humidity environment. Capsules are shaped like a bullet and come in different sizes ranging from 000 (biggest) to 5 (smallest); their volumes are shown in **Table 10-3**.

The bulk densities of typical API and excipients are within the range of 0.4–0.8 g/cm^3 or, for an average, 0.6 g/cm^3. The quantity of powder that can be placed into the overfill capacity of an empty, two-piece, hard gelatin capsule based on the bulk density is shown in Table 10-3. However, depending on the Carr compressibility index calculated based on the bulk and tapped densities, more powder mix can be placed inside a given size empty capsule as the percentage of compressibility increases. One can thus select the capsule size by comparing the desired weight of the powder mix with the calculated fill-weight based on the tapped density. For example, a 250-mg powder mix based on a bulk density of 0.6 g/cm^3 can be placed in a size 1 capsule, but with a tapped density of 0.75 g/cm^3 (20% compressibility), the same quantity can be placed in a size 2 capsule.

Filling of Hard Gelatin Capsules

The steps in a capsule filling operation are (1) rectification, where the capsules are oriented in the same direction; (2) separation, where the capsule body and cap are separated; (3) *dosing*, where powder blends and granulations are filled; (4) closing and ejection, where capsules are closed by locking cap and body and are ejected, and (5) dedusting and polishing using brushes. Additionally, the capsules may be weighed and inspected for defects.

There are two types of capsule-filling machines: manual and automatic. In the manual machines, all the steps except dedusting and polishing are done manually. These types of machines are good for making small experimental or clinical batches. Automatic machines are used for large clinical studies and for commercial products. Automatic machines are broadly classified into dosator and dosing disk types.

Dosator

It consists of a tube with an open end and a movable piston inside. As the tube plunges inside a hopper containing the drug powder, the powder is drawn inside the tube and, through compaction by a plunger, forms a plug which is then inserted into the capsule. A schematic diagram of a

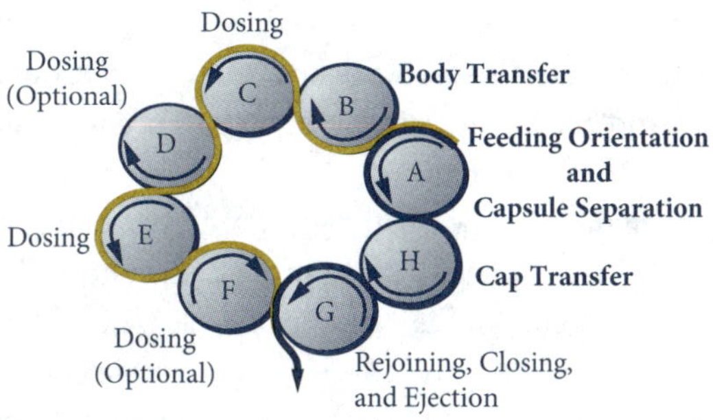

Dosing Capabilities:
Positions *C* and *E*: powder; positions *D* and *F*: tablet

Figure 10-13 Capsule-filling operation.
Courtesy of: MG America.

dosator filling machine is shown in **Figure 10-13**. The machine has the capability of filling capsules of all sizes by using appropriate change parts. It also has optional attachments for inserting tablets into capsules for blinding purposes in clinical trials. It is not necessary to have a free-flowing powder, but a lubricant is needed in the formulation to facilitate plug ejection.

Dosing Disk

This type of machine has a disk with multiple holes. The powder is drawn into the first hole and then is compacted by a tamping pin. Additional powder is added in the second hole followed by tamping and so on until a plug is formed, which is then inserted into the capsule. The capsules are closed and ejected.

The advantages and disadvantages of hard gelatin capsules are summarized in **Table 10-4**.

The hard gelatin capsules are subjected to the same tests as tablets, such as weight variation, content uniformity, disintegration, and dissolution. Enteric coating can also be applied to capsules. Despite concerns related to BSE and dosage form tampering, advances in materials and equipment design have imparted great versatility to this dosage form. Nonanimal materials have been developed for manufacturing capsules, and the concerns about tampering have been solved by adding bands to the capsules and developing new locking mechanisms for cap and body. In short, hard gelatin capsules are still widely used in the pharmaceutical industry.

Drug Release

Uncoated capsules are designed to be water-soluble and provide a quick release of content in the stomach. To facilitate an immediate release of the capsule content, a small quantity of sodium bicarbonate and citric acid, which generates carbon dioxide in water, may be added to help open the capsule. If the drug is water-soluble and a fast release is desired, the excipients should be

Table 10-4 Advantages and Disadvantages of Hard Gelatin Capsules

Advantages	Disadvantages
Capsules dissolve faster than tablets.	Capsule filling is slow compared to tableting.
There is no need to form a hard compact.	Stability could be a problem.
Powders, beads, granules, and even liquids can be filled.	There are concerns related to bovine spongiform encephalopathy (BSE).
They are easy to swallow.	
They can be used for blinding studies.	

hydrophilic, and if a slow release of the water-soluble drug is desired, the excipient should be hydrophobic. The excipients for water-insoluble drugs usually consist of a blend of water-soluble ingredients, such as lactose, and cellulose derivatives, such as microcrystalline methylcellulose (MCC). The relative content of the hydrophilic and hydrophobic blend is known to play a role in drug dissolution. If the drug dose is low (< 50 mg), more hydrophilic excipient is needed to facilitate drug dissolution. For higher drug doses, a more hydrophobic blend is needed to enhance the formulation compatibility. In general, the rate of drug release is delayed as the proportion of the hydrophobic polymer is increased relative to the water-soluble component. These observations serve as a good guideline for formulation. One notes, however, that the release profile for a drug may vary with other formulation factors.

Soft Gelatin Capsules

Soft gelatin capsules are made from more flexible gelatin by adding a higher amount of plasticizer. They contain the same excipients as the hard gelatin capsules and are formed, filled, and sealed in one operation. The soft gelatin capsules can be used to improve bioavailability because the drug is dissolved or suspended, which facilitates dissolution-dependent absorption of the drug. As bioavailability increases, the dose and consequently the dosing frequency can be decreased. They are easy to swallow, hence patient compliance is improved. In addition, soft gelatin capsules can be used as patentable line extensions and are tamper-evident. They have some of the same disadvantages as the hard gelatin capsules. One of the biggest might be the fact that it is a specialized technology and not many companies have it in-house. So the work has to be carried out at a contract facility. But soft gelatin capsules are a good alternative to tablets.

IX. Chapter Summary

The science that deals with the properties of small particles is known as micromeritics. One of the most important properties of solid particles is their flowability/compressibility, which depends on the particle size, shape, porosity, bulk and compressed density, and surface textures. The pharmaceutical processes are based upon changes in these parameters. The subject of micromeritics has been discussed generally. This chapter attempts to explain these properties by describing the processes and evaluating the tableting outcome. It should be emphasized that these processes constitute the basic mechanisms in the development of solid dosage forms that are not only the most widely used, but also the most acceptable dosage forms for the delivery of pharmaceutical and medicinal agents. They are easy to manufacture, as different processing techniques can be used to accommodate changes in desired doses and the physicochemical properties of the drugs.

X. References

1. Pharmaceutical cGMPs for the 21st Century—A Risk Based Approach, U.S. FDA, Sept. 2004.
2. WHO Expert Committee on Specifications for Pharmaceutical Preparations, 1999.
3. Lowenthal W. Mechanism of action of disintegrants. *Pharm Acta Helv.* 48(1):589–609, 1973.
4. Whitaker M, Baker GR, Westrup J, et al. Application of acoustic emission to the monitoring and end point determination of a high shear granulation process. *Int J Pharm.* 205:79–91, 2000.
5. Tok AT, Goh X, Ng WK, and Tan RBH. Monitoring granulation rate processes using three PAT tools in a pilot-scale fluidized bed. *AAPS Pharm Sci Tech.* 9(4):1083–1091, 2008.
6. Carr RL Jr. Evaluating flow properties of solids. *Chem Eng.* 72:163–168, 1965.

XI. Homework Problems

1. Name four of the most important excipients with examples and their usage in compressed tablet formulation.
2. Select the correct answers.
   (*a*) A disintegrant should be hydrophobic in nature.
   (*b*) A disintegrant is water-soluble.
   (*c*) A disintegrant is water-insoluble but has a high affinity for water to produce a swelling effect.
   (*d*) A disintegrant may be one that releases gases in aqueous solution (effervescent).
   (*e*) The concentration of disintegrants in a tablet formulation is 2–5%.
3. Show how you would prepare the following formulation for 100 ibuprofen (200 mg) compressed tablets. Identify the uses of the excipients.

Ibuprofen	45.25%
Caffeine	22.62%
Avicel PH 101	31.67%
Stearic Acid	0.45%

4. Describe the role of a hydrophilic binder (e.g. hydroxypropylcellulose) in the wet granulation process.
5. The height of a powder cone is 20 cm, and the radius is 25 cm. What is the angle of repose? Does the powder have good flow?
6. The bulk density of a powder blend is 0.43 g/cm^3. The tapped density is 0.51 g/cm^3. Calculate the Carr index.
7. For quality control purposes, what are the in-process and postcompression tests for tablet properties?
8. Calculate the percentage friability when the initial weight is 6.238 g and the final weight is 6.235 g.
9. Describe the role of plasticizer in film coating in relation to coating defects.
10. A powder formulation has a bulk density of 0.6 g/cm^3. Calculate the amount of the powder that can be filled into capsules of sizes 0, 1, 2, 3, 4, and 5 (see Table 10-3 for capsule volume capacity).
11. (*a*) Piroxicam is a BCS class II drug with low solubility. For experimental use, hard gelatin capsules (wt of powder = 300 mg) of 20 mg dose are being made using a blend of 75% lactose anhydrous and 25% microcrystalline cellulose (MCC) and stearic acid (2 mg/capsule). If the final powder has a tapped density of 0.62 g/cm^3, select a capsule size and calculate the amount of each ingredient needed for making a batch of 50 capsules. (*b*) If the capsules were made using a blend of 25% lactose anhydrous and 75% MCC, how does the filler affect the drug dissolution rate?
12. What is the physicochemical property that allows hypromellose to be used in making gelatin-equivalent hard capsules?

PART III

PHARMACEUTICAL DEVELOPMENT II: POLYPHASIC SYSTEMS

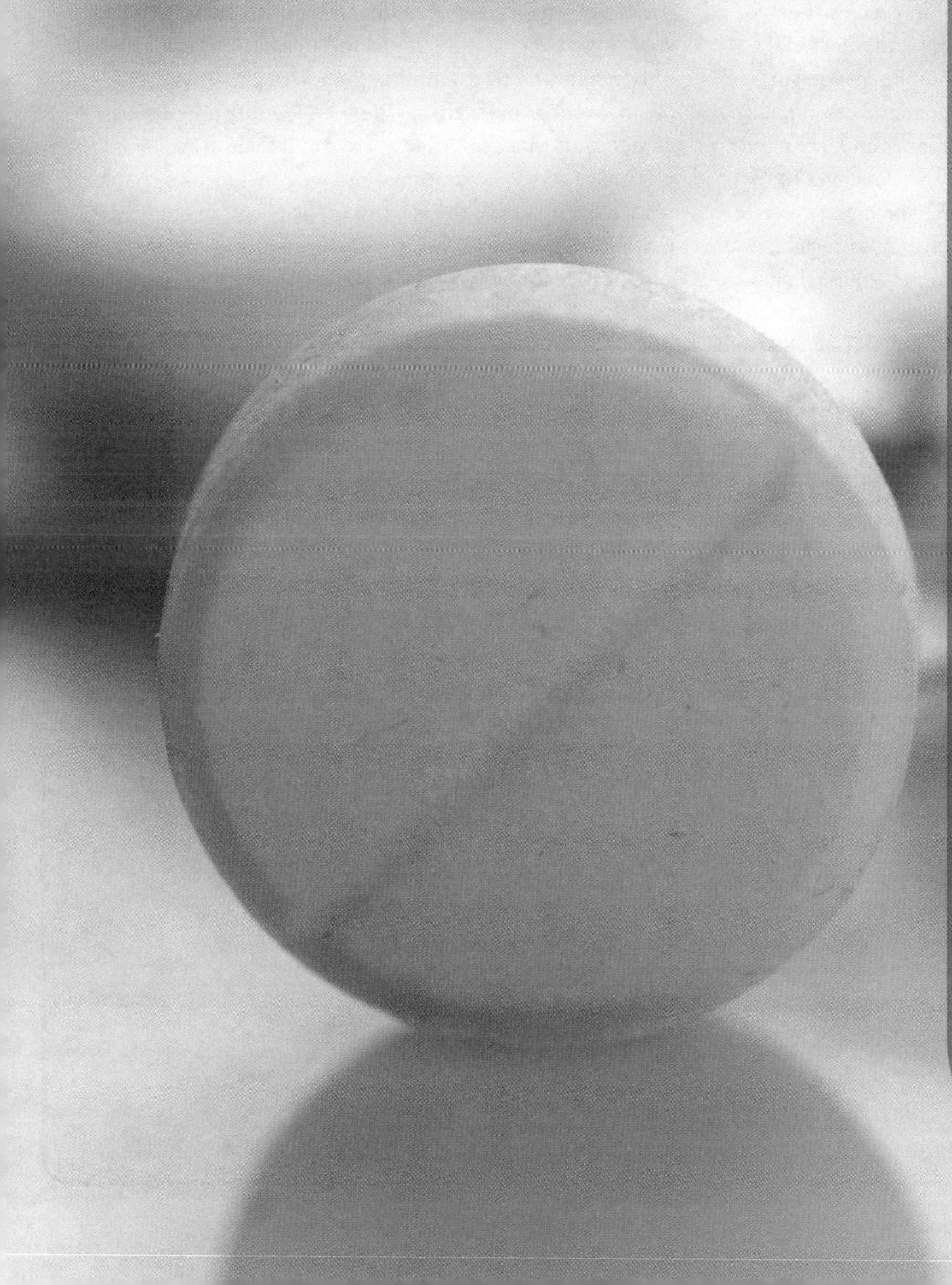

CHAPTER 11

Interfacial Phenomena

The topic of this chapter has wide extensions into pharmaceutical systems such as powders, suspensions, emulsions, colloidal dispersions, and other semisolid dosage forms. Common to all systems is the presence of heterogeneous phases in which solid or liquid particles coexist with the continuous solution. Because the formulation objectives are to create these stable interfaces, knowledge of the interfacial phenomena, such as the properties of molecules situated in the interfacial region, surface energy and interfacial tension, and the effects of solution components on surface properties and energy, is both important and essential. The theories governing the interfacial phenomena include surface chemistry principles derived from changes in surface free energy or surface tension, which plays a major role in determining the stability of a dispersed system, and the electric properties of solid, liquid, and colloidal particles and their interactions with the solution components. One of the principal contributions of surface chemistry to medical science has been the elucidation of drug properties in various heterogeneous conditions, ranging from dosage form development to phase-dependent processes of drug absorption and the passage of drugs across the biological membranes. The plan of this chapter is as follows. First, surface chemistry, one that depends on the surface free energy changes, in pure liquid and in solutions is discussed. This is followed by examining the interfacial processes on adsorption and wetting. We then identify and discuss compounds that are surface-active and their usage in pharmaceutical preparations, and we conclude the chapter with a discussion of the electrokinetic effects of charged particles, a part of surface chemistry that is of special significance to the colloidal system.

CHAPTER OUTLINE

OBJECTIVES

1. Understand the concept of free energy residing at the surface and the expression of such energy with a measurable quantity known as the surface tension.
2. Understand the methods of surface tension measurement.
3. Comprehend the concept and use of the Laplace equation.
4. Understand the Gibbs adsorption equation and the thermodynamic implications of interfacial molecular properties.
5. Describe the wetting process based on surface tension changes at the interfaces.
6. Know the properties of surface-active agents.
7. Know the HLB system and its pharmaceutical applications.
8. Describe the diffuse double layer and zeta potential for charged particles.
9. Understand the electrokinetic effects and the stability of charged solid particles in electrolyte solutions.

I. Principles in Surface Chemistry

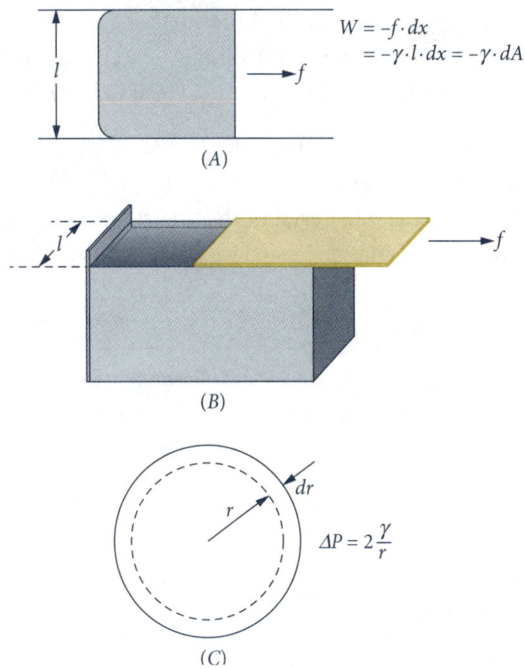

Figure 11-1 Work of maintaining or extending a surface: (*A*) a soap film; (*B*) a liquid surface covered by insert material; and (*C*) a soap bubble.

When two distinct phases exist in a system, the boundary between them is called the interface. The interface may be formed by a liquid or solid phase with, in any combination, other phases (gas, liquid, or solid). Two gases do not form an interface. As we shall learn from discussion that follows, the key parameter in surface chemistry is the *surface tension*, which is measured at the interface that involves air or vapor. When the surface tension is measured at an interface not involving a gas, it is termed interfacial tension. There is no strict rule on what this quantity should be called, but for clarity the interface that it represents is often indicated. The symbol for surface tension is γ, which is often followed by subscripts *S* for solid, *L* for liquid, and *V* for vapor, so that the symbols γ_{LV}, γ_{SV}, γ_{LL}, and γ_{LS} indicate surface or interfacial tension of liquid–vapor, solid–vapor, liquid–liquid, and liquid–solid interfaces, respectively. It is understood, however, that γ_L and γ_S are used to indicate γ_{LV} and γ_{SV}.

Surface Tension and Measurement

The surface tension of a liquid can be looked upon as the property (resulting from cohesional forces) that draws a liquid together to form a liquid–vapor interface, thereby distinguishing the liquid from a gas. Molecules at the interface are in constant motion (average residence time is about 10^{-6} s), indicating that energy resides in the interface, or more specifically, work is required to maintain or to extend this interface.

Surface Tension of Liquids

A common example to demonstrate the work required to increase a liquid–vapor surface is soap films, as they persist long enough to be visualized. If a soap film is formed in a frame one side of which can move freely, an important fact is that the film will spontaneously contract, and to prevent contraction, a force f must be applied (see **Figure 11-1**). If f is decreased slightly, contraction occurs, and if f is increased, the film extends. This contraction and expansion phenomenon demonstrates a reversible process (at constant temperature and pressure); therefore, the work required to maintain or to extend the interface corresponds to a Gibbs free energy quantity. For a small displacement dx of the movable side of the frame, the work done by the film is $W = -f dx$. If the width of the movable side is l, the force can be written as γl, where γ is the force per unit length (dyn/cm in the cgs system) exerted by the film.† Thus,

$$W = -f\,dx = -\gamma l\,dx = -\gamma\,dA \tag{11-1}$$

†Parenthetically, common usage defines γ as the surface tension for one surface. A soap film has two surfaces; hence, f may be written as $f = \gamma(2l)$. But as the area change would now be $2l\,dx$, this still leads to the expression of Equation (11-1).

The parameter γ is called the surface tension. The term $l\,dx$ gives the change in the area (dA) of the film. Hence, in a lesser geometry-specific expression, surface tension is the free energy required to maintain the interface per surface area, with a unit of erg/cm^2.

Now consider a pure liquid covered by a lid that can be slid back and forth to change the amount of liquid surface (see Figure 11-1B). Assuming that there is no interaction between the liquid and the material of the lid, the force on the lid is then γl as before, and the free energy change per change in surface area is also $\gamma\,dA$ under constant pressure and temperature.

Surface Energy

The total possible free energy change of a liquid, according to the first and second laws of thermodynamics and the change in surface area, is

$$dG = V\,dP + \gamma\,dA - S\,dT$$

Under constant temperature and pressure, however, the bulk properties of the liquid are not changed. Thus, *the surface tension is the surface free energy (per unit area)*. By using G^S for surface free energy, the thermodynamic expression of γ is

$$\gamma = (\partial G/\partial A)_{T,P} = G^S$$

The surface entropy, also per unit of area, is the change in free energy as a function of temperature under constant pressure. That is,

$$(\partial G^S/\partial T)_P = (\partial \gamma/\partial T)_P = S^S$$

The standard relationship of free energy, enthalpy, and entropy is

$$H^S = G^S + TS^S$$

Often, as a good approximation, H^S and the surface energy E^S are not distinguished, so the above equation is usually given in the form

$$E^S = G^S + TS^S = \gamma - T\,d\gamma/dT \qquad (11\text{-}2)$$

Equation (11-2) defines the surface energy of a liquid. The surface tension of a liquid decreases with increasing temperature, which makes the term $-T\,d\gamma/dT$ a positive value. Hence, it is understood that the surface tension is somewhat less than that of E^S. *But, at constant temperature and pressure, $T\,d\gamma/dT$ is zero, the surface energy is the surface free energy, and the surface free energy per unit area is the surface tension.*

Curved Interface

Now consider a soap bubble blowing experiment. The physical reality is that the film spontaneously seeks to decrease its total surface free energy by changing the surface area, but, in doing so, shrinks the bubble to the point that the increased pressure (from blowing) prevents further change. This is known as the Laplace theory, which relates the mechanical pressure across an interface to its curvature. Consider a bubble of radius r (see Figure 11-1). The total surface free energy is $4\pi r^2\gamma$, and if the radius were to decrease by dr, the change in surface free energy would be

$$dG^S = -8\pi r\gamma\,dr$$

Because shrinking decreases the total free energy, at equilibrium the tendency to shrink must be balanced by a pressure difference (ΔP) across the film such that the work against this pressure difference is just equal to the decrease in surface free energy. The work is $-f\,dr$, ΔP is force per unit area, and the area is $4\pi r^2$. Hence,

$$W = -(\Delta P)\,4\pi r^2\,dr = -8\pi r\gamma\,dr$$

or

$$\Delta P = 2\gamma/r \qquad (11\text{-}3)$$

Equation (11-3) is the Laplace equation for a spherical interface. An important conclusion is that the smaller the bubble, i.e., the smaller the value of r, the larger is ΔP. Conversely, ΔP becomes zero if r approaches infinity, which corresponds to the case of a plane surface.

Example 11-1: Surface tension and mechanical pressure

To blow a bubble of 2-mm radius using water ($\gamma = 72.8$ dyn/cm) and a soap water ($\gamma = 9.0$ dyn/cm), what are the internal pressures (the Laplace pressure ΔP) needed, given that the density of water or soap water is 1 g/cm^3, 1 atm = 760 mmHg = 1.01325×10^6 dyn/cm^2, and the density of mercury = 13.595 g/cm^3.

Solution:

Water: $\Delta P = 2\gamma/r = 2 \times 72.8/0.2 = 728$ dyn/cm^2

$= 728 \times 760/1.01325 \times 10^6 = 0.546$ mmHg

$= 0.546 \times 13.595/1 = 7.42$ mmH_2O

Soap water: $\Delta P = 2\gamma/r = 2 \times 9.0/0.2 = 180$ dyn/cm^2

$= 180 \times 760/1.01325 \times 10^6 = 0.135$ mmHg

$= 0.135 \times 13.595/1 = 1.84$ mmH_2O

Capillary Rise

If a small-bore tube is partially immersed in a liquid as shown in **Figure 11-2*A***, one usually observes that the liquid rises to a height h above the liquid surface. This phenomenon may be described by the Laplace equation if the liquid wets the wall of the capillary tube, whose radius is r, and the meniscus formed is hemispherical. In this case, $\Delta P = 2\gamma/r$. If, as the figure further shows, P_1 is the atmosphere pressure and P_2 is the pressure just under the meniscus, then $P_1 - P_2 = 2\gamma/r$. This pressure difference is counterbalanced by the hydrostatic pressure of the capillary rise, that is, $P_1 - P_2 = \rho gh$, where ρ is the density of the liquid and g is the standard acceleration of gravity. Hence,

$$\rho gh = 2\gamma/r \qquad \text{or} \qquad h = 2\gamma/\rho gr \qquad (11\text{-}4)$$

Equation (11-4) is exact only to the limit of small r; otherwise corrections are needed.

A general case of the capillary rise is shown in **Figure 11-2*B***, where the liquid meets the capillary wall at a contact angle θ, and the meniscus is part of a large sphere with a radius R. It can be seen that R is related to the radius of the capillary tube by the equation $R = r/\cos\theta$. Hence, Equation (11-4) becomes

$$h = 2\gamma\cos\theta/\rho gr \qquad (11\text{-}5)$$

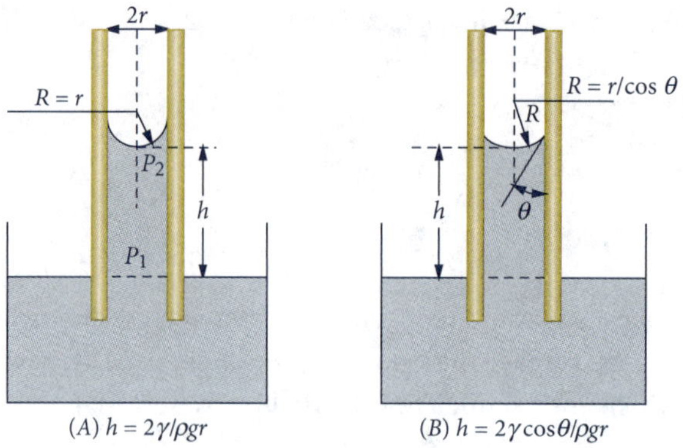

Figure 11-2 The capillary rise with (*A*) a hemispherical meniscus (radius *r*) and (*B*) a curvature (radius $r/\cos\theta$) meniscus.

A liquid making a contact angle of 90° with the wall would show no capillary rise. When the contact angle is greater than 90°, as in mercury ($\theta = 140°$), $\cos\theta$ is negative and so is h, and this would lead to a capillary depression. Equation (11-5) can also be obtained without using the R concept. The spontaneous contractile tendency of a liquid surface acts as though there were a surface force of γ per unit length. In capillary rise, the length is the circumference of the capillary tube, the total such force is $2\pi r\gamma$, and its vertical component is thus $2\pi r\gamma\cos\theta$. This force is balanced by the force exerted by gravity on the column of liquid rise, or $\pi r^2\rho gh$. When one equates these two forces, Equation (11-5) is again obtained.

The surface tension can be determined by measuring the height of a liquid rise, using Equation (11-4) if r is sufficiently small and $\cos\theta = 1$. For example, pure ethanol was shown to rise to a height of 5.88 cm at 20°C in a capillary tube with an inner diameter of 0.02 cm. The density of ethanol is 0.78932 g/cm^3. Using Equation (11-4), one obtains

$$\gamma = \rho ghr/2 = 0.78932 \times 980.67 \times 5.88 \times 0.01/2 = 22.78\,\text{dyn/cm}$$

The capillary rise phenomenon is not only the basis for an absolute measurement of surface tension but also one of its major manifestations. The phenomenon accounts for the general tendency of liquids and gases to enter pores and fine cracks. As seen earlier, the combination of vapor pressure–induced surface free energy change and the Laplace curved interface concept leads to the Kelvin equation, which gives a basic model for the measurement of pore sizes and capillary channels. Waterproofing of fabrics is another example involving a direct application of Equation (11-5). Fabrics are porous materials, where the spaces between fibers amount to small capillary tubes. Coated fibers on which water has a contact angle of greater than 90° provide a Laplace pressure that opposes the entry of water into the fabric. Only when this pressure is exceeded (as by rubbing the wet fabric) will water penetrate freely through the filled capillary channels.

Measurement of Surface Tension by Detachment

A very simple relationship of surface tension and weight can be reached if one considers the fall of a liquid drop from the tip of a tube. If the drop of liquid formed is allowed to grow by delivering liquid slowly through the tube, a size is reached such that the surface tension can no longer support the weight of the drop, and it falls. From the ideal weight of the drop (W_{ideal}), the surface tension is calculated as

$$W_{\text{ideal}} = 2\pi r\gamma \tag{11-6}$$

where r is the radius of the tube tip. But as the detached drop always leaves behind a considerable residue of liquid, the actual weight of a drop that is measured will need to be corrected by a factor f in that

$$W_{actu} = W_{ideal} f$$

This factor is expressed as a function of $r/V^{1/3}$, where V is the volume of the drop, and the values have been tabulated.[1] The correction is considerable, but the method is shown to be accurate and convenient. In practice, a sufficient number of drops can be collected to provide an accurate determination of the drop weight.

A number of methods similar to the drop weight measurement have been used for surface tension measurement. The du Nouy tensiometer uses a platinum wire ring immersed at the surface or interface. The weight of liquid pulled out of the plane is immediately determined before the ring becomes detached. In this case, the detached ideal weight is $W_{ideal} = 4\pi R\gamma$, where R is the radius of the ring, allowing for both the inside and outside meniscus depending on how liquid wets the ring. As with the drop weight method, rather large corrections using tabulated correction factors are involved.[1,2] If, instead of a ring, one uses a metal (platinum) flag as in the Wilhelmy balance method, the ideal weight can be directly determined without using a correction factor. The Wilhelmy balance also allows measurement of surface tension as a function of surface area and is a popular instrument for surface tension measurement.

Surface Tension of Solutions—Gibbs Adsorption Phenomenon

Many behavioral aspects of interfacial systems come about simply because of the relatively large amount of surface within the system. As matter is subdivided, the free energy of the system increases proportionally to the amount of new surface created. The laws of thermodynamics, however, dictate that the system will seek the lowest energy state that is possible under the circumstances. This phenomenon can be illustrated as follows. Consider a container of oil and water in which the oil is floating above the water and the two phases are separated by a surface of minimum area and minimum free energy. Upon vigorous shaking of the container, the oil phase is now dispersed in the water phase as droplets, and the total surface of the oil–water interface is greatly increased. IIowever, when allowed to stand at rest, the droplets join to form increasingly larger drops of oil, each having less surface than the sum of the surfaces of individual droplets that formed it, thereby reducing surface free energy. This behavior continues until the whole mass of oil is again floating above the water phase. It is known that some "surface-active" agents can be used to maintain the increased surface area resulting from the dispersion, thereby increasing the stability of the dispersed system. Why is this so, and what are the surface-active agents? The answers may be found from the work of J. W. Gibbs, and the result is known as the *Gibbs adsorption equation*.

Gibbs Adsorption Equation

A two-component aqueous solution can be described consisting of an interfacial phase between the surface of the solution and the vapor above it and a bulk phase of the solution itself. It is recalled that under constant temperature and pressure, the surface free energy of a pure liquid involves only surface tension. Because there are two components in a solution, the thermodynamic functions must now include the amount of each component as a variable. In fact, at constant temperature and pressure, neither temperature nor pressure contributes to free energy change. Thus, at the interface, the free energy includes only the chemical potential of the components and the surface tension, i.e.,

$$G^S = n_1^S\mu_1^S + n_2^S\mu_2^S + \gamma A \tag{11-7}$$

where n is the number of molecules in moles, μ is the chemical potential, A is the surface area, subscripts 1 and 2 denote solvent and solute, respectively, and the superscript S indicates the interface. For the bulk phase, it follows that the free energy change only includes the chemical potential of the components in that

$$G = n_1\mu_1 + n_2\mu_2 \tag{11-8}$$

These free energy expressions can be used to determine the distribution of the solute between the interfacial region and the bulk solution under equilibrium conditions, which is the main objective of the Gibbs adsorption theory.

The distribution of the solute and solvent at equilibrium may be deduced as follows. For simplicity, first let us consider the bulk phase. Upon differentiation of Equation (11-8), we obtain

$$dG = n_1\,d\mu_1 + n_2\,d\mu_2 + \mu_1\,dn_1 + \mu_2\,dn_2 \tag{11-9}$$

The chemical potential is the free energy change of a system per mole of an added component, when other conditions are held constant. This makes the quantity μ a coefficient of the change dG for a small increment of dn. Hence, again at constant temperature and pressure, the change in free energy dG can be written as

$$dG = \mu_1\,dn_1 + \mu_2\,dn_2 \tag{11-10}$$

Comparison of Equations (11-9) and (11-10) gives

$$n_1\,d\mu_1 + n_2\,d\mu_2 = 0 \tag{11-11}$$

Now, for the interface, one can obtain an equation similar to Equation (11-11) as

$$n_1^S\,d\mu_1^S + n_2^S\,d\mu_2^S + A\,d\gamma = 0 \tag{11-12}$$

One of the important concepts of the chemical potential of a reversible process is that when equilibrium (between the bulk and interfacial phases) is reached, the chemical potential of any given component will be the same in each phase. Thus, at equilibrium, $d\mu_1 = d\mu_1^S$ and $d\mu_2 = d\mu_2^S$. If we now multiply Equation (11-11) by a factor of n_1^S/n_1 and then combine the modified equation with Equation (11-12), the resulting expression is

$$-\frac{d\gamma}{d\mu_2} = \frac{n_2^S - n_2(n_1^S/n_1)}{A} = \Gamma_2 \tag{11-13}$$

Equation (11-13) is one form of the Gibbs adsorption equation. The quantity Γ_2 is the negative change in surface tension per change of chemical potential. It also indicates the difference between the number of moles of solute residing at the surface and that in the bulk solution of a comparable area. Here n_2^S is the moles of solute at the surface where the number of solvent molecules is n_1^S, whereas $n_2(n_1^S/n_1)$ is the moles of solute in a bulk region that contains n_1^S solvent molecules. For this reason, Γ_2 is known as the algebraic *surface excess* of the solute at the interface over the number of moles that would be present in a bulk region containing the same number of moles of solvent.

The chemical potential can be expressed in terms of the activity of the solute (a_2) at equilibrium, that is, $d\mu = RT\,d\,(\ln a_2)$, and for a dilute solution, the activity is taken to be the concentration C. These substitutions lead to a common form of the Gibbs equation:

$$\Gamma_2 = -(C/RT)\,d\gamma/dC = [n_2^S - n_2(n_1^S/n_1)]/A \tag{11-14}$$

Here, as the equation indicates, if the solute prefers to concentrate at the interface, Γ_2 will be positive and the surface tension will decrease with increasing concentration. Conversely, if Γ_2 is a negative excess, as in electrolyte solutions, then the surface concentration of electrolytes will be less than it is in solution and $d\gamma/dC$ assumes a positive value. Thus, *compounds having a tendency to reside at the interface will reduce the surface tension of the liquid and are thus called surface-active.* Small electrolytes are not surface-active and tend to move away from the surface. In the case of 1 *M* sodium chloride, the negative surface excess is equivalent to a surface layer of pure water about one molecule deep.

Surface Monolayer and Pressure

The surface excess Γ_2 may be measured directly or calculated based on the Gibbs equation as a means to assess the behavior of the surface-active agent at the interface. Studies by McBain and Swain[3] using a fast-moving knife blade (a microtome) have shown that the surface sample collected from an 0.053 *m* solution of phenol contained 2.52×10^{-6} g more of phenol per gram of water than did the bulk solution. The calculated Γ_2 value is 2.77×10^{-10} mol/cm^2, which is in good agreement with the Gibbs adsorption phenomenon (see Example 11-2 for calculations). Although the value of Γ_2 is a very small number, it corresponds to about 80 Å^2 per molecule, or about twice the value for a close-packed monolayer of molecules lying flat on the surface. This example suggests that molecules of a surface-active agent will assume a close-packed structure as in gas adsorption that led to the formation of a monomolecular layer at the interfacial surface.

Example 11-2: At 20°C, a 3.2-g sample collected by a microtome experiment from the surface of a trough containing an 0.053 *m* solution of phenol (mol wt = 94) and having a surface area of 310 cm^2 contained 2.52×10^{-6} g more of phenol per gram of water than did the bulk solution.

(*a*) Calculate the surface excess Γ_2 from the experimental data.

(*b*) Determine the surface excess Γ_2, using the Gibbs adsorption equation.

(*c*) What is the surface pressure (π) of the solution of 0.05 *m* phenol?

(*d*) If the depth of the phenol molecule is 4×10^{-8} cm on the liquid surface, calculate the equivalent three-dimensional pressure (π/h).

The surface tension of water and that of 0.05 *m* and 0.127 *m* solutions of phenol at 20°C are 72.7, 67.7, and 60.1 dyn/cm, respectively.

Solution: $\Gamma_2 = -(C/RT)\, d\gamma/dC = [n_2^S - n_2(n_1^S/n_1)]/A$

(*a*) $\Gamma_2 = (2.52 \times 10^{-6})(3.2)/(94)(310) = 2.77 \times 10^{-10}$ mol/cm^2

(*b*) $-d\gamma/dC$ may be estimated as $-\Delta\gamma/\Delta C$, which is 100 between 0 and 0.05 *m* and 98.7 between 0.05 and 0.127 *m*; average value = 99.4.

$$\Gamma_2 = -(C/RT)\, d\gamma/dC$$

$$= (0.053)(99.4)/(8.3143 \times 10^7)(293.2) = 2.16 \times 10^{-10} \text{ mol/cm}^2$$

(*c*) $\pi = \gamma^o - \gamma = 72.7 - 67.7 = 5.0$ dyn/cm

(*d*) $\pi/h = 5.0/(4 \times 10^{-8}) = 1.25 \times 10^8$ dyn/cm^2

$$= 1.25 \times 10^8/(1.01325 \times 10^6) = 123 \text{ atm}$$

The formation of a monolayer by surface-active compounds gives the Gibbs adsorption equation another view of the surface behavior known as surface pressure. In sufficiently dilute solution, the surface tension lowering is proportional to solute concentration, i.e.,

$$\gamma = \gamma^o - bC$$

where γ^o is the surface tension of the pure solvent and b is a proportional constant. Differentiation of the above equation gives $-C d\gamma/dC = \gamma^o - \gamma$. The Gibbs adsorption Equation (11-14) can thus be reduced to

$$\Gamma_2 = (\gamma^o - \gamma)/RT$$

It is now convenient to introduce the quantity of π *as* $\gamma^o - \gamma$, which is called the surface pressure, and the quantity of σ, which is taken to be $1/\Gamma_2$, as the surface area occupied by 1 mol of molecules. With these substitutions, the Gibbs adsorption equation becomes

$$\pi\sigma = RT \qquad \text{where } \pi = \gamma^o - \gamma \text{ and } \sigma = 1/\Gamma_2$$

or $$\pi A = nRT \qquad (11\text{-}15)$$

where A is the area occupied by one molecule. As can be seen, this equation represents the state of a two-dimensional ideal gas, suggesting that molecules at the liquid–vapor interface behave as anchored two-dimensional gas. The surface pressure does in fact correspond to a two-dimensional pressure. In the case of 0.05 m phenol, π is calculated to be 5 dyn/cm (see Example 11-2). This value may seem small, but when one considers the depth of the molecule (4×10^{-8} cm), the equivalent three-dimensional pressure would be 1.25×10^8 dyn/cm^2, or 123 atm, which is quite appreciable at the molecular level. Equation (11-15) also shows that the surface pressure is inversely proportional to the area. As σ decreases, π will increase until a close-packed monolayer is formed, at which point, further attempts to decrease the area will result in first a sharp increase in surface pressure and then a collapse of the monolayer.

Liquid Films and Film Balance

For an insoluble surfactant, its surface behavior may be studied by direct spreading of the material onto the liquid surface, usually water, to form a monolayer film. Because the concentration of the surfactant in water is zero, Γ_2 is known directly as the amount placed on a known area of surface, and so is its reciprocal value σ (area/mole of molecules), or A (area/molecule). The surface or *film pressure* is usually obtained from surface tension measurements. The study of liquid films can be carried out using a film balance, which consists of a water trough with calibrated surface area, a moving compressing barrier, and a fixed floating barrier with a tensiometer for force measurement. When a surfactant is added onto the water surface and is compressed against the floating barrier, the compressive force per unit area is known as the surface or film pressure ($\pi = \gamma^o - \gamma$). Such experiments enable the determination of the monolayer and the area and volume of the surfactant molecule that make up the monolayer. These data are of significance in determining the quantity of the surfactant for various applications.

Fatty acids, such as stearic acid, $CH_3(CH_2)_{16}COOH$, that contain a hydrophilic group which, through partial immersion, aids in spreading the molecule across the water surface and a long hydrocarbon chain that prevents the molecule from dissolving, are ideal for liquid film studies. The film balance experiment is usually carried out by adding a measured amount of surfactant onto the water surface and gradually advancing the movable barrier toward the fixed floating barrier. As the surface area is reduced by pushing forward the movable barrier, the force exerted

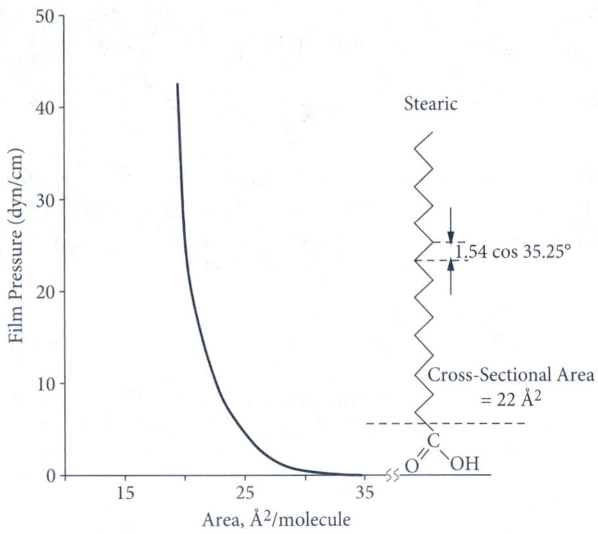

Figure 11-3 Illustration of a pressure–area isotherm and molecular orientation of stearic acid at the air–water interface.
Data from: GM Barrow, *Physical Chemistry*, 2nd ed., McGraw-Hill, Inc., 1966, p. 756 and Herman E. Reis Jr. of Standard Oil Company of Indiana, Whiting, Ind.

on the fixed barrier is recorded by the tension device. The collected data are then analyzed by a plot of the force in dynes per centimeter on the fixed barrier versus the surface area per molecule of the surfactant, i.e., the surface area covered divided by the number of molecules in the sample. A typical force–area plot is shown in **Figure 11-3**. The initial slow increase in film force with decreasing surface area (from right to left) indicates that the surface is not completely covered by the surface-active film. The beginning of a steep increase in force at a lower value of area per molecule is then taken to correspond to the completion of the monolayer film. Further decrease in surface area must compress the film itself, and a large increase in force is necessary. The film, however, will ultimately buckle and fold, and the area can be increased without any increase in force. The film balance study is employed to measure the surface area of a monolayer, which is then used to determine the dimensions of the molecule based on the following relationship:

Molecular volume = height of molecule × cross-sectional area

$$M/\rho N = hA$$

where M is the molecular weight, ρ is the density, N is Avogadro's number, h is the length of the molecule or thickness of the film, and A is the cross-sectional area of one molecule (see Example 11-3 for calculation).

Example 11-3: (*a*) The cross-sectional area for stearic acid was determined by film balance to be 22 Å^2. Determine the length of the molecule. (*b*) For comparison, calculate the cross-sectional area of stearic acid based on molecular information. (For stearic acid, $M = 285$, $\rho = 0.85\ \text{g/cm}^3$.)

Solution:

(*a*) $h = M/\rho AN = 285/(0.85 \times 22 \times 10^{-16} \times 6.02 \times 10^{23}) = 25.3 \times 10^{-8}\ \text{cm}$, or 25.3 Å

(*b*) $M/\rho N = 284/(0.85 \times 6.02 \times 10^{23}) = 550\ \text{Å}^3$

h = (# of carbon)(bond length)$(\cos\theta)^{\dagger}$ = 17 × 1.54 cos 35° = 21 Å

A (cross-sectional area) = 550/21 = 26 Å^2

†The length of the alkyl chain is estimated based on the vertical length of the C—H bond. Assuming tetrahedral structure, the C—H bond (1.54 Å) rises with an angle of 35.25°. The calculated A is in good agreement with the value determined by film balance, thus indicating the existence of a monolayer on the liquid surface.

Table 11-1 Molecular Cross-Sectional Area and Thickness in Surface Films

Surfactant	Formula	Film Thickness, Å (Length of Molecule)	Cross-Sectional Area, Å^2
Stearic acid	$C_{17}H_{35}COOH$	25	22
Oleic acid	$C_{17}H_{33}COOH$	11.2	46
Cerotic acid	$C_{25}H_{51}COOH$	31	25
Tristearin	$(C_{18}H_{35}O_2)_3C_3H_5$	25	66
Triolein	$(C_{18}H_{33}O_2)_3C_3H_5$	13	126

A number of organic acids have been studied by film balance, and the measured molecular dimensions are given in **Table 11-1**. For stearic acid, the cross-sectional area was shown to be 22 Å^2. Notice that oleic acid and triolein give cross-sectional areas that are about twice those of stearic acid and tristearin, but have a film thickness that is about one-half of the stearic counterparts. Oleic acid and derivatives contain a double bond at the midpoint of the hydrocarbon chain. It is suggested that the double bond(s) is (are) polar and remains in contact with water, hence, only one-half the length of the hydrocarbon chain is vertically oriented above the water surface. This arrangement thus increases the cross-sectional area but decreases the thickness of the monomolecular film. In film balance studies, it is worth noting that the original spread of the surfactant corresponds to a two-dimensional gaseous state; but as the area is condensed, so does the packing structure. The surface-active agent thus undergoes changes from gaseous state to liquid and even to two-dimensional solid state as the surface pressure increases.

II. Interfacial Interaction

Adsorption of Solute by Solid Particles

The topic of gas adsorption by small particles has been discussed. A very important but not well-understood process is the adsorption of solute of a solution onto a solid adsorbent. This process is involved, e.g., in the decolorizing of solutions using activated charcoal, chromatographic separation of solutes based on adsorption, and wetting of suspending particles.

Adsorption Isotherms

The process of adsorption from solution appears to be limited to the formation of a monolayer, with any further addition of solute being strongly opposed by the power of solvation. A fairly satisfactory empirical isotherm, which can be applied to gas adsorptions at low pressures, was introduced by Freundlich for the adsorption from solution. If y is the weight of solute adsorbed per gram of adsorbent and c is the concentration of the solute in solution, the *Freundlich isotherm* is given by

$$y = kc^{1/n}$$

where k and n are empirical constants. The equation is usually used in the logarithmic form

$$\log y = \log k + (1/n)\log c \quad (11\text{-}16)$$

Experimental results that conform to Equation (11-16) will yield a straight line for the plot of log *y* versus log *c*. The constants can then be determined from the slope and intercept.

Example 11-4: The data on the adsorption of acetic acid by activated charcoal (1 g) in aqueous acetic acid solution at 25°C are as follows. Plot the data according to the Freundlich equation, and determine the constants given in Equation (11-16).

Concentration (*M*)	*y*	y_{calc}	Concentration (*M*)	*y*	y_{calc}
0.0181	0.467	0.462	0.4711	2.040	2.027
0.0309	0.624	0.590	0.8817	2.480	2.689
0.0616	0.801	0.806	2.7850	3.760	4.533
0.1259	1.110	1.114	3.5250	3.900	5.043
0.2677	1.550	1.569			

Solution:

The plot of *y* versus *c* is given in **Figure 11-4*A***, and the plot of log *y* versus log *c* is given in **Figure 11-4*B***. The straight line of Figure 11-4*B* gives

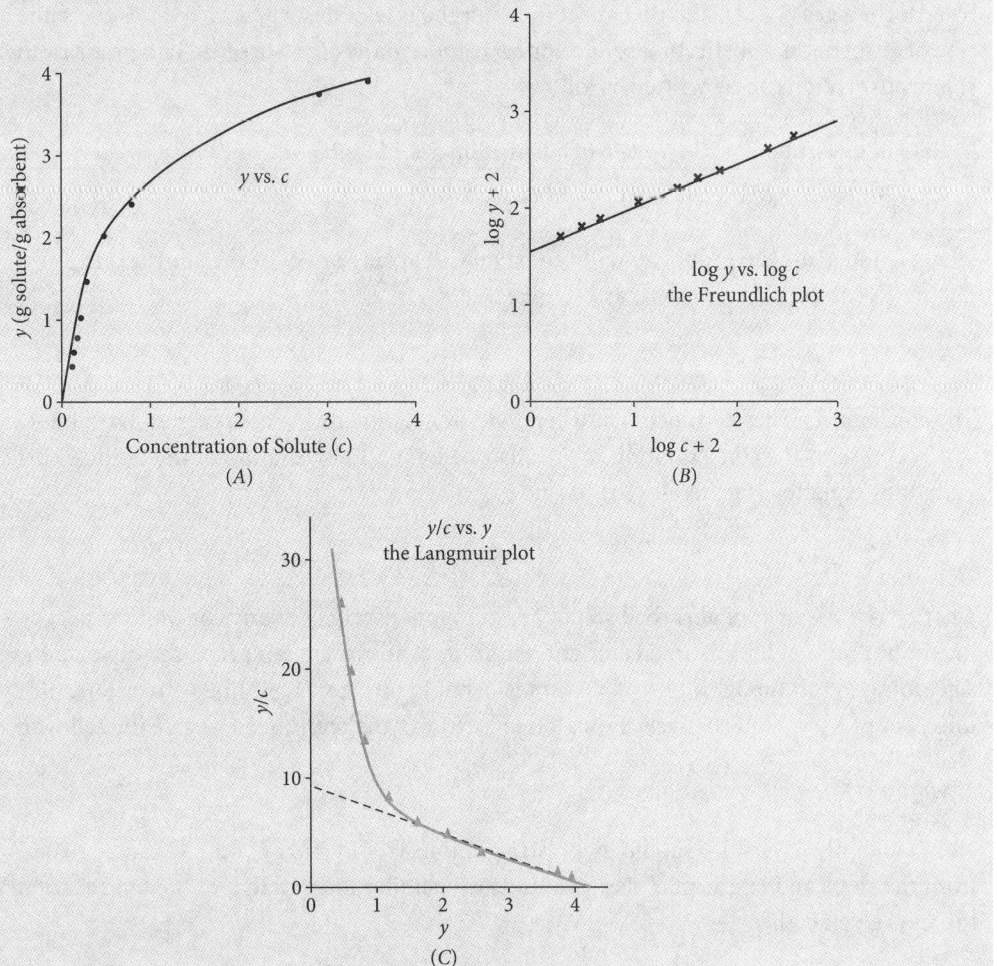

Figure 11-4 Adsorption of acetic acid by activated charcoal at 25°C: (*A*) plot of *y* versus *c*, (*B*) the Freundlich plot (Equation (11-16)), and (*C*) the Langmuir plot (Equation (11-19)).

$k = 2.85 \qquad 1/n = 0.453$

Hence, the isotherm can be expressed as $y = 2.85c^{0.453}$.

The calculated y values (y_{calc}) using the determined constants are obtained and are given in the above table for comparison. As can be seen, at relatively low concentrations, the calculated value corresponds well with the experimental results.

Example 11-4 shows that the Freundlich equation is applicable at relatively low concentrations of the solute. The physical meanings of the constants are not apparently known. The Freundlich equation also does not account for the concentration effect on the possible saturation of the surface sites. As the concentration of the solute increases, the adsorption isotherm usually gradually reaches a plateau similar to that of the *Langmuir isotherm* for gas adsorption. Thus, one can also use the Langmuir equation to study the adsorption of solute onto the particle surface, which is in fact more applicable to isotherm data in the region of near saturation.

It is recalled that the Langmuir model for gas adsorption is based on the theory that the rate of desorption is proportional to the fraction of the surface covered with gas (θ), whereas the rate of adsorption is proportional to the amount of gas present and the fraction of the surface not covered by adsorbed gas ($1 - \theta$), and that at equilibrium the rate of desorption becomes the same as the rate of adsorption. Substituting solute concentration for gas pressure, the Langmuir isotherm for solute adsorption can be written as follows:

Rate of desorption = $k\theta$ rate of adsorption = $k'c(1 - \theta)$

At equilibrium: $k\theta = k'c(1 - \theta)$

where k and k' are the proportionality constants. Rearrangement of the above equation and introducing K_d (desorption constant) as k/k' give

$$k/k' = c(1 - \theta)/\theta = K_d \qquad (11\text{-}17)$$

The constant K_d is defined such that when θ is 50%, K_d equals the concentration of the solute, that is, K_d represents the concentration of the adsorbate for 50% saturation of the particle surface. The Langmuir equation is generally written as

$$c/y = K_d/y_m + c/y_m \qquad (11\text{-}18)$$

where y is the weight of absorbed solute per gram of adsorbent at any concentration c; y_m is the maximum ratio of the adsorbed amount per gram of adsorbent; and K_d is the dissociation constant. According to this model, a plot of c/y versus c should give a straight line with a slope of $1/y_m$ and an intercept of K_d/y_m. Alternatively, Equation (11-18) may be rearranged to give the following form:

$$y/c = y_m/K_d - y/K_d \qquad (11\text{-}19)$$

Now, a plot of y/c versus y should give a straight line, from which y_m and K_d can be determined from the slope and intercept. This equation is in a similar form to that of the binding of drugs to proteins given earlier.

A plot of the data given in Example 11-4 is shown in **Figure 11-4C**. It is seen that at lower solute concentrations, a steep line is obtained, which may indicate the presence of highly active sites on the particle surface. At higher concentrations, the solid surface approaches saturation, and a straight line is obtained that gives $y_m = 4.5$ and a $K_d = 0.592\ M$. Many alkaloids, dyes, fatty acids, etc., are known to be adsorbed from solutions by solids such as activated charcoal, silica gel, and alumina. The adsorption of strychnine, atropine, and quinine on clay from their aqueous solutions has been described using the Langmuir isotherm.

Adsorption Types

The adsorption process in solutions of nonelectrolytes or weak electrolytes may be classified as (1) positive adsorption, in which the solute is adsorbed as a whole molecule; (2) negative adsorption, where instead of the solute, the solvent is being adsorbed; and (3) equal quantity adsorption, in which the solution as a whole is being adsorbed. The adsorption of a solute from a solution is thus a positive adsorption. In strong electrolyte solutions, the adsorption process is complex but includes (1) equal quantity adsorption of both the cation and anion; (2) hydrolytic adsorption that involves strong adsorption of either hydronium or hydroxide ion; and (3) ion exchange adsorption, in which a small amount of a cation or anion is adsorbed through the ion exchange process.

Chromatography

One of the most significant applications of particle adsorption is in liquid chromatography, a method for separating mixed compounds for analytical determinations and/or purification based on adsorption or ion exchange principles. In adsorption chromatography, solid particles may be engineered to exhibit strong affinity toward hydrophilic or hydrophobic compounds. When a solution sample containing a mixture of solutes is applied to a column of such particles (stationary phase), the compounds will be adsorbed onto the particles based on their hydrophobicity. These compounds are then eluted out of the column by means of a solvent (mobile phase) forced through the column. The compounds will be desorbed based on the hydrophobicity of the solvent, relative to that of the particles. As a result, the mixed solutes are separately eluted according to their retention time in the column. When the column is made to withstand high-speed delivery of solvent, the process is known as *high-performance liquid chromatography* (HPLC). Ion exchange columns made using natural and synthetic material are similarly used based on the ion exchange principle for the analysis of ionic species.

The principal factors that influence the adsorption of substances by solid particles are the surface characteristics of the particles, solubility of the solutes, and the pH of the solvent. As mentioned earlier, solid particles may be engineered to exhibit different chemical functionalities. Particles with attached hydrophilic groups, e.g., will have stronger affinity toward more-hydrophilic compounds. When applied in chromatography, the elution of such compounds from the column is made with an organic-based solvent. The process is termed normal-phase chromatography. Conversely, if the particles contain attached long-chain hydrocarbons, they are used to separate compounds based on their hydrophobicity where the mobile phase is an aqueous-based solvent. This is termed the reverse-phase chromatography. In addition to functionality, because the surface area determines the extent of total adsorption, the finer the particle size of the solid adsorbent, the greater the extent of adsorption. In general, the degree of adsorption of a solute is inversely proportional to its solubility in the solvent from which the solute departs. This effect is expected because if adsorption is to occur, the solute–solvent bonding must be broken first. Hence, the greater the solubility, the stronger the solute–solvent attraction and the smaller the extent of adsorption. The pH of the solution affects greatly the adsorption of organic acids and bases by influencing their ionization and aqueous solubility. For particles of strong hydrophobic property, e.g., adsorption will be increased as the ionization of the drug is suppressed and at maximum when the molecules are neutral. In chromatography, separation of compounds is usually achieved by controlling the pH and the composition of the solvent system.

Effect of Adsorption on Drugs

Drug poisoning may be treated by giving orally a mixture of adsorbents of activated charcoal, magnesium oxide (MgO), and tannic acid. Activated charcoal is known to adsorb many drugs such as chlorpheniramine, propoxyphene, diphenylhydantoin, colchicine, and acetylsalicylic acid. In dialysis, the removal of toxic levels of drug from the blood is achieved by transporting blood through a membrane over charcoal and some other active adsorbent. The surface area of the adsorbent is a determining factor in its adsorption capacity of toxic drug concentrations; for oral use, e.g., charcoal tablets are only one-half as effective as the powdered material. Antacids can inadvertently act as adsorbents for drugs taken simultaneously or present in the same formulation.

The adsorption process also occurs in the containers. Drug containers, glass or plastic, are known to adsorb a large quantity of bacteriostatic or fungistatic agents that are added to drug formulations. The process is called sorption, meaning that these molecules can penetrate and have penetrated the wall surface into the plastic matrix. For example, sorbic acid in solution was shown to penetrate plastic container materials including plastic cellulose acetate and cellulose triacetate in a pH-dependent manner. The sorption process was greatly diminished as the pH was increased to values corresponding to complete ionization of the drug. The sorption of local anesthetics by plastic containers, which varied with varying types of plastic materials, also occurred at pH where the drugs were in the neutral form.

The Wetting Phenomena

Wetting of Solid Particles

If the adsorption of pure liquid by solid particle results in the formation of a liquid film over the particle surface, the process is known as *wetting*. Chemically, nonwetting may be due to the failure of the liquid to displace the film of air and/or other substances at the particle surface. Nonwetting is reflected physically by a contact angle (θ) of the liquid at the liquid–solid interface, which ranges from 0° (wetting) to 180° (completely nonwetting, where the particle is in contact with the liquid at one point). Consider a nonwetted particle that floats on top of the water. The water surface at the interface is curved, and the contact angle will be greater than 90°.

As an adsorption process, wetting is accompanied by a change in surface free energy. This surface free energy change can be analyzed based on the wetting process types shown in **Table 11-2**, which include adhesion, spreading, and immersion. The adhesion process involves the loss of surface area of the free solid and free liquid, but a gain in the surface area of the interface. The work required, i.e., the *free adhesion energy* (W_a), is thus equivalent to $\gamma_S + \gamma_L - \gamma_{SL}$. The spreading of a liquid on the solid surface is the next step of the wetting process. This involves the breaking of the cohesive force between the liquid molecules to create new surface area, so that one-half of it

Table 11-2 Surface Free Energy Change Involved in the Wetting Process

Process	Surface Free Energy Change	Work, dyn/cm^2
Adhesion	*Solid/liquid in contact* Lost: $+\gamma_S$; $+\gamma_L$ Gained: $-\gamma_{SL}$	Free adhesion energy (W_a) $W_a = \gamma_S + \gamma_L - \gamma_{SL}$
Spreading	*Liquid on solid surface* Lost: $+\gamma_S$ Gained: $-\gamma_L$; $-\gamma_{SL}$	Spreading coefficient ($S_{L/S}$) $S_{L/S} = \gamma_S - \gamma_{SL} - \gamma_L$
Immersion	*Solid in liquid* Lost: $+\gamma_S$ Gained: $-\gamma_{SL}$	Immersion free energy (F_e) $F_e = \gamma_S - \gamma_{SL}$

will be used for adhesion. The net change in surface area corresponds to a change in surface energy of $-\gamma_L$. The loss of the solid surface area gives a free energy change of $+\gamma_S$, whereas the formation of the solid–liquid interface results in a free energy change of $-\gamma_{SL}$. Thus, the overall work required for this process, which is known as the *spreading coefficient* ($S_{L/S}$), is $\gamma_S - \gamma_{SL} - \gamma_L$. When a solid particle is immersed in the liquid, wetting is complete. The free energy change is known as the immersion free energy (F_e), which corresponds to the loss of the solid surface ($+\gamma_S$) and the formation of a solid–liquid interface ($-\gamma_{SL}$), that is, $F_e = \gamma_S - \gamma_{SL}$.

Accurate measurement of the surface tension of solid–vapor and solid–liquid interfaces is difficult and involves measurements of contact angle and heat of adsorption. But the equations shown in Table 11-2 are quite useful in indicating the requirement for the wetting of solid particles. It should be pointed out first that a positive value of W_a, $S_{L/S}$, and F_e corresponds to a negative change in free energy per change in surface area, and hence indicates a spontaneous occurrence of the process. The term immersion is used to indicate complete wetting. The reasoning is that in order for the wetting to occur, the surface tension at the solid–liquid interface must be lower than the surface tension of the solid, that is, $\gamma_S > \gamma_{SL}$. Because the surface tension of water is, in most cases, considerably higher than that of the organic drugs, wetting is not spontaneous. But, as shall be seen later, surface-active compounds that can significantly lower the surface tension of water at concentrations below their critical micelle concentration can be used as wetting agents. Studies by Zisman[4] have shown that based on contact angle, a critical surface tension γ_c may be determined for various solids that parallels the expected solid–vapor surface tension. It appears to be true for both solid and liquid that the more nonpolar the surface, the lower the surface tension.

Spreading at Liquid–Liquid Interface

Two immiscible liquids form a liquid–liquid interface because (1) the molecules of each liquid are held together by a cohesive force that prevents the liquids from homogeneous mixing and (2) there is an adhesion force between the two liquid phases, manifested by free energy changes. Hence, the surface free energy at the interface can be described as consisting of free cohesion energy and *free adhesion energy*. Consider a drop of an organic liquid (B) such as hexane placed on water (A). Similar to the spread of a liquid on solid, as described earlier, the free adhesion energy or work required to convert the liquid surfaces to a liquid–liquid interface is

$$W_a = \gamma_A + \gamma_B - \gamma_{AB}$$

Because the work of adhesion expressed in surface tension denotes energy per square centimeter, the free cohesion energy should be taken to correspond to work required to destroy 2 cm² of an existing liquid surface. Thus, in order for liquid B to spread on A, the work required to break the cohesion of molecules B ($W_{c,B}$) is

$$W_{c,B} = 2\gamma_B$$

The algebraic combination of the above equations gives the expression of a spreading coefficient for B on A as

$$S_{B/A} = W_a - W_{c,B} = \gamma_A - \gamma_B - \gamma_{AB} \quad (11\text{-}20)$$

The spreading coefficient is a thermodynamic quantity of $-(\partial G/\partial A)_{P,T}$, that is, a change of free energy per change of surface area at constant pressure and temperature. By similar deduction, one can write the spreading coefficient of A on B as

$$S_{A/B} = W_a - W_{c,A} = \gamma_B - \gamma_A - \gamma_{AB} \quad (11\text{-}21)$$

To a first understanding of these equations, it can be said that if the work required to break the cohesion force of the spreading liquid (W_c) is larger than the work gained by spreading (W_a), the liquid will not spread. Thus, a positive value of the spreading coefficient indicates spreading. This is further demonstrated by the relationship $S = -(\partial G/\partial A)_{P,T}$, which shows that spreading is spontaneous if S is positive. The surface tension of liquids and liquid–liquid interfaces can be accurately measured. Water has a high surface tension compared to organic liquids, and the interfacial tension is somewhat less than that of water. This suggests that most organic liquids will spread on water; the lower the value of γ_B, the easier it is for the organic liquid to spread. The reverse, however, is just the opposite: Water will not spread easily on an organic liquid that has a low surface tension, as can be seen from the following calculations involving hexane and water at 20°C:

Hexane on water: $S_{B/A} = \gamma_A - \gamma_B - \gamma_{AB} = 72.8 - 18.0 - 50.8 = 4.0$ dyn/cm

Water on hexane: $S_{A/B} = \gamma_B - \gamma_A - \gamma_{AB} = 18 - 72.8 - 50.8 = -105.6$ dyn/cm

When a liquid is not well spread on another liquid, it appears as a floating drop known as a *lens*. For some liquids, the initial spreading described by the above theory may change with time. The reason is that spreading leads to the formation of a monomolecular film and a reduction of surface tension from the value for pure liquid to some lower value. When sufficient reduction of the surface tension occurs, the spreading coefficient may thus become negative. This is quite likely for the hexane–water system, which has an initial spreading coefficient of only 4.0 dyn/cm. The reversal of spreading can result in the formation or reformation of a lens.

III. Surface-Active Agents

The surface tension of water is quite sensitive to the presence of a solute. In a water–ethanol system, where the difference in surface tension between the two liquids is large, the surface tension of the solution drops rapidly from that of pure water (72.75 dyn/cm; 20°C) over the first 15% of ethanol added and then slowly approaches the value for pure ethanol (22.75 dyn/cm; 20°C). This type of behavior becomes accentuated in the case of a long-chain solute having a polar end group: sodium lauryl sulfate. There is a sharp drop in γ even for very dilute solutions. As shown by the Gibbs adsorption equation, the thermodynamic implication is that such compounds concentrate at the air–liquid interface. With sodium lauryl sulfate, there is nearly a complete monolayer by 0.01 *M* concentration. In contrast, an electrolyte solution of sodium chloride shows a linear increase in γ with increasing concentration of the salt,[5] where the thermodynamic implication is that the surface region is more dilute in electrolyte than the bulk solution, or that negative adsorption occurs at the interface. These long-chain molecules with a polar end group are called *surface-active agents* or *surfactants*.

Chemical Properties

Surfactants are amphiphiles, meaning that they have affinity for both polar and nonpolar solvents. They may be considerably more hydrophilic than lipophilic or vice versa, or have a balanced hydro- and lipophilicity depending on the nature of the polar and nonpolar groups within the molecular structure. The makeup of a lipophilic, or hydrophobic, moiety usually consists of a long-chain alkyl or aryl group. It is the hydrophilic group that varies with different types of surfactants. Hence, it is convenient to classify these compounds based on their hydrophilic moieties. As will be shown later, surfactants are also being categorized based on their relative polarity so that their structural features and surface properties can be identified for different pharmaceutical applications. The polar group of most surface-active agents may be classified as anionic, cationic, amphoteric, and non-ionic. The last group makes up the bulk of the surfactants used in pharmaceutical preparations.

Anionic Surfactants

The anionic surfactants are long-chain molecules of carboxylates, sulfates, or sulfonates. The carboxylates, or soaps, are generally prepared by saponification of natural fatty acid glycerides in alkaline solution, with chain length in the range of 12 to 18 carbons. The cations associated with soaps are sodium, potassium, ammonium, and triethanolamine. The degree of water solubility depends on the chain length and the presence of double bonds. Sodium oleate (18 carbons, double bond), e.g., is quite soluble, compared to sodium stearate (18 carbons), in water at room temperature. Multivalent ions such as Ca^{2+} and Mg^{2+} markedly reduce the compound's aqueous solubility even at low alkyl chain length, making the soaps not very useful in hard water that contains high contents of these ions. Hydrolysis of soap leads to the formation of free acid and hydroxide ions.

Among the alkyl sulfates ($R—OSO_3^-$), the most noted member is sodium lauryl (12 carbons) sulfate, which is widely used as an emulsifier and a solubilizing agent in pharmaceutical preparations. The sulfates are also susceptible to hydrolysis, leading to the formation of the long-chain alcohol. Control of pH is thus essential when one is working with the sulfates. In comparison, some alkyl and alkyl aryl sulfonates ($R—SO_3^-$) have been shown to be less susceptible to hydrolysis, or to precipitation by association with Ca^{2+} or Mg^{2+}. The dialkyl sodium sulfosuccinates are known to be both oil- and water-soluble and form micelles in both phases. Sodium 1,4-bis(2-ethylhexyl) sulfosuccinate, in particular, known as Aerosol OT, has been shown to reduce surface tension to extremely low values and acts as an excellent wetting agent in many types of solid dosage forms.

Cationic Agents

Long-chain cations including amines and quaternary ammonium salts are surface-active in part due to their interactions with negatively charged surfaces such as cell membranes. In general, they are cytotoxic,[6] and the most noted use in pharmaceutical preparations is as antimicrobial preservatives. Benzalkonium hydrochloride, e.g., is an important preservative in the preparation of ophthalmic and nasal solutions. It is adsorbed readily at the cell membrane structure in a nonspecific manner, leading to cell lysis. The quaternary ammonium salt is stable over the entire pH range of the solution, but is incompatible with the presence of anionic agents or drugs. Because of their affinity to cell membrane, cationic surfactants have been used in liposome preparations as a vector for intracellular delivery of therapeutic agents.

Amphoteric Surfactants

These compounds include most of the naturally occurring surfactants in the biological system. They are zwitterions containing either the amino-carboxylic acid or the phosphate-quaternary ammonium salt acid–base conjugations. The former are polypeptides, proteins, and alkyl betaines (such as β-alanine trimethylbetaine: $(CH_3)_3N^+CH_2CH_2COO^-$) whereas the latter group consists of phospholipids such as lecithins and cephalins. They are more surface-active than ionic surfactants having the same group because in effect the oppositely charged ions are neutralized. Phospholipids, which constitute the structure base of cell membranes, form colloidal systems that have been extensively studied for potential use as drug delivery systems.[7] In oral drug absorption, it is recalled that these substances have a strong effect on the in vivo solubility, dissolution, and absorption of water-insoluble drugs.

Non-ionic Surfactants

The list of such compounds is rather long, but basically they contain a small alcohol base such as propylene glycol, sorbitan, or glycerol, to which fatty acids are attached to form the fatty acid esters. In the case of glycerol, mono-, di-, and triglycerides can be formed. Also included in this group of compounds are the fatty alcohols of different chain lengths (lauryl, 12; cetyl, 16; stearyl, 18 carbons; etc.), steroidal alcohols, and cholesterol. The aqueous solubility of these compounds is rather low, which limits the surfactant action at the aqueous interface. For this reason, polyoxy groups, in the form of —$[OCH_2CH_2]_n$— are added through an ether linkage with one of the alcohol groups to enhance solubility. The longer the polyoxy chain, the higher will be the solubility. For internal as well as external applications, the most widely used surfactants are the polyoxyethylene sorbitan fatty acid esters. Closely related are polyoxyethylene glyceryl esters, as well as the comparable polyoxypropylene esters. Polyoxyethylene derivatives of fatty alcohol, such as polyoxyethylene-stearyl ether, have also been made to take advantage of the fact that, unlike the esters, the ethers are quite resistant to acid- and base-catalyzed hydrolysis.

Micelle Formation

The ionic surfactants have been called colloidal electrolytes. Among these, sodium dodecyl sulfate (SDS) has been well studied. In very dilute solution, SDS behaves much as any other uni-univalent electrolyte in terms of colligative and ionic properties. The freezing point depression of SDS, for example, increases linearly with concentration until a "critical concentration" is reached, above which the property of the solution sharply deviates from that of normal electrolytes. This change in thermodynamic properties is paralleled by changes in other physicochemical properties such as the equivalent electrical conductivity. The formation of particles, which are called micelles, becomes apparent at concentrations above this critical concentration. The phenomenon is rather unique in that at concentrations below the critical concentration, although some dimeric complex may be present, the existence of a whole spectrum of particle sizes is not indicated by any available evidence. The fact that the micelles are formed in a rather dramatic sharpness has led to the suggestion that the aggregation of the colloidal electrolytes may represent the appearance of a new phase, which the added colloidal molecules prefer. This is the reason why colloidal electrolytes decrease the surface tension of water very powerfully at very low concentrations, where the interface is a preferred environment for the colloidal electrolytes. As soon as micelles form, however, they provide an alternative favorable environment. Thus, beyond the critical concentration, to which the term critical micelle concentration (CMC) is now given, the surface tension is almost independent of the concentration of the colloidal electrolyte. The concept of a new phase is of interest. If the CMC is regarded as a saturated phase at which the micelles form, then the heat of micelle formation may be written as

$$[\partial(\text{CMC})/\partial T]_P = \Delta H_T^\circ/RT^2$$

An example of the formation of micelles by the potassium salt of fatty acids and the effect of micelle formation on drug solubility are illustrated in Example 11-5.

Example 11-5: The solubility of dimethylaminoazobenzene (mol wt = 225) in some soap solutions at 20°C is determined as follows:

Concentration of Soap, *M*	**0.05**	**0.10**	**0.15**	**0.20**	**0.30**
Solubility of drug, mg/L in					
Potassium decanoate	1	1.5	30	64	120
Potassium dodecanoate	40	110	150	255	350
Potassium tetradecanoate	125	255	350	510	

Determine the critical micelle concentration, and describe the relationship of solubility with the concentration and alkyl chain length of the surfactants.

Solution:

The CMC may be graphically determined by a plot of solubility versus the concentration of the surfactant. The plot for potassium decanoate (10 carbons) shows two distinct straight lines, from which the CMC is found to be about 0.1 *M*.

The plots for potassium dodecanoate (12 carbons) and tetradecanoate (14 carbons) show single straight lines, indicating that CMC diminishes as the chain length increases.

The data also show that for each soap system at concentrations above CMC, the drug solubility increases linearly with increasing micelle concentration. When the solubilities are converted to molar scale, the amounts of dissolved drug per mole of surfactant were determined as 2.8, 5.2, and 9.0 mmol for decanoate, dodecanoate, and tetradecanoate systems, respectively.

It has been suggested that there is a roughly approximate relationship between micelle solubility and the alkyl chain length of the surfactants in that the solubility is proportional to the cube of the chain length. For the decanoate, dodecanoate, and tetradecanoate, the ratio of $(\text{chain length})^3$ is 3.2 : 5.6 : 9.0, which is fairly in line with the measured solubility data.

Hydrophilic–Lipophilic Balance (HLB)

HLB Designation

It is somewhat difficult to differentiate the surfactants based on solely their surface activity and the usefulness of such activity for a particular pharmaceutical application. A mere determination of surface tension does not take into account the overall compatibility of the surfactant in a system. For example, in making an emulsion, the phase in which the surfactant is most soluble will form the continuous phase; thus depending on the type of emulsion to be prepared, different criteria regarding the selection of surfactant will be needed. The most widely used system for classification of surfactants has been the *hydrophilic–lipophilic balance* (HLB) system, originally conceived for non-ionic surfactants. In this system, each surfactant is assigned a number, which represents the percentage weight of the hydrophilic (polyoxyethylene) group divided by 5 in order to limit the range from 0 to 20. Thus, for a 100% hydrophilic molecule, as in polyethylene glycol, the HLB value would be 20. An increase in the polyoxy chain results in an increase in hydrophilicity and hence the HLB value. The advantage of this system is that, to a first approximation, one can compare surfactants having different polar and nonpolar groups and gain an appreciation of their aqueous or nonaqueous solubility. The HLB values are also algebraically additive, so that when a blend of surfactants is needed to obtain a particular HLB value, it can be calculated from the weighted mean of the surfactant mixture. Some commonly used surfactants with their HLB values are shown in **Table 11-3**. The HLB values for surfactants other than the non-ionics have been determined by comparison of their physical chemical properties that reflect the molecular polarity with the surfactants having known HLB values. These properties include aqueous solubility, interfacial tension, and dielectric constant. Surfactants exhibiting values greater than 20, such as sodium lauryl sulfate (HLB = 40), are deemed to have greater hydrophilic behavior than that of the polyoxyethylene groups alone.

Table 11-3 HLB Values of Frequently Used Pharmaceutical Surfactants

Surfactant	Trademark	HLB	Use
Sorbitan trioleate	Span 85	1.8	Antifoaming agents (HLB: 1–3)
Sorbitan tristearate	Span 65	2.1	
Glyceryl monostearate		3.8	
Sorbitan monooleate	Span 80	4.3	W/O emulsifiers (HLB: 4–6)
Sorbitan monostearate	Span 60	4.7	
Sorbitan monopalmitate	Span 40	6.7	
Sorbitan monolaurate	Span 20	8.6	Wetting agents (HLB: 7–9)
Polyoxyethylene lauryl ether	Brij 30	9.6	
Polyoxyethylene sorbitan monooleate	Tween 81	10.0	O/W emulsifiers (HLB: 8–18)
Polyoxyethylene sorbitan tristearate	Tween 65	10.5	
Polyoxyethylene monooleate		11.4	
Polyoxyethylene monostearate		11.6	
Triethanolamine oleate		12.0	
Polyoxyethylene sorbitan monolaurate	Tween 21	13.3	Detergents (HLB: 13–15)
Polyoxyethylene sorbitan monostearate	Tween 60	14.9	
Polyoxyethylene sorbitan monooleate	Tween 80	15.0	
Polyoxyethylene sorbitan monopalmitate	Tween 40	15.6	Solubilizing agents (HLB: 15–18)
Polyoxyethylene sorbitan monolaurate	Tween 20	16.7	
Sodium oleate		18.0	
Sodium lauryl sulfate		40.0	

Pharmaceutical Applications

Surfactants are mainly used as wetting, emulsifying, and solubilizing agents. It was largely due to the experimental work by Griffin[8, 9] that the HLB system was linked to these applications. There is perhaps a required HLB value for a given application. If an oil-in-water (O/W) emulsion is desired, the formulator should use emulsifiers with an HLB in the range of 8–18. In contrast, emulsifiers with HLB values in the range of 3–6 would be desirable for the preparation of water-in-oil (W/O) emulsions. This is in keeping with the fact that for a stable emulsion, the emulsifier must be more soluble in the continuous phase than in the dispersed phase. The concept of a required HLB also stems from the fact that the polarity of the dispersed phase must be considered, because the relative affinity of the surfactant toward the two phases varies with varying materials. For the preparation of O/W emulsion of cottonseed oil, heavy mineral oil, or stearic acid, e.g., the required HLB was shown to be 7.5, 10.5, or 17, respectively. Here, it is seen that the extremely insoluble stearic acid is properly emulsified only with highly hydrophilic surfactants.

The general guideline for the selection of surfactant for pharmaceutical use based on the HLB value is given in Table 11-3. It is apparent that a high HLB value (15–18) is needed for use as a solubilizing agent. As shown earlier, at concentrations above the CMC, the solubility of water-insoluble drugs increases linearly with the surfactant concentration. Micelle may be regarded as a solvent in solvent for organic solutes.[3] Just as the dissolving of more sugar may be achieved by adding more water, the dissolved amount of organic molecules can be increased by adding more colloidal electrolyte that forms the micelles. Wetting of solid particles is a complex phenomenon that involves a reduction of the surface tension of the solvent (water) and interaction of the surfactant at the solid–liquid interface. There is a critical surface tension for a given solid surface, and particles are wetted if the liquid surface tension is reduced to below the critical surface tension. The interaction of surfactant at the solid surface can increase the critical surface tension by making the solid more polar or decrease the critical surface tension by making the surface more nonpolar. The latter occurs if the adsorbed surfactant has its nonpolar group oriented toward the aqueous phase. These facts suggest that the surfactant used should be effective in reducing the surface tension of water at concentrations below the CMC, but with sufficiently high HLB to ensure a relatively polar solid surface. An HLB range of 7–9 has been recommended for wetting agents.

IV. Electrokinetic Phenomena

Electrokinetic phenomena play a dominant role in the stability of suspension and colloidal systems. Although the pharmaceutical systems are presented later, the theory on treating the surface properties of charged particles is presented here, so that a comprehensive view of the interfacial phenomena pertaining to the interfaces and solution components is achieved. Several interesting phenomena may occur if there is relative motion between a charged surface and an electrolyte solution; these are called *electrokinetic effects*. The surface is either that of a solid particle suspended in solution or the solid wall of tube down which the solution flows. What happens is essentially that a charged surface experiences a force in an electric field or that a field is induced by the motion of such a surface in the solution. Thus, if a field is applied to the suspended particles, they will move; or, alternatively, if a solution is made to flow down a tube, an electric field develops. In each case there is a *plane of shear* between the surface and the solution, which lies within the *electrical double layer*. The potential at this plane is lower than that of the surface, and it is called the *zeta potential* ζ. There are four types of electrokinetic effects, depending on whether the solid surface stays stationary or moves and whether the field is applied or induced. Under an applied field, suspended particles move; this process is called electrophoresis. Motion of particles in a centrifugal field, in contrast, induces a sedimentation potential. If the solid surface is that of a wall of a tube, a flow of solution, or electroosmosis, occurs upon application of a potential gradient. Conversely, a forced flow of solution induces a potential gradient known as the streaming potential. We will consider mainly the electrophoretic property as it relates to zeta potential and how charged particles respond to electrolyte solutions.

Surface Charge and Electrical Double Layer

Origin of Charges

There are several reasons why a particle surface is charged. The presence of acidic and basic groups on the particle surface is one that would bring positive or negative charges to surface through ionization. Soaps and some other lyophilic (solvent-loving) colloids carry negative charges in the form of ionic micelles. In the case of proteins, the number and sign of the surface charge will depend on whether the solution is acidic or basic and the protein's isoelectric point. Colloidal particles can also acquire charged surface through preferential adsorption of ions in solution. Inorganic colloids, such as AgCl, a lyophobic (solvent-hating) system, can become negatively charged by preferential adsorption of Cl^- over Ag^+. Particles, such as those of cellulose, that do not carry charges by themselves can become negatively charged in an aqueous medium, due to the adsorption of hydroxide ions, which exhibit greater capillary activity than does the hydronium ion. The nature of the net charges on the colloidal particles is clearly important in processes regarding the tendency of the colloidal particles to come together, or flocculate, as these processes must overcome the electrostatic repulsion between the particles.

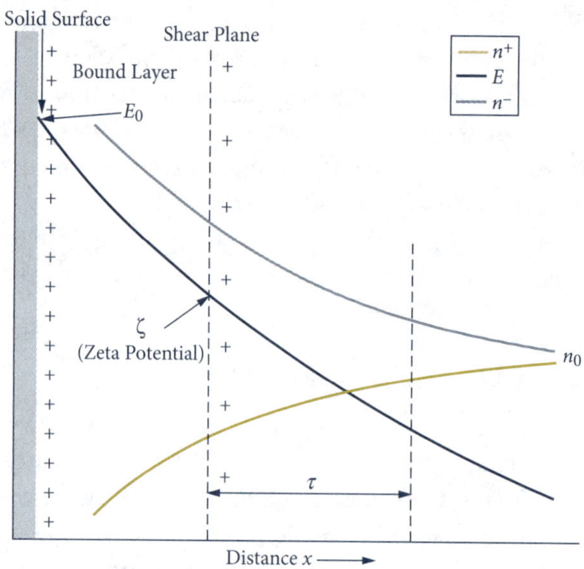

Figure 11-5 The diffuse double layer showing the plane of shear, zeta potential, diffuse layer, and potential and ionic concentration changes.

The Diffuse Double Layer

The effective charge of a particle in an electrokinetic effect is the fixed charge, which is made up of the actual charge of the particle and the ionic charges that are held sufficiently close to the particle that they will remain with the particle as it moves through the solution. This phenomenon is best understood by recognizing that a layer of water molecules is probably very tightly bound to the particle surface, because all ions, to a greater or lesser degree, are hydrated. Because the system as a whole must maintain electrical neutrality, the opposite charge to that of the fixed charge will tend to surround the colloidal particle and form a diffuse layer, which will move with the solution rather than the particle. This situation is illustrated schematically in **Figure 11-5**. Consider a particle with positive surface charge in a uni-univalent electrolyte solution with a concentration of n_o. The particle surface and the bound layer will be positively charged. The neighboring solution will be counterbalanced by the higher concentration of the anion (n^-) and lower concentration of the cation (n^+) of the electrolyte, both of which, however, will change as a function of distance into the solution until n^+ and n^- are equal (to n_o). The particle has a surface charge of σ_o and a corresponding potential E_0, which is generally called the Nernst potential. At the plane of shear, i.e., the boundary of the bound layer, the surface charge is reduced to σ_s, and the corresponding potential is now known as ζ, the zeta, or electrokinetic, potential. The presence of the counterions (or *gegenions*) is diffuse. The physical picture is that at a solution plane further away from the shear plane, the net excess of negative charge is equivalent to the positive charge on the particle surface. This plane is regarded as the electrical "center of gravity" of charge in the solution and, as described by the Debye–Hückel theory, the boundary of the ionic atmosphere. This second layer is the diffuse layer. The ionic atmosphere constitutes the diffuse double layer.

The change in electric potential as a function of distance from the surface can be derived based on the *Poisson theorem* that the rate of change of electrostatic potential at a given point is proportional to the charge density at that point. With this notation, it can be shown that

$$E = E_0 e^{-\kappa x} \tag{11-22}$$

where E is the potential at a solution plane having a distance x from the surface, E_0 is the surface potential, and κ is known as the Debye–Hückel constant. This equation indicates that the potential decays exponentially with distance into the solution. When E drops to $1/e$ of E_0, the distance between the plane and the surface is $1/\kappa$. Now it is appropriate to look at the significance of κ. The Debye–Hückel constant is given as

$$\kappa^2 = 8\pi\mu e^2 N/DRT \tag{11-23}$$

where μ is the ionic strength of the solution, e is the charge of the electron, N is the Avogadro number, R is the gas constant, and D is the dielectric constant of water at constant temperature T. The reciprocal of κ is a distance that defines the boundary of the diffuse double layer. If one imagines a spherical surface on which the charge is $+ze$, then there will be a double layer of solution surrounding the particle where the outer edge will have a net excess charge (from the counterions) of $-ze$ and be located at a distance of $1/\kappa$ from the particle surface. The quantity of this distance can be easily calculated using the simplified equation for aqueous medium at 25°C:

$$d = 1/\kappa = 3.05 \times 10^{-8}/\mu^{1/2} \quad \text{cm} \tag{11-24}$$

There is an immediate application of this equation to the dependency of the diffuse double layer on electrolyte concentration. As can be seen, at 0.001 M of a uni-univalent electrolyte and 25°C, d is calculated to be 96.4 Å; when the concentration is increased to 0.01 M, d = 30.5 Å. When d decreases, it reduces the repulsive force between particles, thus allowing them increased possibility to come together. Any change in d also reflects a change in the zeta potential, which is discussed next.

Electrophoretic Property

An electrokinetic experiment may be set up with a potential gradient in a solution containing charged particles. The motion of the particles will depend on the strength of the field (F), the zeta potential of the particles, and the viscous drag of the electrolyte solution. This can be done even though the size, surface charge, molecular weight if it is a macromolecule, and diffusion rate of the particles are all unknown. From the preceding discussion, it can be deduced that the "center of gravity" of the diffuse double layer is at the point where E has dropped to $1/e$ of ζ at a distance τ from the plane of shear. Hence, as a first approximation, the charge per surface area (σ_s) at the plane of shear can be written as

$$\sigma_s = D\zeta/4\pi\tau$$

The balance of force regarding the motion of the particles involves the electrical force per area of the particle, which is $\sigma_s F$, and the viscous drag per unit area, which is $\eta v/\tau$, where η (eta) is the viscosity and v is the velocity of the particle motion. Thus,

$$v = \sigma_s F\tau/\eta = \zeta DF/4\pi\eta \tag{11-25}$$

Here the velocity is directly related to the zeta potential and the strength of the electric field. If F is measured in volts per centimeter, v is measured in micrometers per second, ζ is expressed in millivolts, then, using known values of D and η for water at 25°C, one obtains the following equation:

$$\zeta = 12.9v/F \tag{11-26}$$

Thus, if a colloidal particle moves 70 μm/s in a field of 10 V/cm, its zeta potential is 90.3 mV. The sign of the zeta potential may be positive or negative depending on the direction of motion relative to the field. The instrument for electrophoretic measurement is called a zetameter.

Most measured zeta potentials are in the range of ±100 mV for lyophobic colloids. The actual values depend on the nature and concentration of the electrolytes and may reverse sign as the

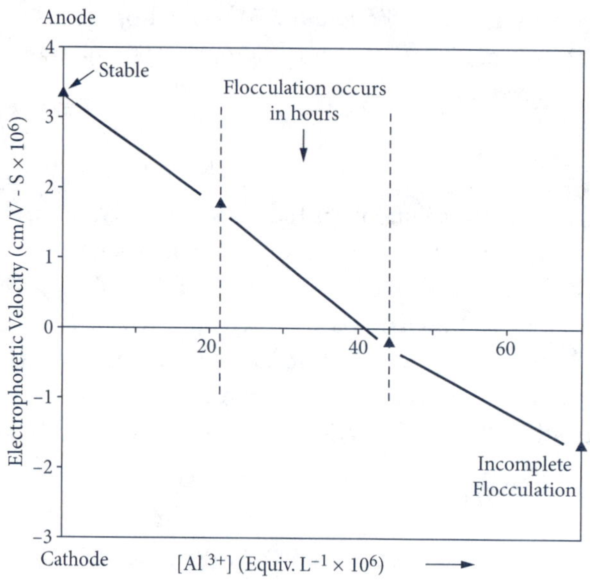

Figure 11-6 Flocculation of gold sol.

concentration of the electrolyte increases. A typical zeta potential–concentration curve is given in **Figure 11-6**. It is seen that at low electrolyte concentration, the electrostatic repulsion is strong and the charged colloidal particle is quite stable. A decrease in zeta potential induces flocculation. At high concentration of the electrolyte, the charge is reversed and the zeta potential is again established, which reduces flocculation.

V. Chapter Summary

The principles of surface chemistry reveal that certain types of molecules prefer the interfacial environment over the bulk solution and, in doing so, render the interfaces more stable by reducing the surface free energy associated with the creation of new surfaces. Despite the passage of time, the classical theories on surface tension, such as those of Laplace, Kelvin, Gibbs, and Young and Dupré (on contact angle), remain the defining concepts for the understanding of interfacial phenomena, and have led to the discovery of surfactants of diverse structural and molecular properties. The interfacial phenomena are by no means fully understood. New phenomena regarding the adsorption and wetting processes continue to surface as the behavior of molecules at the interface is more clearly presented. The spreading of a droplet of surfactant solution over a hydrophobic surface, e.g., is now described as involving the surfactant molecule at the front of the advancing liquid, whose "mission" is to seek out the solid surface and make it more hydrophilic (by increasing its critical surface tension), thus rendering the surface wettable. Such a time-dependent wetting process has been confirmed by theoretical consideration and experimental results.[10,11] In contrast, a surface may be amphiphilic as in some polymeric material or made so by incorporating a surface-active agent. The wetting of such a surface by a polar liquid droplet now involves a rearrangement or overturning of the surface molecular layer so that the hydrophilic moiety is pointing to the advancing liquid front.[12] In adsorption studies, surfactant effects on surface tension both below and above CMC values are being closely studied.[13,14] Some data have shown molecular behaviors that deviate from the Gibbs absorption, indicating that there are yet undefined molecular behaviors at the interface.

More types of particles are being introduced for potential pharmaceutical use and studied via interfacial interactions. The forces acting between particles of colloids and others involve undoubtedly basic types including London–van der Waals, solvation, hydrophobic, and electrostatic forces. Of these, the electric property as defined by the diffuse double layer remains a dominant force in colloidal particle interaction. This concept forms the base through which the effects of surfactants and electrolyte solutions on the colloidal system are being characterized. Pharmacists will likely be involved or see new products developed based on the interfacial sciences. Thus, an understanding of the basic theories is necessary for those entering the field. It is for this reason that this chapter is arranged and written.

VI. References

1. Adamson AW. *Physical Chemistry of Surfaces*. New York, Wiley (Interscience), 1967, 2nd ed.
2. Harkins WD and Jordan HF. *J Am Chem Soc*. 52:1751, 1930.
3. McBain JW and Swain RC. *Proc Royal Soc*. A154:608, 1936.
4. Zisman WA. *Adv Chem Ser*. 43:1, 1964.
5. Evans HB Jr. and Clever HL. *J Phys Chem*. 68:3433, 1964.
6. Wang LY, Ma JKH, Pan WF, Toledo-Velasque D, Malanga CJ, and Rojanasakul Y. *Pharm Res*. 11:513–517, 1994.
7. Liao WP, DeHaven J, Shao J, et al. *Drug Delivery*. 5:111–118, 1998.
8. Griffin WC. *J Soc Cos Chem*. 1:311, 1949.
9. Griffin WC. *J Soc Cos Chem*. 5:249, 1954.
10. Starov VM, Kosvintsev SR, and Velarde MG. *J Colloid Interface Sci*. 227:185, 2000.
11. Zhdanov S, Starov V, Sobolev V, and Velarde M. *J Colloid Interface Sci*. 264:481–489, 2003.
12. Starov VM. *Adv Colloid Interface Sci*. 111:3–27, 2004.
13. Menger FM, Shi L, and Rizvi SA. *J Am Chem Soc*. 131:10380–10381, 2009.
14. Svitova TF, Wetherbee MJ, and Radke CJ. *J Colloid Interface Sci*. 26:170–179, 2003.

VII. Homework Problems

1. The surface tension of a soap solution is 6 dyn/cm. What is the value of ΔP for a soap bubble (with a radius of 2 cm) blown with this solution? (1 atm = 1.01325 dyn/cm².)
2. A sample of dichloromethane (density = 1.326 g/mL) was found to give a capillary rise of 3.85 cm in a capillary having an inner radius of 0.01 cm. What is the surface tension of this liquid?
3. The ideal weight of a drop of benzene formed at the dropping tip having a 3-mm diameter is 27.9 mg. What is the surface tension of benzene at 20°C?
4. The surface tension of an aqueous solution varied with concentration according to the equation $\gamma = 72 - 500C$, provided that C is less than 0.05 *M*. What is the surface excess of the solute at a concentration of 0.02 *M* at 25°C? ($R = 8.3143 \times 10^7$ erg/K-mol.)
5. Consider an immiscible system containing hexane and water. If a powder sample of (*a*) $BaSO_4$, (*b*) PbO, or (*c*) charcoal is added to the system, to what phase will the powder be dispersed? The solids are not soluble in either hexane or water. The surface tension data show the following:

   $BaSO_4$: $\gamma_{HS} \geq \gamma_{WS} + \gamma_{WH}$
   Charcoal: $\gamma_{WS} \geq \gamma_{WH} + \gamma_{HS}$
   PbO: $\gamma_{WH} > \gamma_{WS} - \gamma_{HS}$

   Interfaces: HS: hexane–solid; WS: water–solid; WH: water–hexane.
6. The surface tension and interfacial tension against water at 20°C for a number of liquids are shown in **Table 11-4.**

Table 11-4 The Surface Tension and Interfacial Tension against Water at 20°C for Some Common Liquids

Compounds	Surface Tension, dyn/cm	Interfacial Tension, dyn/cm
Water	72.7	—
Decane	23.9	52.3
Octane	21.8	51.7
Oleic acid	32.5	15.6
Mercury	476	428

(*a*) Which organic liquids would not spread on water? (*b*) Would water spread on mercury?

7. The following results were obtained for the freezing point depression of aqueous solution of sodium octyl sulfate:

ΔT_f, °C	0.3410	0.4071	0.4804	0.5446	0.5437	0.5462	0.5724	0.5462
Molality	0.1000	0.1200	0.1400	0.1600	0.1700	0.1800	0.2000	0.2400

Calculate the osmotic coefficient of the water ($= \Delta T_{f,\text{exp}}/\Delta T_{f,\text{calc}}$) in these solutions, and from these values determine the critical micelle concentration.

8. In order to have a blend of surfactants to give an HLB of 10.5, what must be the weight percentages for the following pairs of surfactants? Span 60 and Tween 60; Span 40 and Tween 40; Span 65 and Tween 60.

9. Calculate the thickness (d) of the diffuse double layer of a charged particle in (*a*) 0.005 *M* NaCl and (*b*) 0.005 *M* $CaCl_2$ solutions at 25°C.

10. What would be the velocity of a colloidal particle of silver iodide, with radius 10^{-5} cm, in water at 25°C in a potential gradient of 10 V/cm, if its zeta potential is 25 mV?

11. If a particle surface has a potential (E) of 50.6 mV in an 0.01 *M* NaCl solution at 25°C, what are the concentrations of Na^+ and Cl^- at the particle surface?

    Information needed to solve the problem: The distribution of ions as a function of potential gradient is

    $$n^+ = n_o e^{-eE/kT} \quad \text{and} \quad n^- = n_o e^{eE/kT}$$

    1 eV is 1.6021×10^{-12} erg, or 1 e(mV) is 1.6021×10^{-15} erg; and kT at 25°C = 1.35805×10^{-16} (erg/deg) × 298.16 deg = 4.05×10^{-14} erg. Thus, when $E = 25.3$ mV, $eE = kT$ at 25°C.

12. Referring to Problem 11, calculate (*a*) the thickness of the diffuse double layer, (*b*) the potential, and (*c*) Na^+ and Cl^- concentrations at the boundary of the diffuse double layer.

13. A silica particle with a radius of 1×10^{-4} cm shows an electrophoretic velocity of 2.5×10^{-3} cm/s at 25°C under a potential gradient of 10.0 V/cm. Calculate the zeta potential of the particle in this medium. Assuming Stokes' law for the viscous drag, what total charge does the particle carry?

    Information needed: If the particle, including its bound layer, has a net charge σ, the terminal velocity under the field strength F will be $v = \sigma F/6\pi r\eta$, if Stokes' law holds. The viscosity of the solution can be taken as 0.01 P (dyn-s/cm^2).

CHAPTER 12

Rheology in Pharmacy

There are some very interesting phenomena regarding the flow of matter. A funnel filled with honey will drop steadily, making a drop-type device a good dispensing system, but the same cannot be said with a funnel full of mayonnaise, for which a scooping method is by far most effective. On display at the University of Queensland in Brisbane, Australia, for over 80 years now, is a funnel full of well-packed molten pitch. The drop rate has been observed to be about one drop every 9.5 years. Then there is Silly Putty (polydimethylsiloxane). At rest, it stays as a lump; when forced by nature and time, it flows to a puddle; when rolled into a ball and bounced, it is an elastic solid; yet when stretched rapidly, it breaks cleanly as a piece of plastic.

The rheological behavior of a material, stemming from its viscoelastic properties, determines how the material should be used. Such behavior is also the result of an internal structure that changes according to applied stress. It is thus possible to change the rheology of a system by taking advantage of certain material that has, or is able to provide, the desired rheological behavior. Rheology is the science of flow and deformation of matter. It extends widely into pharmaceutical preparations ranging from the flow of powders from hoppers to die cavities in tableting to the formulation of stable suspensions, emulsions, colloidal systems, and semisolid products. This chapter describes the theories and application of rheology and includes a section on topical dosage forms.

CHAPTER OUTLINE

OBJECTIVES

1. Understand viscosity as a defining parameter for the flow of liquids.
2. Define elasticity, strain, and elastic modulus.
3. Describe the flow curves; the relationships among stress (τ), rate of shear ($\dot{g}$), and viscosity (η); and the differences in Newtonian and non-Newtonian flows.
4. Describe the effect of temperature on viscosity.
5. Understand all terminologies and processes regarding non-Newtonian systems and their general properties, including plastic, pseudoplastic, thixotropic, and antithixotropic flows; yield stress (τ_y); and zero-shear viscosity (η_0).
6. Understand the term viscoelasticity and its expression via storage (G') and loss moduli (G''), and the phase angle (δ).

(Continues)

(*Continued*)

7. Be familiar with various types of rheological measurements.
8. Discuss and be able to determine how G', G'', $\tan\delta$, η_0, and the linear viscoelastic region (LVR) can be used to formulate stable pharmaceutical suspensions.
9. Understand the concept and mechanisms of topical drug delivery.
10. Discuss the type, preparation, and use of topical pharmaceutical systems in liquid and semisolid dosage forms.

I. Rheological Properties—An Overview

Rheological Behavior and Terminology

Viscosity

Rheology is the science of the flow and deformation of matter, one that is concerned with the mechanics of deformable bodies, primarily those that are describable as liquids, solids, and in-betweens. Consider first the flow property of a liquid. If a liquid is flowing between parallel walls, one ordinarily observes that the material immediately adjacent to the walls is stationary, while the material farther away toward the center of the flowing body moves increasingly rapidly. This is due to the fact that there is a frictional force between moving liquid layers. If the difference in velocity between two liquid layers is dv and the distance between them is dx (see **Figure 12-1**), then the frictional force (f) will be proportional to dv/dx times the area of the moving layer (A), as shown in the following equation:

$$f = \eta A\, dv/dx \qquad \text{or} \qquad f/A = \eta\, dv/dx \tag{12-1}$$

In a forced flow, f/A is the *shear stress* applied to the liquid, and dv/dx is the rate of shear. The proportionality constant η is called the coefficient of viscosity. It is called a coefficient because under a forced flow, as we shall see later, the *viscosity* of some systems will not be a constant. Equation (12-1) is the defining equation for viscosity, known as *Newton's law of viscosity*.[1] It follows that we define a Newtonian fluid as a system whose viscosity coefficient is a constant, independent of the value of dv/dx, that is, independent of shear.

Elasticity

A solid material may be deformed by an applied force but return to its original form or shape when the force is removed (such as the behavior of an elastic band). This characteristic is termed elasticity. The deformation, generally called strain, of an ideal elastic body is proportional to the applied stress (force per unit area), and the ratio of stress to strain is called the elastic modulus. For example, in a stretching process (*Young's elastic modulus Y*), the strain of a stretched filament having a cross-sectional area of A can be expressed as the ratio of the stretched length to its original length. If the length under tension is l_s and the length after the stress is removed returns to the original length l_0, then

$$Y = (f/A)/[(l_s - l_0)/l_0] = fl_0/A(l_s - l_0) \tag{12-2}$$

where $(l_s - l_0)/l_0$ is the strain and f/A is the stress in force per unit of area. This relationship, called *Hooke's law*,[2] applies to real

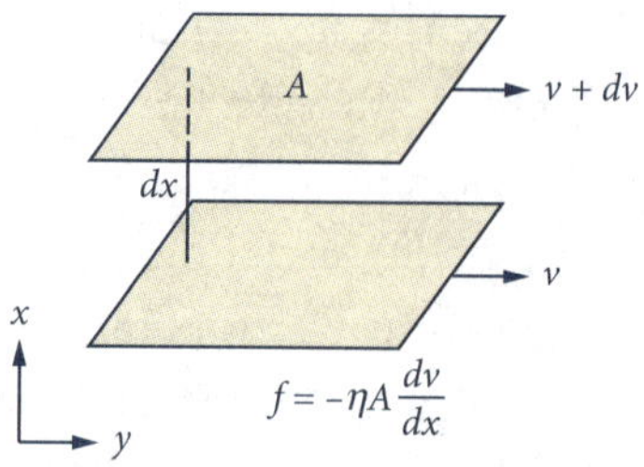

Figure 12-1 The defining model for viscosity.

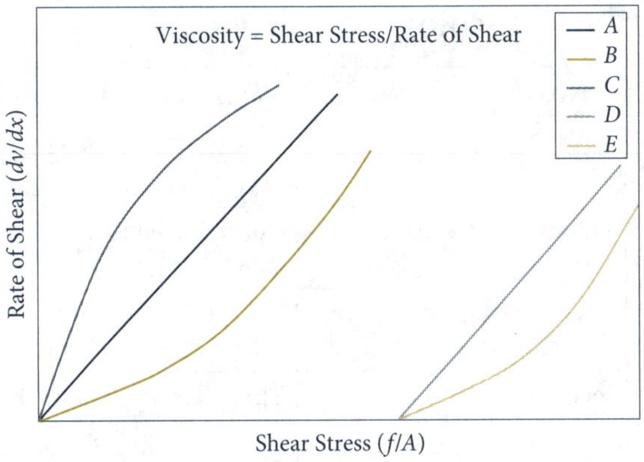

Figure 12-2 Flow curves: (*A*) Newtonian fluid, (*B*) pseudoplastic fluid, (*C*) dilatant, (*D*) Bingham plastic, and (*E*) pseudoplastic solid with a yield value.

solids subjected to moderate stresses for short time. A material of cubic symmetry has, in addition to Young's modulus *Y*, shear or rigidity modulus *G* (change in tangential stress divided by changes in the resulting angle of extension) (see the section in this chapter on viscoelasticity) and *bulk modulus K* (change in hydrostatic pressure divided by the resulting change in volume). A less isotropic solid, compared to a cubic geometry, may have moduli that are different for different directions of stress, up to a maximum of 21 in all.

Flow Curves

The subject of rheology is made more complicated by nonideal behaviors. This is demonstrated by the *flow curves* shown in **Figure 12-2.** The flow curve,† also known as the rheogram or consistency curve, is the plot of the rate of shear (dv/dx) versus the shear stress (f/A) of a liquid or deformable solid. Because viscosity is the ratio $(f/A)/(dv/dx)$, the ideal behavior is indicated by a straight line through the origin (curve *A*), i.e., a constant viscosity with respect to shear stress or rate of shear. This is known as the *Newtonian flow*. A liquid whose viscosity decreases with increasing stress (such as an increasing rate of stirring) is called pseudoplastic (curve *B*); if the viscosity increases with stress, the liquid is *dilatant* (curve *C*). An ideal elastic solid has no shear at any shear stress, but actual solids will yield to stress at a point known as the *yield stress*, beyond which flow occurs. For metals, the yield stress values are in the range of 10–50 kg/mm^2. A solid is known as a *Bingham plastic* if, once flow takes place, the rate of shear increases linearly with increasing shear stress in excess of the yield value (curve *D*), or a pseudoplastic solid if the viscosity decreases with increasing shear stress (curve *E*).

The situation is yet more complicated than described because viscosity can also vary with time. A liquid that becomes more fluid with increasing time of flow is said to be *thixotropic*, whereas if the viscosity increases with time under shear, the material is said to be *antithixotropic*, or *rheopectic*. These variations are summarized in **Table 12-1**.

Rheological principles are readily demonstrated in pharmaceutical suspensions, emulsions, lotions, ointments, pastes, and suppositories. The stability, consistency, and smoothness of these products are achieved through proper use of materials based on their rheological behavior. The flow properties of such products are important in terms of the patient's acceptance and proper use of the product, as these properties can affect the processes of packaging, removal of products from containers, extrusion from a tube, application on skin, or injection through a syringe needle. The viscosity of a product can also have a significant effect on the absorption of drugs and their distribution in the organism.

†In the literature, flow curves are also given as a plot of shear stress versus rate of shear. In this case, the curves are reversed, but the results are the same.

Table 12-1 Viscosity and Rheological Behavior

System	Viscosity	Property or Type of Material
Gases, single-phase liquids	Constant	Newtonian flow
Bingham plastic	Constant[†]	Flows when stress > yield stress
Dilatant behavior	Increases with shear stress	Concentrated and deflocculated suspensions, slurries, emulsions
Pseudoplastic liquid or solid with yield value	Decreases with shear stress	Shear-thinning due to internal structure changes
Rheopectic	Increases with time of flow	Time-dependent gelation enhanced by low stress, such as by tapping
Thixotropic	Decreases with time of flow	Reversible time effect, hysteresis in flow curve, flocculated systems
Antithixotropic	Increases with time of flow	Opposite to thixotropic

[†]Flow is shear stress–dependent; once flow takes place, the rate of shear is proportional to the shear stress in excess of the yield value.

Newtonian Fluids

Viscosity Coefficient

Although Equation (12-1) is the defining equation for viscosity, the experiment corresponding to the defined condition is not a convenient one. The most common manifestation of viscosity in engineering and biological processes is in the flow of a fluid through a cylindrical tube, such as the flow of blood in the vascular system. Hence, we describe the expression of viscosity and its effect on liquid flow in such a situation. Consider the flow of a liquid through a cylindrical tube, with a radius R, for a length l (see **Figure 12-3A**). The viscous drag, in working against the flow, results in a pressure drop over the length of l of the tube. This viscous drag stems from the thin film of fluid that is tightly held to the wall of the tube. If one considers the flowing body as consisting

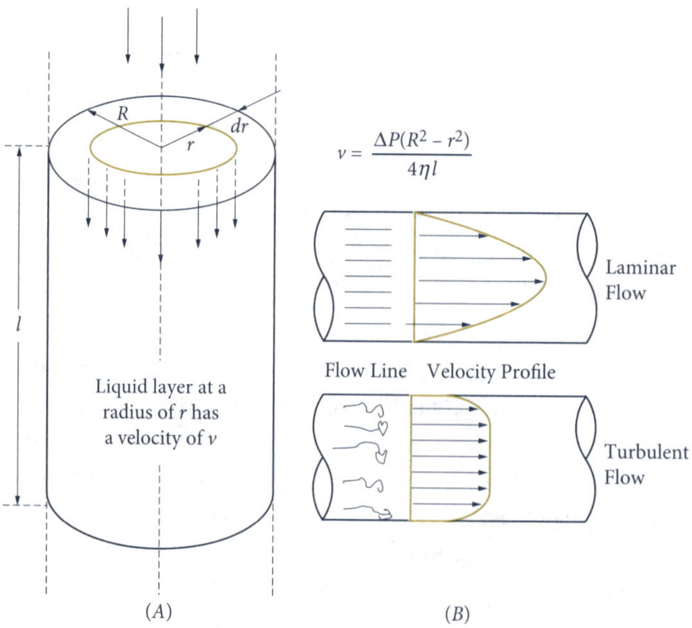

Figure 12-3 (*A*) Flow in a tube with a length l for which the pressure drop is ΔP; (*B*) laminar and turbulent flows and their velocity contour.

of concentric layers of fluid, then each layer will have a different velocity of flow; the rate at the center is the fastest, and that adjacent to the wall is zero. For a given layer with a distance r from the center of the tube, the area of the moving layer is $2\pi rl$. Thus, according to Newton's law of viscosity,

$$f = \eta(2\pi rl)\, dv/dr$$

The force f, which is the result of the viscous drag, corresponds to the pressure drop (ΔP) acting on the area of πr^2. Thus, one can express the viscous drag as

$$\text{Viscous drag} = \Delta P(\pi r^2) = \eta(2\pi rl)(-dv/dr)$$

or $$dv = -(\Delta P/2\eta l)(r)\, dr$$

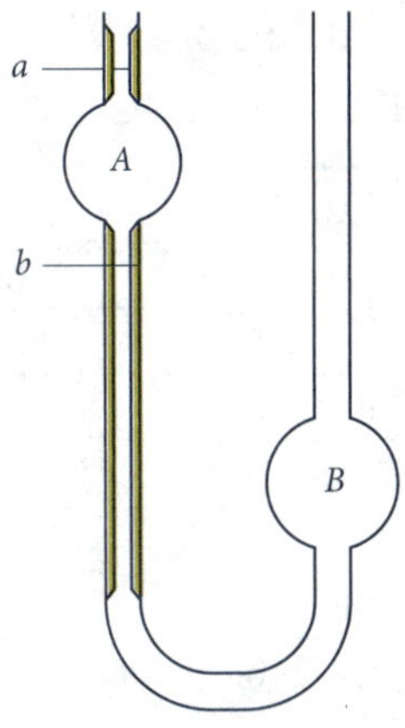

Figure 12-4 An Ostwald viscometer.

The negative sign is inserted to make the drag a positive quantity. Integration now gives the velocity profile as

$$v = \Delta P(R^2 - r^2)/4\eta l \tag{12-3}$$

This equation shows that at the center of the flow, the rate is $\Delta P R^2/4\eta l$; at a radius r, the rate is v; and at the wall of the tube, the velocity is zero. It is now important to mention that the flow of a liquid does not always conform to Equation (12-3). In fact, this equation is only applicable to low flow rates and tubes with rather small diameters, where the velocity contour, as shown in **Figure 12-3*B***, shows a laminar, streamlined, or viscous flow. Counter to the laminar flow is the turbulent flow, which consists of eddies and occurs at higher flow rates or in larger-diameter tubing.

The volume rate of flow of an annulus of thickness dr is $v(2\pi r)\,dr$. Integration of $v(2\pi r)\,dr$ from $r = 0$ to $r = R$ thus gives the total volume rate of flow (V/t) as

$$\frac{V}{t} = \int_0^R \frac{\pi \Delta P(R^2 - r^2)r}{2\eta l}\, dr = \frac{\pi \Delta P R^4}{8\eta l} \tag{12-4}$$

Equation (12-4) was first given by Poiseuille, a French physician who studied the flow of liquids through capillary tubes representative of blood vessels, and it is called the Poiseuille equation.[3] It shows that the blood volume flow through a vessel with a radius R, across a fixed pressure drop, is proportional to R^4. One can relate this equation to the blood flow. For example, if the blood vessel is dilated to exhibit a 5% increase in radius, there will be approximately a 22% increase in blood flow. This equation, with all parameters being measurable, is also the basis through which an absolute value of η for a given liquid is determined.

Ostwald Viscosity Determination

In practice, the viscosity of a liquid is almost always determined by comparing the sample with some reference sample whose viscosity is already known, using the Ostwald viscometer (**Figure 12-4**). This instrument is used to measure the time (t) required for a fixed volume of liquid (from a to b) completely to flow through point b under gravitation. Recognizing that the gravitational force is proportional to the density of the liquid, it can be shown that

$$\eta_1/\eta_2 = \rho_1 t_1/\rho_2 t_2 \tag{12-5}$$

where η_1 and ρ_1 are the viscosity and density of the unknown liquid, respectively, whereas η_2 and ρ_2 are the same parameters of the reference standard. The viscosity of a number of liquids so

Table 12-2 Viscosity Coefficients (cP) of Some Newtonian Fluids

	Temperature, °C					
Liquid	**0**	**20**	**40**	**60**	**75**	**E_{vis}, kcal/mol**
Water	1.792	1.005	0.656	0.469	0.378	4.30
Ethanol	1.773	1.200	0.834	0.592	0.426	3.20
Benzene	0.912	0.652	0.503	0.392	0.335	2.54
Diethyl ether	0.284	0.233	0.197†	0.166†	0.140†	1.65
CCl_4	1.329	0.969	0.739	0.585	0.494	2.50
Glycerin		1500				
Castor oil		1030				

†The viscosity of a liquid at a temperature below its boiling point is measured under a pressure of 1 atm. If a value is given at a temperature above the boiling point as for diethyl ether, which has a boiling point of 34.6°C, the applicable pressure is the vapor pressure of the liquid at that temperature.

determined is given in **Table 12-2**. The unit of the viscosity coefficient, defined using cgs quantities for all parameters, is called the poise (P), named after Poiseuille. Unit analysis of Equation (12-1) or (12-5) shows that the cgs unit of 1 P is 1 dyn-s/cm^2, or 1 g/cm-s. For not so viscous liquids, the viscosity is often expressed in centipoise (cP), in that 1 cP = 0.01 P. Ordinary solvent liquids have viscosities of a few centipoise. Oils, such as heavy lubricating oils, show viscosity in the range of a few poise; glycerin anhydrous has a viscosity of about 15 P at 20°C.

Theory on Viscosity

For liquids of small molecules, the viscosity is a constant at constant temperature, independent of shear stress or the rate of shear. Such liquids conform to the Newtonian flow behavior. In contrast, liquids and solids containing polymeric materials may exhibit non-Newtonian behavior. One reason is that the Newtonian system is free of molecular entanglement, so that a molecule may "jump" through others to get to a nearby hole. For the same reason, it can be seen that viscosity would be temperature-dependent, as the molecule must overcome the liquid structure or an energy barrier to flow past its neighbors. This suggests that the flow of liquid along a tube is a kinetic process analogous to that of a chemical reaction, where the change in the rate of reaction is governed by an energy of activation. Thus, one can also inquire about the rate of a liquid flow by way of an energy maximum encountered by a molecule as it squeezes past its neighbors to a position farther along the tube.

For theoretical purposes, it is more convenient to think in terms of fluidity, i.e., the tendency to flow, rather than viscosity, the resistance to flow. This can be done by defining fluidity (φ) as the reciprocal value of viscosity. The fraction of molecules that have energy in excess of the energy maximum for viscous flow (E_{vis}) can then be used to express the fluidity based on a Boltzmann-type distribution:

$$\varphi = Ae^{-E_{vis}/RT}$$

where A is some undetermined constant. Substituting $1/\eta$ for φ, one obtains

$$\eta = Ae^{E_{vis}/RT} \tag{12-6}$$

or

$$\log \eta = \log A + E_{vis}/2.303RT \tag{12-7}$$

The above equations show that the viscosity of a liquid decreases with increasing temperature, as shown in Table 12-2. The plot of log η versus $1/T$ gives a straight line with a slope of $E_{vis}/2.303R$, from which the E_{vis} value can be determined for various liquids. As shown in Table 12-2, an immediate observation is that for most liquids, the E_{vis} values are 2–3 kcal/mol, except for water, whose value is considerably higher than those of the organic liquids. Classical theories on the structure of water[4] have shown that hydrogen bonding between water molecules may be cooperative, meaning that the formation of a second and third hydrogen bond is made easier or facilitated by the formation of the first hydrogen bond. This leads to the formation of short-lived ($\sim 10^{-10}$ s) clusters, which can include up to 50–100 molecules.[5] A later fluctuation would cause the cluster to break up. The idea is one of "flickering clusters," in that a cluster lasts until fluctuation in the local energy density gives it 4–5 kcal/mol of extra energy; then it breaks up while another cluster is formed elsewhere in the liquid. The E_{vis} value (4.3 kcal/mol) supports the idea of water being a highly structured medium compared to other liquids.

It is also noteworthy that E_{vis} of liquid flow looks rather similar to the energy change for evaporation (ΔE_{vap}), i.e., the energy needed to remove a molecule completely from its neighbors. Both processes involve moving a molecule out of its liquid structure. The flow process seems to require, however, only about one-third of the energy for evaporation. It is possible that a molecule in flow may "squeeze" through space smaller than its size, and thus it has a lower energy level for its "activated state." This idea may be more readily rationalized in the case of liquid metals. Mercury, for example, has an E_{vis} of 600 and a ΔE_{vap} of 13,000 cal/mol. The flow of metal can be thought of as involving the movement of positive ions through a sea of electrons. The much smaller metal ions compared to the atom may thus be an explanation for the much lower energy dependency of the flow process than that of the removal of a metal atom.

II. Non-Newtonian Systems

Pharmaceutical preparations, except those of true solutions, invariably contain polymeric materials in the form of surfactants, lubricants, semisolid bases, solid or liquid particles, and/or macromolecules used as drug delivery matrices. The significance of rheology in pharmaceutical application thus stems from the nonideal rheological behavior of these compounds or the resulting systems. Polymers are complex materials in that they exhibit both viscous and elastic properties under varying conditions of stress, strain, time, and temperature. We begin the discussion of non-Newtonian behavior by examining the flow properties of the pharmaceutical dispersed systems.

Shear Stress–Dependent Flow Properties

Pseudoplastic Flow

Many colloidal systems, especially polymeric solutions of natural and synthetic gums such as tragacanth, methylcellulose, ethylcellulose, sodium carboxymethylcellulose, and sodium alginate, become more fluid as they are stirred faster. The shear-thinning effect is called *pseudoplasticity*.[6] The flow curve of pseudoplastic systems (Figure 12-2, curves *B* and *E*) starts at the origin or at a low shear stress value. Because the slope of the curve corresponds to $1/\eta$, for a curve convex upward, the viscosity decreases as the shear stress increases. Mechanically, it is seen that the stress causes a decrease in viscosity, which then results in an excessive increase in the rate of shear compared to a Newtonian flow.

Polymeric Solution

The molecular structure of a polymer plays an important role in determining its solution viscosity. Linear polymers such as methylcellulose may exhibit an extended or a more compact structure depending on the solvent system. Although it is not very probable to find such molecules in spherical or completely extended configurations, polymeric molecules are shown to exist in random coils of varying tightness in solutions. The distance (from end to end) of the random coils is proportional to the square root of the chain length, but the proportional constant depends on the balance between solvent–chain and chain–chain interactions. In a "good" solvent, the random coil will be extended, whereas in a "poor" solvent, such as methylcellulose in water, the chain prefers its own environment and therefore assumes a compact configuration. The latter promotes molecular aggregation or entanglement, which results in higher viscosity.

The cause of pseudoplastic flow has been described to involve a progressive breakdown of molecular entanglement in the medium by increasing shear stress, counterbalanced by a structure buildup through Brownian motion.[7] Upon applying shear, the randomly coiled, entangled polymer chains tend to disentangle and align themselves in the direction of flow. The shear may affect this development by uncoiling the polymer chain progressively and decreasing the amount of water trapped inside the coils. In contrast, stress also increases the Brownian motion (resulting from the collision of polymer with solvent molecules), which increases the random coiling tendency and intermolecular attraction. When the shear-dependent increases in molecular disentanglement exceed the thermal motion–mediated structural buildup, the viscosity diminishes with increasing shear stress.

Colloidal Particles

The shear thinning of suspended colloidal particles can be understood on the basis of the formation of a macrostructure resulting from the aggregation of small particles. This aggregation involves weak interparticle attractive forces and the formation of flocs that evolve into a space-filling particulate network. The interparticle bonding, however, is weak enough to be broken by the mechanical stress. Thus, under shear stress, the network breaks down in separate flocs, which decrease further in size when the shear stress is increased. Many gels are thus prepared and can be viewed as a weak elastic solid with a yield value. The term yield stress refers to the minimum stress that must be applied to initialize a significant flow and hence a significant drop in viscosity in the shear-thinning behavior. It is often difficult to distinguish between pseudoplastic fluid and pseudoplastic solid with a yield value; the term pseudoplastic is therefore applied without attempting to make the distinction. An example of a colloidal gel is the combination of a nanoemulsion made using a biodegradable polymer and a cationic surfactant with a nanoemulsion of the same polymer made using an anionic surfactant.[8] The electrostatic interaction results in self-assembly of the nanoparticles into a three-dimensional network, which, upon shear stress, breaks down and shows a stress-dependent decrease in viscosity. Hence, a gel that may be extruded or molded into a desired shape can become an injectable liquid upon shear stress. The reversibility of the shear-thinning behavior is discussed later in this chapter in the section on thixotropy.

At extremely low shear rates, the flocs of a system are neither noticeably deformed nor reduced in size by shear, and the system exhibits Newtonian flow. The viscosity at the limit of low shear flow is termed *zero-shear viscosity*, which, in essence, is the viscosity of a system that is at rest and fully recovered from any stress. In pharmaceutical dispersions and semisolids, zero shear or the maximum viscosity of the fluid phase is an important parameter for assessing product stability. For example, high viscosity is normally required in suspensions to prevent sedimentation of particles.

Dilatant Flow

The opposite of pseudoplasticity is the *dilatancy*, or shear thickening, a non-Newtonian behavior where viscosity increases with increasing shear rate (curve C of Figure 12-2). Dilatant systems are rare, but can be developed in concentrated suspensions where the dispersed particles are deflocculated, or show little tendency to form aggregates. When such a concentrated suspension is stirred slowly, there is a sufficient amount of liquid to allow spacing of the particles, so that the viscosity is low and the system appears wet. When high shear is applied, however, the particles tend to form clusters with the liquid being "squeezed" into void spaces, and the suspension becomes more viscous and looks expanded, as if the suspension had dilated. When the shear stress is reduced or lifted, the clustered particles separate, and the viscosity decreases as the suspension appears wet again. This type of suspension will eventually transform to a firm paste. Among systems that exhibit dilatant flow are suspensions of starch (40–50% in aqueous glycerin or ethylene glycol medium) and some inorganic materials such as the deflocculated systems of iron oxide (12%), zinc oxide (30%), barium sulfate (39%), and titanium dioxide (30–50%) in water.[9]

Plastic Flow

The term *plasticity* refers to the propensity of a material to undergo permanent deformation. In concentrated and flocculated suspensions, particles tend to stick together, forming three-dimensional networks throughout the suspension volume, and result in the formation of a solid or paste that has little elasticity. The flow property of such a system depends on the breakdown of the particle agglomeration, thus indicating that the system has an acquired yield stress value. The more strongly flocculated the suspension, the higher the yield stress. It behaves as a rigid body at low stress until the yield stress is reached; then, under a continuing increase in stress, it flows as a fluid with a constant viscosity. Materials that exhibit this type of behavior are called the Bingham plastics or bodies. A common example is toothpaste, which will not be extruded until a pressure is applied to the tube; then it flows out as a plug.

The plastic flow curve does not pass through the origin but shows a linear increase in the rate of shear with the shear stress above the yield stress value (Figure 12-2, curve *D*), indicating that the flowing body has a constant viscosity. The yield stress can be determined from the flow curve by extrapolation of the straight-line plot to the shear stress axis, as indicated in Figure 12-2, whereas the viscosity of the Bingham plastic may be given as

$$\eta_{\text{plastic}} = (\tau - \tau_y)/\dot{g} \quad (12\text{-}8)$$

where τ is the shear stress, $\dot{g}$ is the rate of shear, and τ_y is the yield stress. A plastic is said to be *soft* if the yield stress is low and *stiff* if the viscosity is high. It is now appropriate to point out that before the viscosity is significantly lowered to the constant value at a point above the yield value, the flow curve is nonlinear, which is called a plug flow. Because the system is not quite yet a fluid, it moves in chunks as opposed to the laminar motion of a flowing liquid.

Power Law

The flow curves of non-Newtonian systems are often analyzed to gain quantitative perspectives of the flow using the *Ostwald power law*.[10] In this model, the rate of shear ($\dot{g}$) is empirically taken to be proportional to the shear stress (τ) to the power of n, that is,

$$\dot{g} = K\tau^n \quad (12\text{-}9)$$

or $$\log \dot{g} = \log K + n \log \tau \quad (12\text{-}10)$$

where K is a constant whose unit varies depending on the n value. The n value is an index of deviation from the Newtonian flow; when $n = 1$, K is the reciprocal value of viscosity, and the system is Newtonian. The purpose of the power law is to obtain a linear plot for the curvature relationships between shear stress and shear rate found in pseudoplastic and dilatant flows. If the system fits well to the power law, a plot of $\log \dot{g}$ versus $\log \tau$ will yield a straight line, from which n can be determined. For pseudoplastic flow $n > 1$, whereas for dilatant flow $n < 1$. For accessing pseudoplasticity, the more n differs from unity, the faster the viscosity will be decreased with increasing shear. Many pseudoplastic systems follow the power law with n in the range of 3–4. There are also modified power laws for systems that do not follow the Ostwald model.[11, 12]

Time-Dependent Rheological Behavior

Thixotropy

The term *thixotropy* refers to the decrease in viscosity with time when flow is applied to a sample previously at rest and the recovery of viscosity in time when flow is discontinued.[13] It is one of the oldest documented rheological phenomena, but remains the most challenging problem in colloidal rheology. The essential element of this phenomenon is the reversibility of time-dependent loss and recovery of viscosity, which implies that there is a "memory" associated with the process. The thixotropic behavior has been described on the basis that a macrostructure, formed by relatively weak attractive forces between particles, can be broken into separate flocs by mechanical stresses occurring during flow. The flocs decrease further in size when the strain rate is increased. Reducing the shear rate, in contrast, causes a growth of the flocs, and when flow is arrested, the particle networks rebuild with time. The stress changes correspond to changes in the steady-state formation of microstructures during and after flow. When the structural change requires a finite amount of time, so does the flow-induced stress, thus resulting in thixotropic behavior.

Thixotropic Flow Analysis

A common rheological experiment is a forward-and-backward stress sweep between zero and a maximum value, in which the viscosity is monitored while the stress is increased and then decreased. When the transient data are presented as a flow curve, a thixotropic flow will exhibit a hysteresis loop (**Figure 12-5*A***), where the forward sweep, or the ascending curve, indicates a continuing decrease in viscosity and the formation of microstructure, whereas the backward sweep, or descending curve, indicates the recovery of viscosity and the sample's original structure. The hysteresis is formed because the stress will lag behind the shear rate due to time-dependent recovery of viscosity or the structural state. For example, at the shear rate of $\dot{g}_1$, the stress of the descending curve (τ_d) is lower than that of the ascending curve (τ_a); i.e., the viscosity at the point τ_d is less than that at point τ_a, because the shear-thinning effect has not been sufficiently recovered. If the experiment is performed at a slower cycle time, there will be less difference between the ascending and descending curves at the same shear rate, because the microstructure now has more time to come close to the steady-state one.

The hysteresis loop has been used to characterize the thixotropic behavior of a system. A simple method may be derived via successive shear cycles of a thixotropic liquid, as shown in Figure 12-5*B*. In this case, the ascending curves following the initial run are moving closer to the descending curve because of the time-dependent recovery of viscosity. The rate of the percentage recovery of viscosity at a given shear rate may be estimated as

$$\text{Rate of recovery} = (\tau_a - \tau)/\Delta t(\tau_a - \tau_d)$$

where τ is the shear stress of the ascending curve of a successive run at a given shear rate, to which the initial ascending and descending curves have shear stresses of τ_a and τ_d, respectively, and Δt is the time between successive runs. It should be mentioned that the hysteresis loop results from a combination of shear rate and time effects, and the loop area varies with varying test conditions, shear history, shear rate acceleration, and maximum shear rate. Thus, it provides only a relative measure of thixotropy.

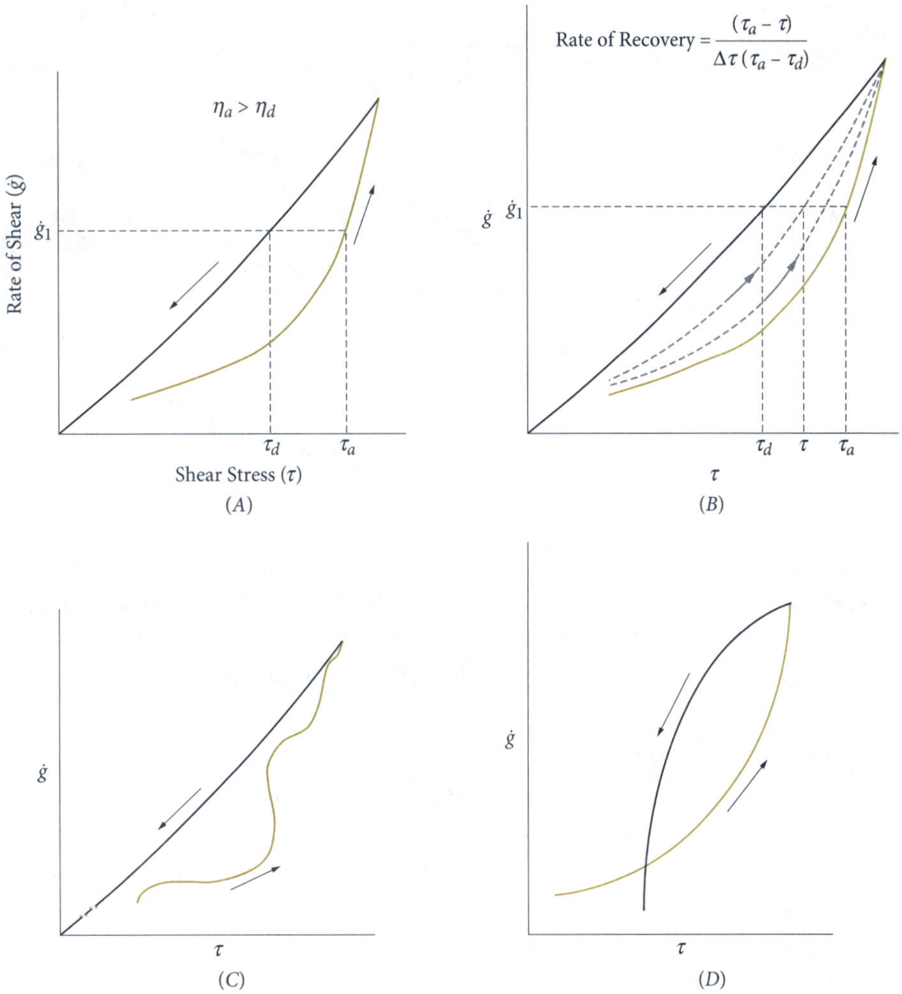

Figure 12-5 Hysteresis loops of (*A*) pseudoplastic and plastic flows, (*B*) successive shear cycles, (*C*) bulging and negative effects, and (*D*) changed zero shear structure.

The shape of the hysteresis loop can provide some information regarding the rheological sample. Two common alternatives are shown in Figure 12-5*C* and *D*. Figure 12-5*C* illustrates a case where the breakdown of the initial structure dominates the time evolution of the stress. Aqueous bentonite gel, e.g., swells under low shear stress, thus showing a bulging ascending curve characterized by a moderate decrease in viscosity. A reduction of stress with increasing shear rate may indicate shear banding (localization of strain to a narrow zone) or heterogeneous shear rate distributions in the sample. At low shear rates, stress may induce structure formation that affects the macrostructure of the system. In this case, the hysteresis loop can take a shape like that in Figure 12-5*D*, which shows a descending curve that is not returning to the origin. The hysteresis loop is a good indication of thixotropy, although irreversible softening of nonthixotropic materials also exhibits hysteresis, but is less effective as a quantitative tool in that shear rate and time effects are not separated in this experiment.

The time-dependent recovery in thixotropy can be illustrated (**Figure 12-6**) via a shear rate step-down experiment. In such an experiment, the transient shear stress is tracked after a sudden reduction in shear rate. A nonthixotropic fluid would react to such a shear change by a decrease of the stress to a lower plateau (Figure 12-6*A*) with time. In contrast, the shear stress in a thioxotropic material would drop instantaneously to a lower value and increase gradually with time to its new steady-state level (Figure 12-6*B*). Many thixotropic materials are also viscoelastic and so may exhibit a time curve showing a relatively fast relaxation before the gradual increase in stress.

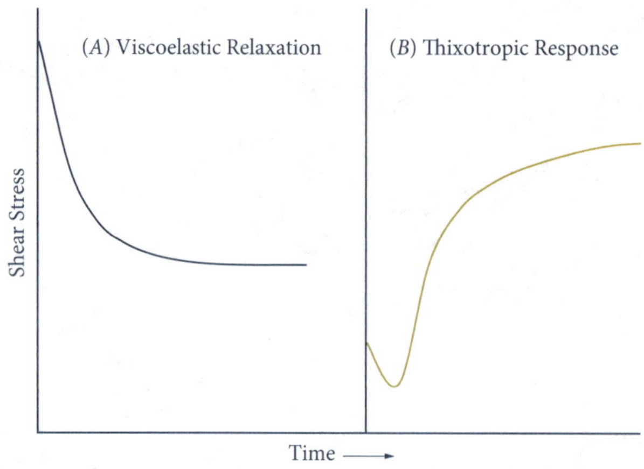

Figure 12-6 Time-dependent responses in shear stress to sudden reduction of shear rate by materials undergoing (*A*) viscoelastic relaxation or (*B*) thixotropic response.

The time-dependent recovery of stress or viscocity in Figure 12-6*B* indicates thixotropy. Such an experiment can be used directly to determine the rate of change in viscosity when the shear rate and the rate of recovery are suddenly changed after cessation of flow.

Structure Characteristics and Preparation

Thixotropy requires a micro- and macrostructural transition that can be reversibly altered by moderate stress, in such a manner that it produces a relatively slow but significant viscosity change. Metastable structures, which balance the hydrodynamic forces of flow by weak interparticle attractive forces, would be suitable for this purpose. Such conditions can be met with nearly all colloidal particles, primarily by reducing the interparticle repulsion forces to enhance particle aggregation. The colloidal systems are stabilized through charge and/or steric effects, and the latter are achieved via particle adsorption of polymeric material. Salts may be used in aqueous systems of low colloidal concentration to bring flocculation, although such a coagulation process may be irreversible. Polymers are used in colloidal systems either to stabilize or to flocculate the colloidal systems. Adsorption of polymeric molecules by particles results in a steric effect between particles, which stabilizes the system. In contrast, polymers such as pactin and xanthan gum and non-ionic surfactants may induce flocculation by bridging the particles through adsorption or by staying in solution to create an osmotic gradient that draws the medium away from the interparticle spaces. The latter is called depletion flocculation.[14] Reducing the layer of thickness of adsorbed polymers by chemical or physicochemical methods can reduce the steric stabilization and lead to flocculation. Polymers that act through either bridging or depletion flocculation provide another route to thixotropic gels.[15, 16] Then there are the particle–particle and particle–medium interactions, including those of acid–base, hydrophobic, and hydrogen bonding, that can be used to achieve flocculation.

There are a few types of particles with which pronounced and reversible time effects can be achieved at very low particle concentrations. These include the fumed silica[17] and carbon black.[18] Silica has been widely used for the preparation of thixotropic colloids. With surface modifications, it can be applied to aqueous as well as nonaqueous media. Colloidal particles may also act as thixotropic agents. Addition of these particles to an emulsion or molten polymer can turn a simple yield stress fluid into a thixotropic material.[19, 20]

It should be mentioned that the transition between macro- and microstructure, two nonequilibrium states, is not easy or even possible under all conditions. The reversibility of a preparation will depend on how well the dispersed system is prepared. Care should be made to ensure that all particles are wetted by the liquid phase, thus avoiding a change in dispersion status during rheological test. Dispersion is usually done by high-shear milling devices, whereas rheological test is carried out in low shear stress. Hence, when properly made, the size of the building blocks for the aggregated structure will be established by dispersion and not changed by rheological test. There is, however, an aging process that may change the microstructure of a colloidal preparation[21, 22] in that the particle structure becomes more rigid and heterogenic with time. The aging process can be reversed by flow, which is known as shear rejuvenation.[23]

Antithixotropy

When flow causes a reversible, time-dependent increase in viscosity, the phenomenon is called antithixotropy, or negative thixotropy. The term rheopexy has also been used to describe the time-dependent phenomenon. Shear thickening may occur in different manifestations. A quasi-instantaneous increase in viscosity with shear rate, i.e., the dilatancy, is irreversible and occurs in concentrated suspensions of deflocculated particles and at sufficiently high shear rates.[24, 25] A time-dependent increase in viscosity during flow is often caused by irreversible aggregation of particles. Such a process would also exhibit the dilatant behavior. Reversible time effects, which are indicated by a reversed hysteresis loop, have been reported in some materials and colloidal suspensions such as magnesia magma.[26, 27] In some colloidal dispersions, the viscosity increases with time at low shear rates after shearing at high shear rate.[28] This behavior has been suggested to be rheopectic but not antithixotropic. The term rheopexy refers to the phenomenon that the gel formation of a system may be facilitated by tapping or low shear compared to keeping the sample at rest. It is not antithixotropy because the reversibility is not defined. Studies on the rheology of bovine synovial fluid and albumin solutions have shown that these fluids are rheopectic (stress increases with time in steady shear), due to protein aggregation and entanglement with the long-chain polysaccharide, sodium hyaluronate, under physiological conditions.[29] The increase in viscosity is consistent with the fluid's lubrication properties. If the protein aggregation were reversible, the fluids would be antithixotropic.

Viscoelasticity

The term *viscoelasticity* refers to a material's viscosity-dependent flow properties as a liquid and its elastic (recoverable deformation) properties as a solid. Such properties exist in many pharmaceutical systems, including ointments, creams, lotions, suppositories, suspensions, and colloidal dispersions. Because the use as well as the performance of such a system is directly associated with mechanical stresses in the form of stirring, dispensing, rubbing, or injecting through needles, the rheological properties are directly linked to its consistency, stability, and effectiveness as a medical product. The concept of the viscoelastic phenomenon is that a microstructure exists as a part of the large continuum that undergoes collective changes in flow and small deformation in response to stress. The various microstructural manifestations may be seen as the lamellar gel phase, interfacial layers, micelles, suspensions, and flocculated systems. The rheological measurements, which are designed to gain information without destroying the structure, can thus be used to quantify the effects of formulation ingredients and process, as well as temperature and aging, on the desired properties of the pharmaceutical system.

Shear Modulus (G)

Consider a small cubical volume of a material. The isotropic shape conveniently limits the elastic modulus to linear modulus Y, shear or rigidity modulus G, and bulk modulus K. The one that applies most to the viscoelasticity of pharmaceutical systems is the shear modulus, which measures the resistance of the material to deformation. The shear-induced deformation of a rectangular

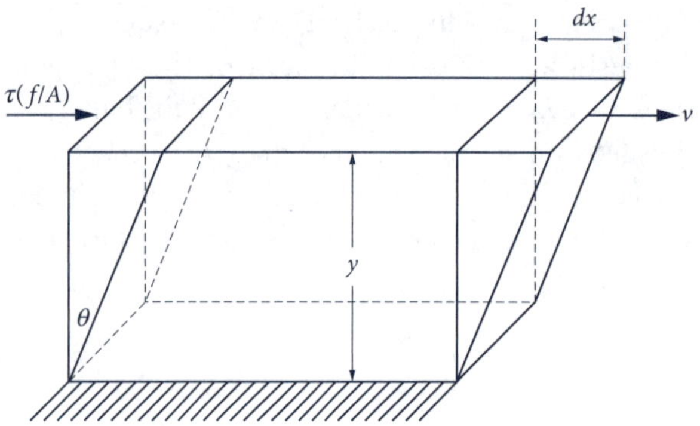

Term	Symbol	Equation
Stress	τ	$\tau = f/A$
Strain	$\hat{S}$	$\hat{S} = dx/y$
Strain rate	$\hat{R}$	$\hat{R} = dx/ydt$
Shear rate	$\dot{g}$	$\dot{g} = dv/y$
Viscosity	η	$\eta = \tau/\dot{g}$
Shear modulus	G^*	$G^* = \tau/\hat{S} = \tau/\tan\theta$

Figure 12-7 Flow and deformation of a viscoelastic body.

body is shown in **Figure 12-7**, where the shear stress (τ) ($= f/A$) is imposed from left to right at the top rectangular plan. At time dt, the velocity at the top surface is dv; if the top surface is moved to the right a distance of dx, forming an angle θ with the base, and the height of the rectangular body is y, then

Rate of shear	$\dot{g} = dv/y$	(unit: s^{-1})
Strain	$\hat{S} = dx/y$	(dimensionless)
Strain rate	$\hat{R} = (dx/dt)/y$	(s^{-1})
Viscosity	$\eta = \tau/\dot{g}$	(dyn-s/cm^2, P, or Pa-s; 1 Pa-s = 10 P = 10 dyn-s/cm^2)
Shear modulus	$G^* = \tau/\hat{S} = fy/A\,dx = \tau/\tan\theta$	(dyn/cm^2, or Pa)

The displacement distance dx can be divided into two components: elastic deformation and slippage. The elastic deformation is recoverable, but the slippage of viscoelasticity is lost to viscous flow. This phenomenon results in a partial recovery of the shape and the elastic energy once the stress is lifted. The overall shear modulus is then called the *complex modulus* (G^*), which consists of a storage modulus (G'), indicating the recoverable energy or elasticity, and a loss modulus (G''), indicating the viscous flow as a result of shear. The relationship among G^*, G', and G'' is

$$G^* = G' + iG'' \tag{12-11}$$

where G^* measures the material's total resistance to deformation, i is the imaginary number $(-1)^{1/2}$, and G'' is nonrecoverable.

Phase Angle

The storage and loss moduli are determined using a simple harmonic, or sinusoidal oscillatory model, known as dynamic testing. In such measurements, an applied oscillatory (sinusoidal) stress (or strain) is responded to by the material with a sinusoidal strain (or stress), where the two waves

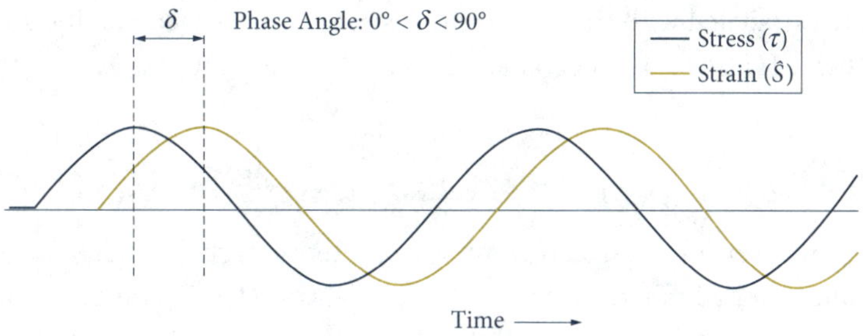

Figure 12-8 Oscillatory stress (τ), material response ($\hat{S}$), and phase angle (δ), by which the force oscillation leads the response oscillation.

are separated by a *phase angle* δ (**Figure 12-8**). From the measured contact stiffness (which is the ratio of the amplitudes of applied and responding waves times $\cos\delta$) and the damping of oscillation by the material (which gives the ratio of amplitudes of applied and responding waves times $\sin\delta$), G' and G'' are determined as a function of the applied frequency. These data are then used for the determination of the phase angle in that

$$\tan\delta = G''/G' \qquad (12\text{-}12)$$

Tan delta ($\tan\delta$), as it is often called, is very useful in quantifying the extent of elasticity in fluids and semisolids. The phase angle has a value from 0° to 90°. A material is elastic (solidlike) if $\delta = 0°$ ($\tan\delta = 0$); it is viscoelastic if the angle lies below 90°, and it becomes a liquid when $\delta = 90°$ ($\tan\delta = \infty$). Studies have shown that $\tan\delta$ may be used to access interparticle association. A value greater than 3 indicates little or no interaction between particles, whereas a value less than 1 indicates significant particle aggregation. In the range of 1 to 3, particles are weakly associated.[30, 31]

The use of G', G'', and δ to evaluate potential particle sedimentation from a suspension is illustrated in **Figure 12-9.** In a gel formulation, G' is consistently higher than G'', and the phase angle is low and is independent of the applied frequency, making it solidlike. For a viscoelastic liquid at low frequencies, $G'' > G'$, and the phase angle approaches 90° near zero frequencies. There is a *crossover frequency* at which G' overtakes G'', marking the transition from viscous to elastic states. Such a formulation is liquidlike at rest; the particles in the system will flow and settle eventually when left alone. In comparison, a viscoelastic solid will have higher G' than G'' at low frequencies. The phase angle can approach 0° at near zero frequency, thus making it a more stable dispersion than even the gel system. As frequency increases, G'' overtakes G' ($\tan\delta$ increases); this results in a transition from the viscoelastic solid to viscoelastic liquid, which can be formulated to match the

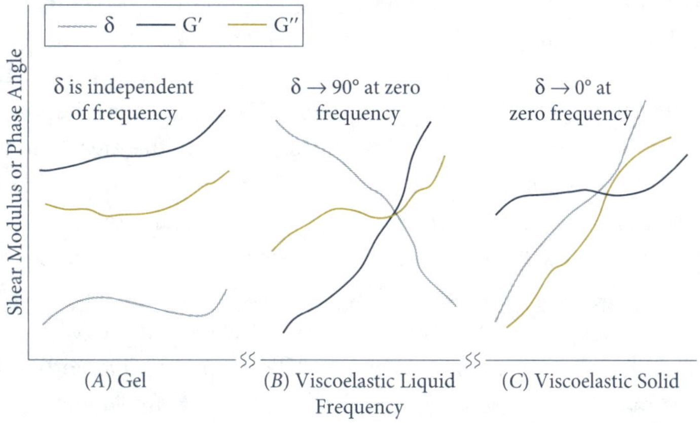

Figure 12-9 Changes in G', G'', and phase angle as a function of frequency in the (*A*) gel; (*B*) viscoelastic liquid; and (*C*) viscoelastic solid systems.

mechanical stresses associated with the use of this system. The microcrystalline sodium carboxymethylcellulose (Avicell CL-611) has been shown to exhibit such properties as a stabilizer for topical creams.[32]

Rheological Measurement

Instruments that provide rheological testing are viscometers and rheometers. The former measure the viscosity of a fluid over a limited shear rate range. A rheometer, in comparison, measures the viscosity over a wide range of shear rates and the viscoelasticity of fluids, semisolids, and solids. In terms of geometry of contact with the sample, the measuring systems utilize rotating concentric cylinders for liquids of very low to medium viscosity, cone and plate for samples of low to high viscosity, parallel plates for low viscosity to soft solids, and rectangular torsion for soft to rigid solids. The rheological behavior can be studied using a number of tests including time sweep, strain, stress, or frequency sweep, creep/recovery, flow, and stress relaxation. Some of these tests and associated terminology are described below.

Oscillatory Time Sweep

Materials (e.g., dispersions and polymers) that undergo macro- and microstructural rearrangement with time should be tested to determine the equilibrium time for the recovery of their structural characteristics. Many factors, including the concentration, particle size and shape, and surface chemistry of the dispersed phase, influence the rheological behavior of dispersions. The true rheological behavior can only be observed if the system is in an equilibrium state. Thus the system should be characterized for its recovery time before data collection. A simple test is the oscillatory time sweep, which monitors how the material properties change with shear by monitoring certain viscoelastic parameters as time advances. The oscillatory procedure uses a conditioning step that applies a preshear controlling shear rate (such as at $100\,s^{-1}$ for 30 s) at controlled temperature. The time sweep is then carried out by applying a constant oscillatory stress or strain. For many viscoelastic liquids, when tested by time sweep such as at a constant oscillation stress, there is an increase in the material's storage modulus before a steady value is obtained within a few minutes, suggesting that the sample should be rested for the time required for reaching the steady value before further testing.

Stress or Strain Sweep

Dynamic stress or strain sweep is a measurement in which the material's response (strain or stress) to increasing amplitude of deformation is monitored at a constant frequency and temperature. In comparison, a frequency sweep is carried out with increasing frequency, where the material's response is monitored at constant amplitude (stress or strain) and temperature. The major application of the stress or strain sweep is to identify the linear viscoelastic region (LVR), which represents one of the important characteristics of a viscoelastic material. **Figure 12-10** shows the stress sweep of an ink sample at two conditions: (1) immediately after preshear and (2) 150 s after preshear. First, it can be seen that the two curves are not identical; the measured G' values for the nonrecovered sample are considerably lower than those from the sample that has been recovered from preshear stress, indicating that the time sweep experiment is important for material characterization. The figure also shows a linear region of G' at low stress values. Upon further increase in stress, a marked decrease in G' occurs, indicating a breakdown of the viscoelastic structure. This phenomenon, which also occurs in a strain sweep, as the magnitudes of stress and strain are linearly related, indicates that if the deformation is small or applied sufficiently slowly, there is a full retainment of the material's viscoelasticity as the molecular arrangements are never far from equilibrium. The mechanical response is then just a reflection of the dynamic processes at the molecular level in the domain of LVR.[33]

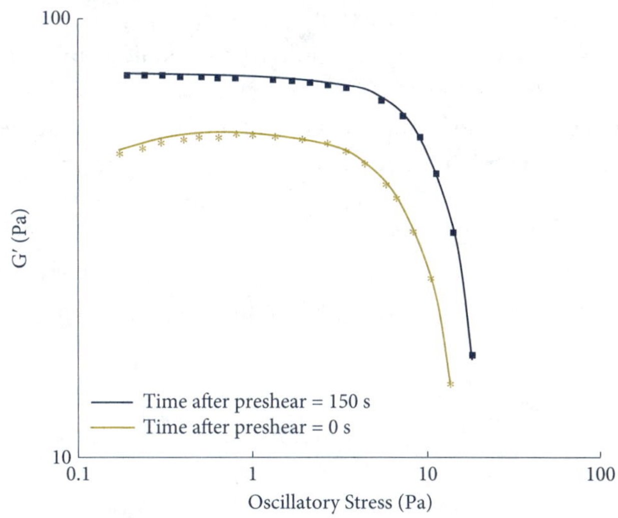

Figure 12-10 Change in storage modulus as a function of stress frequency (in log scale).
Reproduced from: F.A. Mazzeo, "Importance of Oscillatory Time Sweeps in Rheology," TA Instruments, 109 Lukens Drive, Newcastle, DE, USA.

The stress or strain at which the structure begins to break down is known as the critical stress or strain, which gives the length of LVR; the longer the length, the greater the cohesive energy that measures the strength of the internal structure of the viscoelastic body. The cohesive energy can be calculated as

$$E_c = G'\hat{S}_c^2/2$$

where E_c is the cohesive energy and $\hat{S}_c$ is the critical strain. Pharmaceutical formulation with longer LVR will be more resistant to breakdown by stress, such as that encountered during transportation and handling, than one with lesser LVR.

Creep/Recovery Test

A *creep test* is used to determine the strain response of a viscoelastic material under a constant low stress, such as at levels below the yield stress, over time (for example, 500 s). The creep (deformation and flow) is then allowed to recover by removing the applied stress. A typical creep test result is shown in **Figure 12-11**, where a material is subjected to repeated creep tests until the

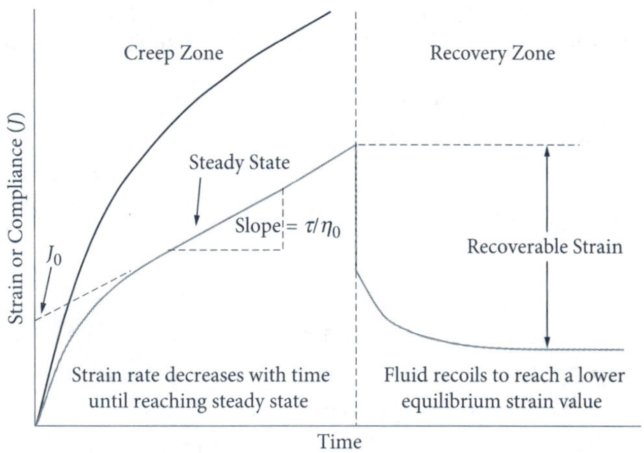

Figure 12-11 Creep test and recovery of a viscoelastic material.

strain rate is decreased (from the solid curve to the steady state curve) to an equilibrated state. The strain may be expressed as a percentage of strain (dimensionless) or as strain per unit of stress (cm^2/dyn), known as the compliance (J). A soft material with low G' compared to a stiffer material having a higher G' is said to be more compliant. In the recovery zone, the viscoelastic material recoils, and the strain decreases, eventually reaching equilibrium at some small value. The recovered strain or compliance reflects the material's elasticity. Two very useful properties may be derived from the creep test: One is the extrapolated J value (J_o) from the equilibrium curve under stress, which is the theoretical limit of recovery; the second is the slope of the equilibrium curve, from which the zero-shear viscosity (η_0) can be determined as

$$\eta_0 = \text{shear stress/slope} \qquad (12\text{-}13)$$

As we shall see later, the zero-shear viscosity is an important parameter for preventing the sedimentation of particles in formulations.

III. Rheology in Pharmacy

The rheological principles are used in pharmacy to (1) gain product stability; (2) achieve desired rheological properties for the use of the products; (3) facilitate processing of pharmaceutical materials in mixing, tableting, and capsule filling, packaging, and transportation of products; and (4) control the release and absorption of drugs from dosage forms. The role of rheology in the stability and use of pharmaceutical systems is described below.

Rheology and Particle Sedimentation

Zero-Shear Viscosity

The sedimentation of particles from a pharmaceutical suspension is given by Stokes' law, provided that the particles are spherical, uncharged, and in dilute quantities, as follows:

$$V_s = d^2(\rho_i - \rho_m)g/18\eta_0 \qquad (12\text{-}14)$$

where V_s is the sedimentation velocity, d is the diameter of the particle, ρ_i and ρ_m are the densities of the particle and medium, respectively, g is the gravitational acceleration, and η_0 is the zero-shear viscosity. The sedimentation velocity can be calculated, and so can the time required for the particle to reach the bottom. If this sedimentation time is longer than the accepted limit for a given application, then the formulation is acceptable. The sedimentation equation can be further divided into shear stress and the rate of shear. The downward stress caused by gravitation is

$$\tau_s = d(\rho_i - \rho_m)g/6 \qquad (12\text{-}15)$$

whereas the maximum rate of shear is

$$\dot{g}_{\max} = 3V_s/d \qquad (12\text{-}16)$$

Thus it is possible to evaluate both the shear stress and the shear rate of the suspension system. Suspensions may be acceptable to sedimentation for two reasons: (1) The material has a sufficiently high zero-shear viscosity that sedimentation occurs in an acceptably slow manner, and (2) the bulk material has a yield stress that is high enough to hold the particles in suspension. The use of the above equations to gain such information is illustrated in Example 12-1.

Example 12-1: If an aqueous suspension has a zero-shear viscosity of 5 P at 20°C, which is comparable to that of 95% glycerin in water, what are the sedimentation rate, rate of shear, and yield stress for this formulation? The drug particles have a density of 1.25 g/cm^3 and a mean diameter of 20 μm. The medium density is 1 g/cm^3.

Solution:

$$V_s = d^2(\rho_i - \rho_m)g/18\eta_0 = (20 \times 10^{-4})^2 \times (1.25 - 1.0) \times 980.67/18 \times 5$$

$$= 1.09 \times 10^{-5}\ \text{cm/s}$$

$$\tau_s = d(\rho_i - \rho_m)g/6 = 20 \times 10^{-4}\ (1.25 - 1.0) \times 980.67/6$$

$$= 0.082\ \text{dyn/cm}^2$$

$$\dot{g}_{max} = 3V_s/d = 3 \times 1.09 \times 10^{-5}/20 \times 10^{-4} = 0.0163\ \text{s}^{-1}$$

Interpretation:

The calculated shear rate is slightly above the range for the sedimentation of fine powders in liquids. The correlation of shear rates with mechanical stresses associated with various activities is shown in **Table 12-3**.

The downward stress may be considered the yield stress for this formulation. The yield stress can be increased by viscoelastic agents to values greater than the calculated value; the formulation, then, would be able to hold the particles in suspension.

Viscoelastic Effects

The zero-shear viscosity can be determined by the creep test, as described. If the material has a yield stress but a weak gel structure, the sample may still give sedimentation during transportation and handling. Thus for stability studies, the LVR of the formulation is also determined using dynamic strain or stress sweep experiments. In addition, the measurement of tan δ also gives a strong indication of the elastic property (see Figure 12-9). The stability of a dispersed system increases with an increase in the elastic portion of the viscoelastic behavior.

Table 12-3 Shear Rates and Common Activities

Action	Shear Rate, s^{-1}	Activity/Product
Sedimentation of fine particles	10^{-6}–10^{-3}	Pharmaceuticals, paints
Leveling by surface tension	10^{-2}–10^{-1}	Paints, printing (inks)
Draining off surface	10^{-1}–10^{1}	Coatings
Extruding, pouring, chewing, swallowing, dip coating	10^{0}–10^{2}	Eating, food and confectionery, painting
Mixing, stirring, pipe flowing	10^{1}–10^{3}	Preparing solutions, pumping, blood flow
Injection, brushing	10^{2}–10^{4}	Hypodermic syringe, painting
Rubbing, nasal spraying	10^{4}–10^{5}	Applying topical products
Spraying	10^{5}–10^{6}	Atomization, spray drying
Lubrication	10^{3}–10^{7}	Bearings, engines

Effects of Particle Size and Distribution on Viscosity

The particle size, as shown by Stokes' law, has a direct effect on the sedimentation rate. In addition, particle size has a significant effect on the viscosity of the liquid, because the latter depends on interparticle interactions that increase with an increasing number of particles. For a given weight of material, a smaller particle size corresponds to a greater number of particles. This results in greater interaction between particles that is necessary for the formation of the macrostructure in pseudoplastic and thixotropic systems, and hence a greater zero-shear viscosity. The effect of particle size distribution may be explained as follows. In a wider distribution, the smaller particles can be easily distributed in void spaces, making the liquid more responsive to shear stress or flow. The viscosity of the system increases with increasing volume fraction of the particles; but at the same volume fraction, the system that has a wider particle size distribution will have lower viscosity than the system having a narrower particle size distribution. Thus, a narrow particle size distribution is preferred over a wider particle size distribution to bring stability to the formulation.

Pseudoplastic and Thixotropic Systems in Pharmacy

The rheological behaviors of pseudoplastic and thixotropic systems are such that the viscosity of the system decreases upon shear. Hence, the equilibrium state of these formulations is usually a viscous liquid or a gel-like system. A pseudoplastic system may or may not be thixotropic, but the recovery of viscosity may be a time-dependent process involving specific mechanisms.[8] For topical formulations, similar advantages may be obtained from both phenomena.

Viscoelastic Materials

Commonly used agents for cream and gel formations include carbomers (Carbopols), cellulose derivatives, poloxamers (Pluronics), and some natural gums such as acacia, xanthan, and tragacanth. Carbomers are high-molecular-weight, water-soluble polymers derived from acrylic acid. When dispersed in hydroalcoholic vehicle, they form solutions in the 2.5–3.5 pH range, but gels when the pH is raised to 5–6. The aqueous gels exhibit plastic flow. When used with lecithin (phosphatidylcholine) in the preparation of liposome hydrogels, carbomer enhances the elasticity of the viscoelastic system.[34] There are, however, changed rheological behaviors when carbomer gels are prepared, as in some topical formulations, using glycerol and/or propylene glycol as solvent. For example, carbomer microgels formed in systems containing water, glycerol, propylene glycol, and triethanolamine (which neutralizes the polymer's carboxylic groups) have been shown to exhibit much more enhanced pseudoplastic behavior than Carbopol in water alone, and modest thixotropy at higher shear rates.[35] It is suggested that glycerol and propylene glycol can alter the rheological behavior by changing the solvent–solvent and solvent–polymer interactions. This phenomenon has also been observed in hydrogels of chitosan, investigated as a polymeric drug carrier, where the gel formation with glycerol gives a plastic flow, but the gel formation with propylene glycol shows thixotropic behavior.[36]

Cellulose derivatives such as methylcellulose, ethylcellulose, hydroxypropyl methylcellulose (HPMC), and carboxymethylcellulose are commonly used gelling agents that exhibit varied viscoelasticity. Ethylcellulose has been shown to form nonaqueous gel with propylene glycol dicaprylate/dicaprate that exhibits a polymer concentration–dependent yield stress and thixotropy. The mechanism was shown to involve the formation of a physically cross-linked three-dimensional gel network, where the solvent molecules affect the formation of gel networks through intermolecular hydrogen bonding between ethylcellulose polymer chains.[37] HPMC is noted as a hydrophilic surface-active agent. A polymer blend of HPMC with hyaluronic acid (HA), a polysaccharide that exhibits pseudoplastic flow, has been tested for its suitability as an injectable drug delivery vehicle. The concept is that HPMC can increase the water-binding property of the polymer blend and lower the yield stress of HA, thus enhancing the injectability and water contact of the system for sustained-release drug delivery.[38] The microcrystalline cellulose with sodium carboxymethylcellulose forms viscous gels that exhibit both elastic and viscous moduli and thixotropic flow.[32, 39] The yield stress and elasticity of the system increase with increasing polymer concentration.

Poloxamers, which are copolymers of polyoxyethylene and polyoxypropylene, have been studied for their pseudoplastic and thixotropic properties. Poloxamers having melting points in the range of 48–58°C have been tested as a continuous phase at 70°C for the dispersion of insoluble drugs using lactose as a model. The molten poloxamer dispersion showed thixotropic and shear-thinning rheology. The dispersion is uniform and exhibits suitable apparent viscosity (0.32–2.8 Pa-s) for liquid filling of hard gelatin capsules.[40] The potential use of poloxamers for injections has also been tested on poloxamer 407–lidocaine HCl gels.[41] Lidocaine, a local anesthetic used for treatment of acute and chronic pain, has a short duration of action; thus, a long-acting single-dose injection would be of clinical value. Such a formulation depends on the rheological property and the sol-gel transition of the system. The study showed that poloxamer 407 gels are pseudoplastic (shear-thinned when deformed) and exhibit both storage and loss moduli in their viscoelastic behavior. The viscosity of the system increases with increasing concentration of the polymer. The sol-gel transition temperature, in contrast, was decreased by increasing the polymer concentration and by the addition of NaCl, NaH_2PO_4, Na_2CO_3, or polyethylene glycol 400, suggesting that fine-tuning of formulation ingredients may allow the development of a suitable injectable dosage form. It would seem to be incomplete without mentioning an agent of opposite rheological behavior. Hence, the acacia gum, a hybrid polyelectrolyte consisting of protein and polysaccharide subunits, is now noted as a dilatant material when used as an emulsion stabilizer.[42] Its usual substitute, the hydrophobically modified starch, is only slightly weaker in dilatancy.

Application in Pharmacy

The shear-thinning effect offers the characteristics of a system that remains dispersed without settling when not in use but becomes fluid on shaking long enough to be dispensed as a medicine. The initial state is then regained at rest after use. This phenomenon applies to many systems. Topical application of pharmaceutical preparations is a mechanically similar operation and illustrates the use of thixotropic products in dermatological care.[43, 44] For bone regeneration using polymeric material with or without incorporated drug, a relatively low viscosity is required at high shear rates in order to apply the product properly; once processed, the material should either stop flowing or flow sufficiently slowly under anticipated low stresses. Thixotropic suspensions and emulsions can also be used for intramuscular injections.[45] A concentrated suspension of micronized procaine penicillin G in water has been shown to demonstrate a high degree of thixotropy.[46] The suspension broke down in thickness when it was passed through the hypodermic needle and produced a drug depot in the muscle at the injection site, resulting in a sustained drug release action. In nasal sprays, most corticosteroid suspensions such as Nasonex, Flonase, Vancenase AQ, Rinocort Aqua, and Nasacort AQ are thixotropic.[47] Using the recommended patient use procedure (shaking for 30 s, spraying, and immediately transferring the sample to a rheometer), the rheological behavior of these products was shown to exhibit the expected pattern in that, when initially shaken and dispensed, they flowed more freely, and a recovery of viscosity then followed that would likely inhibit the suspension from flowing out of the nasal cavity. There are, however, large differences in the degree of thixotropy among the products. Nasonex exhibited the highest yield stress, the largest initial and final viscosities, and the highest thixotropy. The rank order of the measured thixotropy for these products is the same as the order in which they are mentioned above.

IV. Dosage Forms for Dermatologic Applications

The skin is not only the target organ for the treatment of *dermatologic* diseases and conditions, but also one through which drugs may be noninvasively delivered to the systemic system. The latter is known as *transdermal* drug delivery, which has a different requirement in formulation strategy compared to those for localized topical applications. In fact, for dermatological use, it is desirable that the entire dose of drug be localized in the skin, even though one realizes that a small amount of drug may always reach the systemic circulation. We confine the current discussion to the dermatological systems.

Drug Delivery Considerations

Skin Physiology

Human skin is a heterogeneous tissue histologically divided into three distinct layers: the epidermis, the dermis, and the subcutaneous fatty tissue. The thickness of the epidermis, other than on the palms and soles of feet, is approximately 75 to 150 μm, depending on the location. The outermost portion of the epidermis is the stratum corneum, about 15 μm thick, which consists of layers of dead, flattened, dehydrated, and keratinized cells embedded in a lipid bilayer. These cells are constantly replaced by new cells that contain mainly the fibrous keratin (40%), water (40%), triglycerides, fatty acids, cholesterol, and phospholipids produced in the basal portion of the epidermis called the stratum germinativum. The stratum corneum functions as a barrier for the skin to prevent water losses from within and penetration of foreign substances from outside. The dermis is a thick layer (3–5 mm) composed of fibrous proteins (collagen, elastin, and reticulin) embedded in a polymeric, mucopolysaccharide gel. It is responsible for the strength and flexibility of the skin. Blood capillaries and nerve endings rise from the subcutaneous fat tissue into the dermis and up to the epidermis. Hair follicles and sebaceous and sweat glands originated in the dermal and subcutaneous layers extend from the dermis through the epidermis to the surface of the skin. Adjoining the dermis is the subcutaneous layer consisting mainly of connective tissue and fat cells. This layer helps to regulate body temperature and provides some protection from mechanical impacts. This is the site for subcutaneous injections and fat storage and sometimes the accumulation of lipophilic drugs.

The skin is a nonporous barrier to the entry of most chemicals. Being keratinized and rich in lipids, however, the stratum corneum behaves as a semipermeable membrane, allowing passive diffusion by drugs of low molecular weight and high lipophilicity.[48] Once below the stratum corneum, the drug may pass through the deeper epidermal tissues and into the dermis. At the vascular layer, it becomes available for adsorption into the systemic circulation. The systemic absorption of drugs through intact, noninflamed skin, however, is typically less than 5% of the applied drug.[49]

The epidermis is not merely a passive physical barrier between the body and the environment. Studies in the past 20 years have shown the expression of many cytochrome P450 (CYP) superfamily genes in the epidermal layers.[50] The CYP enzymes, some of which are inducible by drugs and by diseases such as psoriasis, play an important role in topical drug metabolism. In fact, most, if not all, drugs available for dermatologic use are substrates, inducers, or inhibitors of this enzyme family. Biotransformation of drugs may render a drug inactive before its therapeutic effect is achieved, but also permit the safe use of drugs that possess systemic toxicity. Topical tazarotene, e.g., is rapidly metabolized to tazarotenic acid and other metabolic products, so the risk of systemic toxicity is relatively low. CYP enzymes have also been targeted for treatment of certain skin disorders.[51, 52] Because of the critical role of CYP in the biochemistry of fungi and protozoa, miconazole and clotrimazole have been developed as skin antifungal agents to block synthesis of ergosterol, a major constituent of the fungal cell membrane, and CYP-dependent demethylation of lanosterol.

On the skin surface, there is also a film of lipophilic material composed of sebum, sweat, and desquamating epidermis cells, which varies in composition and thickness depending on the location. When an applied topical formulation loses its solvent through evaporation, the active drug and nonvolatile materials are mixed with the sebaceous film, creating a "secondary formulation." This formation can aid in the delivery of certain drugs. For example, the dapsone gel (Aczone, Allergan) contains water and the nonvolatile diethylene glycol monoethyl ether (DGME) as a vehicle. The drug is partially dissolved in DGME and as suspended particles. Once water dissipates after skin application, drug particles are concentrated in the residual nonvolatile solvent mixed with the sebaceous film, where the dissolved drug penetrates the skin, while the deposited particles dissolve slowly by sebum over time.

Drug Delivery and Absorption

The rate of drug transport across the skin can be described by Fick's law according to the equation

$$J = KDA\Delta C/h \tag{12-17}$$

where J is the steady-state flux, K is the partition coefficient, D is the diffusion coefficient, and ΔC is the concentration gradient of the drug across the stratum corneum. Also, A is the applied skin area and h is the thickness of the stratum corneum. This equation shows that the rate and extent of drug absorption depend on the drug concentration in the formulation and the surface area of the skin to which the drug is applied. The partition coefficient gives the relative affinity of the drug toward the skin and vehicle. An increase in aqueous drug solubility decreases drug absorption. Indeed, when a polar group is introduced into a steroid molecule, the resulting drug was shown to exhibit lowered lipophilicity, partition coefficient, and rate of diffusion across the stratum corneum.[53] Drug absorption can also be increased by a temporary increase in blood flow, as it facilitates the removal of drug from the absorption site, thus maintaining a high ΔC across the stratum corneum. The blood flow may be increased by raised temperature and by vasodilators such as nitroglycerin, nicotine, or caffeine.

Drug absorption through the skin is normally low, but can be increased by using skin penetration enhancers. The mechanism of skin penetration includes paracellular (between cells), transcellular (through cells), and transappendageal (via hair follicles, sweat, and sebaceous (fat) glands) pathways. Most drugs are absorbed through the tortuous path around cells and the lipid bilayer, i.e., the paracellular pathway. The pilosebaceous route, in contrast, is associated with formulations containing finely suspended particles, such as benzoyl peroxide and dapsone. Drug particles deposited into the follicles may slowly dissolve over time, creating a controlled-release or reservoir effect. In practice, it is likely that combinations of pathways are involved in topical drug absorption.

A skin penetration enhancer may act directly on the stratum corneum, fluidize the lipid channels, or alter the partition of the drug into the skin. The resistance of the stratum corneum to drug transport stems from its intricate structure involving the lipid bilayer, lipoproteins, the water/lipid ratio, and desquamating cells. A change in hydration can produce changes of the lipid-based intercellular structure. Hydration is, in fact, an important tool for modifying topical drug delivery. As epidermal cells swell, the aqueous/lipid ratio within the skin is altered, and these cells can become less resistant to mechanical shear and stress. Hydration also helps maintain normal desquamation via serine protease-mediated hydrolysis of proteins and peptides. In certain disease states such as psoriasis, water encourages cell desquamation and thus enhances drug penetration through thick, scaly plaques.

The commonly used penetration inducers include surfactants and propylene glycol. Surfactants are thought to increase cutaneous permeability through temporary or permanent disruption of the epidermal barrier. Cationic surfactants are toxic to cell membranes. It is not surprising that these molecules produce the largest extent of skin irritation and also the largest extent of skin permeability compared to anionic and non-ionic surfactants. Some non-ionic surfactants, such as oleic acid, have been found suitable for topical preparations. Isopropyl myristate was shown to fluidize the intercellular lipids of the stratum corneum and partially dissolve them,[54] and it is used to produce rapid skin penetration by corticosteroids (e.g., Clobex Spray, Galderma). Propylene glycol (PG) is the most widely used agent in topical formulations, owing to its usage as a solvent, antimicrobial, and penetration enhancer. The mechanism of permeability enhancement by PG varies with concentration and formulation type. PG can promote transepidermal water loss by extracting water from the protein domain, causing a change of the barrier function.[55] While the dehydration impedes drug transport, PG increases the skin partition of drugs solubilized in it and aids the actions of other skin penetration enhancers.[56] At high concentrations, PG may promote desquamation, which enhances drug permeation.

Topical Therapeutic Agents

There are hundreds of dermatological disorders caused by inflammatory, infective, and autoimmune diseases or exposures to allergens and environmental factors. The therapeutic agents used for their treatments can be classified as corticosteroids, antibiotics, antifungals, antipruritics, counterirritants, keratolytics, protectants, and emollients. They are frequently prescribed, second only to oral medicines.

Corticosteroids

Most glucocorticoids are topically active against inflammatory dermatoses, and the activity increases with increasing lipophilicity. The commonly used drugs for treating inflammatory dermatoses include, among others, fluocinolone acetonide (0.025%), alclometasone diproprionate (0.05%), triamcinolone acetonide (0.1%), and hydrocortisone acetate (0.5% or 1%), made in cream and ointment. A patient may respond better to one topical corticosteroid than to another, irrespective of their relative potencies. Topical corticosteroids do not cause systemic effects when used on small areas of skin. When applied to large areas of the body, systemic absorption may occur, especially if the skin is damaged or if occlusive dressings are used. The anti-inflammatory action can mask symptoms of infection, and delayed use of topical steroid until after the infection is controlled with topical antibiotics may be warranted.

Antiacne

Acne vulgaris, a common skin disease with manifestations of seborrhea, comedones, papules, pimples, nodules, and possibly scarring, is caused by hormone-induced blockage in the sebaceous follicles. This blockage leads to hyperkeratinization, enlargement of sebaceous gland, increased production of sebum, and the formation of comedones (plugs of keratin and sebum) in the pilosebaceous units. The acne lesions become more severe and inflammatory when infected by the naturally present Propionibacterium acnes. Noninflammatory acne is treated using benzoyl peroxide and salicylic acid. Benzoyl peroxide (in gels and lotions; 2.5–20%) is the most used drug for the treatment of mild to moderate acne vulgaris. It helps to bleach out dead skin and cell debris from follicles, and it reduces the bacterial count in the infected area. As peroxide, the drug can produce mild side effects such as irritant dermatitis, dry skin, and sensitivity to sunlight. Salicylic acid is a concentration-dependent keratolytic agent. For acne treatment (in lotions and creams; 0.5–2%) it promotes desquamation in follicles of acne-prone skin and reduces pore blockage. At high concentrations, it is formulated as flexible collodion (up to 17%) or plaster (40%) for the treatment of warts, corns, and calluses.

Antibiotics for acne treatment are reserved for more severe cases. Commonly used topical antibiotics include clindamycin (solution, lotion, or gel; 1%); erythromycin (solution, gel, and ointment; 2%); and to a lesser extent, tetracycline. The antibacterial dapsone (diaminodiphenyl sulfone), formulated as a 5% gel (Aczone, Allergan), is also used for the treatment of acne. Topical retinoids, such as tretinoin (Retin-A), adapalene (Differin), and tazarotene (Tazorac), are another class of drugs for acne treatment. The retinoids are thought to influence the cell cycle in the follicular lining and thus prevent cell hyperkeratinization. Retinol, which has similar but reduced effect on acne compared to the retinoids, is used in many over-the-counter moisturizers.

Antibacterials and Antifungals

A wide variety of topical antibiotic preparations, such as gentamicin sulfate cream and ointment (0.1%, Schering) and Neosporin ointment (containing 5000 units/g polymyxin B sulfate, 400 units/g bacitracin zinc, and 3.5 mg/g neomycin, Warner Wellcome), are available for prophylaxis and treatment of skin infections. Neosporin is the first aid triple antibiotic preparation containing bacitracin, which is effective against gram-positive streptococci and staphylococci, and polymyxin B and neomycin, both of which are effective against gram-negative organisms. Among the antifungal preparations, nystatin cream (0.5%, Westwood-Squibb) and miconazole nitrate cream (2%, Ortho) are effective against cutaneous candidiasis. Nystatin is also used to treat infection by *Cryptococcus*, whereas miconazole is used in treatment of tinea infections caused by *Trichophyton species*. Other antifungal agents used in topical applications include benzoic and salicylic acid and undecylenic acid.

Antipruritics

The antipruritics, or anti-itch drugs, are used for the relief of pain and itching due to skin irritation, sunburns, allergic reactions, eczema, psoriasis, insect bites, and urticaria from poison ivy. The active drug usually comes from one of several classes including antihistamines such as diphenhydramine (Benadryl); corticosteroids such as hydrocortisone topical cream; local anesthetics such as benzocaine (Lanacaine) cream and lidocaine ointment (2.5%); and counterirritants including phenol, menthol, camphor, mint oil, and coal tar. The commonly known calamine lotion, which contains zinc oxide and iron(III) oxide, actually has little or no anti-itching effect.

Astringent and Protectives

Zinc oxide is used as an astringent (40%, ointment) for various skin conditions. It absorbs skin secretion and forms a protective barrier against external factors. Zinc oxide is also used in sunscreening, which blocks both type A and type B ultraviolet (uv) radiation. Ultraviolet A does not cause sunburn but increases the risk of malignant melanomas. One of the common skin reactions to chronic exposure to sun rays is actinic or solar keratosis. Actinic keratoses are precancerous, thus suggesting a risk of potential malignant transformation at a later time. A fluorouracil cream (Efudex, Roche) may be used for the treatment of multiple actinic keratoses. Ointments and creams may be prepared to contain materials such as antioxidant, alpha hydroxyl acids, moisturizers, etc., for protection against various external factors. These materials may be either the compounds that make up the base of the preparation or the active ingredients in them.

Emollients, or moisturizers, are preparations used to bring softness to the skin. Such preparations usually contain oils, humectants, petrolatum, and other oleaginous agents. As noted earlier, the skin structure prevents serious loss of water from substratum corneum layers; the key factor for a soft skin is water retention in the stratum corneum. Moisturizers, then, are designed to prevent evaporation of water from the skin surface. Oleaginous compounds are useful, because they can reduce water evaporation through the formation of an occlusive layer on the skin surface. Indeed, for dry and aged skin, the most effective moisturizers are heavy oil– or petrolatum-based products, whereas for normal skin, lightweight oils (cetyl alcohol) or hydrophilic ointments are appropriate.

Topical Dosage Forms

Topical formulations are used (1) to deliver medication to the skin, (2) to protect or heal intact or injured skin from the external environment, and (3) to help moisturize the skin. The Food and Drug Administration (FDA) recognizes topical dosage forms as solution, suspension, lotion, paste, gel, ointment, cream, and others (e.g., foams, aerosols, powders, and patches). Among these, ointments, creams, gels, and pastes are referred to as semisolids. They are less pourable than a liquid and less rigid than a solid.

The advantages of topical drug delivery over systemic drug administration for treating dermatologic disorders are that (1) drug delivery is noninvasive, (2) it provides high drug concentration to the site of action, and (3) it results in little or no systemic drug absorption or toxicity. The disadvantages of topical drug delivery lie mainly in the fact that drug levels cannot be monitored as in systemic drug delivery. Treatment can be assessed only qualitatively with clinical efficacy, which often varies with respect to patients and products. There are also problems associated with self-medication in terms of dose measurement and patient compliance and with skin irritation or hypersensitivity reactions from patients to the drug or the delivery system.

The criteria for an acceptable topical preparation and their relation to application effectiveness are illustrated in **Table 12-4.**

Clearly, regardless of the dosage form type, smooth and homogeneous preparations are essential, and the viscosity of the system plays an important role in determining its physical stability, use, and the extent of therapeutic outcome.[57]

Liquid Formulations

As defined by the Center for Drug Evaluation and Research (CDER) of the FDA, a solution is a liquid preparation that contains one or more chemical substances dissolved in a suitable solvent or mixture of mutually miscible solvent. The dissolved substances may include buffer

Table 12-4 Criteria for Acceptance and Application Effectiveness in Topical Preparation

Dosage Form Quality	Application Effectiveness
Acceptable consistency and uniformity	Drug is evenly distributed in formulation.
Small particle sizes: < 200–300 μm	Product should be nongritty when applied to skin.
Physically, chemically, microbiologically stable	Product is safe for use.
No skin irritation or sensitization	Side effects are minimized.
Controlled viscosity based on intended use	Drug provides even spreading, sustained drug level, and needed duration of drug exposure.
Cosmetically and anatomically acceptable	Patient is in compliance.

agents to maintain pH, surfactants to enhance drug solubility, and polymers to increase viscosity. Solutions spread easily on the skin surface, but they can easily be wiped off as well. Liniments are solutions in oil, alcoholic solutions of soap, or emulsions. These formulations are applied by rubbing and should be used on intact skin. They are used for temporary relief of muscular aches and pains.

Lotions are liquid preparations containing very fine powders of solid materials or dilute dispersed liquid substances. They exhibit high fluidity that enables them to be uniformly applied over a large area of the skin. A thin coating of the particles is left behind on the surface after the vehicle dries, which may provide sustained drug action. These suspensions and emulsions tend to separate on long standing, and they should be well shaken before use. A traditional preparation is calamine lotion, which contains zinc oxide and calamine (each 8%); the latter consists of zinc oxide and a small amount of ferric oxide that gives calamine its pink color. This lotion is prepared by suspending zinc oxide and calamine in bentonite magma and calcium hydroxide solution, followed by adding the calcium hydroxide solution to the desired volume. Calamine lotion is used as a protective preparation against sunburn and other skin conditions. A phenolated calamine lotion, formed by adding liquefied phenol (1%) to the calamine lotion, is antipruritic (anti-itch) because of its anesthetic and antiseptic effects.

Collodion, USP, is a yellowish viscous solution of pyroxylin (~5% w/w) in ether and ethanol. When it is applied to the skin surface, the solvents evaporate, leaving behind a thin film coating, which may be flexible or semirigid, depending on other additives. The flexible collodions, which enhance patient comfort, are made using castor oil, which acts as a plasticizer. Because of the film deposit, the incorporated drug may be kept in contact with the skin for an extended time. The collodions are also used to seal minor cuts and wounds. They are, however, flammable and volatile. Another organic polymeric solution preparation is lacquer, which is applied to nail surfaces. For example, Plenac is an antifungal nail lacquer containing ciclopirox and butyl monoester of poly(methylvinyl ether/maleic acid) in a mixed solvent of ethyl acetate and isopropyl alcohol. The applied lacquer produces a drug–polymer film after the solvents are evaporated, which allows the drug to remain in extended contact with the nail and adjacent skin area.

Ointments and Creams

According to FDA CDER, an *ointment* is a semisolid preparation intended for external application to the skin or mucous membranes, whereas a *cream* is a semisolid dosage form containing one or more drug substances dissolved or dispersed in a suitable base. Ointment and cream may be differentiated by the base from which the semisolid is formed. Traditionally, the definition of cream includes both oil-in-water (O/W) and water-in-oil (W/O) emulsions, which are regarded as more cosmetically acceptable than an ointment made using an oleaginous or anhydrous base.

There are four general categories of bases for ointment and cream preparations: hydrocarbon (oleaginous) base, *absorption base*, water-removable base, and water-soluble base. The absorption bases include those (anhydrous) that absorb water to form W/O emulsions and those that are W/O emulsions. Specific examples of these bases and their properties are given in **Table 12-5**. In general, an oleaginous base is greasy and more difficult to wash off, thus allowing the drug to remain in contact with the skin for a prolonged time. Such a base also forms an occlusive barrier, which can prevent the loss of moisture from the skin's stratum corneum, and thus produces an emollient effect on dry, irritated skin. Creams, in contrast, can be easily applied to skin. W/O emulsions have good emollient properties and provide some degree of occlusion, whereas the O/W emulsions are easily washable.

Table 12-5 Properties of Semisolid Bases for Ointments and Creams

Base	Example	Properties
Hydrocarbon	Petrolatum USP, white ointment USP, white petrolatum, Vaseline	Water-insoluble, will not absorb water; occlusive and emollient
Anhydrous	Hydrophilic petrolatum anhydrous, lanolin, Aquaphor, Aquabase	Water-insoluble; will absorb water-forming W/O emulsion; occlusive; emollient
W/O emulsion	Cold cream USP, Eucerin Hydrous lanolin Hydrocream	Water-insoluble, less occlusive More cosmetically acceptable Useful as emollients
O/W emulsion	Hydrophilic ointment USP Unibase, Dermabase	Water-washable; can be diluted Nonocclusive but cosmetically elegant
Water-soluble	Polyethylene glycol ointment USP	Water-soluble and washable, nonocclusive and nongreasy

Hydrocarbon Bases

These bases include petrolatum, mineral oil, paraffins, and waxes. They have no affinity toward water and are used for protecting the skin from external factors such as diaper rash and preventing moisture loss from the skin by forming an occlusive layer. Petrolatum USP is a yellowish fatty material consisting of a mixture of semisolid hydrocarbons extracted from petroleum, with a melting range between 38 and 60°C. White petrolatum USP is a decolorized petrolatum, which is more aesthetically acceptable than petrolatum in formulations. Mineral oil, or liquid petrolatum, is a mixture of liquid hydrocarbons, which is used for the incorporation of large amounts of solid substances such as zinc oxide, salicylic acid, and talc.

Absorption Bases

When a water-in-oil emulsifier is added to an oleaginous base, the mixture becomes an absorption (anhydrous) base capable of absorbing large amounts of water or hydroalcoholic solution. Hydrophilic petrolatum, e.g., which consists of cholesterol, stearyl alcohol, white wax, and white petrolatum, can absorb water up to 10% of its weight. Aquaphor, a purified hydrophilic petrolatum for the incorporation of water-soluble drugs, has the capacity to absorb water up to 3 times its weight. Lanolin is a fatty, semisolid mass obtained from the wool of sheep containing 25–30% water. The anhydrous lanolin is insoluble in water but absorbs water to form W/O emulsion. The anhydrous bases are less greasy than the oleaginous bases, but are sufficient emollient for the treatment of dry skins. The water absorption property of these bases allows for inclusion of water-soluble drugs with rapid-release characteristics.

W/O Emulsion Bases

Cold cream, a white, W/O emulsion formed in the mixture of cetyl ester wax, white wax, mineral oil, sodium borate, and water, and Eucerin cream, a W/O emulsion formed from petrolatum, mineral oil, mineral wax, wool wax, and alcohol, are members of this group. These bases contain water or hydroalcohol and can absorb water up to 50%. Although less occlusive than the oleaginous bases, they are more cosmetically elegant and easier to spread on the skin. These bases are useful as emollients and as a dosage form for hydrophilic drugs.

Water-Removable Bases

Semisolids based on O/W emulsions are less fatty, more elegant, and more easily removed from the skin than those made in hydrocarbon and absorption bases. A good example is the preparation of hydrophilic ointment USP (see Example 12-2), in which the oleaginous stearyl alcohol and white petrolatum are emulsified into water with the aid of propylene glycol, which assists in obtaining a more intimate dispersion of soap, oils, grease, and other substances in water. Bases of this group present a product of cosmetic-like appearance. This, together with their ease of application and removal, often produces a desirable psychological effect on the patient and ensures better patient cooperation, resulting in more efficacious therapy. These bases are useful for the inclusion of water-insoluble drugs for rapid drug release.

Water-Soluble Bases

The water-soluble bases contain polyethylene glycol (PEG) in the molecular weight range of 400 to 6000. Their consistencies vary from a soft semisolid to a hard, waxy solid formulation, depending on the molecular weights of PEG used. The smoothness of these bases renders them highly acceptable for making hand lotions, suntan creams, and skin creams. A peroxide ointment that is stable may be prepared using polyethylene glycols, whereas oil-type bases inactivate the peroxide. The PEG ointment can also be used in making suppositories. Polyethylene glycol ointment USP consists of PEG 3350 (40%) and PEG 400 (60%). Note that these bases are water-soluble, but do not contain water.

Example 12-2: Describe the function of each ingredient in hydrophilic ointment USP, and show how you would prepare this product.

Methylparaben	25 mg
Propylparaben	15 mg
Sodium lauryl sulfate	1 g
Propylene glycol	12 g (sp gr 1.035; 11.6 mL)
Stearyl alcohol	25 g
White petrolatum	25 g
Purified water	37 g (37 mL)

Solution:

Function:

Petrolatum: to provide smoothness and softening effect when applied to skin
Methylparaben/ethylparaben: preservative blend required for ointments and creams

Sodium lauryl sulfate: oil-in-water emulsifier

Stearyl alcohol: adjuvant emulsifier to add hardness to ointment

Propylene glycol: to impart a smoother dispersion of soap, oil, grease, and other substances in water

Preparation:

1. Melt stearyl alcohol and white petrolatum together on a hot plate (70°C).
2. Dissolve the remaining ingredients in water, and heat the solution to 70°C.

3. Add the oleaginous phase slowly to the aqueous phase, stirring constantly.
4. Remove from heat and stir the mixture until it congeals.

Observation: With an O/W emulsion base, damaged skin is assured of a mist conditioning. Release of drug is enhanced by virtue of a water phase and lowered surface tension on the skin brought about by the surfactants. The keratolytic effects have been shown to take a shorter time with the use of emulsion base than with the use of an oleaginous base type.

Gels

As defined in USP 30/NF 25, gels or jellies are semisolids consisting of suspensions made up of either small inorganic particles or large organic molecules interpenetrated by a liquid. Inorganic gels showing networks of small discrete particles are referred to as two-phase gels. If the particle size of the dispersed phase is large, it is called a magma. Single-phase gels are uniform dispersions of organic macromolecules in a liquid where no apparent boundaries exist between the dispersed molecules and the medium. These gels are made using synthetic polymers or natural gums as the gelling agents. The medium is usually aqueous, but can be alcoholic or oleaginous.

The gelling phenomenon by organic polymers stems from the formation of a three-dimensional matrix due to the high degree of cross-linking or association between hydrated molecules in the solvent. This structure restricts and traps the movement of the solvent, and this results in increased viscosity. The particles in such systems are of colloidal sizes, and the gel systems can behave as a thixotropic body, which undergoes a shear- and time-dependent thinning effect. As nongreasy semisolids, gels containing penetration enhancer are popular for administering anti-inflammatory, antiacne, and antipruritic medications. Organic polymers used for pharmaceutical gel preparations include carbomers, poloxmers, cellulose derivatives, and natural gums such as acacia, tragacanth, and sodium alginate. Among these, the carbomers, which can swell in water up to 1000 times their original volume, are very popular for the preparation of topical gels. Some of these products are benzoyl peroxide (Desquam-X, Westwood-Squibb; carbomer 940) and clindamycin (Cleocin T, Pharmacia-Upjohn; carbomer 934P) for treatment of acne vulgaris; desoximetasone (Topicort, Hoechst Marion Roussel; carbomer 940) and clobetasone (Temovate Gel, Glaxo-Wellcome; carbomer 934P) as anti-inflammatory/antipruritics; and progesterone (Crinone Gel, Wyeth-Ayerst; carbomer 934P) as a vaginal bioadhesive. The viscosity for an 0.5% gel containing carbomer 934P or 940 is 30,000–60,000 cP.

Gels can be prepared using standard laboratory techniques. Dispersion of the gelling agent generally requires a slow, deliberate addition of fine powders to a vortexed medium to prevent clumping of the material. A completely dispersed system will gel with time, up to 24 h for natural gums, and is subjected to the temperature effect. The gelling agents may be prewetted, using agents such as propylene glycol, glycerin, or alcohol. Premixing some gelling agents with other powders often aids the dispersion process. To ensure uniform distribution, all ingredients should be dissolved in the solvent before the gelling agent is added. The gelation can be triggered by temperature changes, such as for the poloxamers[58, 59] and some cellulose derivatives,[60] by pH change such as for the carbomers,[61] or by the presence of cations such as for the alginate.[62] These mechanisms have been tested for the formation of in situ gels that can be injected (intramuscularly) as a liquid but become semisolid under the physiological environment. For example, the pH is an important

Table 12-6 Properties of Some Pharmaceutical Gelling Agents

Compounds	Concentration	Acceptable pH	Properties
Carbomers	0.5–2%	5–10	Maximum viscosity occurs at pH 7.
Carboxymethylcellulose (CMC)	4–6%	2–10	Precipitation occurs at pH 2.
Sodium CMC		5–10	Viscosity decreases at pH below 5.
Sodium alginate	Up to 10%	4–10	Alginic acid precipitates at pH 3 and gels in presence of cations.
Propylene glycol alginate	1–5%	3–6	
Tragacanth		4–8	Powders can be wetted with propylene glycol before dispersion; it gels on cooling.
Poloxamers (Pluronic F-127)	15–50%	Stable in acidic or basic media	Thermal gelation occurs.
Gelatin	10–30%		It is prepared by dispersion in hot water and gels on cooling; gel point: 30°C.
Methylcellulose	1–5%		It gels when heated to 50°C.
Colloidal silicon dioxide		7.5	Viscosity decreases above pH 10.7, due to formation of silicate; viscosity is independent of temperature.

factor for the gelation of carbomer resins. Carbomer (pK_a, ~ 6.0) solution (1%) has pH 2.5–3.0; the addition of a base, typically NaOH or triethanolamine if the system contains alcohol, is required for the gelling process. Maximum viscosity occurs at pH 7, with an acceptable pH range of 5–10. If it is overneutralized, viscosity will be lowered, which cannot be regained by lowering the pH with an acid. Adding alcohol to carbomer gels will decrease the viscosity, which may be overcome by increasing the concentration of the gelling agent. Some basic properties of different gelling agents are summarized in **Table 12-6**. Note that preservatives are generally required for the preparation of pharmaceutical gels.

Pastes

Pastes are prepared to contain a large amount of solids dispersed in a base. They are stiffer than ointment, and when applied to the skin, they remain at the applied site longer than ointments. These formulations can absorb skin secretions and provide a protective barrier for the applied area. Among the few pastes in use today is the zinc oxide paste, which contains zinc oxide (25%), starch, and white petrolatum.

Laboratory Preparation of Ointments and Creams

In making an actual product, the selection of a semisolid base is of prime importance if the finished product is to be effective for the intended use. As a protective ointment, e.g., it is necessary that the ointment neither penetrate the skin barriers nor facilitate the absorption of substances through this barrier. An antiseptic cream, in contrast, is used to destroy or inhibit the growth of bacteria, which may be deep in the skin. A base that has the capacity to deliver the medication effectively is therefore desirable. One can learn the properties of these bases through experiments and, of equal importance, explore the diversity of the bases for different formulation approaches to the same problem.

General Compounding Procedures

The standard laboratory wares include an ointment slab (pill tile), ointment pad, and large stainless steel spatulas. Ointment slabs are either ground glass or porcelain plates, which provide a hard, nonabsorbable surface for mixing. Ointment pads placed in the work area allow for easier and quicker cleanup during and after laboratory work. Large metal spatulas are used instead of smaller ones because they have the proper combination of flexibility and strength for adequate shearing and mixing. Black rubber or plastic spatulas are not used in ointment compounding. When heat is used to melt ingredients, a water bath or a low-temperature hot plate (25–120°C) will be needed. Most ointment base materials melt around 70°C. These two heating devices should provide adequate temperature control to prevent overheating of the samples.

The two methods used for the preparation of ointments are incorporation and fusion. By the incorporation method, the ingredients and the ointment base are mixed via geometric dilution. Because the amount of drug to be incorporated into the ointment is much less than the amount of ointment, geometric dilution begins by incorporating the drug into an amount of ointment of approximately the same size. A second amount of ointment approximately equal to the first mixture is then added and mixed. This stepwise dilution is continued until all of the ointment has been used.

The reduction of particle size of a powder material before it is incorporated into an ointment base is an important step for ointment compounding, especially when a large quantity of the solid is used. This is done by levigating (mixing) the solid material in a nonsolvent (of same volume as the solid), using a mortar and pestle, to form a smooth dispersion. The levigating agent should be physically and chemically compatible with the phase into which the drug is dispersed. Usually, mineral oil is a good levigating agent for drug distributed in an oleaginous base. If the drug is to be dispersed into an aqueous phase, liquid such as glycerin or propylene glycol can be used as the levigating agent.

Some ointment base materials, such as beeswax, paraffin, stearyl alcohol, and high-molecular-weight PEGs, cannot be easily used unless they are melted. The method of choice is then fusion, in which a procedure of melting, mixing, cooling, and stirring is logically carried out. When a number of ingredients are melted, the one with the highest melting point is melted first. The heat is then reduced, and the ingredient with the next-highest melting point is added and melted. The process continues until all ingredients have been added. This ensures that the ingredients are exposed to the lowest possible temperature. When an oil phase and an aqueous phase are being mixed together to make an ointment by fusion, both the oil and aqueous phases are heated and mixed at the same temperature. It is helpful if the aqueous phase is heated a few degrees higher than the oil phase prior to mixing, because the aqueous phase tends to cool faster than the oil phase and may thus cause premature solidification of some ingredients. The temperature, however, should be the lowest possible, so that the time of heating is shortened and the quantity of water loss through evaporation is minimized.

Cooling is an important part of the ointment compounding process. Accelerated cooling, such as by putting the melt on water or ice, can and will change the consistency of the final product, making it stiffer than desired. The addition of volatile ingredients, such as oils, flavors, or drugs, should be done when the system is cooled but is still fluid enough for adequate mixing. Ointments should be cooled until just a few degrees above solidification before they are poured into tubes or jars, although this is not the preferred method of packing, as it takes several hours for most bases to achieve their final consistency and texture after compounding.

Preparation of Ointments

The various types of ointment bases can all be made using the fusion method. The preparation for each type of base is illustrated in Example 12-3. These bases differ from one another based on their water content and affinity. The oleaginous base is void of water. They are poor dosage forms for drug release, but are excellent protective and emollient ointments. The anhydrous (absorption) base can absorb water to form W/O emulsion with stearyl alcohol as the stabilizer, whereas the W/O emulsion base has 20% water. Similar to the W/O emulsion base, the water-removable (O/W emulsion) base is hydrous and contains about 40% water. The polyethylene glycol base is water-miscible, but it *does not contain water*.

Example 12-3: Procedures for making 100 g of different ointment bases.

(*a*) Hydrocarbon base (white ointment)

White wax	5%
White petrolatum	95%

Procedure:

1. Melt the white wax (5 g) on a hot plate (70–75°C).
2. After the wax has completely melted, add petrolatum, and allow the entire mixture to remain on the hot plate until liquefied.
3. Remove from heat and stir the mixture until it has congealed.

(*b*) Anhydrous base

Cholesterol	3%
Stearyl alcohol	3%
White wax	8%
White petrolatum	86%

Procedure:

1. Melt the stearyl alcohol, white wax, and petrolatum together on a hot plate.
2. Add cholesterol to the mixture; stir until completely dissolved.
3. Remove the mixture from the hot plate, and stir until congealed.

(*c*) W/O emulsion base (cold cream)

White wax	12.0%	
Cetyl esters	12.5%	
Mineral oil	56.0%	(sp gr 0.9; 62.2 mL)
Sodium borate	0.5%	
Water	19.0%	(19 mL)

Procedure:

1. Melt the white wax and cetyl esters on a hot plate.
2. Add the mineral oil to this mixture, and bring the temperature to 70°C.
3. Dissolve the sodium borate in water, and heat the solution to 70°C.

4. At the desired temperature, remove both phases from the hot plate and add the aqueous phase, slowly and with constant stirring, to the oil phase.
5. Stir briskly and continuously until congealed.

(*d*) O/W emulsion base: See Example 12-2.

(*e*) Water-soluble base

Polyethylene glycol 400	60%	(sp gr 1.12, 53.6 mL)
Polyethylene glycol 3350	40%	(40 g)

Procedure:

1. Melt PEG 400 and PEG 3350 on a hot plate.
2. Warm the mixture to about 65°C.
3. Remove from the hot plate and stir until congealed.

Incorporation of Drugs into Ointment

The methods for drug incorporation into different ointment bases are discussed below. When appropriate, the formulation of a 2% salicylic acid ointment will be considered to assess the properties of the ointment dosage forms. Salicylic acid, at 2%, is used for topical treatment of acne vulgaris.

Hydrocarbon (Oleaginous) Bases

To incorporate an insoluble drug into these bases, levigate the powder with mineral oil, using a mortar and pestle, and incorporate the wetted powder into the ointment base. If the drug is soluble in the base, it can be incorporated into the base by fusion. In this case, the base is liquefied and the drug is added to the molten base. The mixture is then allowed to cool with occasional stirring.

Anhydrous (Absorption) Bases

The inclusion of drug into these bases can be done by incorporation or fusion. The selection of levigating agent will be based on the phase (internal or external) in which the drug is incorporated. If the drug resides in the internal phase (aqueous), the levigating agent should be water-miscible (glycerin, ethanol, water, or propylene glycol). If the drug resides in the external phase, mineral oil should be used. For highly water-soluble drugs, a small amount of aqueous solution can be added directly and incorporated into the base. Incorporation of a larger quantity of water can be difficult, which may require heating and/or adding more emulsifier. The solubility of salicylic acid in water is about 1 g in 460 mL, suggesting that this drug can be incorporated easily in the external phase, but not so easily in the internal phase.

W/O Emulsion Bases

Water-insoluble drugs can be directly incorporated into the external phase using a spatula. The levigating agent should be mineral oil, which is miscible with the oil phase. The same considerations for incorporating water-soluble ingredients into the anhydrous bases also apply to the W/O emulsion bases. Salicylic acid can be incorporated into the external phase. An alternative would be to use the salt of salicylic acid for incorporation into the aqueous phase.

O/W Emulsion Bases

Insoluble powders, as in salicylic acid, or a small quantity of aqueous solutions (for water-soluble drug) can be incorporated into the external phase, using a mortar and pestle. The levigating agent for an O/W emulsion base should be water, Propylene glycol (PG), glycerin, or other liquid that is miscible with water. One can consider the use of a soluble form of the drug, as in sodium salicylate for incorporation into the external phase. A small quantity of oil can be directly incorporated into the base. If a large amount of an oil is to be added, the addition of more emulsifier would be necessary.

Water-Miscible Bases

Water-soluble drugs can be dissolved in a small quantity of water and incorporated into the base. Insoluble powders will require a water-miscible levigating agent such as glycerin, propylene glycol, or polyethylene glycol 400. Oils can be added into these bases by first mixing the oil with glycerin or propylene glycol and then incorporating the mixture into the base. Heat may be necessary if a large amount of the liquid is to be added. Salicylic acid can be incorporated as an insoluble powder.

Effect of Ointment Bases on Drug Release

The partition of water-insoluble drug into the skin may decrease in an oleaginous phase due to the drug's affinity toward the formulation. Hence, neither the hydrocarbon nor the anhydrous base is a good system for the release of a lipophilic drug. Using salicylic acid as an example, the release of the drug from the oleaginous bases would be slow. Drug release can be significantly increased when the ointment base shows an increased water affinity. The water-soluble and water-removable bases would be the choices for a rapid release of drugs such as salicylic acid. The water-soluble base is also useful for drugs that undergo hydrolytic degradations, as formulations can be made with the water soluble base that contains no water. For hydrophilic drugs, the anhydrous and W/O emulsion systems can provide greater drug release rates, as the base has low affinity for the drug and also absorbs water, thus allowing easier passage of the drug through the ointment matrix.

Tests, Packaging, Storage, and Labeling

For extemporaneous compounding, the following should be determined and recorded: weight and volume of final product, color, odor, appearance, texture, homogeneity, pH, and viscosity. Semisolid preparations are packaged either in large-mouth ointment jars or in metal (tin) or plastic tubes (collapsible tubes) and tested for minimum fill to ensure that the net weight or volume is properly labeled. Ointments should be kept at room temperature and away from excessive heat. The product label should contain information usually required for pharmaceutical products and, as specified by USP, the type of base used in the formation. Ointments and creams are susceptible to contamination by *Pseudomonas aeruginosa* and *Staphylococcus aureus*. This requires that preservatives be added to the topical formulation, which can be the parabens, phenols, benzoic acid, quaternary ammonium salts, or sorbic acid.

V. Chapter Summary

The central theme of this chapter is viscosity, a liquid property that goes, in fact, contrary to what a liquid can do best—flow. When the viscosity of a liquid increases, the system becomes increasingly solidlike, giving rise to various forms of viscoelastic bodies in lotions, creams, gels, ointments, and pastes. We have studied the science that describes these changes, namely, the rheology, to ascertain how viscosity changes with shear stress and time, and we correlated the viscosity changes with changes in molecular structure, whether it be inorganic particles or organic macromolecules in a dispersed system. This knowledge allows us to develop methods for the preparation of stable liquid and semisolid systems, so that their rheological behaviors can be utilized for the purposes of drug delivery and treatment. Topical therapeutic agents are frequently prescribed, second only to orally administered medicines. In addition, numerous topical products, with or without medication, are sold over the counter. There is a unique perspective about such products in that the patient's acceptance of them is often persuaded by the pharmacist's knowledge of their physical properties. We have discussed the principles, use, and preparation of these products in this regard. Traditionally pharmacists not only should know these medications, but also should be able to prepare such a product in pharmacy or in the laboratory setting.

VI. References

1. Newton I. "The resistance which arises from the lack of slipperiness of the parts of the liquid, others things being equal, is proportional to the velocity with which the parts of the liquid are separated from one another—*Newton's law of viscosity*," in *Principia Mathematica*, 1687.
2. Hooke R. "For relatively small deformation of an object, the displacement or size of the deformation is directly proportional to the deforming force or load. Under these conditions the object returns to its original shape and size upon removal of load—*Hooke's law of elasticity*, 1678," Britannica Online Encyclopedia.
3. Pfitzner J. Poiseuille and his law, *Anaesthesia*. 31:273–275, 1976.
4. Nemethy A and Scheraga HA. *J Chem Phys*. 36:3382, 1962.
5. Gelman-Constantin J, Carignano MA, Szieifer I, Marceca EJ, and Corti HR. *J Chem Phys*. 133:024506, 2010.
6. Wilkinson WL. *Non-Newtonian Fluids*. New York, Pergamon, 1960.
7. Mujumbar A, Beris AN, and Metzner AB. *J Non-Newtonian Fluid Mech*. 102:157, 2002.
8. Wang Q, Wang J, Lu G, Defamore MS, and Berkland C. *Biomaterials*. 31:4980–4986, 2010.
9. Fischer EK. *Colloidal Dispersions*. New York, Wiley, 1950.
10. Sherman P. *Industrial Rheology*. New York, Academic, 1970.
11. Yakatan GJ and Araujo OE. *J Pharm Sci*. 57:155, 1968.
12. Sgangraw R, Grim W, and Mattocks AM. *Trans Soc Rheology*. 5:247, 1961.
13. Mewis J and Wagner NJ. *Adv Colloid Interface Sci*. 147–148:214–227, 2009.
14. Blijdenstein TB, Veerman C, and van der Linden E. *Langmuir*. 20:4881–4884, 2004.
15. Chung B, Ramalrishnan S, Bandyopadhay R, et al. *Phys Rev Lett*. 96:228301, 2006.
16. Helgeson ME, Wagner NJ, and Vlasopoulos D. *J Rheol*. 51:297, 2007.
17. Mewis J, Spaull AJB, and Helsen J. *Nature*. 253:618, 1975.
18. Dullaert K and Mewis J. *J Rheol*. 49:1213, 2005.
19. Montes S and White JL. *J Non-Newtonian Fluid Mech*. 49:277, 1993.
20. Ragouilliaux A, Ovarlez G, Shahidzadeh-Bonn N, Hertzhaft B, Palermo T, and Coussot P. *Phys Rev E Stat Nonlin Soft Matter Phys*. 76:051408, 2007.
21. Leheny RL and Nagel SR. *Phys Rev B*. 57:5154, 1998.
22. Willenbacher N. *J Colloid Interface Sci*. 182:501, 1996.
23. Viasnoff V and Lequeux F. *Phys Rev Lett*. 89:069701, 2002.
24. Laun HM, Bung R, and Schmidt F. *J Rheol*. 35:999, 1991.
25. Barns HA. *J Rheol*. 33:329, 1989.
26. Keller DS and Keller DV Jr. *J Rheol*. 34:1267, 1990; Samyn JC and Jung WY. *J Pharm Sci*. 56(2):188–191, 1967.
27. Chong CW, Eriksen SP, and Swintosky JV. *J Am Pharm Assoc*. 49:547–552, 1960.
28. Kani H and Amari T. *Rheol Acta*. 34:303, 1995.
29. Oates KM, Krause WE, Jones RL, and Colby RH. *J R Soc Interface*. 3:167–174, 2006.
30. Jones DS, Woolfson AD, and Brown AF. *Pharm Res*. 15:1131–1136, 1998.

31. Rohn CL. J. *Water-borne Coatings*. 10:12–17, 1987.
32. Adeyeye MC, Jain AC, Ghorab M, and Reilly WJ. *AAPS Pharm Sci Tech*. 3:E8, 2002.
33. Apter JT and Graessley WW. *Biophys J*. 10:539–555, 1970.
34. Dragicevic-Curic N, Winter S, Stupar M, Milic J, Krajisnik D, Gitter B, and Fahr A. *Int J Pharm*. 373:77–84, 2009.
35. Islam MT, Rodriguez-Hornedo N, Ciotti S, and Ackermann C. *Pharm Res*. 21:1192–1199, 2004.
36. Matusova D, Vilkova Z, Truplova E, and Herdova P. *Pharmazie*. 65:523–524, 2010.
37. Heng PW, Chan LW, and Chow KT. *Pharm Res*. 22:676–684, 2005.
38. Hoare T, Zurakowski D, Langer R, and Kohane DS. *J Biomed Mater Res A*. 92:575–585, 2010; Silver FH, LiBrizzi JJ, and Benedetto D. *J App Biomater*. 5:227–234, 1994.
39. Dolz-Planas M, Roldan-Garcia C, Herraez-Dominguez JV, and Belda-Maximino R. *J Pharm Sci*. 80:75–79, 1991.
40. Kattige A and Rowley G. *Drug Dev Ind Pharm*. 32:981–990, 2006.
41. Ricci EJ, Bentley MV, Farah M, Bretas RE, and Marchetti JM. *Eur J Pharm Sci*. 17:161–167, 2003.
42. Erni P, Windhab EJ, Gunde R, Graber M, Pfister B, Parker A, and Fischer P. *Biomacromolecules*. 8:3458–3466, 2007.
43. Boylan JC. *J Pharm Sci*. 55:710–715, 1966; Rowe RC and Sadeghnejad GR. *Int J Pharm*. 38:227–229, 1987.
44. Lippacher A, Muller RH, and Mader K. *Eur J Pharmac Biopharmac*. 58:561, 2004.
45. Boylan JC. *Bull Parenter Drug Assoc*. 19:98–109, 1965.
46. Ober SS, Vincent HC, Simon DE, and Frederick KJ. *J Am Pharm Assoc (Baltim)*. 47(9):667–676, 1958.
47. Sharpe SA, Sandweiss V, Tuazon J, Giordano M, Witchey-Lakshmanan L, Hart J, and Sequeira J. *Drug Dev Ind Pharm*. 29:1005–1012, 2003.
48. Friend DR. *Crit Rev Ther Drug Carrier Syst*. 7:149–184, 1990.
49. Morganti P, Ruocco E, Wolf R, et al. *Clinical Dermatol*. 19:489–501, 2001.
50. Ahmad N and Mukhtar H. *J Invest Dermatol*. 123:417–425, 2004.
51. Cauwenbergh G. *Acta Derm Venereol*. 121:147–153, 1986.
52. Vecchini F and Michel S. *Eur J Dermatol*. 4:583–588, 1994.
53. Scheuplein RJ, Blank IH, Brauner GJ, et al. *J Invest Derm*. 52:63–70, 1969.
54. Leopoid CS and Lippold BC. *J Pharm Pharmacol*. 47:276–281, 1995.
55. Shah DK, Khandavilli S, and Panchagnula R. *Methods Find Exp Clin Pharmacol*. 30:499–512, 2008.
56. Evrard D, Touitou E, Kolusheva S, Fishov Y, and Jelinek R. *Pharm Res*. 18:943–949, 2001.
57. Ivens UI, Steinkjer B, Serup J., et al. *Br J Dermatol*. 145:364–367, 2001.
58. Bochot A, Fattal E, Gulik A, and Couarraze G. *Couvreur Pharm Res*. 15:1364–1369, 1998.
59. Desai S and Blanchard J. *J Pharm Sci*. 87:1190–1195, 1998.
60. Lindell K and Engstom S. *Int J Pharm*. 95:219–228, 1993.
61. Srividya B, Cardoza RM, and Amin PD. *J Control Release*. 73:205–211, 2001.
62. Al-Kassas RS and El-Khatib MW. *Drug Deliv*. 16:145–152, 2009.

VII. Homework Problems

1. The viscosity of a viscoelastic material is measured to be 10 Pa-s. Convert this unit to poise (P), centipoise (cP), and dyn-s/cm^2. What are the units for shear stress and shear rate if the viscosity is expressed in pascal-seconds?
2. Select the best answer. Strain is defined as (*a*) the percentage change in length, as in Young's modulus (Equation (12-2)), (*b*) the ratio of shear stress to elasticity (modulus), (*c*) dimensionless, and (*d*) all of the above.

3. At 37°C, water has a viscosity of 0.696 cP, and the densities of water and blood are 0.993 and 1.061 g/mL, respectively. Using an Ostwald-type viscometer, the time required for the blood to flow between marks through the capillary at 37°C is 215 s, whereas for water the time is 40 s. What is the viscosity of the blood?
4. (*a*) In a 2-cm length of a blood vessel (R = 0.20 cm), the pressure drop is 7.5 mmHg. Calculate the blood flow rate, using the viscosity value determined above. (*b*) What is the blood flow rate if the vessel is 50% blocked (R' = ½R)? (*c*) What may be the factors for blood flow resistance according to the Poiseuille equation? (1 atm = 1.01325 dyn/cm^2.)
5. From the following data, determine the activation energy of viscosity (E_{vis}) for glycerin.

Temperature, °C	0	15	20	25	30
η, P	121.10	23.30	14.90	9.54	6.29

6. What is the difference between a pseudoplastic liquid and a pseudoplastic solid?
7. From the following data obtained for a semisolid preparation, (*a*) plot the flow curve and determine the yield stress and viscosity if applicable and (*b*) describe the flow property (plastic or pseudoplastic).

Shear rate, s^{-1}	75	150	225	325	450	625
Shear stress, dyn/cm^2	10,000	11,000	12,000	13,000	14,000	15,000

8. (*a*) How do you determine if a material is thixotropic? (*b*) In what types of therapeutic applications would a thixotropic system be of value?
9. How would you define the terms *storage* and *loss moduli*. If the measured tan δ for a semisolid preparation is unity (tan δ = 1) at a given applied shear stress, what is the recoverable deformation for this product?
10. Select the correct answers. In the linear viscoelastic region (LVR), (*a*) G' is maximum and constant; (*b*) strain and stress are linearly related; (*c*) tan δ is low; (*d*) the cohesive energy is proportional to the critical shear stress or strain at the point where the LVR no longer exists.
11. A semisolid preparation was subjected to a creep test under a constant stress of 8 Pa. The equilibrium curve (compliance J versus time in seconds) gives the following data:

J, cm^2/dyn × 10^{-3}	1.0	1.13	1.38	1.55
Time, s	240	300	420	500

Calculate the zero-shear viscosity for this preparation.

12. What zero-shear viscosity is necessary to prepare a suspension of drug particles having a sedimentation shear rate of 10^{-3} s^{-1} or slower if the particle size is (*a*) 10 μm or (*b*) 0.1 μm? The densities of the drug particle and the medium are 1.30 and 1.05 g/mL, respectively.
13. Show how you would prepare the following prescription order.

Rx Lidocaine HCl	4%
Epinephrine HCl	50 mg
Tetracaine HCl	500 mg
Ascorbic acid	1.7%
Hydroxyethylcellulose (5000 cP)	1.75%
Preserved water qs	100 mL

14. Show how you would prepare the following prescriptions.

(*a*)

Rx Salicylic acid	1 g
Propylene glycol qs	
Hydrophilic ointment	50 g

(*b*) Protective hand cream (100 g)

Dimethicon	4.0%
Stearic acid	6.0%
Cetyl alcohol	1.5%
Mineral oil, light	2.2% (sp gr 0.88)
Triethanolamine	1.5%
Propylene glycol	1.8% (sp gr 1.035)
Methylparaben	200 mg
Purified water	82.8%

15. Which one of the ointment bases would provide a rapid release of a hydrophilic drug?

16. A prescription calls for a topical preparation of a hydrophilic antibiotic for moderate and continuous release of a drug. The skin area is severely irritated and needs a preparation that is easy to apply and remove. What ointment base would you use and why?

17. Describe briefly which ointment base you would use for the formulation of a lipophilic drug that undergoes hydrolysis in aqueous solutions for a rapid and predictable drug release.

Suspensions, Emulsions, and Colloids

CHAPTER 13

Jun Shao

In the box below is a formulation that, when proper technique is used, will yield a homogeneous mixture of the oil and water, known as an emulsion. The obvious ingredient that makes this emulsification work is acacia, which contains principally calcium, magnesium, and potassium salts of the polysaccharide Arabic acid. By what properties and mechanism(s) does acacia facilitate and stabilize the emulsion system? We address this question by close examination of the science and technology involved in making such products.

The Formulation of an Emulsion

Mineral oil	50 mL
Acacia	12 g
Purified water, q.s.	100 mL

Often pharmaceutical preparations are made to contain two immiscible phases, known as the dispersed systems. A dispersed system consists of a dispersed phase and a continuous or dispersion phase, with the latter normally being an aqueous medium. Depending on the nature of the dispersed phase, the dispersed systems can be classified as suspensions (when solid particles are dispersed into a liquid), emulsions (when a drug-containing liquid is dispersed as droplets into an immiscible liquid), and colloids (when the size of the dispersed particles or droplets is 1–500 nm). The traditional use of dispersed systems for pharmaceutical purposes was, in part, born of necessity, as many drugs do not exhibit certain properties for easy formulation into solid and liquid dosage forms. Voluminous studies, employing principles of chemistry and physics on interfacial phenomenon, micromeritics, and rheology, have made this field particularly applicable for pharmaceutical preparations; and new approaches, such as in the development of micro- and nano-dispersed systems, have emerged for the development of advanced drug delivery strategies. This chapter discusses the theories and technology from which the traditional and new dosage forms may be prepared or developed.

CHAPTER OUTLINE

OBJECTIVES

1. Understand the principles and uses of suspension dosage forms, and be able to prepare suitable suspension formulations.
2. Understand the theory of surface free energy and surface tension.
3. Understand the principles and uses of emulsion dosage forms, and be able to prepare suitable emulsion formulations.
4. Understand the principles and uses of different colloidal systems, and be able to prepare suitable colloidal formulations.
5. Understand the applications and potentials of nanopreparations for drug delivery.

I. Suspensions

Physicochemical Properties of Suspensions

Suspension as a Dosage Form

Most times a suspension is prepared when the drug has a limited solubility in the vehicle (usually water), in that a sufficient dose cannot be dissolved in the desired volume of the vehicle. In some cases, however, a suspension is prepared for reasons other than low solubility. For example, the suspensions usually provide better chemical stability of the drug than the solutions, as in the solution the drug is dispersed as single molecules, which are more accessible to degradation by chemical reactions. The contact of the drug with the taste buds is much less in suspension than in solution. Therefore, taste masking is easier to achieve in suspension than in solution. The drugs should be dissolved from the particles in the suspension before they can be absorbed. Therefore, drug absorption from suspensions is usually slower than from solutions, thus providing a mechanism for prolonged action. Insulin injections are available as solution and suspensions. The solution has a quick action but short duration (of a few hours). In comparison, the suspensions have a slower onset of action, but a sustained drug effect that lasts for about 12–24 h or even longer depending on the formulation.[1]

As a pharmaceutical dosage form, a suspension preparation should meet the following criteria:

- The drug should be chemically stable.
- The drug particles should be physically stable in terms of crystal forms, shapes, and sizes.
- The drug should be dissolved within a certain time period after administration to ensure the desired treatment profile.
- The drug particles should be easily resuspended because the sedimentation of the particles is usually unavoidable.
- The sedimentation rate should be slow enough for even pouring of single doses.
- The suspension should be easily poured by having a desired viscosity.
- The pH of the dispersion media should be consistent.
- The preparation should meet microbial limits.

If the suspension is intended for injection, ophthalmic use, or inhalation, it should also meet the requirements of tonicity and sterility.

Sedimentation Rate and Stokes' Law

The sedimentation of particles in a suspension preparation is usually unavoidable as long as there is a density difference between the dispersed phase and the dispersion media. The particle sedimentation rate V can be described by Stokes' law:

$$V = d^2(\rho_i - \rho_e)g/(18\eta) \qquad (13\text{-}1)$$

where d is the diameter of the particle, ρ_i and ρ_e are the density of the particle and media, respectively, g is the gravitational acceleration, and η is the viscosity of the media. Equation (13-1) is derived for particles that are of perfect spherical shape and a dispersion system in which the medium is stationary and there are no collisions or interactions between the particles. Even with these stipulations, the principles of Stokes' law can still be applied to many pharmaceutical preparations.

From Equation (13-1), we can learn that three variables affect the particle sedimentation rate: the particle size, the density difference between the particle and the medium, and the viscosity of the medium. Each of these variables, therefore, can offer a means to slow down the sedimentation

Table 13-1 Viscosity (cP) of Some Pharmaceutical Liquids

	0°C	25°C	50°C	75°C
Water	1.793	0.895	0.549	0.380
Ethanol	1.790	1.09	0.698	0.476
Benzene	0.900	0.604	0.436	0.335
Ethylene glycol	—	16.1	6.554	3.340
Propylene glycol	248	40.4	11.3	4.77
Glycerol	—	934	152	39.8

rate, which is one of the main challenges in preparing suspensions. As seen from Stokes' law, the smaller the particle size, the slower the sedimentation rate. The reduction of drug particle size can be achieved through certain pharmaceutical processes such as dry milling, which can reduce the particle size to 10–50 μm, and jet milling, which can produce a particle size less than 10 μm. Control of the crystallization process can also result in a particle size in the range of several micrometers. Stokes' law also indicates that a smaller difference in density between the particle and media leads to a slower sedimentation rate. Therefore, minimizing the density difference is another approach to slow down the rate of sedimentation. Although this is not easy to achieve, some success may be realized by using glucose as an inert excipient, which increases the density of the medium. The density of the particle is usually difficult to control.

The last, but perhaps the most useful, variable to achieve suspension is the *viscosity* of the media, which, as shown by Stokes' law, is inversely proportional to the sedimentation rate. For a flowing liquid, viscosity, or the internal friction, represents the pressure (dyn/cm^2) needed to force a difference in flow rate between two parallel liquid planes. If the two planes are separated by 1 cm and the difference in flow rate is 1 cm/s, then the viscosity of the liquid has a cgs unit of 1 poise (P). As a reference, water has a viscosity of 0.00895 P, or 0.895 centipoise (cP) at 25°C (see **Table 13-1** for the temperature effect on the viscosity of some common liquids).

It is not difficult to increase the viscosity of the media. Many pharmaceutical excipients can significantly increase the viscosity of an aqueous medium at relatively low concentrations. These agents are thus called suspending agents, which include, among others, methylcellulose, sodium carboxymethylcellulose, and carbopol 934P. Carbopol 934P, for example, can yield a viscosity of about 300 P at a concentration of 0.5% at pH 7.5. The use of particle size and viscosity to alter the sedimentation rate is illustrated in Example 13-1.

Example 13-1: What is the sedimentation rate (in cgs units†) of a suspension with spherical particles in water if (*a*) the diameter and density of the powder are 5 μm and 1.33 g/cm^3, respectively (the viscosity of water is 0.9 cP); (*b*) the diameter of the powder is reduced to 1 μm; and (*c*) the viscosity is increased to 4.5 cP while maintaining the particle size at 5 μm?

Solution: According to Stokes' law,

$$V = d^2(\rho_i - \rho_e)g/(18\eta)$$

(*a*) With particle size = 5 μm,

$$V = (5 \times 10^{-4}\ \text{cm})^2\ (1.33\ \text{g/cm}^3 - 1.0\ \text{g/cm}^3)\ (980\ \text{cm/s}^2)/(18 \times 0.9 \times 10^{-2}\ \text{P})$$

$$V = 5.0 \times 10^{-4}\ \text{cm/s}$$

(*b*) When the particle size is reduced to 1 μm,

$$V = (1 \times 10^{-4}\,\text{cm})^2 (1.33\,\text{g/cm}^3 - 1.0\,\text{g/cm}^3)\ (980\,\text{cm/s}^2)/(18 \times 0.9 \times 10^{-2}\,\text{P})$$

$$V = 2.0 \times 10^{-5}\,\text{cm/s}$$

(*c*) When particle size = 5 μm and $\eta = 4.5\,\text{cP}$,

$$V = (5 \times 10^{-4}\,\text{cm})^2 (1.33\,\text{g/cm}^3 - 1.0\,\text{g/cm}^3)\ (980\,\text{cm/s}^2)/(18 \times 4.5 \times 10^{-2}\,\text{P})$$

$$V = 1.0 \times 10^{-4}\,\text{cm/s}$$

---

†*Note*: Usually the cgs instead of the SI unit system is used when dealing with viscosity. In the cgs system, length is in centimeters, mass is in grams, time is in seconds, force is in dynes, and energy is in ergs. The unit of viscosity is poise (P) or dyn-s/cm², but commonly viscosity is expressed in centipoise (cP). 1 cP = 0.01 P.

Stokes' sedimentation equation can be further divided into shear stress and the rate of shear. The downward stress (τ_s) caused by gravitation is

$$\tau_s = d(\rho_i - \rho_e)g/6 \qquad (13\text{-}1a)$$

whereas the maximum rate of shear ($\dot{g}_{\max}$) is

$$\dot{g}_{\max} = 3V/d \qquad (13\text{-}1b)$$

Thus it is possible to evaluate both the shear stress and the shear rate of the suspension system. Suspensions may be acceptable to sedimentation for two reasons: (1) The material has a sufficiently high zero-shear viscosity that sedimentation occurs in an acceptably slow manner, and (2) the bulk material has a yield stress that is high enough to hold the particles in suspension. The use of the above equations to gain such information is illustrated in Example 13-2.

The particle size, according to Stokes' law, has a direct effect on the sedimentation rate. Rheological measurements show that both the size and the distribution of particles also have a significant effect on the viscosity of the liquid. For a given weight of material, a smaller particle size corresponds to a greater number of particles. This results in greater interaction between particles that is necessary for the formation of the macrostructure in pseudoplastic and thixotropic systems, and hence a greater zero-shear viscosity. The effect of particle size distribution may be explained as follows. In a wider distribution, the smaller particles can be easily distributed in void spaces, making the liquid more responsive to shear stress or flow. The viscosity of the system increases with increasing volume fraction of the particles, but at the same volume fraction, the system that has a wider particle size distribution will have lower viscosity than the system having a narrower particle size distribution. Thus, a narrow particle size distribution may increase formulation stability through its increasing effect on viscosity.

Example 13-2: If an aqueous suspension has a zero-shear viscosity of 5 P at 20°C, which is comparable to that of 95% glycerin in water, what are the sedimentation rate, rate of shear, and yield stress for this formulation? The drug particles have a density of 1.25 g/cm³ and a mean diameter of 20 μm. The medium density is 1 g/cm³.

Solution:

$$V = d^2(\rho_i - \rho_e)g/18\eta_0 = (20 \times 10^{-4})^2 \times (1.25 - 1.0) \times 980.67/18 \times 5$$
$$= 1.09 \times 10^{-5}\,\text{cm/s}$$
$$\tau_s = d(\rho_i - \rho_e)g/6 = 20 \times 10^{-4}\,(1.25 - 1.0) \times 980.67/6$$
$$= 0.082\,\text{dyn/cm}^2$$
$$\dot{g}_{\max} = 3V/d = 3 \times 1.09 \times 10^{-5}/20 \times 10^{-4} = 0.0163\,\text{s}^{-1}$$

Interpretation:

The calculated shear rate is slightly above the range for the sedimentation of fine powders in liquids. The correlation of shear rates with mechanical stresses associated with various activities is shown in **Table 13-2**.

The downward stress may be considered the yield stress for this formulation. The yield stress can be increased by viscoelastic agents to values greater than the calculated value; the formulation, then, would be able to hold the particles in suspension.

Caking and Flocculation

In the above discussion, we learned that reduction of the particle size can reduce the sedimentation rate. However, the particle size should not be too small because very fine particles tend to form a compact cake at the bottom of the container over a prolonged time. Once the cake is formed, it is not easy to be broken up or resuspended to the original status. Basically, the suspension preparation is destroyed in such a case. The formation of cake depends on both the particle size and the particle shape. Needle-shaped particles are more prone to form cake than spherical or barrel-shaped particles. To avoid caking, one of the methods is to induce the formation of loosely bound particle aggregates, known as *flocs* or *floccules*. In floccules, the particles are held together through weak bonds, such as via van der Waals forces, in a lattice structure in which all the particles' positions are fixed relative to one another. Such loose aggregations prevent the particles from forming tight aggregation that may eventually lead to cake formation. The physical characteristic of the floccules is such that they settle down quickly but with a high sedimentation volume, which is in

Table 13-2 Shear Rates and Common Activities

Action	Shear Rate, s^{-1}	Activity/Product
Sedimentation of fine particles	10^{-6}–10^{-3}	Pharmaceuticals, paints
Leveling by surface tension	10^{-2}–10^{-1}	Paints, printing (inks)
Draining off surface	10^{-1}–10^{1}	Coatings
Extruding, pouring, chewing, swallowing, dip coating	10^{0}–10^{2}	Eating, food and confectionery, painting
Mixing, stirring, pipe flowing	10^{1}–10^{3}	Preparing solutions, pumping, blood flow
Injection, brushing	10^{2}–10^{4}	Hypodermic syringe, painting
Rubbing, nasal spraying	10^{4}–10^{5}	Applying topical products
Spraying	10^{5}–10^{6}	Atomization, spray drying

direct contrast to the irreversible caking process. The sedimentation volume refers to the volume the particles occupy after the sedimentation is completed. A high sedimentation volume of loosely aggregated particles allows easy resuspension.

Floccules can be prepared, depending on the particles' nature, by different methods with the aids of flocculating agents (flocculants). Electrolytes such as multivalent cations (for example, Al^{3+}, Ca^{2+}) can effectively neutralize the negative charges on the surface of the particles, so that they can be used to reduce the repulsion force between particles and to promote particle association in the formation of floccules. Clays such as bentonite magma and polymers such as chitosan and gelatin can also be used as flocculating agents.

Zeta Potential

In suspensions, particles usually exhibit electric charges depending on the nature of the composition. It is recalled that the electric potential on the surface of the particle to the electrically neutral zone in the bulk medium is the *Nernst potential*. There is an aqueous layer wrapping around and moving together with the particles. In this immediate aqueous layer, due to the electrostatic attraction, more ions with charges opposite to the Nernst potential are present than ions with charges the same as the Nernst potential. As a result, the electric potential from the surface of the immediate aqueous layer to the electrically neutral zone in the bulk medium will be less than the Nernst potential. This potential is called the zeta potential. Because the immediate aqueous layer moves together with the particles, it is the zeta potential rather than the Nernst potential that determines the electrostatic interaction between the particles. Thus, when certain electrolytes are added into the suspension, the zeta potential of the particles will be reduced, and as the zeta potential is reduced to a critical value, the attraction force will become larger than the repulsion force between the particles. At this point, particles start to aggregate to form floccules.

Preparation of Pharmaceutical Suspensions

Suspension Composition

In addition to the drug particles and the dispersion medium, which is usually water, the following ingredients are usually added into the suspension formulation: a suspending agent (such as methylcellulose, hydroxypropyl methylcellulose) to increase the viscosity; a wetting agent (such as sodium lauryl sulfate, Tween 80, glycerin, alcohol) to make the hydrophobic particles easily in contact with water so that they can be suspended in the medium instead of being afloat on top of the medium; stabilizing agents (such as antioxidant sodium bisulfate and chelator EDTA) to prevent auto-catalyzed and metal ions–catalyzed oxidation of the drug; preservatives (such as parabens, benzoic acid) to inhibit microbial growth; flavorants (such as orange oil, vanillin) to provide a pleasing flavor; sweeteners (such as syrup, sorbital) to provide a sweet taste; colorants (FD&C colorants) to provide a suitable color; and a buffering system to stabilize the pH. The commonly used suspending agents (with final concentration range in parentheses) include acacia NF (2.0%–5.0%), sodium carboxymethylcellulose USP (0.5%–1.5%), colloidal silicon dioxide NF (1.5%–3.5%), carbomer resins NF (0.5%–5.0%), methylcellulose (0.5%–5.0%), and tragacanth NF (0.5%–2.0%). In the final concentration range, both methylcellulose and sodium carboxymethylcellulose have been shown to yield a viscosity up to 800 cP in water.

The selection of a suspending agent depends on the intended use and the desired rheological characteristics of the final formulation. For stability, one can select a non-Newtonian flow property for the suspension by using an agent that produces a pseudoplastic (shear-thinning) or thixotropic (time-dependent thinning during shear) flow. A thixotropic characteristic, e.g., can increase the physical stability of a suspension in that the suspension thickens while standing to slow down sedimentation but becomes thinner when shaken, which makes pouring and application easier.

Preparation

To prepare the suspension, first the drugs are triturated, with or without a wetting agent, to a certain particle size. Then the medium (usually water) containing other ingredients is added. The whole mixture is then blended to achieve a homogeneous status. It is noteworthy that some special procedures are required for the preparation of suspending agents. When the powder of a suspending agent is added into water as a bulk, it usually forms big clumps. The outer layer of the clump is hydrated to form a very viscous layer, hindering the penetration of water into the clump. Then it will take a very long time for the whole clump to become hydrated (dissolved). A good practice would be to sieve (sprinkle) the powders a small quantity at a time onto the surface of the medium with stirring to avoid the formation of clumps. Some suspending agents such as methylcellulose are more soluble in cold water than in hot water, and others such as sodium carboxymethylcellulose are more soluble in hot water than in cold water. Carbomers, such as Carbopol 943P, will yield acidic pH when dissolved in water. Adjusting the pH is thus necessary when carbomers are used.

Extemporaneous Compounding

Preparations of suspensions in a pharmacy or laboratory can be carried out in a way similar to the procedure described above. Usually, the principal active ingredient (the drug) should be triturated to reduce the particle size, or to break down the aggregation of particles. This is especially important when the source of the drug is in the form of tablets or capsules. A mortar and pestle can be used to crush and grind the tablets or the contents of capsules (the capsule shell should be removed and discarded). Note that modified-release tablets or capsules (such as sustained-release products) should not be used for extemporaneous compounding of suspension, because the compounding process will alter the drug release profile and absorption process, and thus the pharmacological outcome expected from the original product. The ground drug can be mixed with a wetting agent if needed. After this, the suspension medium (the vehicle) can be added and mixed thoroughly. The vehicle is usually an aqueous medium. Depending on the drug's physicochemical properties and its intended use, the vehicle can be as simple as purified water or syrup, or as a formulated medium such as the vehicle for oral suspension, NF, which contains suspending agents, preservatives, buffering agents, etc. (see Examples 13-3 and 13-4 for more details). It should be pointed out that no preservatives, alcohols, flavorants, or colorants can be added if the extemporaneous preparation is intended for neonates, and no sugar should be added to the formulation for diabetic patients.

Example 13-3: What is the intended use of the sorbitol solution in the following formula of an antacid oral suspension?

Aluminum hydroxide	326.8 g
Sorbitol solution	282.0 mL
Syrup	93.0 mL
Glycerin	25.0 mL
Methylparaben	0.9 g
Propylparaben	0.3 g
Flavor	q.s.
Purified water, to make	1000.0 mL

Solution: In the preparation of oral suspensions, the pharmacist should become knowledgeable about the ingredients used in the formulation. Per our discussion in the text, wetting agents are sometimes needed for proper dispersion of the suspended drug particles. In general, alcohol, glycerin, and other hydroscopic liquids are used as wetting agents in an aqueous medium. The sorbitol solution USP is an aqueous solution containing about 70% w/w D-sorbitol with small amount of mannitol and other isomeric polyhydric alcohols. This solution is neutral and syruplike, and it is used to replace alcohol and glycerin as a wetting agent and as a suspending agent.

Example 13-4: What is missing in the following formulation for the barium sulfate suspension?

Barium sulfate	90.0 g
Sodium saccharin	0.04 g
Lemon flavorant	1.0 mL
Purified water, q.s.	350.0 mL

Solution: One can see that in this suspension formulation there are the dispersed phase (barium sulfate) and dispersion media (water) with flavorant (lemon flavorant) and sweetener (sodium saccharin). Clearly the dispersed phase will quickly settle down at the bottom. Therefore, the key component, the suspending agent, is missing. The original formulation contains 2.0 g of sodium carboxymethylcellulose, which can be replaced by other suspending agents such methylcellulose.

Dry Powders for Suspension

A drug such as amoxicillin is unstable when exposed to water; thus a dry powder form for suspension is manufactured instead of the final suspension form. The dry powder form contains all the ingredients except the dispersion media. This approach allows a long shelf life. For example, amoxicillin powder for suspension is a mixture of dried powders containing, in addition to amoxicillin, the inactive ingredients of colloidal silicon dioxide, FD&C Red #40, fruit granulated sugar, natural and artificial fruit gum flavor, sodium benzoate, sodium citrate, and xanthan gum. Upon dispensing, the pharmacist will add the dispersion medium (usually purified water) in a suitable quantity. The final suspension is supposed to be administered to the patient over a short period (per the predetermined shelf life) and, after that, discarded due to the loss of drug potency via chemical degradation.

II. Emulsions

The Emulsion Process

Emulsification

When a liquid is dispersed into another immiscible liquid, such a system is called an emulsion. The dispersed liquid (phase) is called the internal phase, which exists in small droplets, whereas the dispersion vehicle (phase) is called the external phase, which is continuous. When an oil phase is dispersed into water, the internal phase is oil, and the system is called an oil-in-water (O/W) emulsion. When a water phase is dispersed into oil, the internal phase is water, and the system is called a water-in-oil (W/O) emulsion. Common sense tells us that two immiscible phases (such as oil and water) cannot be mixed well. Therefore, to prepare an emulsion that is a well-dispersed homogeneous mixture, a third phase should be used to facilitate and stabilize the dispersion. This third phase is known as the *emulsifier*. Emulsifiers can interact with both oil and water phases, meaning that they have a certain affinity toward both oil and water, serving as a solvation agent for the nondissolvable liquid particulate at the oil–water interface. Emulsifiers are usually surfactants, which are surface-active compounds.

The emulsion technology has found its way into many applications in pharmaceuticals as well as in other areas such as cosmetics and food. Many drugs are not soluble in water, but are soluble in oils and other hydrophobic substances. Because an oily solution is not suitable for consumption, O/W emulsion where the water-insoluble drug is dissolved in the oil phase has become a useful approach in drug formulation considerations. The taste of the drug—as we know, most drugs taste bad—can be covered up to a certain extent when the drug is localized inside the internal phase of the emulsion. Emulsions have been found to enhance drug absorption because the oil phase is closer to the biological membrane in chemical nature than water and thus can be more readily absorbed. This facilitates the absorption of drug that is incorporated in the oil droplets. The emulsifiers, as surfactants, can also improve drug absorption through biological membranes to various degrees.

Surface or Interfacial Free Energy

The mechanism by which an emulsifier stabilizes the dispersion of the oil phase into water phase, or vice versa, can be examined by noting the surface free energy changes. When the oil phase is dispersed into the water phase, a large interface between the oil and water is created. This results in an increase in the surface energy (or, more accurately, surface free energy) of the system and renders the system unstable, as the energy change is opposite to a spontaneous process (a natural process without external energy) that moves from a high to a low energy state. For example, a subject placed at a higher position (with higher energy potential) will fall to a lower position (with lower energy potential) if the support, which counteracts with the energy system, is removed at the high-energy position. Thus, one can see that the action of an emulsifier is to reduce the interfacial energy created by the emulsion process.

What is surface free energy? Consider the surface of water in a beaker. The water molecules at the surface are bound to water molecules beneath them through an association force (F_1), which is likely the hydrogen bonding. This force tends to pull the top layer of water molecules downward into the bulk of water and away from the air, resulting in a decrease of the surface area. The top layer water molecules are also subject to forces in the air (F_2), which tend to pull the water molecule upward into the air. The sum of these two forces collectively determines the *surface tension of water*, which can be defined as the work (energy) needed to overcome the association force, resulting in an increase of a unit area of the liquid surface. In other words, surface tension is regarded as the surface energy per unit of surface area, and the surface free energy is the product of the surface tension and the area of the interface. In a similar definition, the tension between two immiscible liquid phases is called the interfacial tension.

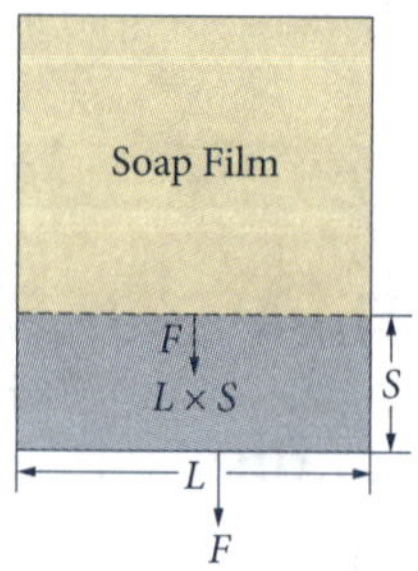

Figure 13-1 Surface free energy–surface tension relationship of a soap film.

Consider a soap film of a single-molecule layer on a rectangular frame (**Figure 13-1**). The film can be expanded, due to the surface tension between the film and the air, by pulling the bar with a force F. This force is dependent on the length (L) of the bar: the longer the bar, the bigger the F. The surface tension (γ) is defined as the force per unit length. Because both the front and the back of the film are exposed to the air, the effective length of interaction should be $2L$. Therefore, the surface tension γ in this case can be written as

$$\gamma = F/(2L) \qquad (13\text{-}2)$$

When the bar moves a distance S, the work (W) is $F \times S$. This work translates into the form of surface free energy. From Equation (13-2), we know that $F = \gamma \times 2L$. Therefore,

$$W = \gamma \times 2L \times S$$

Here, the quantity of $2L \times S$ is the total increase in the surface area ΔA (which includes area changes for both sides). Therefore,

$$W = \gamma \times \Delta A \qquad (13\text{-}3)$$

or Surface free energy change = surface tension × surface area change

Example 13-5: If the surface tension between the soap film and air is 50 dyn/cm, what will be the minimum force needed to pull the 2-cm bar? How much is the increase of surface free energy if the bar is pulled down by 1 cm?

Solution: $F = \gamma \times 2L$, thus

$$F = 50\,\text{dyn/cm} \times 2 \times 2\,\text{cm} = 200\,\text{dyn}$$
$$W = F \times S = 200\,\text{dyn} \times 1\,\text{cm} = 200\,\text{erg}$$
or $$W = \gamma \times \Delta A = 50\,\text{dyn/cm} \times 2\,\text{cm} \times 1\,\text{cm} \times 2 = 200\,\text{erg}$$

Answer: The minimum force to pull the bar is 200 dyn, and the surface free energy increase is 200 erg.

The concept of surface free energy as a function of surface area can be used to predict whether an oil droplet can be spread out onto the surface of water. Let us go back to the beaker with water. The surface area between water and air is A, and the surface tension of water is γ_W. If a droplet of mineral oil (surface tension is γ_O) is now placed on top of the water, as shown in **Figure 13-2*A***, can the mineral oil droplet spread out onto the whole surface of water as shown in **Figure 13-2*B***? To answer this question, one can examine the interfacial area change, as the area change is related to surface free energy and the only energy change over this process is the surface free energy. If the mineral oil droplet spreads out, certain surface areas will disappear while other areas will be created. These changes can be summarized as shown in **Table 13-3**.

As can be seen, the lost area after spreading is mainly the interface between the water and air. In comparison, the areas of the oil droplet–water and the oil droplet–air interfaces are very small and negligible. The created surface areas include mainly the interface between the oil layer and air and the interface between

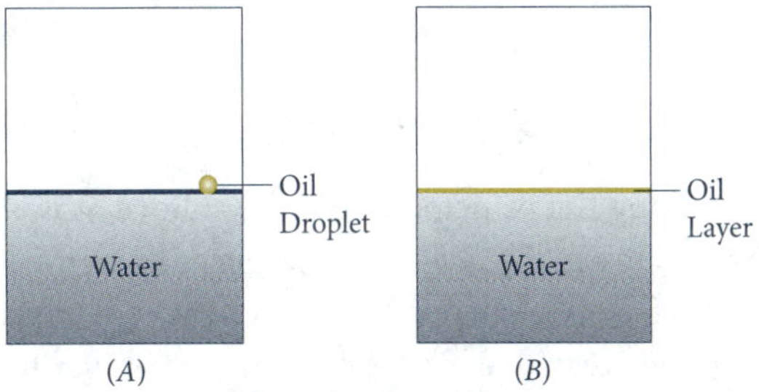

Figure 13-2 Spreading of an oil droplet on the surface of water: (*A*) a drop of oil on water; (*B*) the drop spreads on and covers the surface of water.

Table 13-3 Surface Free Energy

Loss of Interfacial Area	Free Energy Change	Gain of Interfacial Areas	Free Energy Change
Water–air	$\gamma_W A$	Oil–air	$\gamma_O A$
Oil droplet–air	Negligible	Water–oil	$\gamma_{WO} A$
Water–oil droplet	Negligible	Oil–beaker	Negligible

the oil layer and water. One can also see an interface between the edge of the oil layer and the beaker wall, but that will be very small and negligible. Thus, one can write the surface free energy changes as $\gamma_W A$ for the lost interface after spreading, and $\gamma_O A$ and $\gamma_{WO} A$ for the gained interfaces as a result of spreading, where γ_{WO} is the interfacial tension between the water and oil. The change in surface free energy due to the spreading of the oil droplet is then

$$\Delta W = \gamma_O A + \gamma_{WO} A - \gamma_W A = A(\gamma_O + \gamma_{WO} - \gamma_W)$$

The above equation shows that if $\gamma_W - (\gamma_O + \gamma_{WO}) > 0$, the surface free energy change will be negative, and the spreading process will occur spontaneously. If, in contrast, $\gamma_W < (\gamma_O + \gamma_{WO})$, the surface free energy increases with the spreading, then the process of spreading will not happen spontaneously. This difference in surface and interfacial tension between two states, that is, $\gamma_W - (\gamma_O + \gamma_{WO})$, is called the spreading coefficient.

It is interesting to note that although oil and water are immiscible, there is a limited solubility between the two, which can lead to saturated solutions in both phases. As a result, both γ_W and γ_O may change, and consequently, the spreading coefficient may change as well. If the initial spreading coefficient changes from positive to negative, the oil droplet will initially spread out onto the water and then contract into a droplet after a while.

Example 13-6: Can a mineral oil droplet spread out onto water at room temperature, when the surface tension of water and mineral oil are 73 and 30 dyn/cm, respectively? (Assume the water–oil interfacial tension is 55 dyn/cm.)

Solution: Spreading coefficient $= \gamma_W - (\gamma_O + \gamma_{WO})$

$$= 73\ \text{dyn/cm} - (30\ \text{dyn/cm} + 55\ \text{dyn/cm})$$

$$= -12\ \text{dyn/cm}$$

Answer: Because the spreading coefficient is negative, the oil droplet cannot spontaneously spread onto the water surface.

Theories of Emulsification

Applying the principles described above, it is clear that when an oil phase is dispersed into a water phase, the formation of thermodynamically stable droplets depends on a negative change in surface free energy. In such a system, a large interfacial area between the oil and water phases is to be created, which is considerably larger than the combined area of all interfaces in the initial state (before emulsion). The surface free energy increased after emulsion is thus $\gamma_{WO} A$, where A is the interfacial area between the water and the oil droplets. The higher this energy, the less stable the emulsion. Because the purpose of emulsion is to create small oil droplets (in nanometer to micrometer size), *A* is usually not adjusted to regulate the surface free energy. Hence, the main approach to produce a stable emulsion is to reduce the interfacial tension using emulsifiers.

An emulsifier is a surface-active agent that, as an amphiphilic molecule, generally consists of a polar and a nonpolar moiety. These two moieties are often described as a structural feature that contains a hydrophilic head and lipophilic long chain (such as the polar choline phosphate group and nonpolar alkyl chains in phospholipids), so that the hydrophilic and hydrophobic interactions of the emulsifier at the water–oil interface can be easily understood. The interactions of the emulsifier with the interfacial molecules (water or oil) reduce the internal pulling force by the like molecules, and therefore the interfacial tension. This stabilizes the interface and hence the emulsion. It has been proposed that in emulsions, the emulsifier molecules will arrange in a special orientation. For example, in O/W emulsion, the nonpolar chains of the emulsifier molecules will stick into the oil droplets with the polar heads outward to the surrounding aqueous phase, so that the system can be stabilized. This is termed the *oriented-wedge theory*. Another theory, known as the *interfacial film theory*, suggests that the emulsifier molecules form films between the two phases, or wrap around the dispersed droplets, to reduce the interfacial tension.

Preparation of Pharmaceutical Emulsions

HLB Values

Depending on the chemical structure, some *emulsifiers* show greater affinity toward polar molecules than nonpolar molecules, and they are said to be hydrophilic emulsifiers, whereas others show the opposite property (lipophilic emulsifiers). A hydrophilic–lipophilic balance (HLB) system has been developed for the measurement of the hydrophilic and lipophilic properties of the surfactants, based on an arbitrary scale from 0 to 20, calculated based on the portion of the hydrophilic moiety in the molecule. A molecule consisting of only lipophilic moiety will have an HLB of 0. A molecule consisting of only hydrophilic moiety will have an HLB value of 20. Depending on the actual structure, the individual surfactant will have an HLB value between the two extremes in that a greater HLB value corresponds to a greater hydrophilicity of the surface active agent. For O/W emulsions, more hydrophilic surfactants are required as the emulsifiers, and for W/O emulsions, more lipophilic surfactants are required as the emulsifiers. **Table 13-4** shows the correlation of the HLB values and utilities of the surfactants.[2] It should be pointed out that the HLB range in the table can be expanded 1–2 units on both sides for most of the groups; and some surfactants, such as sodium lauryl sulfate, exhibit multifunctional properties that allow them to be used as a solubilizer, detergent, wetting agent, and emulsifier.

Table 13-4 HLB Values and Utilities of Surfactants†

HLB Value	Utilities	Examples
0–3	Antifoaming agents	Mineral oil, fatty alcohol, wax
4–6	W/O emulsifiers	Span 80, lanolin
7–18	Wetting agents	Brij 30, docusate sodium
8–18	O/W emulsifiers	Tween 20, Cremophor A25
13–15	Detergents	Alkyl benzene sulfonates
10–18	Solubilizers	Sodium lauryl sulfate

†Modified from: Griffin, 1954.

To form a stable emulsion, certain oil phases need emulsifiers with special HLB values. Many times, a single emulsifier cannot meet the requirement of a specific HLB value, and a mixture of emulsifiers is thus needed to provide the desired HLB value. The overall HLB value of a mixture of surfactants can be calculated as

$$HLB_{mixture} = f_1(HLB_1) + f_2(HLB_2) + f_3(HLB_3) + \cdots \quad (13\text{-}4)$$

where f_i is the weight fraction of the surfactant having a value of HLB_i. When multiple emulsifiers are used, the chemical compatibility of the emulsifiers should be examined. In general, an anionic emulsifier is not compatible with a cationic surfactant one, as the interaction of the opposite electric charges can lead to precipitation and/or loss of emulsifying function. The same caution should be paid to the potential chemical incompatibility between the surfactant(s) and the active or other ingredients in the formulation.

Emulsifiers

As shown in Table 13-4, many compounds have been developed as excipients in the making of pharmaceutical emulsions. These agents can be classified into four groups: natural emulsifiers, semisynthetic emulsifiers, synthetic emulsifiers, and fine solids. Acacia is a natural emulsifier with an HLB of 8.0, and it is primarily used for O/W emulsions. It is also used as a viscosity-enhancing and suspending agent that yields a viscosity of 600 cP at a concentration of 35%. Acacia is a mixture of sugars and hemicelluloses with a molecular weight range of 240–580 kD. It is soluble in water but not in alcohol (95%). Lanolin is a natural emulsifier used for W/O emulsions. It is a refined mixture of fat from sheep wool. It is not soluble in water. However, it can absorb water to form W/O emulsions. Lecithin is also a natural emulsifier used primarily for O/W emulsions. It is a mixture of phosphatides, mainly including phosphatidylcholine, phosphatidylethanolamine, etc. It is insoluble in water, but can be easily hydrated to form emulsions. Examples of semisynthetic emulsifiers are methylcellulose and sodium lauryl sulfate. Methylcellulose is produced by the partial substitution of —OH groups in long-chain cellulose with $—OCH_3$. Its molecular weight varies in the range of 10–220 kD. It can be used for O/W emulsions. It can function as an emulsifier, viscosity-enhancing agent, and emulsion stabilizer. It disperses in water to form a colloidal system. Sodium lauryl sulfate is a mixture of sodium alkyl sulfates mainly containing sodium lauryl sulfate $[CH_3(CH_2)_{10}CH_2SO_4Na]$. It has very high HLB value, is freely soluble in water, and can be used for O/W emulsion and as a wetting agent and detergent. Spans and Tweens are probably the most commonly used synthetic emulsifiers. Spans are sorbitan fatty acid esters suitable for use in preparing W/O emulsions. Depending on whether it is mono-, di- or triesters and on the length of the alkyl chain, Span can have an HLB value in the range of 2–9. For example, sorbitan monostearate (Span 60, with a 17-carbon chain) has an HLB of 4.7, sorbitan tristearate (Span 65, with three 17-carbon chains) has an HLB of 2.1, whereas sorbitan monolaurate (Span 20, with a 12-carbon chain) has an HLB of 8.6. Spans are insoluble but dispersible in water. Tweens are polyoxyethylene sorbitan fatty acid esters with HLBs of 10–17, usually used for O/W emulsions. Tweens have four polyoxyethylene chains that are hydrophilic. These chains can form mono-, di-, and triester with fatty acids. The HLB value of a Tween is mainly determined by the polyoxyethylene chains and the fatty acid chain(s). Tweens are soluble or dispersible in water. Tweens and Spans are often used together to form both O/W and W/O emulsions, which are usually more stable than that formed only with one emulsifier. Fine solids such as bentonite and magnesium stearate are sometimes used to form emulsions. Bentonite is basically hydrated aluminum silicate, which is mainly used as a suspending and viscosity-enhancing agent. It also can be used to form O/W emulsions or as a stabilizer for such an emulsion. Magnesium stearate is very hydrophobic, mainly used as lubricant in the tableting process, but can be used to stabilize W/O emulsions.

Preparation of Emulsions

Emulsions are usually prepared by mixing or blending. In laboratory or pharmacy, the commonly used equipment for emulsion preparation is mortar and pestle for small-quantity preparation. Wedgewood or porcelain mortar rather than glass mortar should be used, in order to provide enough friction to break up the internal phase into small droplets. High-speed homogenizers are useful in preparing small-size emulsions. In industry, the emulsion can be prepared by high-volume, high-speed blenders. The common ingredients in emulsions, similar to those of the suspension formulation, may include, in addition to the oil and water phases and emulsifiers, flavorants, preservatives, colorants, thickening agents, antioxidants, and buffering agent.

There are four conventional methods for emulsion preparation: continental method, English method, bottle method, and in situ soap method. The continental method is also called the *dry gum* method in which the emulsifier is first thoroughly mixed together with the oil phase through trituration (it is dry, no water at this stage), and then the aqueous phase is added all at once with further trituration. Other ingredients except those that are already dissolved in oil and water are added later (see Example 13-7). Certain ingredients, such as alcohol, may interfere with the stability of the emulsion. Thus, they should be added last with a slow speed and sufficient agitation to prevent possible damage to the formed emulsion. The continental method can produce smaller, more uniform oil droplets compared to other procedures, but is not suitable for preparing emulsions with high viscosity. When one is preparing a mineral oil in water emulsion using acacia as the emulsifier, a weight ratio of 4 : 2 : 1 for oil : water : emulsifier is known to produce an emulsion with suitable quality and stability.

In the English method, also called the wet gum method, first the emulsifier is mixed with water, and then the oil phase is slowly added with enough agitation to form the emulsion. This method is suitable for the viscous oil phase. Once the emulsion is formed, the excipients other than those already dissolved in the water or oil phase can be added with agitation. Again, the excipients that may interfere with the stability of the emulsion should be added last with a slow speed and sufficient agitation.

Example 13-7: Show how you would prepare the following emulsion.†

Mineral oil emulsion NF:	Mineral oil	500 mL
	Acacia, in very fine powder	125 g
	Syrup	100 mL
	Vanillin	40 mg
	Alcohol	60 mL
	Purified water, q.s.	1000 mL

Solution: Using the continental method,

(1) mix mineral oil (500 mL) with acacia (125 g) in a dry mortar;

(2) add purified water (250 mL) all at once and emulsify the mixture to form the primary emulsion;

(3) dissolve vanillin (40 mg) and purified water (50 mL) in alcohol (60 mL), and mix with 100 mL of syrup;

(4) add the mix in divided portions, triturate after each addition, to the prime emulsion;

(5) add sufficient purified water to make 1000 mL and mix well.

†*Note*: The primary emulsion is formed with a ratio of oil : water : emulsifier of 4 : 2 : 1. In this dry gum method, the oil and the hydrocolloid (acacia) is rapidly mixed, after which water is added all at once with rapid trituration. Alternatively, the wet gum method may also be used. In this case, the ratio of oil : water : emulsifier will be again 4 : 2 : 1, but first a mucilage is made by adding a small amount of water to acacia and the mixture is triturated until uniform. Then, mineral oil is added in small quantities via rapid trituration. This mixture is thick and viscous, and more water is added slowly but under rapid trituration to complete the emulsion.

Mineral oil emulsion NF can be used as a laxative for constipation. It can also be used to soften or cleanse skin. For internal use, heavy mineral oil, which is less likely to cause "leakage," should be used for the preparation.

The bottle method is usually used for extemporaneous preparation of emulsions with volatile or low-viscosity oils. In this method, the emulsifier is added to the oil or the water phase in a capped bottle. After shaking to gain a thorough mix of the two, the other phase is added, where the internal phase is dispersed by shaking. Other ingredients are added after the formation of the emulsion. This method is not suitable for viscous oils, and usually it yields larger droplets of the internal phase than methods that use the trituration technique.

The in situ soap method utilizes the reaction of certain ingredients to form surfactants. For example, when calcium hydroxide, $Ca(OH)_2$, is mixed with oleic acid, $CH_3(CH_2)_7CH{=}CH(CH_2)_7COOH$, calcium oleate is produced. In aqueous solution, calcium oleate will dissociate to form the oleate anion that has sufficient hydrophilicity (through the carboxylate) as well as lipophilicity (through the carbon chain) to act as an emulsifier. In comparison, the carboxylic group in oleic acid is protonated, which does not exhibit the amphiphilic characteristics of a surface-active agent.

Emulsion Stability

Type of Instability

As discussed above, emulsions are not physically stable systems. The following unstable phenomena may occur:

Aggregation: The droplets of the dispersed phase form large aggregates but not yet larger droplets; the aggregated droplets can be easily dispersed again by gently shaking.

Coalescence: The droplets of the dispersed phase come together and merge into large droplet or droplets; the merged droplets cannot be dispersed into small droplets by gentle shaking.

Phase inversion: The original internal and external phases are reversed to become the external and internal phases, respectively, due to the use of a large volume of the internal phase in the original formulation and/or misuse of the emulsifier(s).

When the small droplets flocculate via loose aggregation, they become concentrated in one specific part of the emulsion. This is known as creaming, which causes the drug to be distributed unevenly in the preparation. It occurs because the oil is generally less dense than the water phase. Coalescence is an irreversible process, in which the emulsifier-stabilized interface is destroyed. The occurrence of coalescence may result from insufficient viscosity of the continuous phase and/or a high ratio of the internal volume to the total volume of the emulsion. Phase inversion may occur when a large volume of the internal phase is used or in systems containing cationic species. For example, monovalent cations tend to form O/W emulsions, whereas divalent cations tend to form W/O emulsions. The addition of a calcium salt to a system emulsified using sodium stearate may thus convert an O/W emulsion to a W/O emulsion.

Phase inversion or the types of emulsion (O/W versus W/O) can be determined by staining, dilution, and conductivity methods. In the staining method, a dye that is soluble only in water or oil is added into the emulsion, and the stained emulsion is observed under the microscope, from which the type of emulsion can be determined. In the dilution method, a drop of emulsion is added to water in a beaker or test tube with or without very gentle shaking. If the drop remains, the external phase of the emulsion is taken to be the oil. If the drop is dispersed into the water, the external phase of the emulsion is water. In the conductivity method, the electric conductivity of the emulsion is measured. A high conductivity corresponds to an external phase made of aqueous medium, as oil is highly electric-resistant.

Prevention of Emulsion Defects

In general, an emulsion is deemed physically stable when it retains its original appearance, odor, and color and exhibits no creaming or coalescence. Several methods can be used to prevent these unstable phenomena from happening. First, appropriate emulsifying agents with suitable HLB value and sufficient quantity should be used. Often, the addition of a second emulsifier that has an HLB value significantly different from that of the prime emulsifier can help to stabilize the emulsion (see Example 13-8). Second, the size of the droplets should be reduced to minimize the sedimentation or floating rate. Third, the difference in density of the two phases should be reduced, if possible. Fourth, a viscosity agent can be used to increase the viscosity of the preparation to prevent the aggregation of the droplets. Exposure to hot or cold temperature can cause phase separation (aggregation or coalescence), which should be avoided.

Example 13-8: Describe the purpose of using cetostearyl alcohol for the following formulation.

Mineral oil	300 mL
Sodium lauryl sulfate	10 g
Cetostearyl alcohol	90 g
Purified water, q.s.	1000 mL

Solution: O/W emulsions of mineral oil stabilized with surfactant like sodium lauryl sulfate are fluid liquids. Their low viscosity may lead to creaming and coalescence.

The use of a fatty alcohol works in concert with the ionic surfactant in stabilizing the emulsion. The concentration of cetostearyl alcohol in the above formulation exceeds its solubility in mineral oil. The preparation of the emulsion involves melting of the fatty alcohol (60–70°C) and mixing it with mineral oil at that temperature. When mixed with water, the alcohol interacts with the aqueous surface to produce a liquid crystalline phase with gel-like network structure. On cooling, the alcohol may solidify and cause a thickening of the emulsion to provide a viscoelastic effect. This rheological property prevents creaming of the oil droplets, which are trapped or immobilized by the gel-like structure.[3]

The optimum ratio of cetostearyl alcohol to surfactant is 9:1. At lower concentrations of the fatty alcohol, the emulsions are fluid and prone to creaming and coalescence.

III. Colloids

Properties of Colloids

Particle Size

In a commonly used definition, the colloidal system is a dispersed system in which the size of the dispersed phase is 1–500 nm. The dispersion medium can be liquid, solid, or gas. When the dispersion medium is a gas or solid, the system is termed aerosol or solid sol, respectively. When the dispersion medium is liquid, it is usually called a *sol* if the dispersed phase is solid, or a nano- or microemulsion if the dispersed phase is liquid. Traditionally, the term microemulsion is used to describe emulsions with droplet size of 1–100 nm. There is, however, a need to expand this size range to the whole colloidal size limit, as an emulsion with a droplet size of 100 nm is similar to an emulsion with a droplet size of 300 nm in terms of thermodynamic properties. Also it is observed sometimes that the droplet size will increase when the emulsion is diluted with the external phase. For example, the average droplet size of a microemulsion consisting of oleic acid, labrasol, transcutol P, and water (8 : 50 : 16 : 26) increases from 104 to 210 and 300 nm after diluted 10 and 25 times with water, respectively. It is perhaps more appropriate to use nanoemulsion, rather than microemulsion, to describe emulsions with droplet sizes in the lower colloidal range (1–100 nm). For many macromolecules of high molecular weights, when "dissolved" in solution, the size of the single molecules can be several nanometers. Such solutions, strictly speaking, are thus colloidal dispersions rather than true solutions. The difference between a true solution and a colloidal dispersion is that the latter scatters light whereas the former does not.

Light-Scattering and Colloid Stability

The light-scattering phenomenon in a colloidal system is described by the Tyndall effect. To observe the Tyndall effect, you can set a beam of light passing through a solution in a dark room and observe the light in the vertical direction. Because a true solution does not scatter the light, as the size of the solute molecule is too small compared to the wavelength of the light, the light will pass through the solution in front of you, undetected. In the case of a colloid, however, the size of the dispersed phase is large enough to scatter the light, and some of the light rays will be deflected toward the direction of your observation. The light-scattering effect is the result of the Brownian motion of the colloidal particles, which is brought about by the collision of the particles with the constant and random movement of the solvent molecules. According to the molecular kinetic theory, particles or droplets suspended in a medium will experience constant collisions with the random moving solvent molecules. However, in coarse dispersions, such as suspensions and emulsions, the masses of the particles and droplets are sufficiently large that the impetus from the collisions with solvent molecules does not cause noticeable motion. Only with a sufficiently small size, such as in the colloidal size range, may the particles be pushed to one direction and quickly to a changed direction by the solvent particles. The importance of this phenomenon is that although both suspensions and emulsions have stability issues such as sedimentation, aggregation, and coalescence, the colloidal systems are thermodynamically stable, meaning the two phases are not susceptible to separation. As a consequence, these small particles or droplets can remain suspended in the medium.

Colloidal Systems in Pharmacy

Lyophilic Colloids

The colloidal systems formed by dissolved single molecules of hydrophilic macromolecules, such as proteins, carbomers, methylcellulose, gelatin, and acacia, are called the *lyophilic* (solvent-loving) *colloids*. The dispersed particles (single molecules) are covered with a solvent sheath. The lyophilic colloids can be readily prepared by mixing the two phases (such as gelatin and water) well and letting the mixture stand for a certain time until the dispersed phase (gelatin) is hydrated (swelled) and dispersed into the dispersion medium. If the concentration of the dispersed phase is high enough, the system can become semisolid, known as a gel or, in the case of inorganic particles, magma. Gels are more physically stable than a liquid form because the relative movement of the dispersed phase and dispersion media in the dispersion system is prohibited, making phase separation unlikely. Many viscosity-increasing agents such as carbomer, methylcellulose, and agar can be used as gelling agents.

Some of the gels can become liquid under certain shear force such as by shaking, but return to semisolid form slowly after the shear force is removed. Recall that this phenomenon indicates a thixotropic response of the gel to shear stress. One example is the 5% bentonite magma, NF. It is thought that under the shear force the binding force between the dispersed particles is disrupted, so that the system can flow. When the shear force is removed, binding between the molecules resumes and the gel is reformed by a slow restoration process. This provides some advantages as a pharmaceutical preparation. First, the semisolid status prevents the phase separation seen in many liquid preparations, so that the preparation is more physically stable. Second, its change to the liquid form and its slow restoration upon shearing allow enough time for dispensing a single dose, or making an injection.

Certain gel formations have been shown to exhibit temperature-dependent changes in their physical properties. These gels exist in liquid form at room temperature (25°C), but become semisolid at the body temperature (37°C). This kind of gel has unique pharmaceutical applications. The liquid form allows easy application (such as by spray), and once it is applied to the body parts, it quickly turns to a gel to provide a longer contact period than liquid and thus enhanced drug absorption. The prolonged contact with the absorption mucosa is of particular importance when the drug is delivered through nasal, buccal, or ophthalmic routes. The liquid form at room temperature also allows the preparation to be injectable. After injection such as into muscles, it is gelled to provide a sustained-release mechanism for the delivery of the drug. Polymers such as poloxamer 407 (a copolymer of ethylene oxide and propylene oxide), poly(*N*-isopropylacrylamide), and low-molecular-weight PLGA-PEG-PLGA (copolymer of poly(lactic-*co*-glycolic) acid and polyethylene glycol) can be used to form thermosensitive gels. The release of the drug from the gels is usually still too fast but can be modified by formulation. For example, carrageenan has been used as a gelling agent to improve the sustained release of drug from poloxamer-based gels,[4] whereas a sustained release of GLP-1 (glucagon-like peptide 1), which enhances glucose lowering in type II diabetes, was achieved using the in situ gel of low-molecular-weight PLGA-PEG-PLGA and Zn-precipitated GLP-1 as a drug delivery system.[5]

Lyophobic Colloids

Different from the lyophilic colloids, the dispersed phases in the *lyophobic* (solvent-hating) *colloids* have little affinity, if any, toward the dispersion medium. The dispersion process hence will not be spontaneous. Examples of these materials are hydrophobic polymers such as poly(lactic-*co*-glycolic acid) (PLGA) and ethylcellulose and inorganic particles such as silver, gold, and sulfur. Because they cannot be spontaneously dispersed, preparation of the lyophobic colloids requires various physical and chemical considerations for the reduction of particle size to the colloidal range. For direct dispersion, the coarse particles are reduced to small particles by various methods such as high-intensity ultrasonic generators, colloidal mills, etc. The change of particle size can be made by a condensation and precipitation process, through which one can use an initial supersaturation condition followed by crystallization and precipitation to form colloidal-size particles. For example, when a large amount of water is mixed with concentrated sulfur solution in ethanol, sulfur will immediately precipitate to form colloids. Another example is to dissolve a polymer (such as PLGA) in an organic solvent such as acetone, followed by dropping the polymer solution into water containing polyvinyl alcohol (PVA) as an emulsifier, with stirring and sonication. An O/W emulsion is initially formed. As the acetone diffuses out from the inner phase into the external aqueous phase, the PLGA will precipitate out to form particles within colloidal size range. This method is also called the spontaneous emulsification solvent diffusion method.[6] Another similar method of double emulsion–solvent evaporation can be used also. In this method, a W/O emulsion is prepared with the drug in the aqueous phase and the polymer in the oil phase; then this emulsion is mixed with a large amount of water to form W/O/W emulsion. Under certain conditions, the oil phase is removed by evaporation, and the water-insoluble polymers precipitate out to form nanoparticles. This method requires the oil phase to be easily evaporated. Methylene chloride is commonly used as the oil phase in such a method.[7] Chemically, lyophilic materials can be cross-linked to form colloidal-size particles that are water-insoluble. For example, gelatin, when dissolved in water, can be precipitated by acetone with vigorous stirring to form colloidal particles. The precipitated gelatin can then be cross-linked with glutaraldehyde and redispersed in water to form a particulate colloidal system.[8] Polymers with certain charges can be cross-linked with poly counterions, a method known as ionic cross-link. For example, cationic chitosan can be cross-linked by anionic tripolyphosphate (TPP). When an alkaline phase (pH 7–9) containing TPP is added to an acidic phase (pH 4–6) containing chitosan, nanoparticles will be immediately formed through inter- and intramolecular linkages created between the TPP phosphate and chitosan amino groups.[9] Lyophobic colloids have also been made using a polymerization method, in which first an emulsion containing some monomers in the internal phase is prepared, and then a polymerization initiator is added to trigger the polymerization of the monomers within each droplet to form nanoparticles. For certain polymerization reactions, the reaction can be initiated by high temperature.[10]

Micelles, Liposomes, and Nanoemulsions

When the concentration of a surfactant solution is increased to a certain point, the surfactant molecules (usually having a lipophilic chain and polar head) will begin to associate with one another to form a spherical particle with the lipophilic chains forming the core of the sphere and the polar heads orienting outward to the surrounding aqueous environment. These particles are called micelles, and the sizes of micelles are in the range of colloids. The minimum concentration for a surfactant to form micelles is called the critical micelle concentration (CMC). Below CMC, the surface tension of the solution will decrease with increasing surfactant concentration. The minimum value of surface tension occurs at the CMC, and it will not decrease further with further increase in surfactant concentration. Surfactants are known to enhance the solubility of hydrophobic drugs by incorporating the drug into the hydrophobic wall and/or inside the micelles. Therefore, the surfactant concentration for such purposes should be CMC or above.

The phospholipids can form bilayer (like the cell membrane) or multilayer aggregations. When these aggregations are dispersed into water, they are known as liposomes. Because the membranes of liposomes are similar to the cell membrane, liposomes as a drug delivery system can enhance the cellular absorption of drugs loaded inside the liposomes. Although the science on liposomal drug delivery has received great attention in recent years, several issues regarding its pharmaceutical applications remain unresolved. Namely, the loaded drugs may leak out of the formulation, which is undesirable in many of its proposed uses, and methods for the manufacture of stable and unisize liposomes with sufficient drug loading as well as for scaled-up production are still a major challenge to pharmaceutical scientists.

When appropriately formulated, i.e., with suitable emulsifiers and a suitable ratio of emulsifier to oil to water, emulsions can be made as colloidal droplets, or nanoemulsions. Such preparations have been used to enhance drug absorption through various routes, such as transdermal, intranasal, and oral administration. Recently, a self-nanoemulsifying drug delivery system (SNEDDS) has been developed.[11] In this technique, a preconcentrate consisting of the oil, surfactant with or without cosurfactant is first prepared. When added to water, the preconcentrate can spontaneously form nanoemulsions with droplets of 10–100 nm. The choices of oils and surfactants and cosurfactants are basically empirical. Oils with medium chain of certain hydrophilicity (HLB 4–6) and surfactants of high HLB value around 15 are preferred. Compared to nanoemulsions, SNEDDS provides several advantages. First, the preconcentrate is more physically stable and less affected by the environmental factors such as temperature. Second, the drug loaded in the preconcentrate is more chemically stable over the storage period due to the absence of water. Third, the preconcentrate can be filled in capsules due to their anhydrous nature, providing a convenient and more patient-compliant approach. **Figure 13-3** is a phase diagram of the mixture of an oil, water, and emulsifiers for a SNEDDS preparation. In this study, the preconcentrate is prepared by mixing the oil (lauroglycol FCC), surfactant (Cremophor EL), and cosurfactant (Transcutol HP), where the ratio of Cremophor EL to Transcutol HP is kept constant at 4 : 3. The area marked by NE (nanoemulsion) indicates the region (composition of oil, water, and emulsifier) where the SNEDDS is formed, and a phase inversion depending on the content of water. As can be seen, when the ratio of oil to (surfactant + cosurfactant) falls in the range of 1 : 8 to 1 : 1, W/O nanoemulsion starts to form when 10% water (from phosphate buffered saline) is added to the preconcentrate. When the weight of water is increased to 25–30%, however, the nanoemulsion becomes O/W, indicating that the SNEDDS system is dynamic and can be used to prepare W/O as well as O/W nanoemulsions.

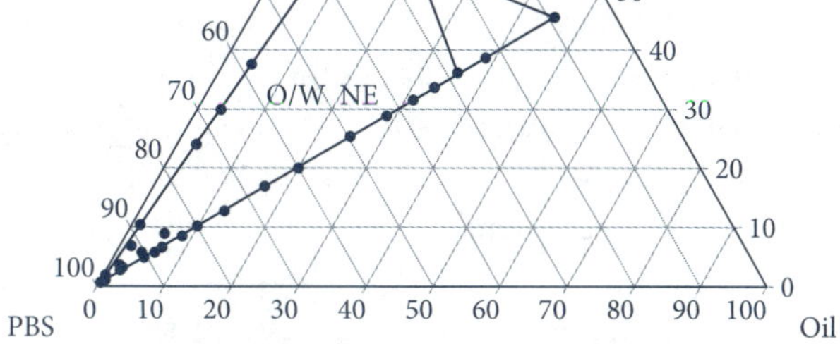

Figure 13-3 Phase diagram showing the formation of SNEDDS nanoemulsion (NE) with oil (lauroglycol FCC), surfactant (SA, Cremophor EL) and cosurfactant (CoSA, Transcutol HP) and water (PBS) at room temperature. The ratio of SA to CoSA is 4 : 3.[11]

IV. Applications of Nanopreparations in Drug Delivery

Research on nanopreparations such as nanoparticles, nanoemulsions, and liposomes has been significantly advanced in the past two decades. These preparations can be used to achieve various objectives in drug delivery, such as to enhance the absorption of drugs, to stabilize the drugs by preventing the drugs from contact with the harsh environment, to deliver the drugs to a special tissue or organ by certain targeting approaches, and to provide controlled-release mechanisms.

Enhancing Absorption

Biological membranes are usually not permeable to hydrophilic drugs such as proteins and peptides. The absorption of these drugs is very minimal. Studies have shown that insulin-loaded liposomes can enhance the pulmonary absorption of insulin,[12] and chitosan-coated PLGA nanoparticles can enhance pulmonary absorption of calcitonin.[13] Chitosan is a natural cationic polymer that can adhere to absorption mucosa and can open the tight junctions between the epithelial cells of the membrane, thereby enhancing drug absorption. Studies have also shown that when loaded in the preconcentrate of O/W SNEDDS nanoemulsion, the oral absorption of beta-lactamase (a protein) can be improved.[14] It is thought that some of the fine oil droplets can be easily absorbed intact in the GI tract, and thus the loaded drugs will be absorbed simultaneously. The challenge here is the loading of hydrophilic protein into the oil phase. In this study, first the protein is incorporated into a solid dispersion with amphiphiles such as hydrogenated soy phosphatidylcholine. Then the solid dispersion is dissolved into the preconcentrate of SNEDDS. It is believed that the amphiphilic molecules wrapping around the protein molecules help the protein stay inside the preconcentrate, and then stay inside the oil droplets when the preconcentrate is diluted with water.

The water-insoluble drugs pose a big challenge for delivery because the drugs must be in a solution form before they can be sufficiently absorbed. Nanoemulsions can be used to solve this problem. The water-insoluble drug can be dissolved in a suitable oil medium and then made to form O/W nanoemulsions or SNEDDS. These preparations mimic the solution form, as the drug is highly dispersed. Such preparations will significantly enhance the absorption based on the following three possibilities: (1) The drug may be absorbed with the fine oil droplets; (2) the emulsifiers in the preparation may interact with the absorption membrane to make it more permeable; and (3) if the oil phase is digested, such as in the case of oral administration, the drug may precipitate out in very fine amorphous forms that can be quickly dissolved in the biological fluid to warrant enough absorption. Or the drug may remain inside the micelles formed by the partially digested product of the oil phase, which may enhance the absorption. Many studies have shown that nanoemulsions or SNEDDS can significantly enhance the oral bioavailability of water-insoluble drug.[15,16,17] The marketed product, Neoral, a nanoemulsion preparation of cyclosporine, a water-insoluble drug, is an example of such a strategy.

Reducing Degradation and Elimination

Many drugs are susceptible to enzymatic or chemical degradation. Once loaded inside the nanopreparations, the drugs are isolated from the harsh environment and thus protected from potential degradation. Insulin-loaded nanoparticles made of chitosan and hydroxypropyl methylcellulose phthalate have been shown to improve the oral bioavailability of insulin 10-fold compared to the solution form due to the reduced degradation in the GI tract and the mucoadhesive and permeation-enhancing properties of chitosan.[18] Liposomes coated with chitosan or chitosan–aprotinin conjugate (aprotinin is an enzyme inhibitor) have been shown significantly to enhance the pharmacological activity of orally delivered calcitonin by 11-fold and 15-fold, respectively, compared to the solution dosage form.[19] Indocyanine green (ICG) is a diagnostic agent and has the potential to be used for photodynamic treatment of cancer. It is not stable in water, and once injected into the blood circulation, it is bound to the plasma proteins and quickly eliminated from the circulation (half-life of about 2–4 min). Studies have shown that once it is loaded in PLGA nanoparticles, the half-life in water is improved by about 4 times.[20] The ICG-loaded PLGA nanoparticle can significantly prolong the circulation time of ICG in the blood system, and thus enhance the ICG deposit into various tissues.[6, 20]

Targeting Delivery

Nanopreparations can also be developed for targeting delivery of drug to tumors. It has been found that the vasculature systems in most of the solid tumors have higher permeability than that in normal tissue, and the lymphatic drainages in the tumor tissues are slow, resulting in long retention of macromolecules. This enhanced permeability and retention (EPR) effect provides a passive targeting mechanism. To utilize the EPR effect, small-molecule anticancer agent can be loaded into nanopreparations. High amounts of deposit into tumor can be achieved if the nanopreparation has a sufficiently long half-life in the blood circulation, as this kind of passive targeting through EPR needs time. Conventional polymeric nanoparticles are rapidly removed from the bloodstream after intravenous administration by the reticuloendothelial system (RES). One of the commonly used methods to prolong the circulation time of nanopreparations is to modify the surface with PEG.[21, 22] PEG, a hydrophilic polymer, can help the nanoparticles avoid being recognized by the RES and thus have a prolonged residence in blood. PEG-modified doxorubicin-loaded liposome (Doxil) has been shown to enhance the blood circulation of doxorubicin, a chemotherapeutic agent, and reduce the distribution volume of doxorubicin by limiting its presence mainly in blood circulation, thus enhancing the uptake of the drug by solid tumors through the EPR effect. Doxil also has fewer adverse effects such as cardiotoxicity compared to the solution form of free doxorubicin.[23]

In addition to the passive targeting through EPR, the surface of the nanopreparations can be further modified to achieve an active targeting mechanism. For example, the high-affinity folate receptor is overexpressed on the cell surface in many epithelial carcinomas such as breast cancer and ovarian cancer, but it occurs in only a limited number of normal tissues with low to moderate levels. Modification of nanopreparations with surface attached folic acid can make the systems actively target the tumors with overexpression of folate receptor.[24, 25] Studies have shown that surface modification of ICG-loaded PLGA nanoparticles with both folic acid and PEG can achieve double or more anticancer effect compared to the single modification with folic acid or PEG, and 3-fold or more ICG deposit into tumor compared to the unmodified PLGA nanoparticles. These studies show that the nanopreparations clearly represent an important approach in current drug targeting research.

V. Chapter Summary

This chapter describes the dosage forms of suspensions, emulsions, and colloidal systems as well as the principles and methods to prepare these common pharmaceutical dosage forms. The main issue with suspensions and emulsions is the phase separation, but the colloidal systems do not have this problem and are thermodynamically stable. Suspensions are usually prepared for drugs with limited water solubility. Sometimes drugs are prepared as suspension in order to have a sustained-release profile to prolong the drug action. Emulsions usually employ surfactants to make a relatively stable homogeneous mixture of oil and water, so that various water-soluble and oil-soluble drugs and ingredients can be mixed well for easy administration. Colloidal systems such as nanoparticle dispersions and nanoemulsions have emerged as important delivery systems providing some unique advantages in enhancing drug absorption and stability and targeted drug delivery.

VI. References

1. Defelippis MR, Bakaysa DL, Bell MA, et al. Preparation and characterization of a cocrystalline suspension of [LysB28, ProB29]-human insulin analogue. *J Pharm Sci.* 87:170–176, 1998.
2. Griffin WC. Calculation of HLB values of non-ionic surfactants. *J Soc Cos Chem.* 5:259, 1954.
3. Talman FAJ and Rowan EM. *J Pharm Pharmacol.* 22:338, 1970; Barry BW, et al., *J Pharm Sci.* 62:1954, 1973.
4. Liu Y, Zhu YY, Wei G, and Lu WY. Effect of carrageenan on poloxamer-based *in situ* gel for vaginal use: Improved in vitro and in vivo sustained-release properties. *Eur J Pharm Sci.* 37:306–312, 2009.
5. Choi S, Baudys M, and Kim SW. Control of blood glucose by novel GLP-1 delivery using biodegradable triblock copolymer of PLGA-PEG-PLGA in type 2 diabetic rats. *Pharm Res.* 21:827–831, 2004.
6. Saxena V, Sadoqi M, and Shao J. Polymeric nanoparticulate delivery system for indocyanine green: Biodistribution in healthy mice. *Int J Pharm.* 308:200–204, 2006.
7. Damgé C, Maincent P, and Ubrich N. Oral delivery of insulin associated to polymeric nanoparticles in diabetic rats. *J Control Release.* 117:163–170, 2007.
8. Bajpai AK and Choubey J. Design of gelatin nanoparticles as swelling controlled delivery system for chloroquine phosphate. *J Mater Sci Mater Med.* 17:345–358, 2006.
9. Dung TH, Lee SR, Han SD, et al. Chitosan-TPP nanoparticle as a release system of antisense oligonucleotide in the oral environment. *J Nanosci Nanotechnol.* 7:3695–3699, 2007.
10. Wu M, Dellacherie E, Durand A, and Marie E. Poly(*n*-butyl cyanoacrylate) nanoparticles via miniemulsion polymerization (1): Dextran-based surfactants. *Colloids Surf B: Biointerfaces.* 69:141–146, 2009.
11. Rao SVR and Shao J. Self-nanoemulsifying drug delivery systems (SNEDDS) for oral delivery of protein drugs. I. Formulation development. *Int J Pharm.* 362:2–9, 2008.
12. Huang YY and Wang CH. Pulmonary delivery of insulin by liposomal carriers. *J Controlled Release.* 113:9–14, 2006.
13. Yamamoto H, Kuno Y, Sugimoto S, Takeuchi H, and Kawashima Y. Surface-modified PLGA nanosphere with chitosan improved pulmonary delivery of calcitonin by mucoadhesion and opening of the intercellular tight junctions. *J Control Release.* 102:373–381, 2005.
14. Rao SVR, Yajurvedi K, and Shao J. Self-nanoemulsifying drug delivery system (SNEDDS) for oral delivery of protein drugs. III. *In vivo* oral absorption study. *Int J Pharm.* 362:16–19, 2008.
15. Araya H, Tomita M, and Hayashi M. The novel formulation design of O/W microemulsion for improving the gastrointestinal absorption of poorly water soluble compounds. *Int J Pharm.* 305:61–74, 2005.
16. Kawakami K, Yoshikawa T, Hayashi T, Nishihara Y, and Masuda K. Microemulsion formulation for enhanced absorption of poorly soluble drugs. II. In vivo study. *J Control Release.* 81:75–82, 2002.
17. Shah NH, Carvajal MT, Patel CI, Infeld MH, and Malick AW. Self-emulsifying drug delivery systems (SEDDS) with polyglycolyzed glycerides for improving in vitro dissolution and oral absorption of lipophilic drugs. *Int J Pharm.* 106:15–23, 1994.
18. Makhlof A, Tozuka Y, and Takeuchi H. Design and evaluation of novel pH-sensitive chitosan nanoparticles for oral insulin delivery. *Eur J Pharm Sci.* 42:445–451, 2011.
19. Werle M and Takeuchi H. Chitosan–aprotinin coated liposomes for oral peptide delivery: Development, characterisation and in vivo evaluation. *Int J Pharm.* 370:26–32, 2009.

20. Saxena V, Sadoqi M, and Shao J. Enhanced photo-stability, thermal-stability and aqueous-stability of indocyanine green in polymeric nanoparticulate systems. *J Photochem Photobiol B: Biol.* 74:29–38, 2004.
21. Avgoustakis K, Beletsi A, Panagi Z, et al. Effect of copolymer composition on the physicochemical characteristics, in vitro stability, and biodistribution of PLGA-mPEG nanoparticles. *Int J Pharm.* 259:115–127, 2003.
22. Gref R, Domb A, Quellec P, et al. The controlled intravenous delivery of drugs using PEG-coated sterically stabilized nanospheres. *Adv Drug Deliv Rev.* 16:215–223, 1995.
23. Gabizon A, Shmeeda H, and Barenholz Y. Pharmacokinetics of PEGylated liposomal doxorubicin: Review of animal and human studies. *Clin Pharmacokinetics.* 42:419–436, 2003.
24. Leamon CP and Low PS. Folate-mediated targeting: From diagnostics to drug and gene delivery. *Drug Discov Today.* 6:44–51, 2001.
25. Miki K, Oride K, Inoue S, et al. Ring-opening metathesis polymerization-based synthesis of polymeric nanoparticles for enhanced tumor imaging in vivo: Synergistic effect of folate-receptor targeting and PEGylation. *Biomaterials.* 31:934–942, 2010.

VII. Homework Problems

1. What are the physicochemical parameters that define the physical stability of (*a*) a suspension or (*b*) an emulsion?
2. (*a*) From Equation (13-1), determine the cgs unit for viscosity. (*b*) What is the cgs unit for surface tension?
3. A drug powder with a true density of 2.25 g/cm^3 and a mean diameter of 50 μm is dispersed in a vehicle containing 1.9% carboxymethylcellulose (medium viscosity) having a solution density of 1.02 g/cm^3 and a zero-shear viscosity of 800 cP. Using Stokes' law, calculate the sedimentation rate of this suspension.
4. If, in the above suspension, the particle size is reduced to 10 μm, calculate the sedimentation rate, the stress caused by gravitation, and the maximum rate of shear using Equations (13-1), (13-1*a*), and (13-1*b*). Check Table 13-2 and see if this sedimentation is acceptable as a pharmaceutical preparation.
5. The following is the formula for the vehicle for oral suspension, NF. Describe the function of each ingredient and show how the formula should be prepared.

Cellulose, Microcrystalline (MCC)	800 mg
Xanthan gum	200 mg
Carrageenan	150 mg
Carboxymethylcellulose Sodium (High Viscosity)	25 mg
Citric Acid	250 mg
Sodium Phosphate, Dibasic	120 mg
Simethicone	0.1 mL
Potassium Sorbate	100 mg
Methylparaben	100 mg
Purified water, a sufficient quantity to make	100 mL

6. What are floccules? Name three kinds of flocculating agents with examples.
7. Describe how flocculation occurs in suspensions containing charged particles.
8. The required HLB value for mineral oil to form a stable O/W emulsion is 12. If Tween 20 (HLB 16.7) and Span 60 (HLB 4.7) are used as the emulsifiers, what should be the weight ratio of the two emulsifiers? If 20 g are needed to prepare 100 g of the emulsion, calculate the amount needed for each emulsifier.
9. **Table 13-5** shows the required HLB for some lipid materials used as the oil phase for either W/O or O/W emulsions.

Table 13-5 Required HLB Values for the Oil Phase Materials Used in O/W and W/O Emulsions

Lipid	O/W	W/O
Beeswax	9–12	4
Castor oil	14	6
Cetyl alcohol	15	
Cottonseed oil	6–10	5
Lanolin anhydrous	10–12	8
Mineral oil	11–12	5
Oleic acid	17	
Olive oil	14	6
Paraffin wax	10–11	4
Petrolatum	8–12	5
Stearic acid	15	6

Using these data, calculate the required HLB value for the following formulation.

Rx	Mineral oil	25 g
	Cetyl alcohol	10 g
	Petrolatum	10 g
	Emulsifier	1.5 g
	Preservatives	2.0 g
	Purified water, q.s.	100 g

10. How does a surfactant work as an emulsifier?
11. Would a droplet of decane or oleic acid spread on water at 20°C? The surface tension data are as follows:

	γ, dyn/cm	γ_{LL}, dyn/cm
Water	72.8	
Decane	23.9	
Oleic acid	32.5	
Water–decane		52.3
Water–oleic acid		15.6

12. Describe the potential stability problems associated with emulsions and methods to enhance emulsion stability.
13. Why is the colloidal system thermodynamically stable whereas the macroemulsion system is not?
14. Describe the property of a lyophilic colloid that exhibits (*a*) thixotropy and (*b*) thermal sensitivity.
15. What are the core materials used in making (*a*) nanoparticles, (*b*) nanoemulsions, (*c*) liposomes, (*d*) micelles, and (*e*) polymeric micelles?
16. Name the potential applications of the nanosystems in pharmaceutical drug delivery.
17. Why is the nanosystem particularly suited for passive targeting of drug to the tumor site in anticancer chemotherapy?

CHAPTER 14

Transdermal Drug Delivery

Sudjit Luanpitpong and Yon Rojanasakul

Transdermal drug delivery offers several advantages over oral and parenteral routes of administration. However, the physiological skin barrier, which is attributable to the unique structure of the stratum corneum, limits its permeability to only certain drugs and drug candidates. Expanding the use of the transdermal route to a larger group of drug candidates remains a major challenge in transdermal drug development. Currently, several pharmaceutical, chemical, and physical approaches have been developed to overcome the barrier function of the skin and to enhance drug absorption. These enhancement methods have been employed in several drug products currently in use and in clinical trials. This chapter describes the basic principles of transdermal drug delivery, skin barrier properties, and routes of drug penetration. Also discussed are the various *penetration enhancement* methods and transdermal delivery systems as well as some examples of commercial products and their use.

CHAPTER OUTLINE

OBJECTIVES

1. Describe the skin barrier to drug penetration.
2. Describe the advantages and limitations of transdermal drug delivery.
3. Describe the physicochemical factors affecting drug penetration across the skin.
4. Describe various means of penetration enhancement and its mechanisms of action.
5. Describe the principle and basic components of transdermal patches.

I. Transdermal Delivery Routes

Terminology

Transdermal delivery is the movement of compounds (drugs) across the skin into the systemic circulation. *Epidermis* is the outer, epithelial portion of the skin. The outermost layer of epidermis called *stratum corneum* poses the major resistance to transdermal transport. Capillary network (blood and lymphatic vessels), nerve endings, pilobaceous units (hair follicles and sebaceous glands) and sweat glands are embedded within the dermis.

Skin presents the largest and most readily accessible organ of the body, accounting for approximately 16% of total body weight and one-third of blood circulating through the body. The skin serves as environmental barrier to prevent the loss of water and body components, protect the body from environmental insults and also has important immune and sensory functions.[1, 2]

Routes of Skin Penetration

Regardless of the dosage forms (e.g., creams, gels, ointments, suspensions, emulsions, and patches), drug molecules that are in contact with the skin may penetrate the skin through three possible pathways: a) appendageal route or shunt pathway via the sweat ducts, hair follicles, and sebaceous glands; b) intercellular route across the stratum corneum via the tortuous route of lipid matrix; and c) transcellular route directly across the stratum corneum (**Figure 14-1**).[3, 4]

Appendageal Route

Skin appendages (sweat ducts, hair follicles, and sebaceous glands) provide a continuous pathway directly across the stratum corneum. However, their influence on drug penetration is limited by a number of factors, including the limited availability of appendages that occupy a relatively small surface area for penetration (approximately 0.1% of skin surface area) and the traveling against the permeant diffusion pathway of secretions. It has been suggested that the appendageal route is predominant only for the pre-steady-state penetration of polar molecules. Its contribution to the steady-state flux of most drugs is minimal, but may influence the flux of large polar molecules or ions that have difficulties diffusing across the stratum corneum. Accordingly, most skin penetration enhancement methods have focused on increasing drug penetration across the stratum corneum.

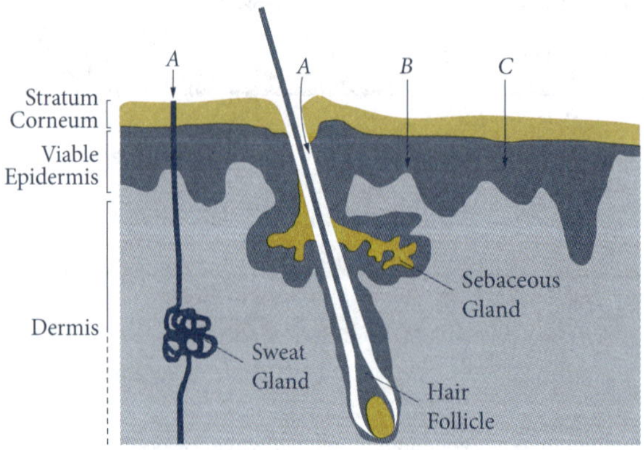

Figure 14-1 A simplified diagram of the cross section of human skin illustrating the various possible routes of penetration: (*A*) appendageal route, (*B*) intercellular route, and (*C*) transcellular route.

Intercellular and Transcellular Route

Intercellular and transcellular routes involve the penetration across the stratum corneum through the tortuous routes of continuous lipid matrix and corneocytes, respectively. To understand thoroughly these routes of penetration, one must study an overview of the stratum corneum's structure and barrier function.

II. Epidermal Barrier

The epidermis itself is divided into several layers, working in concert to provide strength and flexibility to the skin. Just above the dermis is the stratum basale (basal layer), which proceeds upward through the stratum spinosum (prickle layer) and stratum granulosum (granular layer) to the outermost layer, the stratum corneum (horny layer). Keratinocytes are the predominant cell type of the epidermis, existing from the stratum basale to the stratum granulosum at which they transform into corneocytes (inactive, dead keratinocytes) of the stratum corneum. The stratum corneum consists of 10–15 layers of corneocytes depending on the body site and varies in thickness from approximately 10–15 μm (dry state) to 40 μm (hydrated state).[5]

Stratum Corneum Barrier

The stratum corneum is considered the major barrier to transdermal drug penetration. The structure of the stratum corneum is conceptually modeled as *bricks and mortars*.[1,6] The keratin-rich corneocytes with their resistant cell envelope are considered to be the bricks, and the lipid matrixes between the cells (intercellular space) are considered to be the mortars. All the bricks are linked by corneodesmosomes (**Figure 14-2**). Notably, corneocytes are not brick-shaped but are polygonal, elongated, and flat. Both the bricks and mortars of the stratum corneum are produced by keratinocytes in the stratum granulosum at which the granular contents containing proteins and lipids are released into the intercellular space as they are transformed into the corneocytes. During the transformation of keratinocytes, their plasma membranes are replaced with an insoluble protein layer called cornified envelope, which confers its strength and scaffold to attachment of the lipid mortars. Corneocytes contain a natural moisturizing factor (NMF), which is essential to the retention of water.[7] In the intercellular space, lipids including ceramides (converted from glycosyl ceramides of the stratum granulosum), cholesterol, cholesterol esters, and long-chain fatty acids spontaneously organize with water into multiple stacked bilayers between the corneocytes to form a *lamellar* structure (**Figure 14-3**). The lipid lamellar is further complicated by the presence of intrinsic and extrinsic proteins such as enzymes. Accordingly, the lipid-phase behavior of the skin is strikingly different from that of other biological membranes and is vital to its barrier function.[8]

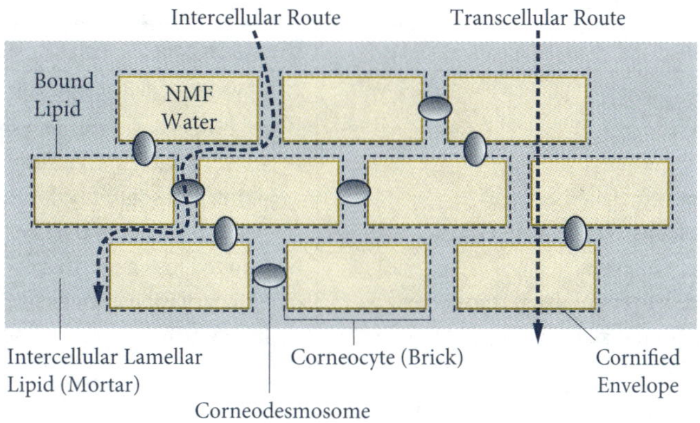

Figure 14-2 Diagrammatic representation of the bricks-and-mortars model of the stratum corneum.

It was earlier believed that hydrophilic molecules would diffuse through the intercellular route while the lipophilic molecules would diffuse through the transcellular route. Recent studies on the stratum corneum structure suggest that it is not that simple to determine the predominant route of drug penetration as each route cannot be viewed in isolation (Figure 14-2). Within the corneocytes is an aqueous environment, but the cells are surrounded by the lipid-bound envelope, which is connected to lamellar lipids. Each corneocyte is separated by approximately 4–20 lipid lamellae. Accordingly, a number of partitioning and diffusion steps are required for the transcellular route. For the intercellular route, which represents a tortuous route winding around the cells and along the lipid lamellae, the distance path is estimated to be much farther than the thickness of the stratum corneum or transcellular route. Additionally, drugs must sequentially partition into and diffuse through repeated aqueous and lipid domains of multiple stacked bilayers (Figure 14-3). Therefore, the physiochemical properties of drugs strongly influence their permeation route.

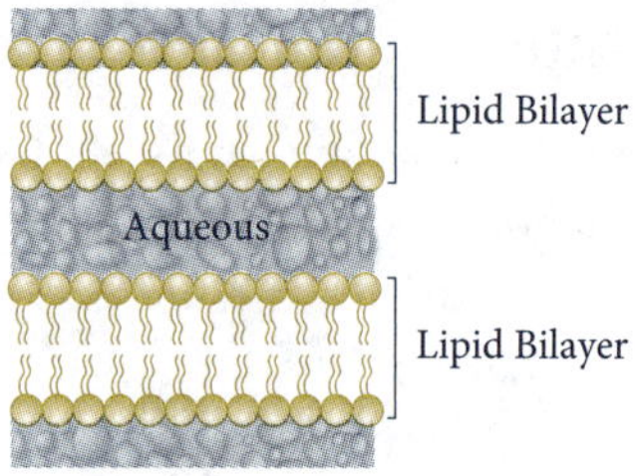

Figure 14-3 Lamellar structure of the intercellular lipid.

III. Advantages and Limitations

As mentioned earlier, the skin has a large surface area and blood supply; therefore it has gained increasing interest as a site for systemic drug delivery. The advantages and limitations of the transdermal drug delivery are summarized in **Table 14-1**.[9, 10]

Several mathematical models have been developed to describe and predict the skin permeation of drugs. *Potts and Guy*[11] correlate skin permeability (P_s) to a drug in an aqueous solution with the drug's molecular weight (MW) and octanol–water partition coefficient by Equation (14-1):

$$\log P_s \cong -2.7 + 0.71 \log K_{O/W} - 0.0061\text{MW} \qquad (14\text{-}1)$$

A similar equation has been proposed by others with the addition of the drug's melting point (MP) to better fit the data[12]:

$$\log P_s = -2.355 + 0.82 \log K_{O/W} - 0.00933\text{MW} - 0.00387\text{MP} \qquad (14\text{-}2)$$

These models provide a quantitative structure–activity relationship (QSAR) between the permeability and the relative solubility of a drug in the octanol–water system, and show that while the permeability increases with increasing log $K_{O/W}$, greater values in molecular volume and melting point result in lowered skin permeability.

Table 14-1 Advantages and Limitations of Transdermal Drug Delivery

Advantages	Limitations
• Easily accessible • Large available surface area • Low proteolytic enzyme activity • Avoidance of first-pass metabolism • Avoidance of variables associated with GI tract, e.g., pH and gastric emptying time • Facilitates sustained delivery of drugs, providing a steady-state plasma profile, reducing dosing frequency and peak-associated side effects • Noninvasive, desirable for long-term treatment • High flexibility for dosing, easily removed in case of toxicity	• Limited to drugs with suitable physicochemical properties, including molecular weight and size, partition and diffusion coefficients, melting point, and solubility, for the penetration of the stratum corneum barrier • Limited to potent drugs • Skin irritation and sensitization in some individuals

IV. Penetration Enhancement

As indicated earlier, the stratum corneum presents the rate-limiting barrier for transdermal drug delivery. Consequently, various approaches have been developed to overcome the stratum corneum barrier.

Drug-Based Approaches

Drug- and vehicle-based approaches are designed mainly to enhance the partitioning of drugs into the stratum corneum. These approaches include the following.

Saturated and Supersaturated Solutions

Drug permeation across the stratum corneum is governed by the passive diffusion process according to Fick's first law of diffusion (Equation 14-3)

$$\frac{dm}{A\,dt} = J = \frac{DC_0K}{h} \tag{14-3}$$

where J is flux or cumulative amount of drug passing the membrane per unit surface area (A), D is the diffusion coefficient of the drug, C_0 is the concentration of the drug in the vehicle, K is the partition coefficient between the stratum corneum and the vehicle, and h is the diffusional path length or thickness of the membrane.

The maximum flux of drug across the membrane (maximum skin penetration rate) is obtained when a drug is at its highest thermodynamic activity, as is the case in saturated or supersaturated solutions. Equation (14-3) can be rewritten in terms of thermodynamic activities as[13]

$$\frac{dm}{A\,dt} = \frac{aD}{\gamma h} \tag{14-4}$$

where a is the thermodynamic activity of the drug and γ is the effective activity coefficient in the membrane. In Equation (14-4), the concentration of drug in the membrane (C_0K) is now expressed as a/γ. The diffusion process is driven by the activity rather than the actual concentration of the drug in the membrane, which can be significantly greater than the activity under supersaturated conditions. *Supersaturation* of the vehicle leads to increased activity in the membrane and a greater increase in concentration. One can view the membrane as becoming saturated or supersaturated under these conditions. Because the concentration of the vehicle is already supersaturated, flux increases as the drug must permeate across the membrane. Supersaturation can be formed by evaporation of volatile solvent or by the cosolvent phenomenon. Briefly, mixing of a saturated solution with a poor solvent or antisolvent could create a supersaturated system. The supersaturated system can also be prepared by cooling a heated saturated solution down to skin temperature or by using moisture from the skin as an antisolvent. An increase in the flux of various drugs from 5-fold to more than 10-fold has been reported by using supersaturated solutions. The limitations of supersaturated systems are that (1) they are thermodynamically unstable and (2) they increase the chance of drug *crystallization*. Such crystallization can be inhibited by antinucleating agents such as polyvinylpyrrolidone (PVP) and hydroxypropyl methylcellulose (HPMC), which are thought to adsorb onto the initial crystals, thus preventing further crystallization.[14, 15]

Prodrugs

Prodrugs are inactive or less active forms of drug substances. Once administered, prodrugs are metabolized into active drugs, which exert pharmacological effects. Prodrugs are designed to improve the partition coefficient or solubility of unfavorable active drugs. Generally, a *promoiety* is covalently linked to an active drug via an ester bond to optimize the balance between lipid and aqueous domain. Prodrugs are cleaved by nonspecific esterases upon reaching the viable epidermis to release the active drugs. A good example is the increase in the penetration of a very polar drug, 6-mercaptopurine, up to 240-fold higher than its parent form, using S^6-acyloxymethyl and 9-dialkylaminomethyl promoieties.[16]

Ion Pairs

Charged drugs do not readily penetrate the stratum corneum. Formation of ion pairs with oppositely charged species to the charged drugs would neutralize the charges and improve the drug's partition into the stratum corneum. The ion pairs then dissociate in the viable epidermis, releasing the parent charged drugs that subsequently diffuse into the deeper skin layers. The ion pair strategy has been used to enhance the skin penetration of various drugs, including ibuprofen, diclofenac, and lidocaine.[17]

Eutectic Mixtures

As mentioned earlier, the melting points of drugs influence their skin permeability. In general, lowering the melting point increases the solubility of the drug in a given solvent, including skin lipids. A eutectic mixture or a mixture of two components at a certain ratio that inhibit the crystallization of each other could lower the melting point of the two components compared to each component alone. The phase diagram of the eutectic composition and temperature for a binary system is shown in **Figure 14-4**. At or above the eutectic temperature, which is lower than the melting point of either solid A or solid B, there exists solid A in liquid, solid B in liquid, or solution of A and B, depending on the composition of the two components. At the eutectic composition, both solids melt at the eutectic temperature. However, not all systems can form eutectic mixtures. Many studies reported the use of chemical penetration enhancers as the second component, e.g., ibuprofen with terpenes, and propranolol with fatty acids.[17]

Vehicle-Based Approaches

Liposomes are thermodynamically stable vesicles consisting of lipid bilayers surrounding aqueous central cores. Both compartments are capable of encapsulating or entrapping drugs, depending on their biphasic nature (lipophilic or hydrophilic) and solubility. Conventional liposomes are composed of phospholipids, often with cholesterol to stabilize the system. Recent studies have shown that conventional liposomes and the entrapped drugs generally accumulate in the stratum corneum and upper skin layers, with minimal drugs penetrating into the deeper tissues, thus having minimal value as a drug delivery carrier. Highly deformable, elastic liposomes, the transfersomes, have been developed to address this issue.[18] In addition to the phospholipid component, transfersomes contain 10–25% of surfactants such as sodium cholate, deoxycholate, Span 80, Tween 80, or dipotassium glycyrrhizinate. Surfactants act as an edge activator that permits elasticity

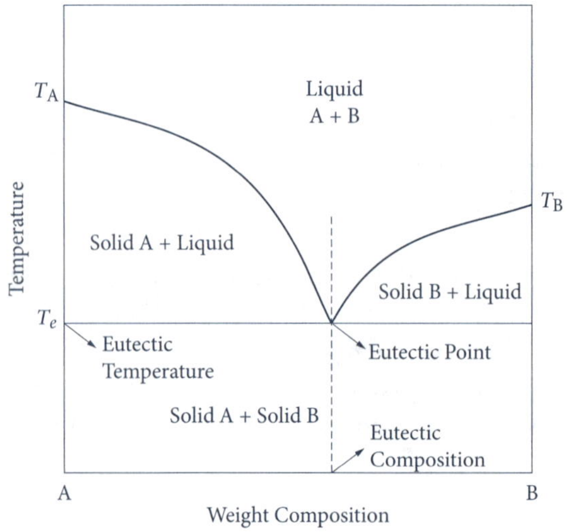

Figure 14-4 A simplified binary phase diagram. Abbreviations: T_A, melting point of solid A; T_B, melting point of solid B; T_e, the eutectic temperature.

and deformation of the bilayer structure. Transfersomes are said to squeeze through small channels sized only 10% of their diameter. This great flexibility allows them spontaneously to penetrate the stratum corneum (intercellular route) and avoid dehydration and instability caused by evaporation at the skin surface. Once in the lipid lamellar, the osmotic gradient from the difference in water content at the stratum corneum (~20% of water when dehydrated) and the viable epidermis (~100% of water at the basement layer) is suggested to be the driving force of transfersomes penetration into the deeper region. Recently, ketoprofen in transfersomes gel (Diractin) has been shown to be more efficacious in relieving muscle pain than a placebo gel or an oral ketoprofen.[19]

Ethosomes are liposomes that have a high ethanol content (20–45%). Ethanol, a well-known penetration enhancer, fluidizes the ethosomal lipids and confers high flexibility to the ethosomes. It has been proposed that ethosomes facilitate transdermal drug delivery by (1) the ethanol effect as ethanol initially disrupts the stratum corneum lipid and (2) the ethosomal effect, which allows the squeezing of ethosomes through the disrupted lipid membrane into the deeper skin layers.[20] Ethosomes have been used as a drug delivery carrier for various systemic drugs, including minoxidil, zidovudine, testosterone, and salbutamol.

Micellar nanoparticles (MNPs) are multiphasic nanoemulsions that can accommodate a range of compounds with varying physicochemical properties.[21] MNP formulation requires at least an oil, stabilizer or surfactant, solvent that usually assists drug solubilization, and an aqueous medium. MNPs are reported to have rapid skin penetration, attributable to their small size (< 100-nm diameter) and a structure which is complementary to the skin structure. The first transdermal commercial product utilizing the MNP technology is Estrasorb for estrogen replacement therapy. Other MNP formulations containing nicotine, oxybutynin, fentanyl, raloxifene, and cetririzine have also been developed and have shown promising results.

Other nanoparticulate systems have been adopted for transdermal drug delivery applications, including solid lipid nanoparticles (SLNs)and nanostructured lipid carriers (NLCs). Both SLN and NLC are lipid-based nanoparticles that, due to their solid matrix structure, can encapsulate drugs and control their release. It is assumed that the high surface area of these nanoparticulate systems facilitates the contact of encapsulated drugs with the stratum corneum, thus providing the occlusion effect that helps promote drug penetration. Recently, SLN and NLC dispersions of the anti-inflammatory flurbiprofen have been incorporated into hydrogels. The formulations show sustained release and increased bioavailability of the drug compared to oral administration in animal models.[17]

Stratum Corneum Modifications

Substances that reversibly decrease the barrier function of the stratum corneum to promote the skin penetration are known as chemical penetration enhancers. Ideal properties of the chemical enhancers include the following: They (1) are pharmacologically inactive; (2) are nontoxic, nonirritating, and nonallergenic; (3) are compatible with other ingredients in the formulation; (4) have rapid and reproducible permeability-enhancing effect; and (5) allow the skin barrier to recover rapidly after removal. Many classes of chemical enhancers have been tested for their enhancing activity.[22] The activity of enhancers can be expressed as enhancement ratio (ER)[23]

$$ER = \frac{\text{drug permeability coefficent after enhancer treatment}}{\text{drug permeability coefficent before enhancer treatment}} \quad (14\text{-}5)$$

Chemical enhancers promote the penetration of drugs across the skin through various mechanisms as described below.

Hydration

The water content of the stratum corneum is approximately 15–20% of its dry weight, depending on the external environmental humidity and body area. Hydration of the stratum corneum has been shown to increase the penetration of both hydrophilic and lipophilic drugs.[24, 25] It is assumed that high water content alters the solubility and partitioning of drugs as well as loosens up the skin structure. A small amount of water is present at the head group region of lipids, resulting in loosened lipid packing. A larger amount of water could exist as a separate phase in the intracellular space and cause corneocyte swelling. Hydration can be achieved by soaking the skin, using formulations with high water content (e.g., oil-in-water emulsions), and by occlusion with (1) hydrophobic ointments or water-in-oil emulsions containing paraffins, oils, or waxes that prevent transepidermal water loss (TEWL); (2) dressings; (3) plastic films; and (4) transdermal patches.

Lipid Disruption and Fluidization

Depending on their molecular structure, penetration enhancers can disrupt or fluidize the lipid organization by one or more of the following mechanisms: (1) intercalation into the lipid lamellae; (2) disruption of the lipid packing; (3) formation of separate domains in the lamellae; and (4) disappearance of the lamellar phase, resulting in the increase in diffusion coefficient (D) and permeation rate of drugs (refer to Fick's first law, Equation (14-3)).[26] Lipid disruption is believed to be the major enhancement mechanism of various chemical enhancers.

Fatty Acids

The penetration enhancing effect of fatty acids is dependent on their molecular structure, such as the chain length, polarity, saturation, and functional groups. The optimal structure was reported as saturated fatty acids with C10–C12 chain lengths attached to a polar head group, or C18 for unsaturated fatty acids.[27, 28] It has been suggested that short alkyl chains or unsaturated alkyl chains disrupt the packing of long, saturated alkyl chains of the stratum corneum lipids. Comparisons have been made with branched versus unbranched saturated fatty acids, and *cis* versus *trans* unsaturated fatty acids. In some but not all cases, the branched saturated fatty acids are more effective than the unbranched fatty acids in enhancing the skin penetration, whereas *cis* and *trans* unsaturated C16–C18 fatty acids are equally effective.[29] Among the various fatty acids, oleic acid is one of the most commonly used for penetration enhancement. With a double bond located halfway along the C18 chain in the *cis* configuration, oleic acid has a kinked or bent structure that helps disrupt the intercellular lipid packing and facilitates drug partitioning in the skin.[30]

Azone

Azone, 1-dodecylazacycloheptan-2-one, or laurocapram is a well-known C12 penetration enhancer. Its enhancing activity is believed to relate to its soup-spoon conformation, in which the seven-member ring lies in the plane of lipid polar head groups. However, Hadgraft et al. suggest that its intercalation into the stratum corneum lipid bilayers provides resistance to the existence of soup-spoon conformation.[31] Instead, based on the examination of a zone and five analogs, they suggest the influence of hydrogen bonding between the polar head groups of the compounds and ceramide molecules as an alternative mechanism. This bonding stabilizes the ceramide molecules, resulting in the penetration-retarding effect shown in the analog N-0195 of azone.

Surfactants

Surfactants are amphiphilic molecules composed of a hydrophilic head and lipophilic tail, usually an alkyl chain. Surfactants are classified by their charged head group as cationic (positively charged), anionic (negatively charged), and nonionic (uncharged) surfactants. Generally, the penetration enhancing effect of surfactants is concentration dependent. One of the most commonly used surfactants is sodium lauryl sulfate (SLS), an anionic surfactant. SLS disrupts the stratum corneum lipids and proteins in a partially reversible manner when used at 1% concentration. Such effect presumably is caused by the ability of SLS to absorb water, resulting in increased water content in the stratum corneum and subsequent expansion of the intercellular spaces.[17] Surfactants can also directly remove the stratum corneum lipids and decrease the skin barrier function.[1]

Terpenes

Terpenes are lipophilic nonaromatic substances found in essential oils. Several terpenes have been classified as Generally Recognized As Safe (GRAS) by the Food and Drug Administration (FDA) and have been shown to have a reversible enhancing effect. The penetration enhancement of terpenes is related to their physicochemical properties. For example, terpenes containing oxygen have a strong enhancing effect, whereas bicyclic terpenes have a weak effect.[17]

Alcohols

Ethanol is the most commonly used alcohol for penetration enhancement. Due to its versatile characteristics, various enhancement mechanisms of ethanol have been reported. As a solvent, ethanol increases the solubility of drugs. Once evaporating at skin temperature, ethanol may lead to supersaturation of drugs, thus improving their transport across the skin. In addition, ethanol is said to extract lipids and form aqueous channels in the stratum corneum, thus increasing skin permeability.[32]

Pore-Forming Peptides

Magainin is a known pore-forming peptide in bacterial cell walls. Kim et al. reported enhanced skin permeability through the administration of magainin with the chemical enhancer *N*-lauroylsacrosine in 50% ethanol (NLS-ethanol) from 15-fold with NLS-ethanol alone to 47-fold with the addition of magainin.[33] Structural analysis of the skin showed that NLS-ethanol disrupts the stratum corneum lipids and magainin potentiates the effect. Magainin alone, however, has no effect on the lipid disruption, probably due to its poor penetration into the stratum corneum.

Interaction with Keratin

Certain chemicals such as dimethylsulfoxide (DMSO), pyrrolidones, and urea interact with keratin in the corneocytes and alter skin permeability. DMSO has been extensively studied due to its ability to enhance the penetration of both hydrophilic and lipophilic compounds as well as its ease of formulation. The effect of DMSO is concentration-dependent with the effective concentration at $> 60\%$. At such a high concentration, DMSO interacts and binds with keratin filaments of the corneocytes, resulting in disruption of the filamentous structures.[23] Other mechanisms of DMSO have been attributed to its lipid-extracting ability and disorganization of intercellular structures. Topical application of high-concentration DMSO causes skin irritation, erythema, scaling, contact urticaria, and burning. DMSO analogs with greater applicability include dimethylacetamide, dimethylformamide, and decylmethylsulfoxide.

Pyrrolidone carboxylic acid is a component of the natural moisturizing factor (NMF), which regulates stratum corneum hydration. Accordingly, several pyrrolidone analogs have been developed and tested for their penetration-enhancing activity. Of those, *N*-methyl-2-pyrrolidone (NMP) and 2-pyrrolidone (2P) are most promising. At low concentrations, NMP and 2P interact with keratin filaments of the stratum corneum. At high concentrations, they interact with the polar head of lipid bilayers, displacing water molecules from the head region and generating large solvation shells that disrupt lipid packing.[30] Pyrrolidones improve the skin penetration of hydrophilic drugs but have minimal effect on lipophilic drugs. Skin irritation, including dermatitis and erythema, is the major factor limiting the use of pyrrolidones.

Urea is another component of NMF. Due to its hygroscopic and keratolytic properties, urea has long been used in clinical dermatology to treat psoriasis, neurodermatitis, and other hyperkeratotic skin conditions. Its penetration-enhancing activity is attributed to its interaction with keratin (keratolytic property) and hydration of the stratum corneum (hygroscopic property). However, the application of urea as penetration enhancer is limited by its hydrolytic instability and skin irritation, partly as a result of its keratolytic effect.[4]

Increasing Drug Partition and Solubility in the Stratum Corneum

According to Fick's first law of diffusion (Equations (14-3) and (14-4)), increasing drug partitioning and solubility in the stratum corneum would enhance the drug permeation rate, especially if the solubility parameter† of the stratum corneum lipids (δ_s) were changed to become closer to that of drugs in the stratum corneum (δ_i).[23] Therefore, a solvent capable of distributing within the stratum corneum may act as a penetration enhancer by altering the solubility parameter of the lipids from the inherent value ($\delta_s \sim 10$) to that of the drugs. An example of such a solvent is propylene glycol, which enhances the skin permeability of metronidazole ($\delta_i \sim 13.5$) while changing the solubility parameter of skin lipids to 14.8.

†The Hildebrand solubility parameter (δ) is the square root of the cohesive energy density of a substance, i.e., $\delta = [(\Delta H_v - RT)/V]^{1/2}$, where ΔH_v is the heat of vaporization, and V is the molecular volume. This parameter represents the energy needed to remove a unit volume of molecules from their neighbors for a complete separation, and provides a numerical estimation of interactions between materials. Compounds with similar values in solubility parameter will interact with each other, resulting in solvation and miscibility.

Combined Mechanisms

Fick's first law of diffusion indicates several physicochemical factors influencing drug penetration. A synergistic effect could be obtained by exploiting the combination effects, i.e., on drug diffusion (D) and partitioning (K). Examples are the various combinations of propylene glycol and azone, terpenes, oleic acid, NMP, or urea.

Stratum Corneum Bypassed

Tape Stripping

Repeated application of adhesive cellophane tape to the skin surface could remove layers of the stratum corneum over the repetitions, resulting in the loss of skin barrier function. However, tape stripping shows poor reproducibility and patient compliance, and therefore its use is limited.[17]

Stratum Corneum Ablation

In general medicine, ablation is the removal of a part of biological tissues. Stratum corneum ablation is classified according to the method used for the stratum corneum removal.[17, 34]

Laser Ablation

Laser ablation creates pores in the stratum corneum by matching the laser energy wavelength to the main absorption peak of water (2790 nm) or tissue proteins (2940 nm). The matching wavelength causes vibrational heating, formation of a high-pressure region, and subsequent micro-explosion. Laser ablation has been used successfully to enhance the skin penetration of various drugs, including 5-fluorouracil, indomethacin, and hydrocortisone, as well as macromolecules such as peptides and nucleic acids.

Suction Ablation

Suction ablation is the use of vacuum to produce a small blister on the skin, followed by removal of the blister's upper surface to provide a pathway for drug penetration. Although penetration enhancement is achieved, this method has poor patient compliance and is not suitable for routine use due to its multistep, time-consuming process.

Thermal Ablation

Radio-frequency thermal ablation is performed by the insertion of needlelike electrodes into the skin with an alternating current at radio frequency (100 kHz). Ions within the skin follow the change in direction of the alternating current, resulting in frictional heating and cell ablation. Microchannels approximately 30 μm in diameter and 70 μm deep are generated. This technique has been used to improve the transdermal delivery of diclofenac and granisetron in vitro and in vivo.

Microscissioning

Microscissioning involves the use of sharp micrometer-sized particles, e.g., aluminum oxide particles, under an accelerated condition of pressurized nitrogen stream directed toward the skin. The high-velocity particles cut the skin, forming micrometer-sized pores, while the surrounding skin is protected by a Teflon or polyimide mask. Drug formulation is then applied after the microscissioning. This technique raises a safety concern related to particle deposition in the skin and potential infections.

Microneedle Array

A microneedle array is a device containing numerous micrometer-sized needles, which can be fabricated with different materials, lengths, and diameters.[34] These pain-free devices have been shown to penetrate the stratum corneum into the viable epidermis, producing microchannels. Based on their structure, microneedles are classified into two types: solid and hollow needles. Solid needles require the removal of the device prior to application of drug formulation to the skin. Solid needles can also be coated with drugs that remain deposited in the skin after device removal. Alternatively, erodible solid needles that dissolve in the skin can be used. Drugs could be either incorporated into the soluble needles or applied after device removal. Hollow needles are needles with a centered cavity. Upon skin insertion, the hollow center creates a direct channel to the lower skin layers. Due to their more sophisticated fabrication design, solid needles have gained greater interest. Microneedle technology has been used successfully to enhance the penetration of a wide range of drugs and macromolecules, including diclofenac, erythropoietin, insulin, plasmid DNA, and anthrax vaccine.

Energy-Driven Methods

Ultrasound

The use of ultrasound to enhance the transdermal delivery of drugs is known as sonophoresis or phonophoresis. Frequencies ranging from 20 kHz to 16 MHz have been used; however, significant transdermal delivery enhancement was reported at low frequencies (< 100 kHz) with the delivery of macromolecules up to 48 kDa.[35, 36] Ultrasound can have multiple effects on the skin, including (1) the local heating effect, which could increase drug solubility, enhance blood flow, and accelerate drug diffusion; (2) the cavitation effect, which is caused by the growth and oscillation of gaseous cavities. The cavitation effect is more potent in penetration enhancement as it is believed to disrupt the stratum corneum. The safety profile of this technique has not been fully addressed. However, studies have indicated that high-intensity ultrasound can cause second-degree burns.

Iontophoresis

Iontophoresis is the method whereby a low level of electric current (< 10 V) is applied to the skin to generate an electrical potential gradient that drives the solute molecules across the skin. The penetration enhancement can be attributed to one or more of the following mechanisms: (1) electrorepulsion for charged solutes, where like charges repel one another; (2) electroosmosis for uncharged drugs, resulting from the movement of ionic species in the skin that creates osmotic flow of water; and (3) electroperturbation for both charged and uncharged drugs.[34] The appendageal route of skin penetration is believed to be the major transport pathway for iontophoretic drug delivery.[3] Factors that affect the system include electrode type, current type and intensity, pH of donor solution, buffer concentration, and competitive ion effect. The limitations of iontophoresis are the limited amount of current (< 0.5 mA cm^{-2}) that can be used safely, possible skin damage, and difficulty in enhancing the penetration of large molecules (> 7 kDa).

Electroporation

Electroporation involves the use of high-voltage pulses (10–1000 V), usually ≥ 100 V, for a very short time (milliseconds). When applied to the stratum corneum, these electrical pulses induce transient formation of aqueous pores in the lipid bilayers. Therefore, penetration enhancement by this method is closely related to pulse properties such as waveform and frequency. Electroporation has been used successfully for the delivery of molecules varying in size and lipophilicity. Macromolecules such as proteins and nucleotides can be delivered by this method without the 7-kDa limit, as is the case in iontophoresis.[37] Furthermore, electroporation can be used in combination with iontophoresis to increase drug flux, as demonstrated for some peptide drugs.

Jet Injection

Jet injection is a needleless injection to overcome the limitation of needle-based injection, such as needle phobia and accidental needle stick injury. The method uses a high-pressure jet (> 100 m/s) to pierce the skin to deliver drugs. Jet injectors are divided into liquid and powder injectors. For liquid injectors, repeated injections of tiny liquid volumes (10–15 nL) are made to the skin to minimize the pain and bruising associated with conventional injections. Studies using excised human skin indicate that there is a lag time (approximately 48 pulses) for the vehicle to penetrate the epidermis. After that, drug solution can be delivered at the rate of 1 μL/min.[17] For powder injectors, drug is formulated as a fine powder (20–100 μm in diameter). Dry powder formulations have the advantage of being more stable. This is particularly useful for the delivery of biopharmaceuticals such as vaccines that often require cold chain maintenance while in liquid formulations. However, high shear stress during injection could adversely affect the physical integrity of the molecules.

In addition to the methods described above, several other techniques have been proposed and used for the enhancement of transdermal drug delivery. These techniques include the use of pressurized pulses termed photochemical waves, heat-generating patches called controlled heat-assisted drug delivery, the magnetic field termed magnetophoresis, and unidirectional or multidirectional tension (0.01–10 mPa) termed skin stretching.[34] Furthermore, a combination of these methods such as iontophoresis and chemical enhancer, and ultrasound and iontophoresis, could be used to provide a synergistic effect.[38]

V. Transdermal Patches

Transdermal patches are dosage forms designed to deliver therapeutic drugs through the skin. Drugs are formulated in the patch, which is worn on the skin for an extended time. Properties that influence transdermal delivery from patches are (1) diffusion of drug from the vehicle through a rate-limiting membrane or polymer matrix to the stratum corneum; (2) sorption by the stratum corneum and penetration through the viable epidermis; and (3) uptake of drug by capillaries in the dermis.

Basic Components

Several basic components of the transdermal patches are listed below.[39, 40]

Polymer Matrix or Drug Reservoir

Polymers are the backbone of patches that control the release of drugs. Drugs can be dispersed in a polymer matrix, which can be liquid, solid, or semisolid. Polymers utilized for transdermal patches should be biocompatible, chemically stable and inert, and compatible with the drugs and other components. They are classified as natural polymers (e.g., celluloses, gelatin, gums, chitosan, and starch), synthetic elastomers (e.g., polybutadiene, polysiloxane, silicone rubber, butyl rubber, nitrile, and neoprene), and synthetic polymers (e.g., polyvinyl alcohol (PVA), polyvinylpyrrolidone (PVP), polymethylmethacrylate (PMMA), polyethylene (PE), polypropylene (PP), and polyamide).

Drugs

Not all drugs are suitable for transdermal delivery. Drugs that have the following physicochemical properties are good candidates for transdermal patches: uncharged (non-ionic), low molecular weight (< 500 Da), adequate solubility in both oil and water (log P, or log $K_{O/W}$ of the octanol–water system, between 1 and 3), low melting point (< 200°C), and most importantly high potency, requiring low doses to have a therapeutic effect.[39]

Permeation Enhancers

Permeation enhancers are used to promote drug permeation across the stratum corneum.

Pressure-Sensitive Adhesives

Pressure-sensitive adhesives (PSAs) are materials that adhere to a substrate with a small amount of pressure, usually not more than applied finger pressure. They should adhere over an extended time without irritating the skin or leaving residues when removed. PSAs can be on the face (reservoir system) or at the periphery (matrix system) of the patches to help maintain the intimate contact between the patch and skin. Polyacrylates, polyisobutylene, and silicone are the most widely used PSAs. The selection of PSAs largely depends on the patch type. For example, for the reservoir system employing face PSAs, drug penetration must not interfere with the adhesive property.

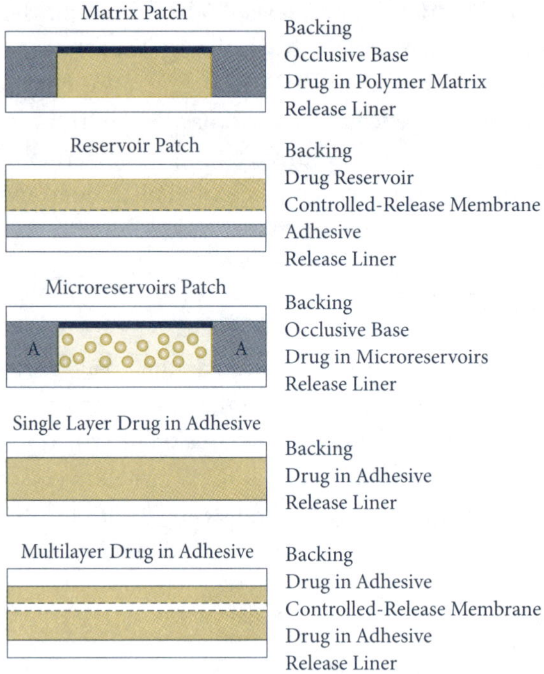

Figure 14-5 Different types of transdermal patches (A = adhesive).

Backing Laminates

Backing laminates prevent the drug from leaving the dosage form. They should be inert and compatible with the drugs and excipients in the formulation. For patient comfort, the backing laminates should be flexible and have high oxygen and moisture transmission rates. Examples of the backing materials used in transdermal patches are polyethylene, polyester, and vinyl polymers.

Other Excipients

Plasticizers such as dibutylphthalate, triethylcitrate, polyethylene glycol, and propylene glycol are used to provide plasticity and flexibility to the patches. In addition to the dosage form, release liners, which are considered part of the primary packaging, also require some special considerations. Release liners cover the patches during storage and are removed prior to use. Due to their prolonged contact with the patches, release liners should be inert and impervious to water and other ingredients.

Types of Patches

There are many types of transdermal patches, but they can be classified into four main categories[40–43] as depicted in **Figure 14-5** and described below.

Matrix Patches

In this system, drug solution or suspension is homogeneously dispersed in a polymer matrix and molded to form a medicated film, which is then overlaid by an adhesive polymer and mounted onto an occlusive base and impermeable backing. Therefore, the matrix-containing drug is in direct contact with the release liner. The advantages of matrix patches include avoidance of dose dumping and the interfering effect of the adhesive on drug release. Polymers commonly used for the matrix patches are cross-linked polyethylene glycol, polyacrylates, ethyl cellulose, PVP, and HPMC.

Reservoir Patches

Reservoir patches are characterized by their inclusion of a viscous liquid compartment containing drug solution or suspension separated from the release liner by a rate-controlling membrane and adhesive. The release rate of drugs from the patch is dictated mainly by drug solubility and thickness of the rate-controlling membrane. Thus far, ethylene vinyl acetate (EVA) is the most commonly used membrane for hydrophilic drugs as its permeability can be easily modified by adjusting the vinyl acetate content in the polymer. Lipophilic drugs poorly permeate the EVA membrane; therefore, polyurethane is more commonly used for this type of drug. The main advantage of reservoir patches is the constant drug release (zero-order) pattern. Some patches combine the reservoir and matrix types in one system, i.e., by replacing the liquid reservoir in the former with a polymer matrix such as polyisobutylene in the latter. This combination system is referred to as the membrane matrix hybrid patch, which offers a greater control of drug release.

Microreservoir Patches

Drug suspension in an aqueous solution is homogeneously dispersed in a polymeric solution by a high-shear mechanical force, forming thousands of drug microreservoirs. The thermodynamically unstable dispersion is then stabilized by cross-linking the polymer in situ, which produces a medicated disk. Drug loss from the disk is prevented by the occlusive base and backing material.

Drug-in-Adhesive Patches

Drugs and other excipients are directly incorporated in the adhesive. Therefore, the adhesive also serves as the formulation base under a single backing layer and is involved in controlling the drug release. Multilayer drug-in-adhesive patches can be fabricated by the addition of a membrane between the two drug-in-adhesive layers. Normally, the multilayer systems contain one immediate drug release layer and another controlled release layer, which is modulated through the membrane. Polymers suitable for the drug-in-adhesive patches are polysiloxanes, polyacrylates, and polyisobutylene. Because these polymers are hydrophobic, hydrophilic drugs are preferred in this drug-in-adhesive system.

VI. Transdermal Products

An increasing number of transdermal products have been approved by the FDA. Currently, approximately 20 drugs and drug combinations have been approved.[43] Some of these products are listed in **Table 14-2**.

Transdermal products in clinical trials include Diractin (ketoprofen in transfersome gel) for pain relief, Intanza (influenza vaccine using microneedle delivery device), Durhalieve (topical triamcinolone acetonide using Azone TS as chemical enhancer) for dermatoses, and Phosphagenics' insulin (insulin in targeted penetration matrix) for diabetes.

Table 14-2 Some Transdermal Products, Method of Delivery, and Indications

Drug	Trade Name	Manufacturer	Method	Indications
Scopolamine	Transderm-Scop	Novartis	Patch (membrane matrix hybrid)	Motion sickness
Nitroglycerin	Nitrodisc	Roberts Pharmaceutical	Patch (microreservoirs)	Angina pectoris
Clonidine	Catapres-TTS	Boehringer Ingelheim	Patch (membrane matrix hybrid)	Hypertension
Estradiol	Estrasorb	Graceway Pharmaceuticals	Topical emulsion (micellar nanoparticles)	Estrogen replacement therapy
Fentanyl	Duragesic	Janssen Pharmaceuticas	Patch (reservoir)	Chronic pain
Fentanyl HCl	Ionsys	Alza	Iontophoresis	Acute postoperative pain
Lidocaine	Sonoprep	Echo Therapeutics	Ultrasound	Local dermal analgesia
Rivastigmine	Exelon	Novartis	Patch (matrix)	Alzheimer's disease
Oxybutynin	Oxytrol	Watson Pharma	Patch (matrix)	Overactive bladder
Nicotine	Nicotrol	Cygnus Inc./McNeil Consumer Product	Patch (drug in adhesive)	Smoking cessation
Buprenorphine	Butrans	Purdue Pharma	Patch (matrix)	Pain relief

VII. Chapter Summary

Although the skin presents the largest and most readily accessible organ of the body, drug penetration via the transdermal route is very limited. The major transport barrier of the skin is the stratum corneum, which consists mainly of dead keratinocytes. Due to its inactive nature, drug permeation across the skin barrier occurs primarily through the passive diffusion process. Hence, most skin permeation enhancement methods are based on modifying the factors governing passive diffusion as presented in Fick's first law of diffusion. Several other methods have been attempted including the physical methods, such as laser ablation and microneedles, and energy-driven methods, such as iontophoresis and jet injection. Additionally, several combination methods such as physical and chemical enhancers have been attempted and may prove to be more effective in delivering drugs transdermally. However, safety concerns of these methods need to be addressed, especially those that involve alterations of the stratum corneum.

VIII. References

1. Wickett RR and Visscher MO. *Am J Infect Control.* 34:S98–S110, 2006.
2. Potts RO and Franoeur ML. *Proc Natl Acad Sci.* 87:3871–3873, 1990.
3. Prausnitz MR, Mitragotri S, and Langer R. *Nat Rev Drug Disc.* 3:115–124, 2004.
4. Trommer H and Neubert RHH. *Skin Pharmacol Physiol.* 19:106–121, 2006.
5. Ya-Xian Z, Suetake T, and Tagami H. *Arch Dermatol Res.* 291:555–559, 1999.
6. Nemes Z and Steinert PM. *Exp Mol Med.* 31:5–19, 1999.
7. Robinson MH and Wickett RR. *J Cosmet Sci.* 55:211–212, 2004.
8. Downing DT, Stewart ME, Wertz PW, Colton SW, Abraham W, and Strauss JS. *J Invest Dermatol Suppl.* 88:2s–6s, 1987.
9. Brown MB, Martin GP, Jones SA, and Akomeah FK. *Drug Deliv.* 13:175–187, 2006.
10. Soni M, Kumar S, and Gupta GD. *J Pharm Res.* 2:1184–1190, 2009.
11. Potts RO and Guy RH. *Pharm Res.* 9:663–669, 1992.

12. Barrat MD. *Toxic in Vitro.* 9:27–37, 1995.
13. Higuchi T. *J Soc Cosmet Chem.* 11:85–97, 1960.
14. Ma X, Taw J, and Chiang C. *Int J Pharm.* 142:115–119, 1996.
15. Krishnaiah YSR, Bhaskar P, and Satyanarayana V. *Pharm Dev Tech.* 9:63–74, 2004.
16. Saab AN, Sloan KB, Beall HD, and Villaneuva R *J Pharm Sci.* 70:1099–1104, 1990.
17. Morrow DIJ, McCarron PA, Woolfson AD, and Donnelly RF. *Open Drug Deliv J.* 1:36–59, 2007.
18. Benson HAE. *Exp Opin Drug Deliv.* 3:727–737, 2006.
19. Rother M, Seidel EJ, Clarkson PM, Mazgareanu S, Vierl U, and Rother I. *Drug Design Dev Ther* 3:143–149, 2009.
20. Verma P and Pathak K. *J Adv Pharm Tech Res.* 1:274–282, 2010.
21. Lee RW, Shenoy DB, and Sheel R. In *Handbook of Non-Invasive Drug Delivery Systems*, Burlington, Elsevier Inc., 2010, 1st ed, pp 37–58.
22. Singh S and Singh J. *Med Res Rev.* 13:569–621, 1993.
23. Benson HAE. *Curr Drug Del.* 2:23–33, 2005.
24. Behl CR, Flynn GL, Kurihara T, et al. *J Invest Dermatol.* 75:346–352, 1980.
25. McKenzie AW and Stoughton RB. *Arch Dermatol.* 86:608–610, 1962.
26. Bouwstra JA, van den Bergh BAI, and Suhonen M. *J Recept Signal Transduct Res.* 21:259–286, 2001.
27. Aungst BJ, Rogers NJ, and Shefter E. *Int J Pharm.* 33:225–234, 1986.
28. Yamada M, Hashida M, and Sezaki H. *J Pharm Sci.* 77:418–424, 1988.
29. Aungst BJ. *Pharm Res.* 6:244–247, 1989.
30. Barry BW. *J Control Release.* 6:85–97, 1987.
31. Hadgraft J, Peck J, Williams DG, Pugh WJ, and Allan G. *Int J Pharm.* 141:17–25, 1996.
32. Hadgraft J. *Int J Pharm.* 224:1–18, 2001.
33. Kim YC, Ludovice PJ, and Prausnitz MR. *J Control Release.* 122:375–383, 2007.
34. Brown MB, Traynor MJ, Martin GP, and Akomeah FK. *Methods Mol Biol.* 437:119–139, 2008.
35. Mitragotri S. *Adv Drug Deliv Rev.* 56:589–601, 2004.
36. Guy RH. *Pharm Res.* 13:1765–1769, 1996.
37. Danet AR, Vanbever R, and Preat V. *Adv Drug Deliv Rev.* 56:659–674, 2004.
38. Mitragotri S. *Pharm Res.* 17:1354–1359, 2000.
39. Gordon RA and Peterson TA. *Drug Deliv Technol.* 3:1–7, 2003.
40. Patel DM and K K. *Int. J Pharm Sci Rev Res.* 6:83–90, 2011.
41. Foco A, Hadziabdic J, and Becic F. *Med Arch.* 58:230–234, 2004.
42. Davis SS. *J Pharm Pharmacol.* 44:186–190, 1992.
43. Prausnitz MR and Langer R. *Nat Biol* 26:1261–1268, 2008.

IX. Homework Problems

1. What is the major transport mechanism of drugs across the skin?
2. What is the major barrier to transdermal drug delivery?
3. Briefly describe the structure and function of the stratum corneum.
4. Describe the advantages and limitations of transdermal drug delivery.
5. Describe drug factors affecting skin permeation.
6. Explain how a supersaturated solution enhances the penetration of drugs across the stratum corneum.
7. What is transfersome?
8. Describe the main mechanisms of skin permeability enhancement.
9. What is the difference between iontophoresis and electroporation?
10. What are the advantages of matrix over reservoir patches?

DRUG DELIVERY AND NOVEL DRUG DELIVERY SYSTEMS

PART IV

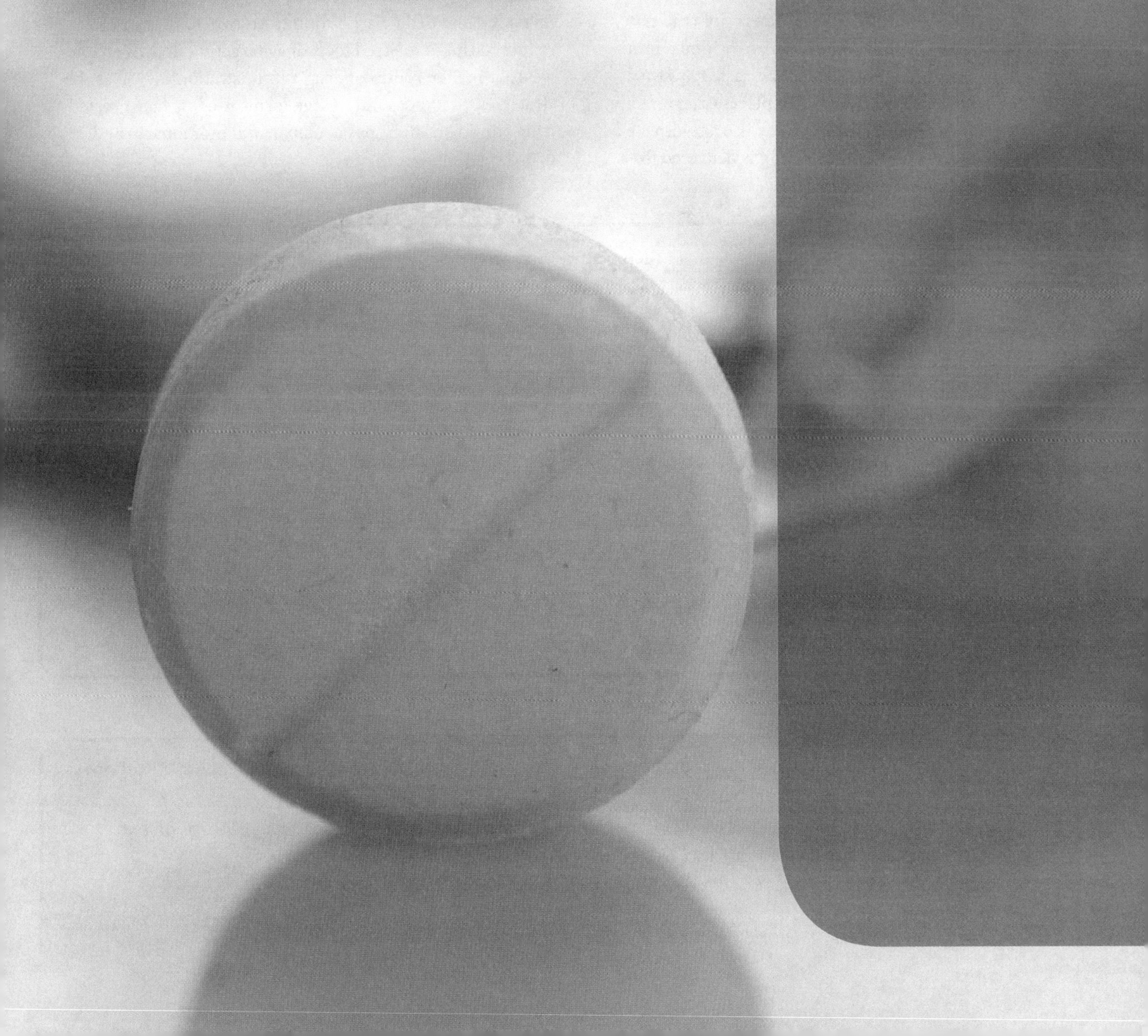

CHAPTER 15

Drug Delivery and Targeting

The physicochemical principles of solids, liquids, semisolids, solutions, and dispersion systems form the basis from which pharmaceutical dosage forms are developed. Drug delivery requires the use of a dosage form that is properly matched with a specific route of drug administration in order to achieve the therapeutic effect. Systemic drug delivery, through which drug is absorbed into the bloodstream, has been proved efficacious for most drugs based on the pharmacokinetic principles. The major delivery routes to achieve systemic absorption are by oral administration, where drug is absorbed at the gastrointestinal sites, and parenteral injection, which places drug directly into the systemic circulation. There are also site-directed administrations, through which a drug is delivered for a localized treatment or, if the system permits, for a systemic drug effect. The latter includes transdermal, intranasal, and intrapulmonary delivery strategies. Drug delivered into the systemic circulation is distributed throughout the body and can pose serious toxic side effects. Creation of special delivery systems has been the main approach in current pharmaceutical research to improve the delivery of drug at a specific site, so that the drug level at the active site is increased and drug distribution to elsewhere in the body is reduced. This is referred to as drug targeting. In this chapter, we examine the routes of drug administration as well as the strategies, methods, and dosage forms used in site-directed drug administration (nasal, ocular, and pulmonary) and drug targeting.

CHAPTER OUTLINE

OBJECTIVES

1. Understand the physiological factors associated with various drug delivery routes and their applications for local or systemic drug delivery.
2. Describe the potential use of the nasal route for local, systemic, and intrathecal drug absorption and permeability factors associated with the nasal epithelium.
3. Be knowledgeable about the nasal products for systemic drug delivery.

(Continues)

(Continued)

4. Understand the mechanisms of ocular drug absorption and methods for pericorneal and intraocular drug delivery.
5. Understand the role of sterility, isotonicity, pH, buffer, viscosity, and preservatives in ophthalmic preparations; perform isotonicity calculations.
6. Describe the lung physiology that governs particle distribution and drug absorption through pulmonary epithelia.
7. Understand the basics of aerosol formulations including MDIs, DPIs, and nebulizers and the proper uses of these products.
8. Describe the roles of vapor pressure, propellants, and surfactants in the formulation of MDIs.
9. Describe the objectives of targeted drug delivery and the concepts of passive and active drug targeting.
10. Understand the concept of a prodrug approach and its use in molecular targeting via receptor-mediated endocytosis, ADEPT, and GDEPT.
11. Describe the types of nanocarriers in passive and active targeting of drugs to tumor cells as well as the physicochemical structures and functions of liposomes and polymeric micelles.
12. Be knowledgeable about drug products for targeted drug delivery, prodrugs, or nanocarriers; and be able to assess the targeting specificity based on experimental data on cellular uptake, drug release, drug absorption, and bioavailability.

I. Routes of Drug Delivery

Transport Barriers

Drug absorption through different routes of administration depends on the physicochemical properties of the drug and the physiology of the tissue system. The design of a dosage form other than the injectable and implantable forms thus must meet the criteria that can be used to deliver the drug or to overcome the barrier resistance of the absorption site to drug transport. The common routes of drug administration are summarized in **Table 15-1**; each of these systems consists of an epithelial transport barrier. A comparative study of the epithelial permeability of various epithelia isolated from rabbits showed that all epithelia possess a relatively high degree of permeation barrier as measured based on their electrical conductance, which is inversely proportional to the membrane resistance to permeation, and the flux using a hydrophilic molecule (6-carboxy fluorescein).[1] The intrinsic membrane permeability of various epithelia to drug transport, in decreasing rank order, is

Intestinal (duodenal/jejunal/ileal/colonic) ≈ nasal ≥ bronchial ≥ tracheal

> vaginal ≥ rectal > corneal > buccal > skin

All epithelia were also found to have relatively constant charge selectivity toward positively charged species. These results show that for drug delivery purposes—especially for tissues that are strongly resistant to drug transport such as the corneal, buccal, and skin—permeation-enhancing methods by either increasing tissue permeability or modifying drug-membrane charge selectivity are generally necessary. The nasal and pulmonary mucosae are nearly as permeable as those of the intestinal epithelia, suggesting that these sites may be exploited as alternative routes for systemic drug delivery.

Table 15-1 Routes of Drug Administration

Route	Absorption Epithelium	Drug Distribution	Dosage Form
Oral	Duodenal/jejunal/ileal/colonic	Systemic	Solid dosage forms, oral solutions, suspensions, emulsions
Parenteral	Intravenous/intramuscular/ subcutaneous systemic	Systemic	Solutions, colloidal systems
Transdermal	Epidermal	Systemic	Patches, topical emulsions
Site-directed:			
Sublingual	Under the tongue	Systemic	Sublingual tablets, tablet triturates, troches
Nasal	Respiratory	Local/systemic	Solutions, sprays, inhalants, semisolids
Inhalation	Bronchial/tracheal alveolar	Intrapulmonary systemic	Aerosols/inhalation powder
Vaginal	Vaginal mucosa	Local	Solution, vaginal inserts, semisolids, tablets
Rectal	Rectal	Local	Suppository, solutions, ointments
Ocular	Corneal	Local	Solutions, inserts, topical formulations
Buccal	Buccal mucosa	Systemic	Slow-release tablets, patches
Topical	Epidermal	Local	Solutions, lotions, semisolids

Major Absorption Routes

Oral Administration

By nature, oral drug delivery is considered to be conventional due to the relative ease with which the intestinal epithelia allow permeation of drugs and nutrients into the systemic system. The GI tract is ideally suited for solid dosage forms formulated for immediate release (tablets or capsules), delayed release (such as enteric-coated tablets), or extended release (tablets or capsules) of drug, as well as liquid formulations. Some drugs, however, are simply not well suited for oral administration. This is true for peptides and proteins, which are degraded by digestive enzymes; very large hydrophobic molecules, where solubility is the defining issue; highly water-soluble drugs that exhibit poor membrane permeability; and drugs that are extensively metabolized in the the gut wall or liver.

Significant metabolic transformation of the drug may occur at the intestinal epithelia. More importantly, drug absorbed through the GI tract enters into the hepatic portal system, which does not directly join the inferior vena cava, the large vein that returns blood to the heart. Instead, the hepatic portal vein collects veins from the stomach and intestine and carries the products absorbed from the digestive tract directly to the liver for processing, storage, or detoxification before the drugs gain access to the general circulation. The liver is organized into functional units known as lobules; each contains a central vein and branched hepatic portal vein, hepatic artery, and bile duct; and the last transports the bile from the liver to the duodenum. In this structure, a drug may be metabolized or eliminated through biliary excretion. For many drugs, the fraction of dose eliminated on the first pass through the liver is substantial, and the first-pass elimination is not limited to any particular pharmacological or chemical group of drugs. In comparison, all other routes of drug administration bypass the the first-pass elimination through the liver.

Parenteral Injection

The principal alternative to oral administration is parenteral injection, which, in addition to circumventing problems associated with oral drug delivery, is especially applicable in emergency use for obtaining a rapid drug response or for patients who are unconscious or otherwise incapacitated. Parenteral administration includes *intravenous* (IV), *intramuscular* (IM), and subcutaneous (SC) injections. Conditions such as acute pain, cardiovascular crisis, and seizures require rapid drug action via IV injection of medication. Intravenous infusions further offer the advantage of providing a relatively constant level of drug therapy over prolonged periods.

Intramuscular injections of medication are used either to achieve rapid absorption of drugs without the need for venous access or as a drug depot to maintain therapeutic blood levels over prolonged periods. The principal sites of injection are the gluteal (buttocks), deltoid (upper arm), and vastus lateralis (thigh) muscles. In general, the injection volumes are limited to 2 mL in the deltoid and thigh muscles and up to 5 mL in the gluteus maximus. Intramuscular injections result in lower but more sustained blood levels than IV administrations, due to the required transport of drug from tissue to the blood circulation. The injected formulation may be considered as a drug "depot" inside the muscle, acting as a repository for the drug. The rate of drug absorption depends on the physiological factors such as the depth of injection, local blood flow, etc., and the formulation factors that control drug release. Poor absorption can occur if the injection is made into the fatty tissue rather than the deeper muscle tissue. Aqueous solutions typically provide the fastest absorption possible from the IM depot, whereas drugs formulated as suspensions, oil-in-water (O/W) or water-in-oil (W/O) emulsions, or solids provide sustained drug release. An example of rapid drug absorption is fosphenytoin, a prodrug of phenytoin for the treatment of epilepsy that is made highly water-soluble by conjugating phosphate moieties to the parent drug. When given IM, the prodrug results in a more rapid and consistent absorption of phenytoin into the bloodstream than the injection of phenytoin itself. Depot injectables are suspension, solid, or oil-based dosage forms. An example of depot injection is Depo-Provera (medroxyprogesterone acetate), which provides a sustained drug release for birth control for a 3-month period.

Subcutaneous injection is an important therapy in self-medication, as in insulin injections by diabetic patients. The rate of drug absorption is slower than that of IM because the drug is injected into the fatty tissue beneath the skin where the blood flow is slow. The slow absorption has been countered with improved drug design, such as by using insulin lispro, to achieve rapid absorption. Subcutaneous depot injections are useful in the delivery of recombinant proteins and peptides for treatment of chronic diseases. An example is Zoladex (goserelin acetate implant) used in hormonal therapy by prostate and breast cancer patients.[2] Zoladex contains a synthetic decapeptide analog of luteinizing hormone-releasing hormone (LHRH) and acts as a potent inhibitor of pituitary gonadotropin secretions and hormone-sensitive tumors. It is supplied as a sterile, biodegradable product containing an equivalent amount of 3.6 mg of goserelin, designed for subcutaneous injection with continuous release over a 28-day period. The formulation consists of drug dispersed in a poly(D,L-lactic and glycolic acids) (PLGA) matrix, made as a 1-mm-diameter cylinder and preloaded in a special single-use syringe with a 16-gauge × 36- ± 0.5-mm siliconized needle with protective needle sleeve (SafeSystem syringe). The absorption of free drug through SC was rapid, with peak blood levels occurring between 0.5 and 1.0 h after dosing. In comparison, Zoladex had a half-life of 12–15 days in male and 8–22 days in female subjects. Goserelin is released from the depot at a much slower rate initially for the first 8 days, following diffusion-based drug-release kinetics, and then at an accerated rate of drug release for the remainder of the 28-day dosing period, due to the biodegradation of the PLGA matrix.

Transdermal Delivery

Some drugs are subjected to extensive first-pass hepatic metabolism via oral absorption, but are able to cross the skin and reach the circulation due to their high lipophilicity. The skin, as a route of drug delivery, has the appeal of being the largest and most readily accessible organ of the body. Transdermal delivery is noninvasive, making it suitable for long-term therapy, highly flexible for dosing or its removal in case of toxicity, and may be used as an alternative to oral drug administration to avoid the first-pass metabolism. In addition, transdermal delivery can facilitate sustained drug release, providing a steady-state plasma profile, reducing dosing frequency- and peak-associated side effects. But, due to the high resistance of the skin barrier, few drugs exhibit the necessary physicochemical properties, e.g., molecular size, partition and diffusion coefficients, melting point, and solubility, to penetrate across the stratum corneum. The stratum corneum consists mainly of dead keratinocytes. Due to its inactive nature, drug permeation across the skin barrier occurs primarily via the passive diffusion process. Hence, most permeation enhancement methods are based on modifying the factors governing passive diffusion as presented in Fick's law of diffusion. Other methods that have been attempted include the physical approaches in laser ablation and microneedles and energy-driven strategies such as by iontophoresis and jet injection. Examples of drugs given by transdermal therapy include, among others, Nitrodisc (nitroglycerin patch, microreservoirs), Estrasorb (estradiol, polymeric micelles), and Ionsys (fentanyl, iontophoresis).

Buccal and Sublingual Absorption

The buccal and sublingual oral mucosae have been used for systemic drug delivery of a few potent drugs, such as nitroglycerin, to avoid drug loss to digestive enzymes and first-pass liver metabolism. Drug delivery through these routes is limited by the small surface area (~100 cm^2) available for absorption and the bitter taste associated with most drugs. The buccal epithelium is highly resistant to drug transport, second only to the stratum corneum of the skin among various epithelia. As a result, the dosage forms usually require the use of penetration enhancers that reversibly alter the permeability of the barrier. These compounds include solubilization agents (propylene glycol, cyclodextrins, sulfoxides, etc.), phospholipids, and surfactants. The relatively high permeation resistance makes the buccal mucosa more useful for sustained release, as it normally produces a low rate of absorption and low bioavailability. In contrast, the sublingual mucosa exhibits relatively high permeability for many drugs and contains a profusion of capillaries beneath the epithelium, allowing for rapid drug absorption and an onset of drug action within a few minutes. A comparison of buccal and sublingual tablets of nitroglycerin shows that for sublingual absorption, a dose of 0.3–0.5 mg usually produces an onset of action in 2–5 min and a short duration of action of about 30 min, whereas for buccal absorption, the same onset of action requires a dose of 1–3 mg, which has a 5-h duration of action. The most commonly used dosage form for sublingual absorption is a small tablet, which dissolves promptly in water to produce a rapid therapeutic effect. Buccal and sublingual tablets are flat, oval tablets to be placed in the buccal pouch or beneath the tongue. Whereas the buccal tablets are designed to erode slowly, tablets for sublingual use are dissolved promptly. Tablet triturates are small, cylindrical tablets containing sucrose and lactose as the diluents. They are compressed with a minimum amount of pressure and are readily soluble in water. In addition to the nitroglycerin sublingual tablets used for acute anginal attacks, some hormones, such as dehydroepiandrosterone and melatonin have been shown to exhibit better absorption via the sublingual route than via oral administration.

Site-Directed Administration

Drug delivery to the skin for topical use and to various anatomical sites with mucosal surfaces (see Table 15-1) involves a large group of medications, most of which, but not all, are intended to treat the disease conditions at the site of delivery. In ocular drug delivery, e.g., practically all medications formulated for ophthalmic drug delivery are intended to work there, due to the small volume of dose that can be delivered and the high resistance of the cornea to drug permeation. In inhalation, the developed medications are primarily used to treat asthma, chronic obstructive pulmonary disease, and other respiratory disorders. Although the lung epithelia have been shown to exhibit excellent permeability for systemic drug absorption, only a few such preparations have been under clinical development (e.g., calcitonin, nafarelin, insulin). There is, however, an increasing interest in the systemic absorption of drugs through intranasal drug delivery. Although locally acting drugs such as decongestants and allergy or infective agents still dominate the product field, medications that provide systemic drug actions, such as migraine drugs, nicotine replacement, and peptide-based pharmaceuticals, have emerged as a new development. The nasal epithelium is similar to the intestinal epithelia in drug permeability and is well vascularized and readily accessible, suggesting that nasal drug delivery may yield rapid systemic drug absorption without the loss of drug due to the first-pass effect.[3] The methods of drug delivery through nasal, ocular, and pulmonary drug administration are discussed in sections that follow.

II. Intranasal Drug Delivery

Advances in biotechnology have made available protein and peptide drugs for the treatment of various diseases. These drugs are unsuitable for oral administration because they are significantly degraded by digestive enzymes in the GI tract or by the first-pass liver metabolism. For small-molecule drugs, when a fast drug action is desired, oral administration is usually ineffective. The parenteral route is inconvenient, especially for long-term therapy. For these reasons, intranasal drug delivery has been extensively invstigated as an alternative to oral or parenteral administration for systemic drug delivery. The nasal absorption characteristics and the feasibility of using the nasal route for systemic drug delivery are discussed below.

Nasal Mucosa

Respiratory Epithelium

The nose is divided into two cavities via the nasal septum; each side, about 7.5 mL in volume, opens at the face via the nostril and connects with the mouth at the nasopharynx (**Figure 15-1**). There are three functional regions in the nose: the vestibular, respiratory, and olfactory regions. The lateral wall of each nasal cavity shows a folded structure that enlarges the surface area to about 75 cm^2.[4] This folded structure includes three turbinates: the superior, the median, and the inferior. The

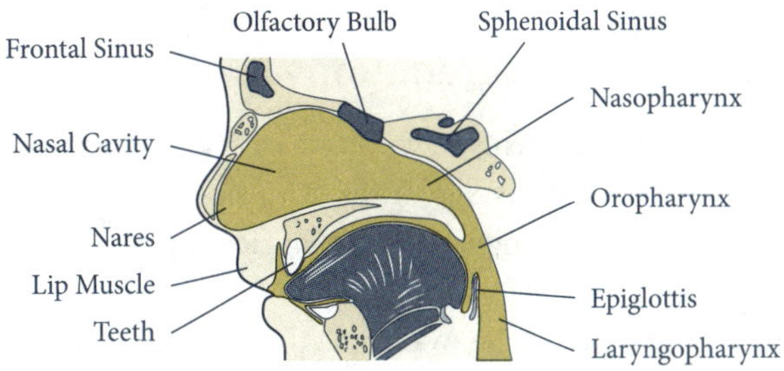

Figure 15-1 The nasal cavity.
Adapted from: Dean Hess, Neil R. MacIntyre, Shelley C. Mishoe, William F. Galvin, and Alexandar B. Adams. *Respiratory Care: Principles and Practice, Second Edition*. pg. 387, Figure 19-9. Jones & Bartlett Learning, Burlington, MA.

nasal vestibule is lined with skinlike cells, but the respiratory region has a typical airway epithelium, consisting of basal, mucus-containing goblet, ciliated columnar, and nonciliated columnar cell types. Basal cells are poorly differentiated cells and act as stem cells to replenish other cell types. The goblet cells, in conjunction with nasal glands, produce secretions that form the mucus layer. The proportions of the ciliated and nonciliated columnar cells vary in different regions: in the anterior lower turbinate area, about 15–20% of the cells are ciliated and 60–70% nonciliated. Toward the nasopharynx, the number of ciliated cells increases while that of the nonciliated cells decreases. The ciliated cells are responsible for transport of mucus and entrapped particles to the pharynx for ingestion; the nonciliated cells, each exhibiting 300–400 microvilli, provide a large surface area for drug absorption. Below the epithelium is the lamina propria, where blood vessels, nerves, and the serous and mucus glands reside.[5] It has a dense network of capillaries; thus drug absorbed through the respiratory epithelium enters the systemic circulation. The mucus layer covering the nasal epithelium is renewed every 10 to 15 min, where the pH of the mucosal secretion ranges from 5.5 to 6.5 in adults and from 5.0 to 6.7 in children.[6] The nasal cavity contains many enzymes including lysozymes responsible for keeping an aseptic environment, phase I and II enzymes (cytochrome P450s, glutathione-*S*-transferases, etc.) for small-molecule metabolism, and aminopeptidases for peptide degradation.

Olfactory Region

The olfactory region is located on the roof of the nasal cavities, just below the cribriform plate of the ethmoid bone that separates the cranial from the nasal cavities. The olfactory tissue covers about 10 cm^2 of the human nasal mucosa. The nerve cells of the olfactory epithelium project into the olfactory bulb of the brain, and this provides, through the nasal cavities, a direct connection of the brain to the external environment. Drug transport through the olfactory epithelium to the brain can occur either by slow transport inside the nerve cells to the olfactory bulb or by faster transfer along the perineural space surrounding the olfactory nerve cells into the cerebrospinal fluid (CSF) in the brain.[7] Thus, the olfactory route could theoretically be used, and has been shown by many studies,[8] to deliver drugs to the central nervous system, bypassing the blood–brain barrier (BBB). But whether sufficient dose can be delivered through this route to the human brain remains to be demonstrated.

Drug Absorption Through Nasal Epithelium

Physiological Barriers

The absorption of hydrophilic, high-molecular-weight drugs (proteins and peptides) is limited by (1) enzyme degradation, (2) mucociliary clearance, and (3) low permeability of the nasal mucosa.

Enzymatic Degradation

Peptides and proteins in the nasal cavity may be enzymatically degraded in the lumen of the nasal cavity or during passage through the epithelial barrier. These sites contain exopeptidases such as mono and diaminopeptidases that cleave peptides at their N and C termini and endopeptidases that attack internal peptide bonds.[9] The use of enzyme inhibitors and/or saturation of enzymes may be approaches to overcome this barrier.

Mucociliary Clearance

The nasal absorption process involves drug passage through the mucus layer. Small, uncharged particles can easily pass through this layer, whereas large or charged particles will be retained in the mucus. Mucin, the principal glycoprotein in the mucus, has the capacity to bind to solutes, thus hindering diffusion. A formulation could also induce pH and temperature changes in the mucus layer, resulting in changed viscosity and binding activity.[10] Because the turnover time of the mucous layer is about 15–20 min, the applied dose can be readily cleared from the nasal cavity by the *mucociliary clearance* mechanism. This is especially true if the drug is not absorbed rapidly across the nasal mucosa. Studies have shown that for liquid and powder formulations, which are not bioadhesive, the half-life for clearance is about 15–30 min.[10] The use of bioadhesive excipients in the formulation is a viable approach to overcome rapid mucociliary clearance. It is also possible to reduce mucociliary clearance by depositing the formulation in the anterior, where fewer cells are ciliated.[11]

Low Permeability

Once through the mucus, drug may cross the epithelium via simple diffusion-based transcellular pathway, paracellular transport via movement between cells, and transcytosis as aided by vesicle carriers. The paracellular pathway for hydrophilic drugs is slow and passive, and it involves passage of drug through aqueous channels between cells. There is a correlation between decreased nasal absorption with increased molecular weight of the drug in a log-log scale. Good systemic bioavailability after nasal administration can be achieved for drugs with an upper molecular weight limit of 1000 daltons (Da) without using permeability enhancer.[12] The transcellular diffusion pathway accounts for the transport of lipophilic drugs that depends on the drug's lipophilicity.

The bioavailability of hydrophilic drugs through nasal absorption is about 10% for low-molecular-weight, water-soluble drugs and 1% or less for peptides such as calcitonin and insulin, due to low membrane permeability. Studies have shown that drug permeability by active transport via carrier-mediated endocytosis or through the tight junctions is also limited by the molecular size. Although tight junctions can be opened and closed to a certain degree, the mean size of these channels is less than 10 Å, which limits the transport of larger molecules.[13] Larger peptides and proteins can be delivered using the endocytotic transport process but only in low amounts.[14] These studies show that membrane permeability is the limiting step for developing nasal formulations, and the use of permeability enhancers is generally necessary.

Physicochemical Barriers

The resistance to drug transport by the nasal epithelium can be assessed based on the physicochemical properties of the drug, to gain insight into the permeation process. These properties include lipophilicity, ionization, molecular weight, and solubility.

Lipophilicity

The primary route of drug transport through the nasal epithelium is via the transcellular diffusion (lipoidal) pathway, where the lipid bilayer provides the epithelial barrier function. Lipophilic molecules can cross the membrane via transcellular diffusion, as they are able to partition into the lipid bilayer of the cell membrane, and diffuse into and traverse through cell cytoplasm. Hydrophobic drugs such as naloxone, buprenorphine, testosterone, and propranolol are completely, or nearly so, absorbed through nasal administration in animal models, whereas hydrophilic compounds such as metoprolol are not.[15] There is a quantitative relationship between the partition coefficient of drugs and their nasal absorption constants.[16] Chemical modification of drug can be used to achieve increased lipophilicity. For example, the nasal absorption of the carboxylic acid esters of L-tyrosine has been shown to be significantly greater than that of L-tyrosine.[17]

Ionization

The pH-mediated ionization of acids and bases can significantly alter their lipophilicity and hence their absorption through the nasal mucosa. Absorption of weak electrolytes such as salicylic acid and aminopyrine by nasal epithelium was found to be highly dependent on their degree of ionization. For aminopyrine, the absorption rate increased with increasing pH as more drug molecules attained the neutral form; the absorption of salicylic acid, however, showed substantial deviation from the theoretical profile,[17] and this has led to the suggestion of an alternative pathway by which ionic species may cross the nasal epithelium. Indeed, studies have shown that benzoic acid is significantly absorbed (~10%) through the nasal mucosa at pH 7.19 when the drug is 99.9% ionized,[18] indicating that aqueous channels may be present in the nasal epithelium, allowing transport of ionized or hydrophilic drugs.

Molecular Weight (MW)

For lipophilic drugs, increased MW is often associated with increased lipophilicity and permeability. For hydrophilic drugs, the permeation of small molecules (< 300 Da) through aqueous channels is not significantly influenced by the molecular weight, but for compounds with MW > 300, the permeability is highly sensitive to the molecular size. Good absorption can be achieved for molecules having MW up to 1000, when no enhancer is used. This limit may be increased to 6000 Da with the aid of a permeation enhancer.[19]

Solubility

Drug solubility is an important factor for the delivery of powders and suspensions. Rapid dissolution of drug particles is necessary to avoid mucociliary clearance and to ensure membrane permeation, which, as previously described, depends on drug solubility, polymorphism, and size and distribution of the particles.

Formulation Considerations

Solution Factors

The roles of solution pH, osmolarity, viscosity, and drug solubility in nasal drug absorption have been well characterized. The pH of the formulation, as well as that of nasal surface, can affect a drug's permeability. To avoid tissue irritation, when possible, the pH of nasal formulations should be adjusted to 4.5–6.5, conforming to that of the mucus.[6] This acidic pH is well suited for the delivery of acidic drugs and preserves the bactericidal activity of lysozyme found in nasal secretions, which is inactivated in alkaline pH. Nasal preparations are generally administered in small volumes ranging from 25 to 200 μL. Nasal secretions can thus alter the pH of the administered dose, suggesting that an adequate buffer capacity may be required to maintain the formulation pH for absorption purposes. Osmolarity is of importance in preserving the integrity of the nasal epithelium. Studies in rats have shown that the absorption of secretin reached a maximum at a sodium chloride concentration of 0.462 *M*,[20] which was hypertonic and resulted in shrinkage of the nasal epithelium. Studies using sorbitol as an osmotic regulator produced the same results. The permeation of secretin, however, was subsequently decreased due to damage of the epithelium.[20] Hence, isotonic solutions are usually preferred for nasal administration.

Viscosity may be altered to increase the contact time between the drug and the nasal mucosa, thereby increasing the time for permeation. However, highly viscous formulations can interfere with the normal mucociliary function and result in altered drug permeability. Increased viscosity is usually achieved using polymers such as polyacrylic acid, carboxymethylcellulose, Carbopols, etc., which in addition to modifying the solution viscosity also act as *bioadhesives* with the mucus layer. The viscosity-prolonged residence time does not necessarily lead to increased absorption. This concept has been illustrated using insulin solutions containing Carbopol or carboxymethylcellulose having similar viscosity, in that Carbopol enhances the absorption of insulin, but carboxymethylcellulose does not. The latter is due to a slowed diffusion of drug through the mucus matrix by increased viscosity, whereas in the former, Carbopol offers the advantage by opening the epithelial tight junctions for improved permeation.

The aqueous solubility of drugs and excipients is always a concern in nasal drug delivery. Enhancement of solubility is often achieved using propylene glycol, small alcohol, Transcutol, medium-chain glycerides, and saturated polyglycolyzed glycerides. Surfactants or cyclodextrins, used in combination with lipophilic permeability enhancers, are also found in nasal preparations. Most nasal solutions are aqueous based and need preservatives to prevent microbial growth. Benzalkonium chloride (which also enhances drug permeability), parabens, phenyl ethyl alcohol, EDTA, and benzoyl alcohol are some of the preservatives used in nasal formulation.

Dosage Form Considerations

The nasal drug delivery systems are designed based on the properties of the drug, intended therapeutic effect, and patient and marketing preferences. The delivery of drugs is usually made using the following systems.

Nasal Drops

Nasal drops are solutions; they are easy to use but lack dose precision. Therefore, nasal drops may not be suitable for delivery of prescription drug.

Nasal Sprays

The formulations are either solutions or suspensions, delivered by metered dose pumps and actuators with an exact dose from 25 to 200 μL. The particle size and morphology (for suspensions) of the drug and viscosity of the formulation determine the choice of pump and actuator assembly. Solution and suspension sprays are preferred over powder sprays because powder results in mucosal irritation.

Nasal Gels

Nasal gels are viscosity-thickened solutions or suspensions. They offer the advantages of reduced postnasal drip due to high viscosity, reduced taste impact due to less swallowing, reduced anterior leakage of the formulation, reduced irritation due to emollient effects, and targeted delivery of drug to mucosa for better absorption.

Nasal Powders

This dosage form is useful if solution and suspension dosage forms cannot be developed due to stability issues. The suitability of the powder formulation depends on the solubility, particle size, aerodynamic properties, and nasal irritancy of the drug and/or excipients. It has been shown that particle sizes greater than 10 μm are deposited in the nasal cavity; those with size in the range of 2 to 10 μm can enter the lungs, whereas particles less than 1 μm are exhaled. Powders offer the advantage of a localized drug application, but nasal mucosa irritancy and metered dose delivery remain challenges in the product development.

Enhancement of Drug Absorption

The basic methods that can be used to improve drug absorption through nasal administration include chemical modification of drug to improve its permeability, increased residence time of drug in the nasal cavivity, inhibition of enzyme-mediated drug degradation, and the use of *permeability-enhancing* molecules.

Chemical Modification

Structural changes should be made without altering the drug's pharmacological activity. In general, a drug may be chemically modified to increase the drug's solubility or permeability, depending on the need to achieve the overall drug abosrption. Conversion of drug to the salt form increases drug solubility but may lead to lowered permeability, whereas ester derivatives of a weak acid can significantly increase drug permeation through the nasal epithelium. For organic drugs, chemical modifications leading to changed molecular size, solubility, and physical constants (for example, pK_a) are quite feasible, but for proteins and peptides, it is generally less successful to use derivatization to improve permeability, although ion pairing may be used to enhance their lipophilicity.

Nasal Residence Time

The mucociliary clearance acts to remove foreign substances from the nasal mucosa as quickly as possible. As mentioned ealier, viscosity-inducing agents can enhance the residence time of drugs, but not necessarily drug absorption because of the multiple effects of viscosity on drug transport. Hydroxypropyl cellulose, e.g., was found to improve the absorption of low-molecular-weight drugs but not peptides and proteins, because of the effect that increased viscosity impedes the diffusion of macromolecules across the mucosa. Instead, a number of studies have shown that bioadhesive starch microsphere (SM) system can be used to enhance peptide drug absorption.[21, 22] The mechanism was thought to involve four steps: First, drug-containing SMs are deposited in the anterior part of the nasal cavity where only a few ciliated cells are present, allowing the microspheres to reach the nasal epithelium slowly; second, the formulation is retained in the nasal cavity for an extended period due to its bioadhesive nature; third, the gelled system provides a local high drug concentration in close contact with the epithelial surface; fourth, the absorption of water by the SMs from the mucus layer could enhance the passage of the drug through the epithelial tight junctions.

Permeability Enhancers

Peptides and proteins do not cross the nasal mucosa efficiently because of their molecular size, lack of lipophilicity, and potential degradation by nasal enzymes. To overcome these permeability barriers, penetration enhancers may be used to improve drug permeation, whereas enzyme inhibitors may be added to prevent drug degradation. Although not always attainable, an ideal permeability enhancer should be (1) effective in small quantity to promote permeability, (2) temporary and reversible in its effects on the membrane, (3) nonirritating and nontoxic, and (4) compatible and working in concert with the drug during permeation.

Permeability enhancers are compounds capable of modifying the nasal mucosa through chemical and physical processes, with the former often being irreversible. The major permeability enhancing mechanisms include

1. Opening of tight junctions between epithelial cells

2. Disruption of membrane through extracting membrane components or creating disorders in the lipid bilayer, resulting in increased membrane fluidity
3. Bioadhesion through gel formation to increase residence time

Examples of chemical enhancers are solubilizing agents, chelating agents, bile salts, and natural and synthetic surfactants.[22] Gel-forming polymers, such as chitosan and Carbopols, can enhance drug absorption by decreasing nasal clearance and by acting on the tight junctions of the epithelial membrane. Some commonly used permeability-enhancing agents and their functions are summarized in **Table 15-2**. As an example, polyoxyethylene-9-lauryl ether (BL-9) has been shown to improve the nasal absorption of hydralazine in both in situ and in vivo nasal absorption studies in rats. Polysorbate 80 (1%) was shown to promote nasal absorption of atropine and hyoscine in solutions. A formulation of meclizine (50 mg/mL) prepared in propylene glycol and 10% glycerol results in 50% absorption of the nasally administered drug, which is, in dosage, comparable to IV therapy. Gentamicin (60 mg/mL in saline solution) was also well absorbed in humans (with peak concentration time of 30–60 min) through nasal administration, with the aid of glycocholate (1%). These studies show that systemic absorption of small-molecule drugs is achievable through nasal drug delivery.

The systemic bioavailability of most peptides and proteins through nasal absorption is about 1–2% when administered as simple solutions.[23] This relatively low absorption can be significantly increased by using permeability enhancer or a combination of enhancing agents. When calcitonin was given intranasally to rats and rabbits using formulations containing different cyclodextrins, its activity, as monitored in decreased serum calcium levels, was significantly increased compared to formulations without added cyclodextrin.[24] Similar effects by cyclodextrins on intranasal insulin delivery were also observed.[25] Studies have also shown that insulin absorption can be enhanced by prolonged contact with the nasal mucosa, using biodegradable starch microspheres (SMs), which gel on absorption of water at the nasal mucosa, thus significantly delaying the clearance of the administered drug.[21, 26] In a study where sodium human insulin was intranasally administered to sheep as either solution or SMs, Illum et al.[21] showed that the SM formulation resulted in a

Table 15-2 Nasal Absorption Enhancing Agents

Type of Compound	Examples	Function and Use
Bile salts (and derivatives)	Sodium deoxycholate, sodium glycocholate, sodium taurodihydrofusidate	Disruption of tight junctions Inhibition of enzyme activity
Surfactants and fatty acids	Sodium lauryl sulfate, saponin, polyoxyethylene-9-lauryl ether, sodium caprylate, sodium laurate, phospholipids (lecithin, lysolecithin)	Membrane disruption
Chelating agents	EDTA, salicylates	Opening of tight junctions
Enzyme inhibitors	Bestatin, amastatia	Enzyme inhibition
Solubilizing agents	Cyclodextrins	Disruption of membranes and tight junctions
Bioadhesive materials:		
Powders	Carbopol, starch microspheres, chitosan	Delayed nasal clearance, opening of tight junctions
Liquids	Chitosan, Carbopol	Reduce nasal clearance, opening of tight junctions

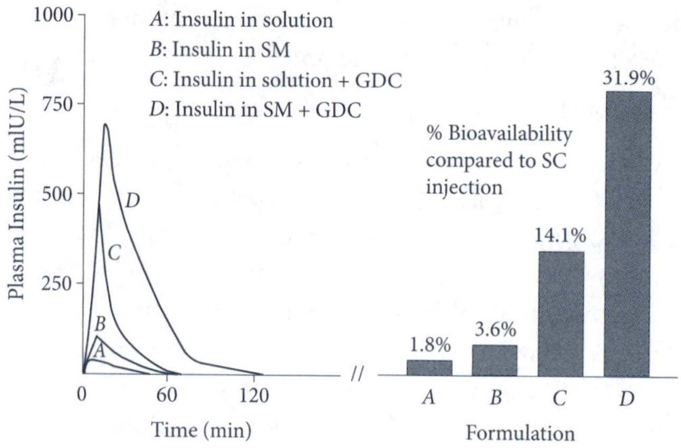

Figure 15-2 Enhancement of nasal absorption of insulin in sheep using bioadhesive starch microspheres and sodium glycodeoxycholate (GDC). Reprinted from: *International Journal of Pharmaceutics*, Vol 222/Issue 1, L. Illum, A.N. Fisher, I. Jabbal-Gill, S.S. Davis, Bioadhesive starch microspheres and absorption enhancing agents act synergistically to enhance the nasal absorption of polypeptides, Pages No. 109–119, Copyright 2001, with permission from Elsevier.

two-fold bioavailability to that of the insulin solution. When sodium glycodeoxycholate (GDC) was incorpated into the formulations as a penetration enhancer, the systemic bioavailability (as compared to subcutaneous injection) increased from 1.8% to 14.1% for the solutions, and from 3.6% to 31.9% for the SM formulations (see **Figure 15-2**). Insulin was rapidly absorbed through the nasal mucosa with a t_{max} within 5 min for all formulations. The pharmacokinetic data were closely mirrored by the pharmacodynamic results as measured in plasma glucose reduction. These results suggest that bioadhesion may work cooperatively with permeability enhancement to facilitate nasal drug absorption.

Microspheres for Nasal Drug Delivery

In addition to the starch microspheres, the use of the microsphere system in nasal drug delivery has been developed using the polymer chitosan, a linear polysaccharide consisting of deacetylated and *N*-acetylated glucosamine units. Microspheres composed of sodium alginate and chitosan were used for intranasal delivery of metoclopramide hydrochloride (an antiemetic).[27] These particles showed good swelling and gelling properties at the nasal mucosa and retained their shape, thus providing a controlled drug release. Drug permeation through the nasal mucosa from the chitosan-containing microspheres was significantly higher than from those consisting of alginate alone, because chitosan also acted on opening the tight junctions of the epithelium, as revealed by transmission electron microscopy. The chitosan microsphere system is thus very attractive for nasal drug delivery, as it can prolong residence time through bioadhesive properties and enhance permeability by opening up the epithelial tight junctions.

Nasal Products for Systemic Drug Delivery

The nasal drug products are developed based on the properties of the drug, the intended therapeutic effect, and patient, and marketing preferences. Certain types of drugs, such as antiemetics, antimigraines, etc., are more preferable than others. In current product lines, nasal sprays for local effects are common. For systemic effects, antimigraine nasal sprays have been developed to provide a fast effect and to avoid the nausea associated with oral administration. Peptide drugs are also available as nasal sprays, in this case to avoid drug degradation

Table 15-3 Nasal Drug Products for Systemic Drug Delivery

Product	Drug/Treatment	Dosage Form	Manufacturer
Miacalcin	Calcitonin-salmon/osteoporosis	200 U/spray	Novartis Pharma
DDAVP	Desmopressin acetate/diabetes insipidus	0.01% solution/spray	Sanofi-Aventis
Suprefact	Buserelin acetate/prostate cancer	100 mg/spray	Sanofi-Aventis
Synarel	Nafarelin acetate/endometriosis	0.2-mg base/spray	Pfizer
Migranal	Dihydroergotamine mesylate/migraine	0.5 mg/spray	Valeant
Zomig	Zolmitriptan/migraine	5 mg/spray	AstraZeneca
Imitrex	Sumatriptan succinate/migraine	5 and 20 mg/spray	GlaxoSmithKline

by GI and hepatic enzymes. A list of the nasal products for systemic drug delivery is given in **Table 15-3**. The nasal absorption of certain drugs has been found superior to the absorption of the oral delivery. Desmopressin, e.g., is available for both nasal and oral administrations. The bioavailability of the oral tablet is 0.1% whereas that of the nasal spray is 3–5%.[28] Miacalcin is a solution of salmon calcitonin (and benzalkonium chloride) for nasal spray, which is recommended for long-term use in the treatment of postmenopausal osteoporosis. The absorption is about 3% of the IV dose.

The nasal epithelium is highly vascularized and has a large surface area readily accessible for drug absorption. Low-molecular-weight lipophilic drugs, such as propranolol, progesterone, etc., are well absorbed across the nasal cavity even without the use of permeability enhancer. These drugs can reach circulation within a few minutes after dosing; their systemic bioavailabilities are often comparable to those obtained from intravenous injection. In fact, many drugs administered intranasally show faster and more efficient absorption than orally administered doses, resulting in a faster onset of action. The application of intranasal drug delivery is likely to expand in the future to include drugs such as anesthetics, antiemetics, and sedatives that benefit from a fast onset of action, and vaccines, peptides, and proteins for immunization, hormonal therapy, and osteoporosis.[29]

III. Ophthalmic Drug Delivery

Ocular Drug Absorption

Human Eye

The eye is a fluid-filled sphere enclosed by three specialized tissue layers. From outermost to innermost they are (1) the sclera/cornea, (2) the choroid/ciliary body/iris, and (3) the retina (see **Figure 15-3**). Most of the eyeball is covered by a tough layer of connective tissue, the *sclera*, which forms the "white" portion of the eye. Anteriorly, the outer layer consists of the transparent cornea through which light rays pass into the interior of the eye. The cornea can be divided into several prominent layers; they are, from the external surface to the interior, epithelium, Bowman's layer, stroma, Descemet's membrane, and endothelium. The epithelium consists of five or six layers of cells, with a thickness of 60–65 nm. The epithelium, together with Bowman's layer (about 12 μm in thickness), which contains fibrils running parallel to the external surface, forms a strong barrier to resist transport of chemicals across the cornea. The stroma makes up 90% of the cornea, which contains layers of collagen fibrils in an aqueous environment. Descemet's layer (10 μm) is formed by secretions from underlying endothelial cells that mark the inner boundary of the aqueous stroma.

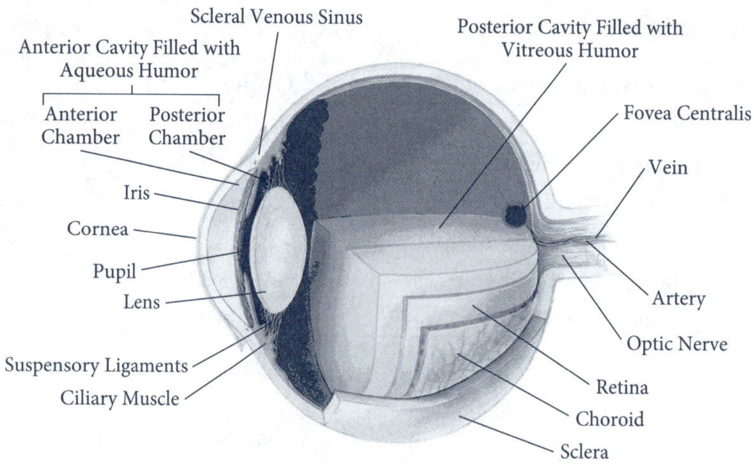

Figure 15-3 The human eye.
Adapted from: Moini, *Anatomy and Physiology for Health Professionals*, pg. 163 Figure 10-11. Jones & Bartlett Learning, LLC.

The middle layer underneath the sclera is the highly pigmented choroid, which contains many blood vessels that nourish the retina. The choroid layer becomes specialized anteriorly to form the ciliary body and iris. The iris is a colored, circular membrane suspended behind the cornea. It is connected to the ciliary body, forming the boundary between the anterior and posterior chambers of the eye. It controls the pupil, located in the middle of the iris, through contraction and relaxation, and it determines the amount of light that enters the eye. The lens is positioned behind the iris, and it refracts the light entering the pupil and focuses it on the retina. The retina is the innermost layer under the choroid, which consists of an outer pigmented layer and an inner nervous tissue layer that contains the photoreceptors to convert light energy to nerve impulses. The light-absorbing pigments in the choroid and retina function to prevent reflection or scattering of light within the eye.

The eye is filled with fluids. Attached to the back of the eyelids and the outer surface of the sclera is the conjunctiva, which is flexibly connected so that the eyes can move with freedom. For cleansing and lubrication, the corneal and conjunctival surfaces are covered by a clear and watery precorneal film secreted by the conjunctival and lacrimal glands, known as tears. There are three layers in the precorneal film: the outer lipid layer (about 0.1 μm), middle aqueous layer (about 7 μm), and inner mucoid layer (0.02–0.05 μm). The film contains salts, glucose, and lysozymes, with an average pH of 7.3–7.7. It is produced at a rate of about 1.2 μL/min.

The interior of the eye consists of two fluid-filled cavities separated by the *lens*; both are transparent to permit passage of light from the cornea to the retina. The anterior cavity between the cornea and lens contains a watery fluid, the aqueous humor, and the large posterior cavity between the lens and retina contains a jellylike substance (about 3.9 mL, pH 7.5), the vitreous humor, which serves to maintain the spherical shape of the eyeball. The aqueous humor (about 300 μl) carries nutrients for the cornea and lens, as both, by design, lack blood supply. This fluid is produced at a rate of 5 mL/day by a capillary network within the ciliary body via ultrafiltration of the blood. The secreted fluid then moves from the posterior chamber to the anterior chamber at a rate of about 3 μL/min and is drained into a canal at the edge of the cornea and returned to the blood. If aqueous humor is not drained as fast as it is formed, excess aqueous humor will accumulate in the anterior cavity, resulting in raised intraocular pressure. This condition is known as glaucoma, where the excess aqueous humor pushes the lens backward into the vitreous humor, which in turn pushes against the inner neural layer of the retina. In humans, the normal intraocular pressure is about 12–20 mmHg. Sustained elevation to 25–30 mmHg can cause retinal damage and lead to blindness if it is not treated.

Drug Delivery Considerations

The eye is anatomically protected from chemicals topically by the cornea and systemically by the retina–blood barrier. Drug absorption through the cornea is also limited by physiological factors. The normal volume of the precorneal film is 7–10 μL. The maximum volume of the conjunctival sac or cul-de-sac is about 30 μL, whereas the normal commercial eyedropper dispenses 50–75 μL of solution; thus more than one-half of the dose may be lost from the eye by overflow. The ideal volume of a solution dose would be 5–10 μL, but such microliter eyedroppers are not usually available to patients. The precorneal film, which flows from the lacrimal gland across the eye and drains into the lacrimal canaliculus, has a turnover time of 2–3 min. This rapid washing and turnover accounts for about 75% loss of the ophthalmic dose. The canaliculi terminate in the lacrimal sac, which directs the drainage toward the nose via the nasolacrimal duct, from which the drug may be absorbed systemically or through the pulmonary route. Topically applied drug can also enter into the systemic circulation through conjunctival absorption, which contains substantial blood supplies, or corneal absorption, where the drug reached in the aqueous humor is drained with the fluid into the systemic system. These factors limit the contact time of ophthalmic solutions to about 1–2 min and their bioavailability to generally less than 10%.

To achieve a sufficient concentration in the back of the eye presents even greater challenges. It is possible for a drug given systemically to produce an ocular effect, if the drug can reach the retina or enters the interior of the eye via the aqueous humor. A few drugs (e.g., tetrahydrocannabinol) do produce an ocular effect when administered systemically, but this requires the use of very high doses. Drug injection into the back of the eye is an alternative, but such treatment is traumatic, and the injected drug may be quickly removed by the circulatory process, thus requiring frequent injections.

Corneal Permeability

Drugs that are used for therapeutic intervention of the interior structures of the eye (iris, pupil, ciliary body, etc.) must be absorbed through the cornea. The major structure of the cornea includes the epithelium, stroma, and endothelium. The epithelium is composed of flat and tightly fitting squamous cells, which show a high degree of resistance to paracellular transport, surpassed only by the skin and buccal epithelia.[1] The stroma accounts for 90% of the total corneal thickness and is composed of 78% in water interspersed with collagen fibrils. Its aqueous nature allows for free diffusion of ionized drugs through the stroma matrix. Similar to the epithelium, the endothelium is selective for passage of lipophilic or un-ionized drugs. This structure characteristic has been demonstrated by studies using excised rabbit cornea, where the percentages of resistance to drug transport by the structure components are correlated to the lipophilic/hydrophilic properties of drugs.[30] For lipophilic drugs, the epithelium of the cornea offers relatively little resistance to transport compared to the stroma. As drugs become more hydrophilic, however, varying degrees of resistance to drug transport are seen in the epithelium, stroma, and endothelium. For hydrophilic drugs, the epithelium layer is shown to be the major penetration barrier; once in the cornea, the stroma and endothelium offer little resistance to drug passage into the anterior chamber. These effects are illustrated in **Table 15-4** via the absorption of β-blockers of varying lipophilicity (as indicated by log P, the logarithm of octanol/buffer partition coefficients).[30]

Table 15-4 Percentage Contribution of Each Corneal Barrier to Drug

		Percentage Resistance to Passage		
Drug	**log $P^{\dagger}$**	**Epithelium**	**Stroma**	**Endothelium**
Penbutolol	2.53	1	46	53
Bufurolol	2.31	18	50	32
Bevantolol	2.19	7	44	49
Propranolol	1.62	7	45	48
Levobunolol	0.72	58	15	27
Oxprenolol	0.69	45	21	34
Cyclophosphamide	0.38	72	10	11
Metoprolol	0.28	48	18	34
Acebutolol	0.20	91	1	8
Nadolol	−0.82	95	1	4
Phenylephrine	−1.00	95	1	4
Sotalol	−1.25	95	1	4
Atenolol	−1.52	97	1	2

†Octanol/buffer (pH 7.65) partition coefficient.

In ophthalmic solutions, the salt form of a drug is often used to increase drug solubility. When a solution is administered, the buffering action of the precorneal film will bring the pH of the solution to the physiological range. At this point, drug exists in equilibrium between neutral and ionized forms where the un-ionized drug (such as a free base) will penetrate the cornea. Once the drug passes the epithelium, the free base is protonated depending on the pH condition, and the ionic species moves across the aqueous stroma. At the junction of the stroma and endothelium, it is again the neutral species that exhibits greater permeability through the endothelium into the aqueous humor. The acid–base equilibrium is also crucial for the transport of drug from the aqueous humor into the iris and ciliary body, where ionized drug can be lost to systemic circulation. This absorption process is a microcosmic representation of the general phenomena through which an acid–base drug moves through biological membranes throughout the body.

The above discussion shows that the eye is anatomically and physiologically well protected, which makes drug delivery difficult. Ophthalmic formulations thus must be optimized to exhibit good corneal permeability, prolonged contact time, and desired rheological properties, in order to overcome the ocular absorption barrier.

Therapeutic Categories

Most ophthalmic preparations are intended for local treatments. Drugs are delivered on the eye, into the eye, or onto the conjunctiva where local activity occurs. The various types of drug categories and their therapeutic use are summarized in **Table 15-5**.

Dosage Forms

Ophthalmic preparations are made using the same standards and precision as those of the parenteral products. The dosage forms, for topical and intraocular use, include solutions, suspensions, gels, ointments, inserts, and intraocular injections and implants.

Table 15-5 Ophthalmic Drugs by Various Therapeutic Categories

Drug Category	Therapeutic Use	Examples
Anesthetics	Preoperative and postoperative pain relief	Tetracaine, proparacaine, lidocaine
Anti-infective agents	Local and systemic	Bacitracin, tetracycline
Antifungal agents	Fungal endophthalmitis and fungal keratitis	Amphotericin B, natamycin, flucytosine
Antihistamines	Relief of itching due to allergens	Peniramine
Anti-inflammatory agents (corticosteroids and NSAIDs)	Allergic conjunctivitis nonspecific, superficial keratitis, herpes zoster	Dexamethasone, loteprednol, prednisolone, diclofenac, flurbiprofen, ketorolac
Antiviral agents	Herpes simplex virus, cytomegalovirus, retinitis	Trifluridine, idoxuridine, vidarabine, ganciclovir
Astringents	Conjunctivitis	Zinc sulfate
β-Adrenergic blockers	Elevated intraocular pressure, chronic open-angle glaucoma	Betazolol, timolol
Miotics	Glaucoma, accommodative esotropia, myasthenia gravis	Pilocarpine, echothiophate, demecarium, latanoprost
Mydriatics and cycloplegics	Dilation of pupil	Atropine, homatropine, phenylephrine, cyclopentolate
Protectants and artificial tears	Eye lubrication	Cellulose derivatives, polyvinyl alcohol
Vasoconstrictors	Minor eye irritations	Naphazoline, oxymetazoline, tetrahydrozoline

Solutions

Ophthalmic solutions have the advantage of being highly acceptable by patients as they interfere very little with vision, but they are washed out quickly from the cul-de-sac, thus requiring frequent applications. The preparation of an ophthalmic solution requires careful consideration of the following factors: sterility, particulate matter, pH and buffering, isotonicity, and viscosity.

Sterility

The most important requirement of all ophthalmic formulations is the sterility. Contaminated products can result in eye infections that could cause blindness, especially if the *Pseudomonas aeruginosa* microbes are involved. The gram-negative bacillus can cause complete loss of sight in 24 to 48 h. A sterile ophthalmic solution in a multiple-dose container can become contaminated during or after use by the patient. The tip of the dropper while out of the container can touch the surface of a table if laid down, or can be in contact with the eyelid or eyelash of the patient during administration. To maintain the sterility of products, antimicrobial preservatives are generally included in multiple-dose formulations. The commonly used preservatives include benzalkonium chloride (0.004–0.01%), phenylmercuric acetate (0.004%), benzethonium chloride (0.01%), and chlorobutanol (0.5%). The sometime ineffectiveness of these agents (at tolerable concentrations) against some strains of *P. aeruginosa* has led to the use of benzalkonium chloride (0.01%) in combination with either polymyxin B sulfate (1000 USP U/mL) or disodium ethylenediaminetetraacetate (EDTA) (0.01–0.1%), which are shown to be effective against most strains of *Pseudomonas*. EDTA is a chelating agent, which renders strains of *P. aeruginosa* more sensitive to benzalkonium chloride. Ophthalmic preparations packaged in single doses do not contain preservative.

pH and Buffer

Formulations based on the pH of the tear fluid (7.4) are safe and nonirritating to the corneal tissue. However, this pH is often not attainable because of the pH dependency of a drug's solubility and chemical stability, which may require the solution to be buffered at a different pH. This approach is workable if the administered solution is quickly diluted by the highly buffered tear fluid and yields to the physiological pH of the eye. Indeed, a fairly wide range of pH (from 4.5 to 11.5) has been noted in ophthalmic solutions,[31] and pH 6.5–8.5 has been deemed useful in preventing corneal damage.[32] To maintain the pH for solubility and stability purposes, several buffer systems have been developed primarily for ophthalmic formulations.[33] Sörensen's modified phosphate buffer (see **Table 15-6**) is satisfactory for many ophthalmic preparations but is not suitable for pilocarpine, scopolamine, and homatropine salts due to instability of the salt form in the phosphate buffer. Other systems such as the Palitzsch buffer (boric acid/sodium borate) and the Atkins and Pantin buffers (boric acid/sodium carbonate, with NaCl) are based on the borate and bicarbonate systems. Ophthalmic solutions, in general, should have a buffer capacity high enough to ensure product stability but low enough to be overcome by the lacrimal fluid, so that the physiological pH of the tissue remains unchanged after applying the solution.

Isotonicity

Ophthalmic solutions should be made isotonic with the lacrimal fluid, which has an osmotic pressure the same as that of an 0.9% solution of NaCl, to prevent unwanted osmosis that could result in tissue damage or pain. A hypotonic solution can produce painful swelling as the lacrimal fluid is diluted, allowing water to penetrate the tissue. Conversely, hypertonic solutions can result in shrinkage of tissue as water from the tissue now undergoes osmosis, moving into the hypertonic solution. The eye can tolerate quite a range of tonicities from 0.6% to as high as 2.0% solution of NaCl.[32] But for safety, an ophthalmic solution is required to be isotonic. The preparation of an isotonic ophthalmic solution is normally done using a buffered isotonic vehicle. Table 15-6 shows the phosphate buffer commonly used in isotonic preparations and the parameters used in determining the amounts of ingredients needed to achieve isotonicity. The usefulness of information given in Table 15-6 is shown in Example 15-1.

Viscosity

The drug action from an ophthalmic solution may be prolonged by increased corneal retention or reduced drainage from the eye, using a viscous solution. The desired viscosity range for ophthalmic solutions is about 15–25 cP. Commonly used viscosity enhancers include cellulose derivatives, polyvinyl alcohol, and polyvinylpyrrolidone. Depending on the grades of the polymer, the desired viscosity of an ophthalmic solution may be achieved with a polymer concentration of 1% or less. For example, if methylcellulose 25 cP is used, a 1% solution will have a viscosity of 25 cP. If methylcellulose 4000 cP is used, an 0.25% solution will provide the same viscosity.

Other Factors

The major chemical degradation reactions in solution are hydrolysis and oxidation. For a stable formulation, hydrolysis is either nonexistent or under control (such as by pH). This leaves oxidation, a potential drug stability problem for ophthalmic solutions; hence, antioxidants are often added to the formulation. Commonly used antioxidants include sulfite, metasulfite, and bisulfate, which are used in high-, intermediate-, and low-pH solutions, respectively. Additionally, it is essential that both the solution and the intended container of an ophthalmic solution be free of particulate matter.

Table 15-6 Parameters and Phosphate Buffers for Isotonic Preparation

Sodium Chloride Equivalent (*E*) and Volume of Water (*V*) per Gram of Drug Needed for Isotonicity					
Drug	***E***	***V*, mL/g**	**Drug**	***E***	***V*, mL/g**
Atropine sulfate	0.12	14.3	Pilocarpine HCl	0.24	26.7
Boric acid	0.52	55.7	Polymyxin B sulfate	0.09	10.0
Cocaine HCl	0.17	17.7	Procaine HCl	0.21	23.3
Ephedrine sulfate	0.20	25.7	Scopolamine HBr	0.12	16.7
Homatropine HBr	0.17	19.0	Sodium borate	0.42	46.7
Neomycin sulfate	0.11	12.3	Zinc sulfate	0.15	16.7

Sörensen's Isotonic/Phosphate Buffered Vehicles[†]			
pH	**0.0667 *M* NaH_2PO_4, mL**	**0.0667 *M* Na_2HPO_4, mL**	**NaCl to Be Added, mg/mL**
6.2	80	20	5.1
6.5	70	30	5.0
6.6	60	40	4.9
6.8	50	50	4.8
7.0	40	60	4.6
7.2	30	70	4.5
7.4	20	80	4.4
7.7	10	90	4.3
8.0	5	95	4.2

[†]From USP XXI, p. 1338.

Example 15-1: Show how you would prepare the following isotonic solutions:

Rx1: Procaine HCl 2%
Aqua. dist. q.s.
Isotonic Buffer (pH 6.6) q.s. ad 30 mL
Make an isotonic solution using the isotonic buffer.

Rx2: Procaine HCl 2%
Sodium chloride q.s.
Make 30 mL of sterile, buffered, isotonic solution at pH 6.6 using the Sörensen's buffer.

Solution:

Rx1 is to be formulated by dissolving the drug in a sufficient amount of distilled water to form an isotonic solution, which is then diluted using an isotonic vehicle to the total volume of 30 mL. This prescription requires 0.6 g of procaine HCl:

Wt of procaine HCl = 30 mL × 2 g/100 mL = 0.6 g

Table 15-6 shows that the volume of water needed to make an isotonic solution of procaine HCl is 23.3 mL/g of drug. Hence for 0.6 g of drug,

$V_{H_2O} = 23.3\,mL/g \times 0.6\,g = 14\,mL$

Thus, to make this solution, dissolve 0.6 g of procaine HCl in 14 mL of distilled water, and then add to the drug solution a sufficient amount (~16 mL) of an isotonic buffer to make a final volume of 30 mL.

Note: Because of the large volume of water used, the final pH and buffer capacity may differ from those of the buffered isotonic vehicle.

Rx2 is to be formulated in a buffered isotonic solution with a pH of 6.6. Table 15-6 shows that a buffer composed of 60 mL of 0.0667 *M* of NaH_2PO_4, 40 mL of 0.0667 *M* of Na_2HPO_4, and 4.9 mg/mL of NaCl is isotonic and gives a pH of 6.6. When procaine HCl is added to this vehicle, the solution is hypertonic.

Hence, the amount of NaCl needed should be reduced to accommodate the inclusion of the drug. This is calculated using the sodium chloride equivalent method:

A (Wt of NaCl for solution without drug) = 4.9 mg/mL × 30 mL = 147 mg

B (NaCl equivalent wt from drug) = 600 mg × E_{drug} = 600 × 0.21 = 126 mg

C (NaCl needed) = 147 − 126 = 21 mg

Because the volume of the prescription is 30 mL and the ratio of the monobasic to dibasic phosphates is 60 : 40, the volume of each solution is calculated to be

V of NaH_2PO_4 solution = 30 × 60/100 = 18 mL

V of Na_2HPO_4 solution = 30 × 40/100 = 12 mL

Hence, to fill this prescription, dissolve 0.6 g of procaine HCl and 21 mg of NaCl in 18 mL of the NaH_2PO_4 solution, and then mix this drug solution with 12 mL of the Na_2HPO_4 solution. The final solution will be isotonic and will have a pH of 6.6.

Suspensions and Ointments

Ophthalmic suspensions are aqueous formulations that contain finely divided particles (10 μm or less) for water-insoluble drugs or drugs whose soluble form is unstable in aqueous solutions. These products have the advantage over solutions of providing more extended corneal contact time. The particle size must be small enough to prevent irritation of the eye and to achieve a desired rate of dissolution. In suspensions, the solution has a concentration equal to the solubility of the drug. As the drug is absorbed, particle dissolution will occur, and it is desirable that the particles have a rapid dissolution rate to maintain saturated concentration within the formulation's residence time in the eye. If the dissolution rate is too slow, a suspension has no more benefit than a saturated solution. Suspensions should not form irreversible aggregates in storage and should be easily dispersed upon shaking. Betoptic (betaxolol HCl), Achromycin (tetracycline HCl, Lederle), and Terra-Cortril (oxytetracycline HCl and hydrocortisone acetate, Roerig) are some examples of ophthalmic suspensions.

Ophthalmic ointments tend to provide a longer contact time with the eye than suspensions but have slower onset of actions and rates of drug release. Ointments must be nonirritating and free from grittiness, which requires that the ointment base be soft (of low yield stress) and the particle size small (micronized). Most ophthalmic ointment bases are a mixture of mineral oil and white petrolatum and have a melting point close to body temperature. The anhydrous lanolin (an absorption base) may be used to incorporate ingredients dissolved in small amounts of water to affect dissolution. Ophthalmic ointments have the drawbacks of blurred vision and oleaginous texture, which cannot be removed easily from the precorneal film. Therefore, ointments are used mostly at night as an adjunctive therapy to eyedrops used during the day. Sterile ointments are prepared by combining individually sterile ingredients under aseptic conditions. Preservatives are required for ophthalmic ointments. The sterile ointment is generally packaged in a small ointment tube fitted with a narrow-gauge tip that permits the extrusion of a fine band of ointment. These ophthalmic tubes are sterilized by autoclaving or by ethylene oxide and may be lined with epoxy or vinyl plastic in cases of metal reactivity or incompatibility. Most ophthalmic ointments are prepared for antimicrobial and/or anti-inflammatory use.

Gels

The generally poor bioavailability exhibited by ophthalmic solutions may be overcome by using a gel system that significantly extends a drug's corneal contact time. For ease of application, ophthalmic gels are formulated as in situ gels, which exist as a liquid in the container but gels on contact with the tear fluid. The gelation can be achieved via thermal (as in Pluronics),[34] pH (as in Carbopols and cellulose acetate phthalate),[35] cation (as in alginates and gellan gum),[36] and lysozyme (as in xanthan gum) mediated mechanisms. Some cellulose derivatives such as hydroxyethyl cellulose, hydroxypropyl methylcellulose, and Carbopol 940 also form mucoadhesive and thermal-sensitive in situ gels. Ophthalmic gels generally require only 5% of the gelling agent, so the gel base is about 95% aqueous. These formulations have been shown to produce a three- to five-fold increase in corneal absorption.

An optimum temperature-responsive gel should have a gel point that is above room temperature but at or slightly below the precorneal temperature (35°C). Studies have shown that some copolymers of Pluronic F-127 with poly(acrylic acid) exhibit this property.[34] Carbopols can form gels at near neutral to alkaline pH; among these Carbopol 940 has been used in the preparation of Pilogel, which contains 4% by weight of pilocarpine HCl. The gellan gum is a microbial polysaccharide produced by the bacterium *P. elodea*. The commercial brand Gelrite—a highly purified, anionic polysaccharide containing glucose, glucuronic acid, and rhamnose moieties—has been used in the product Timoptic-XE (timolol maleate, Merck) for the treatment of elevated intraocular pressure. The gelling mechanism involves interactions of the anionic polymer with divalent cations, such as Mg^{2+}, which promotes chain association. The gel strength increases with increasing cation concentration; thus, it is feasible that a gellan gum solution may gel on contact with tear fluid. Hydroxypropyl methylcellulose has been used in the formulation of a lidocaine gel (Akten, Akron) as a topical anesthetic in conjunction with intravitreous injections and various ocular surgeries. This agent enhances drug absorption and also protects the cornea against drug and surgery-related toxicity to the corneal epithelium.

Ocular Inserts

Ocusert (Alza) is an oval pilocarpine delivering device consisting of a titanium dioxide frame and a pilocarpine core sandwiched between two ethylene–vinyl acetate copolymer membranes. In use, the device is placed under the lower eyelid, where drug dissolves in lacrimal fluid and is released from the device at a controlled rate according to Fick's law. For sparingly soluble drugs, the concentration of dissolved drug in the device is maintained at solubility; hence, the release of drug follows zero-order kinetics. The rate of drug release depends on several factors including the solubility of the drug, the contact surface area, the thickness of the membrane, the diffusion coefficient of the drug through the membrane, and the partition coefficient of the drug between the membrane and the lacrimal fluid. The zero-order release kinetics give a constant rate of drug delivery; e.g., the product Ocusert P-20 delivers a dose of 20 mg/h, which is advantageous for dosage planning. This device, however, which can be lost without being detected, has not been well accepted by patients.[37]

Soluble inserts are preparations that dissolve or erode within 1 h of application. These inserts are made of natural polymers (e.g., collagen), hydroxypropyl cellulose or methylcellulose, or polyvinyl alcohol. The sterile Lacrisert, e.g., is made of hydroxypropyl cellulose for the treatment of moderate to severe cases of dry eye (keratoconjunctivitis sicca). It is a rod-shaped gel formulation, 1.27 mm in diameter and 3.5 mm in length.

Intraocular Dosage Forms

For intraocular injections, parenteral products of anti-infectives, corticosteroids, and anesthetics may be used. The FDA also approved intraocular use of some viscoelastic, antiviral, and miotic preparations and irrigating (balanced salt) solutions that are isotonic with aqueous humor. The viscoelastic preparation (e.g., chondroitin sulfate with sodium hyaluronate and hydroxypropyl methylcellulose) is injected into the anterior segment of the eye during surgical removal of cataracts and corneal implants. An example of an intravitral implant is the ganciclovir tablet with magnesium stearate coated with polyvinyl alcohol and ethylene vinyl acetate (Vitrasert), which is implanted in the vitreous cavity for drug release over a 5- to 8-month period. Vitrasert is used to treat cytomegalovirus retinitis.

A biodegradable implant for controlled ocular drug release has been used in treating postoperative inflammation associated with cataract surgery. Surodex (Oculex Pharmaceuticals, Sunnyvale, CA) is a biodegradable system containing 60 μg of dexamethasone in a poly(lactic-glycolic)-acid (PLGA) matrix, which provides a sustained and controlled release of dexamethasone over 7 days. The biodegradable pellet is implanted into the anterior chamber at the conclusion of cataract surgery. Randomized studies have found Surodex to be as effective as 0.1% dexamethasone eyedrops in the control of postoperative inflammation.[38, 39] The 60 μg of dexamethasone in one pellet is approximately equivalent to that in one drop of the 0.1% solution, indicating that controlled drug release to the target site can significantly reduce the required dose and problems associated with patient compliance. Current concepts in ophthalmic drug delivery also include the use of phospholipid-based liposomes and polymeric micelles formed through self-assembly by non-ionic surfactants. These systems are biodegradable, non-toxic, and nonimmunogenic; they can be used to incorporate both hydrophilic and hydrophobic drugs, protect drug from degradation in solutions, and provide sustained drug release.

IV. Inhalation (Aerosol) Drug Delivery

The pulmonary route is attractive for drug delivery because it offers a large surface area for drug absorption. Because high drug concentration can be delivered directly to the site of action, pulmonary delivery offers greater efficacy and reduced side effects for treatment of pulmonary diseases than systemic drug delivery. The alveolar epithelium is very thin, which permits rapid drug absorption and a rapid onset of action. In addition, pulmonary drug delivery bypasses the GI barriers and the first-pass hepatic metabolism, so that superior therapeutic effect can be achieved at a fraction of the oral dose.

Pulmonary drug delivery is also an attractive alternative to oral or parenteral drug delivery for systemic drug effects. It is noninvasive and is suitable for the delivery of a wide range of drug molecules and types. The lung is the only organ through which the entire cardiac output passes. Drug absorption is regulated by a thin alveolar–vascular permeability barrier, which, in parts of the alveolar region, has an air–blood pathway of less than 0.5 μm.[40] In the adult human lung, the number of alveoli in the deep airways ranges from 200 to 600 million, which results in an enormous epithelial surface area, estimated to be about 140 m^2. Although these alveoli are uniquely adapted for gas exchange via passive diffusion, they also provide a mechanism for effective transport of drugs from the circulation to lung tissues and from lung tissues to the bloodstream. As a result, systemic absorption of drug delivered by aerosol may be many-fold faster than that of the oral administration.[41] Hence, there is a great potential that many drug therapies may be improved via inhalation drug delivery, pending further advances in aerosol technology.

Drug Delivery Considerations

Lung Epithelia

Different terminologies have been used to describe the divisions of the lungs. For simplicity, the pulmonary system may be divided into the upper and lower respiratory tracts (see **Figure 15-4**). The upper respiratory tract is taken to be the airways from the nasal vestibule down to the junction of the larynx and trachea. This includes primarily the nasal cavity, which has been previously described. The lower respiratory tract can be divided into the tracheobronchial, bronchiolar, and alveolar regions. The tracheobronchial region is lined by pseudo-stratified ciliated columnar epithelium, beneath which are mucous glands, connective tissue, cartilage, smooth muscle, and nerves. Various cell types including basal, ciliated, mucous, serous, and Clara cells and migratory lymphocytes are present in this region. The bronchiolar region is characterized by the presence of a columnar epithelium comprising mainly two cell types: the ciliated cells and Clara cells. The alveolar epithelium consists of type I and type II pneumocytes and the presence of surfactants. In addition, a few alveolar macrophages reside within each alveolus. It is worth noting that both the Clara cells and type II pneumocytes contain CYP-450 isozymes and NADPH cytochrome P-450 reductase. High levels of non-CYP-450-dependent enzymes are also present in Clara cells. Type I cells exhibit little or no metabolic activity; thus they are susceptible to drug toxicity. In comparison to the nasal epithelium, which contains various phase I (cytochrome P-450s) and phase II enzymes (glutathione-*S*-transferases) as well as non-CYP-450 enzymes, the lower respiratory tract has considerably less enzyme activity[42] and is thus better suited for drug absorption.

Mucociliary Clearance (MCC)

The tracheobronchial airways are protected by a mucociliary apparatus that serves to entrap and eliminate particles from the lungs via a combined activity of mucous secretion and the beating of cilia protruding from the luminal surface of the columnar cells. The complex but coordinated beating of the cilia moves the mucus layer toward the pharynx, thereby providing a clearance mechanism for the lung. The submucosal glands are found in the trachea and bronchi, and the ciliated cells extend as far down as the terminal bronchioles. Thus, it is the central region of the lung that is protected by the mucociliary apparatus. Once it passes through this central region, a drug has a great potential to be absorbed or to exert a local action in the peripheral (alveolar) lung. MCC is regulated by both cholinergic and adrenergic innervations of the submucosal glands, and each cell type receives fibers from both types of nerve. Serous cells are more responsive to α-adrenergic agonists, whereas mucous cells are more responsive to β-adrenergic agents. Hence, administration of adrenergic drugs is likely to have some effects on the mucociliary apparatus. MCC is under a dual control that includes a neurohumoral-regulated ciliary beating frequency via a β-adrenergic mechanism and the control of the mechanosensitivity of cilated cells mediated through intracellular calcium.[43] The latter may result from a direct stimulation of the ciliated surface or from nervous or hormonal stimulation of mucus secretion leading to increased beating frequency. Thus, a very broad spectrum of stimuli may increase the rate of MCC.

Effects of MCC on Aerosol Drug Delivery

All components of an inhalation aerosol, including particles and its chemical content, may interact with the mucociliary system. The deposition of aerosol particles in the lung depends largely on their mass median aerodynamic diameter (MMAD), which is the measured diameter times the square root of density. Particles show good alveolar penetration if their MMAD is 3 µm or less.[44] Between 3 and 5 µm, the particles are uniformly deposited throughout the lung; above 5 µm, particles are deposited mainly in the conducting airways.[45] Hence, even well-formulated aerosol systems may come into contact with the mucociliary apparatus. A gamma scintigraphic

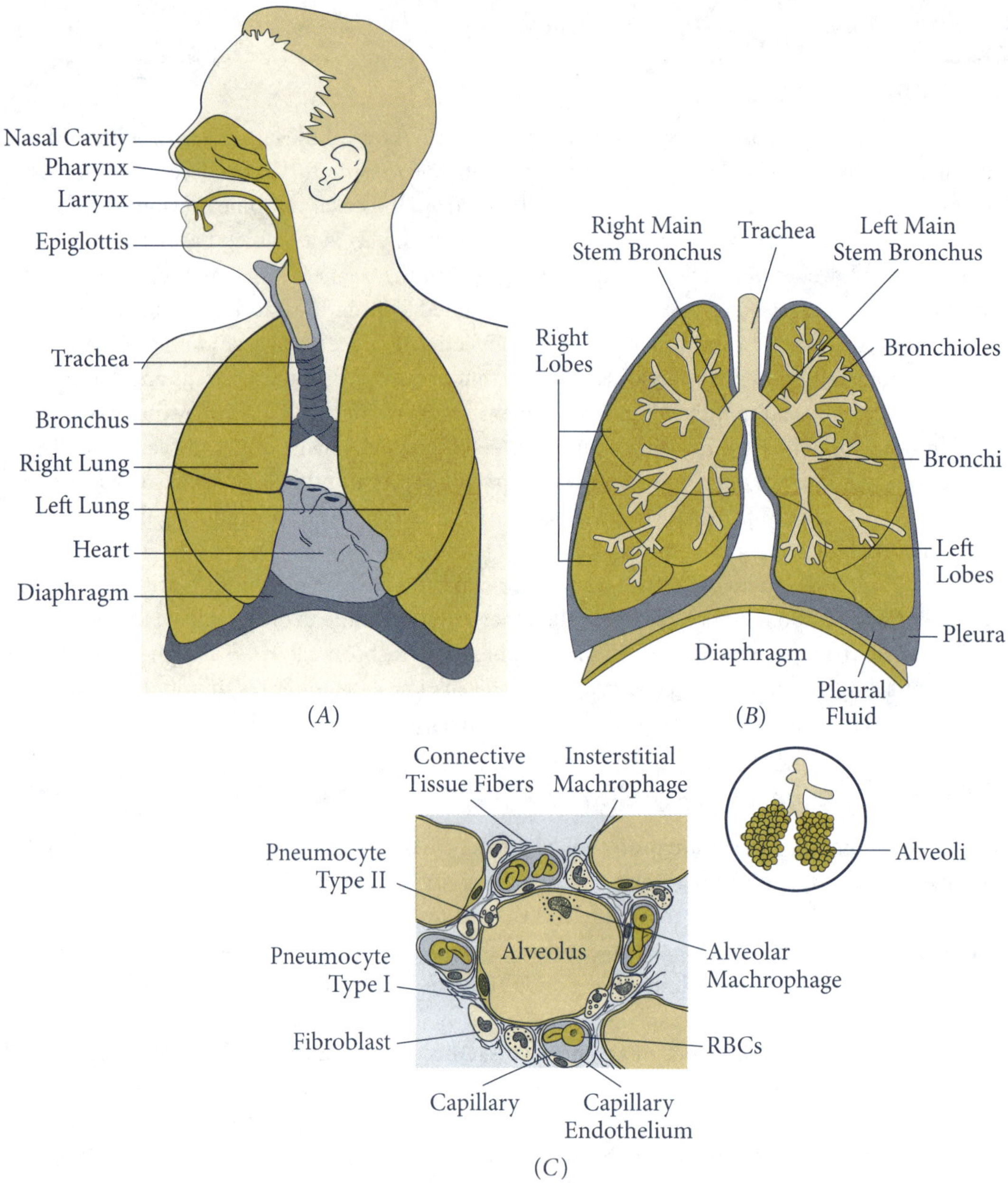

Figure 15-4 The human respiratory system and alveolar epithelium: (*A*) the upper and lower respiratory tracts, (*B*) the lungs, and (*C*) the alveolus.
Sources: © udaix-Shutterstock, Inc., © Anita Potter/Shutterstock, Inc.

study of the effect of MCC on insulin absorption in rabbits showed that aerosol-delivered insulin (2–3 μm) had a peripheral/central lung deposition ratio of 1.52, whereas an intratracheally instilled dose gave a ratio of 0.32.[46] The latter showed a major deposition of drug in the central lung. The measured bioavailability was 57.3% and 5.6% for the aerosolized and instilled drug, respectively, indicating that the MCC of the instilled dose resulted in a 10-fold decrease in bioavailability.

Sympathomimetic drugs in general are known to stimulate mucus secretion, ciliary beating frequency (CBF), and mucociliary transport.[47] Cholinergic drugs, such as acetylcholine and pilocarpine, were shown to increase CBF, and subcutaneous administered bethanecol resulted in a significant increase in the MCC from the proximal airways, which may be attributed to increased mucus secretion.[48] Other drugs, such as aminophylline, have been shown to promote MCC in patients with obstructive airways. Some drugs are known to be strongly ciliotoxic, and these include propranolol[49] and a wide range of pharmaceutical preservatives.[50]

Alveolar Epithelial Permeability

The alveolar wall consists of a specialized epithelium and a closely apposed network of capillaries supported by a delicate interstitial matrix. Nearly 95% of the alveolar surface consists of a single layer of type I pneumocytes joined by tight junctions. These terminally differentiated cells are vulnerable to a variety of injuries, and they have little or no regenerative potential. The type II cells, the other 5%, are more resistant to oxidant injury and are capable of proliferating and repairing the epithelial lesions. Alveolar macrophages are residents of the alveoli and are primarily responsible for the host defense against inhaled pathogens and particles. Studies of the mechanism of drug absorption have shown that the alveolar epithelium, similar to that of the nasal mucosa, is permeable by both hydrophilic and lipophilic drugs.[51, 52] Hydrophilic drugs undergo slow, diffusion-based transport, where the rate of diffusion is inversely proportional to the molecular weight, with pore sizes corresponding to drug diffusion through tight junctions. Lipophilic drugs are transported at rates determined by their partition coefficient via a classical lipoidal transcellular diffusion process. The tight junction permeability is enhanced by many absorption enhancers.[53]

Peptide Degradation

Although some proteins such as interferon undergo little catabolism on passage through the lung, peptides and proteins in general are subjected to hydrolysis in the lung, which is known to exhibit strong aminopeptidase and dipetidyl carboxypeptidase activities.[54] Studies using insulin, ($Asu^{1,7}$)-Eel calcitonin (ECT), and fluorescence-labeled dextrans have shown that pulmonary absorption of the proteins is significantly lower than that of the dextrans with similar molecular weights to the proteins.[55] This was attributed to the enzymatic degradation of the proteins. Indeed, the absorption of intratracheally delivered ECT in the rat lungs, e.g., showed a bioavailability, as measured in hypocalcemic effect, of 2.7% of the intravenous dose when given alone, but approached 100% when given with 20 m*M* bacitracin, a potent aminopeptidase inhibitor that is known to inhibit the enzyme degradation of ECT. Various protease inhibitors have been shown to improve pulmonary absorption of peptides. Examples are captopril and bestatin for enkephalins, phosphoramidon and thiorphan for substance P, bacitracin and sodium glycocholate for calcitonins, and aprotinin for insulin (for details, see Ma et al.[56]). Compounds such as sodium glycocholate and bacitracin not only inhibit protease activity but also enhance the permeability of the protein and peptide drugs. It appears that the peptide degradation problem can be controlled by inhibition of protease activity.

Inhalation Aerosols

Aerosol is a formulation enclosed in a device that functions to vaporize and deliver the content to an applied area. Pharmaceutical aerosols are generally intended for pulmonary, nasal, buccal, and sublingual drug delivery, but can also be used for topical, rectal, or vaginal drug administration. In propellant-driven aerosols, the container is a pressurized package, inside which the pressure is created by the presence of gaseous and liquefied propellants. When the valve of the aerosol is opened, the vapor pressure forces the content of the package out through the opening in the valve. Depending on the formulation and the type of valve employed, the expelled content can take the form of an airborne mist (< 50 μm), as in room disinfectants and deodorizers, known as space sprays, or in larger particles (50–200 μm), known as surface sprays, as in many of the household spraying products. A general comparison of space and surface sprays can be seen from **Table 15-7**.

The inhalation (lung) aerosols used in therapeutics include primarily the *metered-dose inhalers* (MDIs), *dry powder inhalers* (DPIs), and *nebulizers*. Mechanically, the deposition of the delivered drug from these systems is influenced by the inspirational flow and breathing maneuvers of the user and the dynamic factors of the aerosolized drug such as the size, velocity and inertial impaction, and

Table 15-7 General Comparison of Space and Surface Sprays

Content	Space Spray	Surface Spray
Active ingredient	2–30%	20–75%
Propellant	98–70%	80–25%
Pressure (25°C)	30–40 psig[†]	25–55 psig
Particle size	1–50 μm	50–200 μm

[†]Pounds per square inch gauge.

sedimentation of the particles in the airways. Particles with sizes greater than 10 μm deposit primarily in the throat and trachea by impaction, whereas particles of 3 μm or less can reach the deep lung (the alveolar region) by sedimentation. In most inhalation aerosols, drug particles have sizes of 5 μm and less; hence, they are distributed throughout the central and lower regions of the lungs.

Metered-Dose Inhalers

MDIs are propellant-driven inhalers, capable of delivering accurate and reproducible doses of aerosolized drugs to the lungs. The aerosol formulation consists of two components, the product concentrate and the propellant. The product concentrate, in solution or suspension, contains the active drug and additives (e.g., surfactants, protective agents, and solvents) required to make a stable, efficacious product, whereas the propellant aerosolizes the product concentrate and delivers the content in the desired form, size, and distribution.

Product Concentrate

A product concentrate can be a solution or suspension. Solution aerosols are two-phase systems consisting of the product concentrate in a propellant, a propellant blend, or a mixture of propellant and solvent. Solution aerosols can be difficult to formulate because the propellants or propellant–solvent mixtures are often poor solvents for the product concentrate. Ethanol and propylene glycol are among the most commonly used solvents added for making solution aerosols. The percentage of propellant in solution aerosols is of importance in controlling the sprayed particle sizes. As the percentage of propellant increases, so does the degree of dispersion, and the spray becomes very fine. Conversely, a decrease in the percentage of propellant can result in wet and large particles and reduced lower-airway deposition.[57]

Suspension aerosols are made when the product concentrate is insoluble in the propellant or mixture of propellant and solvent. Antiasthmatic drugs, steroids, and antibiotics are delivered as suspension aerosols. Potential problems associated with a suspension formulation may arise from particle size growth, agglomeration, valve clogging, and the moisture content. In dilute suspensions, gravitational phase separation of the dispersed phase is proportional to the square of the particle diameter. Thus coarse suspensions are physically less stable and may exhibit significant content uniformity problems. If the dispersed phase consists of finely milled particles, charge interactions and flocculation can occur, which is also undesirable. An increase in drug concentration can increase the amount of drug delivered, but can also reduce the respirable fraction of the delivered dose. These variables may significantly impact the bioavailability of inhaled drug; thus, a careful consideration of the particle size, concentration, and the surfactants used is generally needed for the formulation of a suspension.

Surfactants generally reduce particle sedimentation and aid in minimizing particle aggregations in suspensions. On the other hand, surfactants that are immiscible with the propellants can decrease the vapor pressure of the aerosol and thus the energy needed to produce "dry" particles.

This results in the formation of coarse aerosols, with decreased capacity to deposit drug in the lower airways.[57] As a consequence, drug may be deposited largely in the trachea but not in the deep lung, resulting in decreased bioavailability.[58] A number of lubricants (isopropyl myristate and light mineral oil) and surfactants (sorbitan trioleate, oleic acid, and lecithin) have been shown to produce fine sprayed particles and overcome the difficulties of particle growth and agglomeration that can lead to clogging of the valve. The moisture content of the formulation is also crucial for producing "dry" particles, and it should be kept below 200–300 ppm.

Propellants

A propellant is a chemical with a vapor pressure greater than atmospheric pressure at 40°C. Propellants in pharmaceutical use include chlorofluorocarbons (CFCs), hydrochlorofluorocarbons (HCFCs), hydrofluorocarbons (HFCs), hydrocarbons, and compressed gases. The three primary propellant systems in MDI products are CFC P-11, P-12, and P-114 (the numerical designation is explained in Example 15-2). The use of these propellants has been limited, since 1996, to the MDI use for the treatment of asthma and chronic obstructive pulmonary diseases, due to their effects on the atmospheric ozone layer depletion. Alternatives to P-12 have since been developed in HFC P-134a and P-227, but there is no alternative for P-11 and P-114. The physical properties of these propellants are shown in **Table 15-8**.

CFCs show good properties for easy liquefaction. For example, P-12 will liquefy when cooled to –21.6°F or when compressed to 84.9 psia at 70°F (psia = pounds per square inch absolute). The liquefied gases have an expansion ratio of about 240 (volume of vaporized gas per 1 mL of liquefied gas), which is much higher than those (3–10) of the compressed gases (e.g., nitrogen, carbon dioxide), making the CFCs excellent propellants for MDIs. In most suspensions, small amounts of P-11 are needed to make a slurry with the active drug and other ingredients. P-11, however, undergoes hydrolysis to yield hydrochloric acid in the presence of water, which can cause corrosion to the container or irritation to applied membranes. Thus, if water is present, P-12 or a blend of P-12 and

Example 15-2: The numerical designation for fluorinated and chlorinated hydrocarbon propellants.

This designation uses a *three-digit* system:

- The digit at the far right refers to the *number of fluorine atoms* in the molecule.
- The second digit from the right represents the *number of hydrogen atoms* + 1.
- The third digit from the right represents *number of carbon atoms* –1; for substituted methane, this third digit is 0 and is omitted; hence, a two-digit number is used.
- The capital letter C is used before the number to indicate the cyclic nature of a compound.
- The small letters following the number are used to indicate decreasing symmetry of isomeric compounds. The most symmetrical compound is given the designated number, and all other isomers are assigned a letter (a, b, etc.) in descending order of symmetry.
- The number of chlorine atoms in a molecule may be determined by subtracting the total number of hydrogen and fluorine atoms from the total number of atoms required for saturation.

The propellant 134a (P-134a) is thus identified as trifluoromonofluoroethane ($F_3C—CH_2F$). In comparison, P-134 is $F_2CH—CHF_2$.

Table 15-8 Vapor Pressure of Some Fluorocarbon Propellants at 70°F (21.1°C)

Chemical Name	Chemical Formula	Numerical Designation	Vapor Pressure, 70°F psia†	Boiling Point, °F (1 atm)	Liquid Density, 70°F (g/mL)
Trichloromonofluoromethane	CCl_3F	11	13.4	74.7	1.485
Dichlorodifluoromethane	CCl_2F_2	12	84.9	−21.6	1.325
Dichlorotetrafluoroethane	$CClF_2CClF_2$	114	27.6	39.4	1.468
Trifluoromonofluoroethane	CF_3CH_2F	134a	85.8	−15.0	1.210
Chlorodifluoroethane	CH_3CClF_2	142b	43.8	14.4	1.120
Difluoroethane	CH_3CHF_2	152a	76.4	−12.5	0.910

†psia (pounds per square inch absolute) = psig (pounds per square inch gauge) + 14.7.

P-114 is used in MDI formulation. The HFCs (P-134a and P-227) differ from CFCs in that they have one or more hydrogen atoms and break down in the atmosphere at a faster rate than the CFCs, thus having a lower effect on ozone depletion. These agents have propellant properties similar to those of P-12, but differ from the CFCs in their surfactant solubility. As a result, surfactants such as oleic acid, sorbitan trioleate, and lecithin used in the CFC systems are not suitable for formulations using the HFC alternatives. Part of the surfactant function is to maximize the fine particle dispersion necessary to facilitate valve operation for dosing reproducibility. The needed surfactant concentration is usually determined by experimentation, which falls typically in the range of 0.01–0.1%, but concentrations as high as 2% have been used. The surfactants listed above have been shown to exhibit a solubility of less than 0.02% in P-134a, and this has led to the search for alternative surfactants that have good solubility in P-134a, such as polyethylene glycol, propoxylated polyethylene glycols, and perfluoroalkanoic acids, or insoluble surfactants that can be used to coat drug particles for easy resuspension.[59] The first drug tested with P-134a was albuterol, which has been shown to be safe and efficient in delivering the medication to the lungs.[60]

MDI System

The essential components of an MDI are the container, metering valve, and actuator. The metering valve (**Figure 15-5**) is designed to deliver a fixed amount of the product concentrate after each actuation. The basic units of a valve assembly are as follows:

1. *Metering chamber*: It has a fixed dimension for valve volume (25 to 100 μL); access to and from the metered chamber is controlled by a dual valve mechanism via the stem.
2. *Stem*: It supports the actuator and is operated through the actuator button to deliver the formulation to the metering chamber from the container or to the actuator from the metering chamber.
3. *Gaskets*: They are placed snugly with the stem to prevent leakage of the formulation in the valve when the system is at rest or in operation.

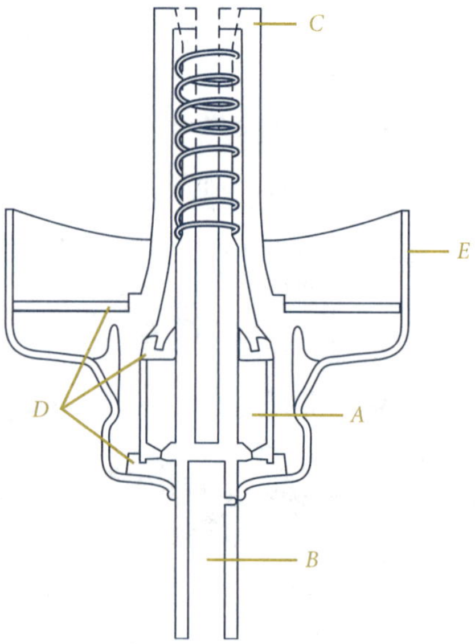

Figure 15-5 Schematic diagram of an inverted metering valve: (*A*) Metering chamber; (*B*) Stem; (*C*) Housing body; (*D*) Gaskets; and (*E*) Mounting cup.

4. *Spring*: The spring holds the gasket in place and provides the mechanism by which the actuator retracts, when actuation is released, to the closed position.
5. *Housing*: A mounting cup is attached to the aerosol container, holding the valve in place; directly below the mounting cup is the housing body, which serves as the link between the dip tube or the stem and the actuator.
6. *Dip tube*: It extends from the housing down into the product concentrate and serves to bring the formulation from the container to the valve. It is used in solution aerosols but not in suspension aerosols.

The metered dose delivered by MDIs is basically regulated through a dual valve mechanism. When the actuator is closed (at rest), a seal blocks the emission from the metering chamber to the atmosphere through the stem orifice, but the chamber is open to the container and is filled with the aerosol content. When the actuator is depressed, the chamber is open to the atmosphere for the release of its contents, but is sealed from the contents of the container. When the actuator is again closed, the chamber is reloaded for the next dose. Two basic types of metering valves are available: one for inverted use and the other for upright use. The latter type is for solution aerosols and contains a thin capillary dip tube. Aerosols containing suspensions are delivered using valves intended for inverted use that do not contain a dip tube. In general, the valve should retain the material in the metering chamber for long periods. It is possible, however, that the material may escape from the chamber after a long period of quiescence because of propellant drainage or suspension instability. This would result in a lower subsequent dose.

MDIs are the major products for inhalation therapy, but are also the most misused devices. It is estimated that 50–60% of patients do not use proper inhaler technique, thus receiving little or no benefit from drug delivered by MDIs. A critical maneuver for the proper use of the MDI is to coordinate the actuation of the aerosol with the patient's inspiration, and for this, the mouthpiece adapter on the MDI has been repeatedly modified to assist patients in receiving the correct dosage when the coordination is not well performed. Larger adapters (called tube spacers) permit the propellant to evaporate before the aerosol reaches the patient. This results in a reduced particle size and velocity, which reduces the inertial impaction and improves the depth of drug deposit in the lungs. The disadvantages of these adapters are the cost, difficulty to clean, and inconvenience to use because of their size. Nevertheless, the correct technique of using an MDI is as follows:

1. Hold the mouthpiece a few inches from the mouth (open-mouth procedure) or into the mouth with closed lips (closed-mouth procedure).
2. Exhale deeply.
3. Start slow, deliberate inhalation and actuate the device.
4. Hold the breath for 5–10 s.
5. Breathe normally.

Dry Powder Inhalers

The DPIs are designed to deliver drug in powder form to the lungs via aerosolization by the patient's inspirational efforts (with a minimum flow rate of 30 L/min). The DPIs have four basic features: (1) a dose-metering mechanism, (2) an aerosolization mechanism, (3) a deaggregation mechanism, and (4) an adapter to direct the aerosol into a patient's mouth. For pulmonary deposition, the particles must have an MMAD of 5 μm or less, hence drugs are milled to desirable sizes prior to formulation. Fine particles do not flow well; one approach to improve aerosolization has been to mix the drug with larger particles such as lactose (60–80 mm) that act as carriers, on which the smaller drug particles are loosely bound. During aerosolization, the deaggregation action of the inhaler causes a stripping of drug particles from the lactose surface, allowing them to traverse through the respiratory tract, while the excipient particles are left behind in the mouthpiece of the device or in the mouth and throat of the patient. In unit dose inhalers, the drug-lactose powder is filled into a hard gelatin capsule.

The DPIs that have been approved for use in the United States are Spinhaler (Intal; disodium cromoglycate; Fisons, Rochester, NY) and Rotahaler (Ventolin; albuterol sulfate; GlaxoSmithKline). The Spinhaler works by inserting the capsule into an impeller in the body of the inhaler. The capsule is pierced by the device when the system is ready to use, and the impeller rotates as the patient breathes through the device, projecting particles into the airstream. The Rotahaler has a mechanism for breaking the capsule into two pieces. The capsule body containing the dose falls into the device, while the cap is retained in the entry port for subsequent disposal. As the patient inhales, an erratic motion of the capsule containing the drug in the airstream causes the dislodged particles to be entrained through a grating system and inhaled. A number of other DPIs are available for use in other countries. The details of these and other medical devices for aerosol delivery can be seen from the studies of Dalby et al.[61]

DPIs are small, portable devices that can be carried in a pocket or purse. In general, less than 20% of the delivered drug reaches the lungs (the same as that of MDIs), with most of the dose deposited within the drug capsule or container. For most drugs available as MDIs, specific DPI delivery devices have also been developed. Studies have shown that, when properly used, there is no difference in efficacy between DPI and MDI in delivering the same drug.[62]

Nebulizers

The nebulizer system converts a liquid formulation into vapor, using energy provided either by a high-velocity airstream, known as a jet nebulizer, or by ultrasonication through the vibration of a piezoelectric crystal, known as an ultrasonic nebulizer. These systems require a nebulizing device, a respiratory solution or suspension, auxiliary tubing, and mouthpieces or face masks. With a controlled airflow rate through the nebulizer, aerosolization of particles or droplets is achieved in 10 to 20 min. Inhalation therapy was once accomplished mostly using nebulizers or atomizers that were restricted to hospital, outpatient clinic, or home use. Declined use of nebulizers coincided with the development of MDI in the mid-1950s, which provided the convenience of portability and accuracy of dosing. There is, however, a resurgence of interest in nebulizers due to their ability to generate small droplets capable of penetrating the deep lung, high-dose delivery capacity, miniaturization of hardware, and the development of high-output nebulizers, permitting shorter treatment time.

The nebulizers are more versatile as a drug delivery system compared to the MDIs and DPIs. Patient coordination, as in MDI use, is not necessary; drug delivery to the lungs is adequate even in severely dyspneic patients regardless of age. The formulation for nebulizers is a solution or suspension, which may be formulated to contain cosolvents for drug solubility if needed, additives to ensure physicochemical stability of the drug, or multiple drugs for combination therapy. Several marketed products for nebulization contain preservatives, stabilizers, sweetener, and salts and acids to adjust the tonicity and pH. These excipients can also be used to facilitate aerosolization or drug absorption. For example, a decrease in pH in an insulin solution from 7.0 to 3.0 improves pulmonary bioavailability of this drug from 13.1% to 41.6%, due to the existence of insulin in the monomeric form at this low pH.[63] While a large fraction (~ 80%) of the nebulized drug dose is entrained in the apparatus, 80% or greater of the inhaled drug is deposited in the lungs.[64] This is quite different from MDIs and DPIs, where a significant fraction of the inhaled drug is swallowed and may contribute to the overall bioavailability through GI absorption. The nebulizers can be used to deliver up to 10 times the dose delivered by MDI or DPI, and they provide combination drug therapy that cannot be done using MDIs and DPIs. The chief drawbacks of the nebulizers are lack of portability, greater costs of drug delivery, and loss of drug to the apparatus.

Inhalation Drug Therapy

Pulmonary Action

Aerosol drug delivery is commonly used for localized treatment of lung diseases including asthma, chronic obstructive pulmonary disease (COPD), chronic bronchitis, respiratory infections, and cystic fibrosis. Depending on the types and disease management, asthma may be treated with (1) β-adrenergic agonists such as albuterol and terbutaline for bronchodilation, (2) anticholinergic agents such as ipratropium bromide (Atrovent), (3) antiallergic and anti-inflammatory agents such as cromolyn and nedocromil, and (4) inhalation corticosteroids such as beclomethasone dipropionate (Beclovent), triamcinolone acetonide (Azmacort), and flunisolide (Aerobid). The exact mode of action of the corticosteroids is unknown, but they are the most effective drugs for the treatment of asthma, presumably because of their broad anti-inflammatory effects. Chronic bronchitis, due to excessive tracheal bronchial mucus production, and emphysema, defined as hyperinflation of the air space at the terminal bronchi with destruction of the alveolar septa, often coexist in patients with COPD. Infections also occur frequently in these patients, making the disease management difficult. In general, theophylline is administered orally to promote bronchodilation, diaphragmatic contractility, and increased MCC. Combined therapy using β-agonists and anticholinergics via MDI has been found to be effective; so is the addition of an inhalation corticosteroid to bronchodilator therapy, in providing improved lung function and decreased frequencies of exacerbations in COPD patients. In treating cystic fibrosis, a potentially useful agent delivered by MDI is the recombinant deoxyribonuclease (rhDNase); this enzyme digests the DNA in the thick mucus, enhances MCC, and improves lung function.

The use of aerosol drug delivery of antibiotics to treat respiratory infections significantly lowered the drug's systemic toxicity. Antibiotic therapy is particularly important in patients with cystic fibrosis, who are susceptible to developing recurrent infections secondary to bronchiectasis. The pulmonary concentrations of antibiotics achieved by aerosols can be 10–40 times greater than those achieved by parenteral administrations.[65] The concentration of aerosolized aminoglycoside, tobramycin, e.g., was shown to be well in excess of the minimal inhibitory concentration necessary to kill most of the organisms in the lungs, and the treatment of gram-negative infections in critically ill patients with aerosolized tobramycin and third generations of cephalosporins has been shown to kill more than 96% of the pathogens colonizing the respiratory tract.[66] Other antibiotics used as aerosols include amikacin sulfate, ciprofloxacin, erythromycin, and amphotericin B.

Systemic Effect

Exubera was developed in 2006 by Pfizer, Sanofi-Aventis, and Nectar Therapeutics as an aerosol for the delivery of human insulin to type I and type II diabetic patients. The drug product was withdrawn in 2007 for not being cost-effective compared to short-acting insulin formulations available as injections. This product showed the feasibility to provide effective and reliable dose of a protein drug through the pulmonary route and, at the same time, some drawbacks that could hamper future product development. Both the formulation and the mechanical device technologies appear to need improvement to meet the therapeutic and cost requirement. From the drug absorption point of view, one significant fact associated with Exubera is that the product is limited to nonsmoking patients who are also free from other existing pulmonary conditions. The clinical data showed that systemic insulin effect in smokers via Exubera is two- to five-fold higher than in nonsmokers, with the former patients experiencing more rapid onset of glucose-lowering action and a greater peak and total effect. This suggests a significant variability in pulmonary drug absorption depending on the condition of the lungs, which is likely an important factor for consideration in future product development, especially for drugs with a narrow therapeutic index.

V. Drug Targeting

Drug targeting refers to the delivery of drug to a specific site, which can be a macromolecule, an organ, a specific cell type, or a subcellular organelle. The overall goal of drug targeting is to achieve increased drug efficacy with reduced drug dose and systemic toxicity. It is worthy to note at the onset that regardless of the methods and approaches used for targeting a drug to a specific site, the dosage form is usually delivered by parenteral injection, a relatively direct route to get the drug to the targeting tissue. Site-specific administration is sometimes possible, but such deliveries typically involve highly invasive procedures. Hence, a targeting dosage form must be suitable for injection without causing adverse effects and must be stable in systemic circulation. A prolonged circulation time often enhances the dosage form's targeting ability.

The need for drug targeting is best exemplified by anticancer chemotherapy, which is necessary for the treatment of cancers that are nonoperative or not suitable for radiation therapy. The bioavailability of anticancer drugs after oral administration is usually low due to reduced absorption. Intravenous delivery of drugs is thus necessary, and the drug is given in high doses that frequently result in high systemic toxicity. Hydrophobic drugs such as paclitaxel are also prepared in solutions containing alcohol and surfactants as solubilizing agents, which add to the toxic side effects of the dosage form. Targeted drug delivery is a promising approach to overcome systemic toxicity, which can be achieved using molecular and particulate targeting systems. Our discussion of drug targeting will be mostly confined to the delivery of anticancer agents.

Prodrug Strategies

Drugs administered parenterally are distributed throughout the body, reaching targeted and nontargeted tissues alike. A drug, however, can be modified to become a part of a complex molecule or polymeric structure that exhibits strong affinity toward certain cell types via antigen–antibody interactions and receptor-mediated endocytosis. This is known as *active targeting*. The molecular approaches of active targeting involve the use of a prodrug that is pharmacologically inactive but is enzyme-activated at the targeting site. These approaches are referred to as carrier-linked prodrug system, antibody-directed enzyme prodrug therapy (ADEPT), and gene-directed enzyme prodrug therapy (GDEPT).

Prodrug Concept

Chemical modification of drugs has been used to improve drug absorption via increased solubility, elimination of first-pass hepatic metabolism, increased biological half-life, and targeted drug delivery. Fosphenytoin, e.g., is a phosphonooxymethyl amine derivative of the anticonvulsant phenytoin. The phosphate attachment increases the aqueous solubility of the drug from 20–25 μg/mL to 140 mg/mL, thus ensuring oral absorption. Once absorbed, fosphenytoin is rapidly converted by alkaline phosphatase ($t_{1/2}$: 7–15 min) to yield the active drug. When acyclovir (an antiviral) is derivatized to yield the L-valylester (valacyclovir), a ligand for the intestinal peptide transporter 1 (PEPT1), the oral bioavailability of the drug is increased from 10–20% to 54%. Peptide transporters are cellular membrane proteins that mediate the uptake of amino acids, small peptides, and other soluble nutrients,[67] which function as nonspecific receptors. Other membrane transporters, such as P-glycoprotein, promote efflux of drugs that results in drug resistance. Drug targeting via PEPT1-mediated uptake is advantageous for oral absorption but lacks cell targeting specificity. Nevertheless, the transporter serves as a targeting moiety.

Carrier-Linked Prodrug Strategy

The design of prodrug targeting systems is schematically illustrated in **Figure 15-6**. A linear model (Figure 15-6*A*) consists of a spacer, usually a peptide, chemically linked to the drug on one end and the targeting moiety on the other end. The targeting moiety can be a monoclonal antibody (mAb), fab fragment, peptide, or aptamer responsive to the antigen or receptor, or a ligand to a specific receptor on the targeted cells. The folate receptor, e.g., is overexpressed on most tumor cells, which provides a selective targeting effect. Linkage between the drug and the spacer can be made via ester, amide, disulfide, or oxime/imine linkage that can be easily cleaved to yield the parent drug. Ideally, any removed moiety should be pharmacologically inactive and nontoxic, while the linkage to active drug must be labile for efficient in vivo activation and, for tumor selectivity, responsive to tumor cell-specific enzyme. An example is folate-vinblastin EC145,[68] a folate-conjugated desacetylvinblastine monohydrazide, in which a hydrophilic peptide spacer is linked to the drug via a reductively labile disulfide linkage. In vivo studies[69] showed that this prodrug is targeted to folate receptor-positive human xenografts in nude mice and exhibits superior antitumor activity and tolerability to the free drug. EC145, under development by Endocyte, is in phase III clinical trials for ovarian and lung cancers.[70] The carrier-linked prodrug can also have a configuration in which the different elements of the targeting system are linked to a polymer backbone (Figure 15-6*B*).

Antibody-Directed Enzyme Prodrug Therapy (ADEPT)

In addition to the tumor targeting moiety, the tumor selectivity of enzyme activation is an important consideration for prodrug strategies. In carrier-linked systems, the prodrugs must be readily transported to the site of action and selectively activated by tumor-specific enzymes. Alternatively,

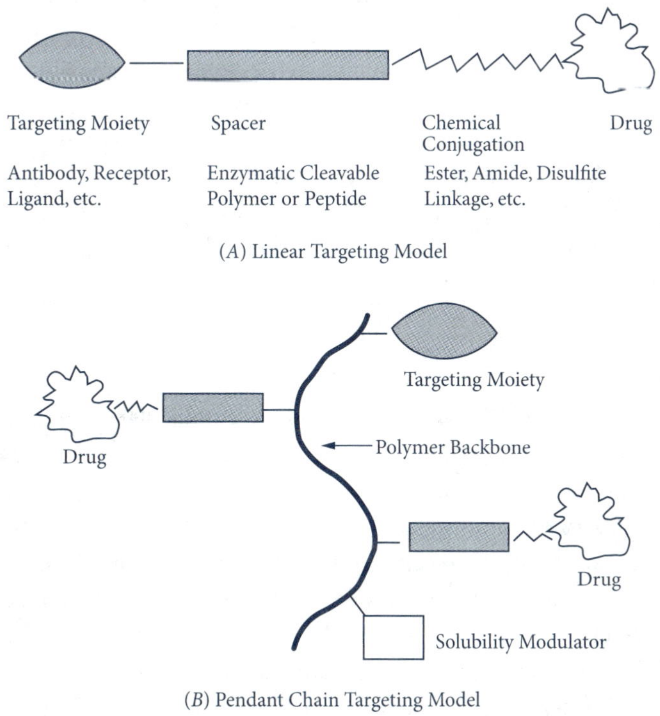

Figure 15-6 Carrier-linked prodrug targeting systems.

a prodrug may be constructed as a bioprecursor, which does not contain a drug-carrier linkage but is chemically modified as a specific substrate to an enzyme, which can be nonmammalian or mammalian, that activates the prodrug by redox reaction or phosphorylation (for antiviral agents). This approach requires first the delivery of the prodrug-activating enzyme to tumor cells using mAb-conjugated enzyme system and then the administration of the prodrug after the excess mAb-enzyme conjugates have been cleared from the blood and normal tissue. The idea is one of a bystander effect, in which the prodrug having the ability to cross the tumor cell membrane is stable and nontoxic but becomes cytotoxic once it reaches the tumor tissue and is activated at the surface and inside the tumor cells by the previously administered enzyme. This is known as the antibody-directed enzyme prodrug therapy. An example of ADEPT in clinical trial is the use of the nitrogen mustard–L-glutamic acid conjugate (ZD2767P) against colorectal cancer.[71] The antibody fragment–enzyme conjugate contains the bacterial carboxypeptidase G2, which converts the prodrug *N*-{4-[*N*,*N*-bis(2-iodoethyl)amino]phenyloxycarbonyl}-L-glutamic acid to the active drug 4-[*N*,*N*-bis(2-iodoethyl)amino]phenol, L-glutamic acid, and CO_2.

Gene-Directed Enzyme Prodrug Therapy (GDEPT)

In this approach, a gene encoding a prodrug-activating enzyme is integrated into a genome of targeted tumor cells or viral vector under the control of tumor-selective promoters. These cells then express the enzyme that activates the prodrug. For effective GDEPT, the system must achieve sufficiently high expression of the enzyme in tumor cells but preferably low or none in other cell types. The activated drug should also exhibit the bystander effect on nontransduced tumor cells. One of the significant applications of GDEPT is in cytochrome P450-based cancer gene therapy that has exhibited substantial potential for improving the safety and efficacy of cancer chemotherapeutics.[72] The primary goal of GDEPT is selectively to increase tumor cell exposure to cytotoxic drug metabolites generated on-site by a prodrug-activating P450 enzyme. This strategy has been exemplified for alkylating agents, cyclophosphamide and ifosfamide, which are activated by select P450 enzymes whose expression is generally high in liver but deficient in tumor cells. Transduction of tumors with a prodrug-activating P450 gene, followed by prodrug treatment, greatly increases the intratumoral levels of cytotoxic metabolites and leads to more efficient killing of the transduced as well as nontransduced tumor cells via bystander effects, without significant increase in host toxicity. The P450 reductase transduction has also been shown substantially to enhance intratumoral prodrug activation and its associated therapeutic effects, and the combined transduction of P450 gene with the gene encoding NADPH-P450 reductase has been shown to achieve an overall 50- to 100-fold increase in tumor cell kill in vivo over that provided by hepatic drug activation alone,[73] indicating that improvements in therapeutic effects can be achieved using an established anticancer drug and combination gene therapy.

Targeting Moiety

The major approaches in cell-specific targeting of drug in a molecular or particulate system are through antigen–antibody and ligand–receptor interactions. In anticancer drug delivery, the attachment of a monoclonal antibody or its Fab fragments, peptides, or aptamer to the targeting system allows the drug carrier to bind specifically to antigens or receptors that are overexpressed on tumor cells. The human epidermal receptor (HER) family of receptor tyrosine kinases offers two highly up regulated targets on tumor cell surfaces: the epidermal growth factor receptor (EGFR) and human epidermal receptor-2 (HER2), both of which mediate cell signaling for growth and proliferation. Trastuzumab, a humanized mAb approved by FDA for targeting metastatic breast cancer, is designed to antagonize HER2 function.[74, 75] Other FDA-approved mAb include rituximab (CD20), bevacizumab (VEGF), cetuximab (EGFR), and alemtuzumab

(CD52). Transferrin receptors are up regulated (2- to 10-fold) in most tumor cells and thus may be exploited for targeting purposes using transferrin or transferrin antibodies as ligands.[76] Aptamers are short DNA or RNA oligonucleotide ligands that are capable of binding to target antigens, analogous to antibodies, with high affinity and specificity.[77] An A10 20-fluoropyrimidine RNA aptamer has been used to target docetaxel-loaded PLGA–PEG nanocarriers to the extracellular domain of the prostate-specific membrane antigen (PSMA), and it was shown significantly to enhance in vitro cellular uptake of the micelle-incorporated anticancer drug and its cytotoxicity.[78]

Rapidly dividing tumor cells have a voracious appetite for certain vitamins, such as biotin, vitamin B12, and folate. Biotin is an essential micronutrient for normal cellular functions and growth, which has been found in significantly higher levels in some cancer cells than in normal tissue.[79] Studies of biotinylated chemotherapeutic agents for cancer cell-specific drug delivery have shown that biotin-conjugated nanoparticles enhanced targeted drug (e.g., paclitaxel) delivery to tumor cells and resulted in greater inhibition of tumor growth in Balb/c mice bearing mammary adenocarcinoma tumors than nontargeted nanoparticles.[80] Folate is an essential vitamin for the biosynthesis of nucleotide bases by proliferating cells,[81,82] and it is largely consumed by cancer cells. As a result, the folate receptor is a highly specific tumor marker, overexpressed by various tumor cells including malignancies of the ovary, brain, kidney, breast, myeloid cells, and lung, but is absent in most normal tissue. For this reason, folate has been extensively used as a targeting ligand for the delivery of anticancer agents.

Active targeting can also be based on ligand–receptor interactions with angiogenesis regulators. When tumor cells cluster and reach a size of around 2–3 mm, diffusion of oxygen and nutrients to the tumor is repressed. This induces angiogenesis, allowing the tumors to grow beyond their diffusion limit. The integrins represent a large group of structurally related receptors for extracellular matrix (ECM) proteins and immunoglobulins that regulate tumor angiogenesis. The $\alpha_v\beta_3$ integrin receptor is for ECM proteins harboring the arginine–glycine–aspartic acid (RGD) sequence. RGD containing peptides can therefore provide strong targeting specificity to integrin-expressing cancer cells.[83] The various targeting moieties mentioned above have all been found effective through in vitro and in vivo tumor-targeting experiments.

Nanocarrier Approaches

Nanoplatforms

Nanosized drug carriers have been paid close attention for their applicability as a drug delivery system. The development of particulate drug carriers stems from early work of microencapsulation in attempts to provide controlled and targeted drug delivery. Pioneer studies by Louis A. Luzzi and coworkers[84–87] are noted here for their contribution to the continuous development of drug-containing microspheres and the more sophisticated systems seen today. The reduction of particle size to the nanoscales (5–100 nm) has made the particulate system extremely attractive, as these systems are readily injectable and are free from solubility considerations associated with the development of parenteral solutions. Furthermore, the nanocarriers can be made for passive and active targeting of drugs to the active sites. With the availability and better understanding of the properties of various polymeric materials, some major forms of nanocarriers have been developed including biodegradable nanospheres, liposomes, polymeric micelles, and dendrimers. A brief description of these nanocarrier types (see **Figure 15-7**) is given below; their general properties are summarized in **Table 15-9**.

Biodegradable nanospheres are drug-polymer matrices made of polymers such as poly(D,L-lactic-*co*-glycolic acid) copolymers (PLGA), chitosan, and cross-linked albumin particles. In PLGA, the biodegradation occurs through random scission of the polymeric chain by hydrolysis,

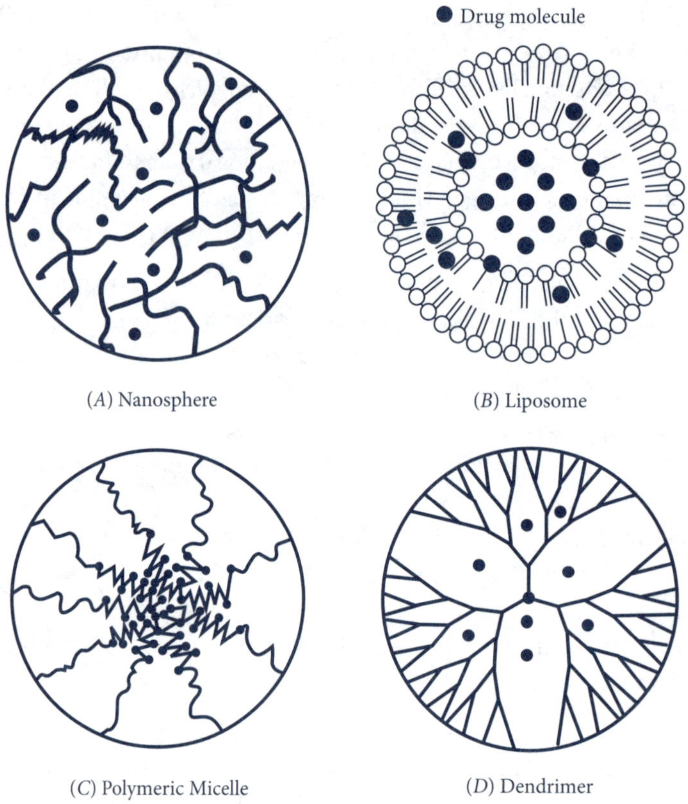

Figure 15-7 Nanocarriers in drug delivery: biodegradable nanosphere, liposome, polymeric micelle, and dendrimer.
Adapted from: Shao P, Wang B, Wang Y, Li J, and Zhang Y. *J Nanomaterials.* 2011: doi 10.1155/2011/389640, 2011.

which leads to the formation of lactic and glycolic acids. These monomers are easily metabolized in the body through the Krebs cycle and eliminated as carbon dioxide and water. In general, the rate of degradation of PLGA increases with increasing content of glycolic acid and shortening of polymeric chain (by lowering the molecular weight). Drug release from the nanospheres may follow a biphasic pattern, first governed by diffusion according to Fick's law and then facilitated by

Table 15-9 Nanocarriers in Drug Targeting

Type	Structure	Size, nm	Drug Release Mechanism
Nanospheres	Biodegradable matrix (PLGA, chitosan, albumin)†	45–400	Diffusion; biodegradation
Liposomes	Unilamellar or multilamellar lipid bilayer(s) with a hydrophilic core (phospholipids; cholesterol)	10–400	Fluidity (lipid exchange); disintegration
Polymeric micelles	Hydrophilic–hydrophobic block copolymer micelles, with a hydrophilic shell and a hydrophobic core (PEG-*b*-PDLLA)†	5–100	Hydration of the hydrophobic core; biodegradation; triggered drug release via pH and thermal sensitive mechanisms
Dendrimers	Unimolecular spheres with hydrophilic, charged, or hydrophobic shell, branched interior and hydrophilic pockets (PAMAM, PPI, etc.)†	~10	Diffusion; decoupling; biodegradation

†PLGA: poly(lactic-glycolic acid); PEG: polyethylene glycol; PDLLA: poly(D,L-lactic acid); PAMAM: poly(amidoamine) dendrimer; PPI: poly(propylene-imine) dendrimer.

polymer degradation. The diffusion process can be approximated using first-order kinetics. Hence, both the biodegradation and the drug release from the nanospheres can be controlled via polymer selection as well as formulation factors that determine the hydrophobicity of the system. PLGA has been used in a variety of pharmaceutical systems (microspheres, implants, films, nanoparticles for targeted delivery, etc.) because of its biodegradability, biocompatibility, and mechanical strength as a drug delivering platform.

Liposomes contain a single or multiple concentric lipid bilayer(s) made of phospholipids and cholesterol and a hydrophilic core, whereas polymeric micelles are made of hydrophilic–hydrophobic block copolymers that contain a hydrophobic core and a hydrophilic shell. Drug release from liposomes depends on the fluidity of the lipid bilayer or their disintegration in the endosomal environment. The diffusion of drug through the lipid bilayer is slow or nonexistent. In polymeric micelles, drug molecules are incorporated in the hydrophobic core through physical entrapment or chemical linkage; their release depends on the hydration of the hydrophobic block or on triggered mechanisms using pH-, temperature-, light-, and ultrasound-sensitive polymers. Detailed discussion of the liposome and micelle platforms is given later.

Dendrimers are repeatedly branched polymers that have a spherical three-dimensional morphology. The name comes from the Greek words dendron and meros, meaning "tree" and "part." They are also called cascade molecules. Dendrimers were first introduced in 1978 by Fritz Vogtle and coworkers.[88] It is synthesized from a starting initiator, such as a nitrogen compound, to which chemical moieties are added by a repeating series of reactions that produce a spherical branching structure. As the process repeats, successive layers are added, and the expanded sphere assumes a structure that consists of (1) an initiator core, (2) interior layers (generations) composed of radically attached repeating units, and (3) terminal functionality groups attached to the outermost generation. The outer layer can be cationic (—NH_3^+), hydrophilic (—OH or PEGylated), anionic (—CO_2^-), or hydrophobic. An example of the various dendrimer types is the poly(amidoamine) dendrimers (PAMAM), which are synthesized by the divergent method starting from ammonia or ethylenediamine as the initiator core. Products up to generation 10 (G10) have been obtained. PAMAN with a molecular weight similar to that of human albumin or hemoglobin (~65,000 Da) has been made for drug delivery purposes. These dendrimers are commercially available under the name of Starburst dendrimers, owing to their starlike pattern when expressed in two-dimensional structure (Figure 15-7).

The physicochemical characteristics of dendrimers, namely, their water solubility, drug entrapment capacity, and large number of functional peripheral groups, make them appropriate candidates as solubilizing agents and carriers for drug delivery. Drug may be incorporated by (1) covalent attachment to the peripheral groups, (2) ionic coupling to the functional groups, or (3) entrapment into the matrix. Dendrimers with a hydrophobic interior and a hydrophilic surface function as unimolecular micelles, which, unlike traditional micelles, do not have a critical micelle concentration. This allows the dendrimers to encapsulate drug at any concentrations. Studies have shown that the solubility of propranolol was increased by two orders of magnitude via conjugation to surface-modified G3 PAMAM dendrimer, which resulted in a significant increase in the drug's oral bioavailability.[89] An increasing number of studies on dendrimers as a drug delivery system are now seen in the drug literature. A system with PAMAM interior and long alkyl chain exterior was shown to deliver 5-fluorouracil with enhanced oral absorption and a two-fold increase in bioavailability in rats, compared to the free drug.[90] Dendrimers with G4-NH_2 function groups are cationic systems that have been shown to provide advantages for intracellular drug delivery and gene targeting.[89] It is likely that the dendrimers will offer new scaffolds for drug delivery, owing to their unique molecular architecture, although potential problems concerning their biocompatibility and toxicity remain to be worked out.

Nanoparticles are particles in which at least one of the particle dimensions is 100 nm or less. In practice, the nanocarriers have a size range of 5–400 nm, which is, nevertheless, within the colloidal size range. Among the nanocarriers, liposomes and polymeric micelles have been extensively studied, and a number of such systems are under clinical investigation or approved for clinical use. Drug-targeting approaches using these two systems will be discussed following a general consideration of the passive and active drug targeting using the particulate systems.

Passive Targeting

Small particles in circulation are normally opsonized (see later discussion) for phagocytosis by cells of the mononuclear phagocytic system (MPS), leading to particle accumulation in the liver and spleen. This would be a form of passive targeting if the liver and spleen or the phagocytes were the intended targets. If not, then it is necessary that the particles be modified to avoid the MPS to gain extended circulation time. Modification of the surface of nanocarriers can be made through adsorption or chemical grafting of materials that are well solvated and flexible to produce a steric effect. Polymers such as poly(ethylene glycol) (PEG) have been used extensively for this purpose, and in polymeric micelle preparations, PEG is often used to form the hydrophilic shell. The term *PEGylation* was coined to describe the modification of a liposome surface by methoxyPEG to create stealth particles in circulation.

A PEGylated particulate system may be passively targeted to tumor cells via the *enhanced permeability* and *retention* (EPR) effect of the highly irregular tumor tissue. Induction of angiogenesis occurs typically in solid tumors because of their high demand for nutrition and oxygen as the cells multiply and cluster. The blood vessels in tumors, however, are irregular in shape, dilated, and leaky due to discontinuous lining of endothelial cells. The perivascular cells and the smooth muscle layers are frequently absent or abnormal in the vascular wall. These defects result in extravasation of blood plasma components and, in drug delivery, the nanocarriers to the tumor tissues. As the tumors progress, the lymphatic drainage in tumor tissues becomes increasingly impaired, which, along with slow venous return, accounts for a high retention of nanocarriers in the tumor tissues. This is referred to as a passive form of targeting, which depends on the size distribution and surface charge of the nanocarriers and the disease pathology. The high permeability of the vasculature and the lack of lymphatic drainage in tumor areas dictate that long-circulating nanocarriers spontaneously accumulate in the targeted tissue via the EPR effect. Extravasation of nanocarriers does not occur from the bloodstream into normal tissues that have tight junctions between capillary endothelial cells.

Active Targeting

Similar to the prodrug approach, nanocarriers can also be modified to contain surface-attached ligands for active targeting based on the concept of antigen–antibody interactions and ligand–receptor interactions. In addition, nanocarriers can be made to contain a drug release triggering mechanism that adds to the controlled release and targeting specificity to tumor tissues. Triggered drug release is achieved through the use of polymers that respond to an internal (e.g., pH- or temperature-sensitive) or external (e.g., ultrasonic- and light-sensitive) triggering factor that is associated with the pathological conditions of the targeted, but not the normal, tissue. The triggering mechanism is attractive and desirable, as the drug is being administered in a manner that precisely matches the physiological needs at the proper site and proper time.

The combination of passive and active targeting as well as triggered drug release makes the particulate systems particularly attractive as a targeting approach. An important element of the particulate system is that the nanocarriers can be made with prolonged circulation time without releasing the drug until they reach the targeted site. This reduces drug distribution to nontargeted tissues and thus the toxic side effects of the drug. As a result, the nanocarriers can offer greater therapeutic benefits over solution therapies, targeted or otherwise. A closer examination of the liposomes and polymeric micelles for improved anticancer chemotherapy is described next.

Liposomes for Drug Targeting

Liposomes are microvesicles composed of one or more bilayers of the biocompatible natural or synthetic phospholipids with an entrapped aqueous core. As a carrier, lipophilic drugs are entrapped exclusively in the lipid bilayer, water-soluble drugs are enclosed in the aqueous core, whereas drugs with intermediate lipophilicity partition between the lipid and aqueous phases and stay in both environments. Their biocompatible nature and their ability to incorporate both water-soluble and water-insoluble drugs make liposomes the most studied colloidal systems for drug delivery purposes. Liposomes are commonly classified, based on their size and lamellarity, into *small unilamellar vesicles* (SUV, 25–100 nm), *large unilamellar vesicles* (LUV, 100–400 nm), and *multilamellar vesicles* (MLV, 200–5000 nm). The unilamellar vesicles have a single lipid bilayer, suitable for the encapsulation of hydrophilic molecules in the aqueous core. MLVs, on the other hand, consist of two or more concentric lipid bilayers that are useful for entrapment of hydrophobic drugs. Liposome drug products are designed to provide one or more of the following functions: (1) extended drug release, (2) delayed drug release, (3) site-specific targeting, and (4) intracellular drug delivery. Extended drug release can enhance drug action at the active site, whereas the purpose of a delayed release is to protect either the drug from chemical and enzymatic degradation in blood circulation or the healthy tissue from the cytotoxicity of the drug. Targeted delivery requires the liposome to retain drug content while in systemic circulation but to release the drug at the active site, preferably inside the targeted cells.

Stability of Liposomes in Circulation

Plain liposomes (without grafted surface material) can be used to protect encapsulated drug from degradation and passively to target the drug to tissues that have a discontinuous endothelium, such as the liver, spleen, and bone marrow. Upon IV administration, liposomes are rapidly captured by MPS and removed from the blood circulation. This phenomenon allows the delivery of antiparasitic and antimicrobial drugs to treat infections localized in the MPS,[91] or the activation of macrophages to produce tumoricidal agents. When the target site is beyond the MPS, however, MPS removal of liposomes from circulation is a key disadvantage of using plain liposomes as a drug delivery system.

Particles such as the liposomes are normally bound by serum opsonins and complement systems, which the MPS cells recognize as markers for phagocytosis. These opsonins include immunoglobulins, fibronectin, beta 2-glycoprotein, and beta 2-macroglobulin.[92, 93] The complement systems are membrane-attacking complexes that induce cell lysis or, in the case of liposomes, the release of their contents, and uptake of lysed cells by MPS phagocytes.[94] The complement-dependent release of liposomal contents is a major factor of the instability of liposomes in circulation. On the other hand, some proteins, such as albumin, can bind to particle surfaces and reduce their recognition by phagocytes.

Interactions of liposomes with the biological system depend on the size, net surface charge, hydrophobicity, and packing of the lipid bilayers.[95] In general, MLVs are eliminated from the blood circulation more rapidly than SUVs, suggesting that small particles may evade MPS cells. Indeed, studies have shown that opsonization of liposomes is size-dependent, and so is the MPS-mediated accumulation of liposomes by the liver.[96] Negatively charged liposomes have a shorter half-life in the blood than do neutral liposomes, whereas the toxic positively charged liposomes are quickly removed from circulation, as a result of the activation of complement systems by the charged liposomes.[97,98] Liposomes can also undergo lipid exchange with high-density and low-density lipoproteins (HDLs and LDLs, respectively) that lead to rapid release of the encapsulated drug. This has led to the use of cholesterol (CHOL) to strengthen the lipid bilayer, which results in closer packing of the phospholipids, enhanced stability, and reduced transfer of lipids to HDL.[99] It has also been shown that liposomes made of phosphatidylcholine (PC) with saturated fatty acyl chains or sphingomyelin (SM) are more stable in the blood than liposomes containing PC with unsaturated fatty acyl chains.[100]

Liposome Drug Products (LDPs)

Currently available LDPs, except Doxil, are all plain liposomes containing neutral and/or negatively charged lipids and CHOL (see **Table 15-10**). AmBisome is a systemic antifungal preparation containing amphotericin B in the form of a lyophilized powder.[101] The product is prepared by mixing hydrogenated soy phosphatidylcholine (HSPC), distearoylphosphatidylglycerol (DSPG), and CHOL (in weight ratio of 4.1 : 1.6 : 1.0) with other ingredients in an aqueous solution; the resulting MLVs were then microemulsified into SUVs (< 100 nm) using a homogenizer. Amphotericin B is intercalated within the lipid membrane, making it an integral part of the lipid structure. DaunoXome is an SUV preparation (45 nm) of single-dose daunorubicin citrate for intravenous infusion. The lipid bilayer of DSPC and CHOL and the drug enclosed in the aqueous core have a molar ratio of 10 : 5 : 1. DaunoXome showed marked difference from conventional daunorubicin injection in pharmacokinetic behavior. It has a steady-state volume of distribution of 6.4 L and plasma clearance of 17 mL/min, whereas the corresponding values for conventional daunorubicin are 1006 L and 236 mL/min, respectively. The elimination half-life of DaunoXome is 4.4 h, which is longer than the distribution half-life (0.77 h), but much shorter than the elimination half-life, of daunorubicin injection (55.4 h).[102] DepoCyt is a cytarabine liposome injection to be delivered intrathecally into the cerebrospinal fluid (CSF) for the treatment of neoplastic meningitis.[103] It is an interesting extended-release formulation, in which the drug is encapsulated in individual cores of nonconcentric lipid bilayers that form a spherical matrix of about 20 μm. The lipid composition is biochemically similar to those of normal human cell membranes. The intrathecal delivery of DepoCyt (50 mg) shows a peak CSF level of free cytarabine of 30–50 μg/mL within 1 h, and a terminal half-life of 5.9 to 82.4 h, without producing a systemic drug effect. Myocet, which encapsulates doxorubicin, is available in Europe. This product is supplied in three separate vials: doxorubicin as dry powder, empty liposomes in citric buffer, and a solution of sodium carbonate. Drug entrapment must be achieved immediately prior to administration.

Table 15-10 Approved Liposome Drug Products

Product Name (Active Agent)	Composition (Type)	Company, Year of Product Approval	Application
Doxil/Caelyx (doxorubicin)	HSPC/CHOL/DSPE–PEG (stealth liposome)	Ortho Biotech, 1995	Kaposi's sarcoma
DaunoXome (daunorubicin citrate)	DSPC/CHOL (SUV)	Galen Limited, UK, 1996	Kaposi's sarcoma
AmBisome (amphotericin B)	HSPC/DSPG/CHOL (SUV)	Astellas Pharma. Inc., 1997	Systemic fungal infection of immuno-compromised
DepoCyt (cytarabine)	DOPC/DPPG/CHOL/ Triolein (bilayer matrix)	Pacira Pharma. Inc., 1999	Lymphomatous meningitis
Myocet/Evacet (doxorubicin)	EPC/CHOL (empty liposome)	Elan Pharma., available in Europe, 2000	Metastatic breast cancer

A number of liposome preparations, using different bilayer systems, have been studied in various stages of clinical trials. For example, Marqibo (Talon Therapeutics) is an SUV liposome injection containing vincristine sulfate and the DSPC-sphingomyelin-CHOL bilayer; Nyotran (for nystatin A1 delivery; Aronex Pharmaceuticals) and Aroplatin (containing an oxaliplatin analog; Antigenics Inc.) are MLVs developed using dimyristoyl phosphatidylcholine (DMPC) and dimyristoyl phosphatidylglycerol (DMPG)[104]; and LEM-ETU (NeoPharm Inc.) is an MLV preparation of paclitaxel using dioleoylphosphatidyl choline (DOPC), CHOL, and the anionic cardiolipin,[105] where liposomes are formed via charge interactions.

Long-Circulating Liposomes

The concept of creating a long-circulating system is based on the incorporation of a hydrophilic polymer with a flexible chain onto the liposome surface. With the flexible chain occupying the space immediately above the surface, binding of plasma opsonins to the liposomes can be excluded, and thus the action of MPS is avoided. Studies have shown that in addition to PEGylation, the action of MPS can be avoided if certain ganglioside, such as GM (ganglioside-monosialic acid) 1, is incorporated onto the liposome surface that mimics the erythrocyte membrane. Hence, two approaches have been used to prepare long-circulating liposomes; one uses gangliosides and related compounds, and the other uses PEG.

GM1 Liposomes

GM1 is a brain tissue–derived monosialoganglioside that, when grafted onto the liposomal surface, extends the blood circulation of the liposomes to several hours in mice. The prolonged circulation and the increased tumor accumulation of GM1 liposomes are correlated to a size range of 90–200 nm, with large liposomes (> 300 nm) showing accumulation in the spleen and smaller vesicles (< 40 nm) penetrating into the liver interstitial spaces.[106] GM1 was shown to reduce the uptake of liposomes by macrophages; a concentration of 10 mol % decreased MPS uptake by 90%, but this effect was abolished when the sialic acid moiety was removed, suggesting that the carboxyl groups on the liposome surface play a role in avoiding opsonization. The cost for the extensive use of sialic acid is prohibitive, and this has led to the use of glucuronic acid as a surface conjugate.[107] These studies showed that palmityl-D-glucuronate–modified liposomes were MPS-avoiding, and resulted in increased tumor accumulation and therapeutic efficacy of adriamicin compared to free drug therapy.

PEG (Stealth) Liposomes

PEG is a biocompatible, hydrophilic polymer that has no significant immunogenic and antigenic activity. The molecular weight or the length of the polymer can be readily modified for specific purposes. When conjugated with therapeutic proteins and peptides, PEG has the capacity to increase drug solubility, stability, and bioavailability with increased half-life[108] and decreased plasma clearance. These benefits have been utilized in the PEGylation of a number of proteins, including PEG–ademase (for immunodeficiency), PEG–aspargase (for leukemia), PEG–interferon-alpha (for chronic hepatitis C), PEG–aldesleukin (PEG–IL-2) (an anticancer agent), and PEG–filgrastim (for chemotherapy-induced neutropenia) for clinical use.[109]

PEG can be incorporated onto the liposomal surface through physical adsorption, incorporation of a PEG–lipid conjugate during liposome formation, or postattachment to premade liposomes. The commonly used method is to anchor the polymer in the liposomal membrane via the PEG–DSPE (distearoylphosphatidylethanolamine) conjugate (see **Figure 15-8**).[110] The presence of PEG on the liposome surface has been shown to produce a strong interbilayer repulsion that counters

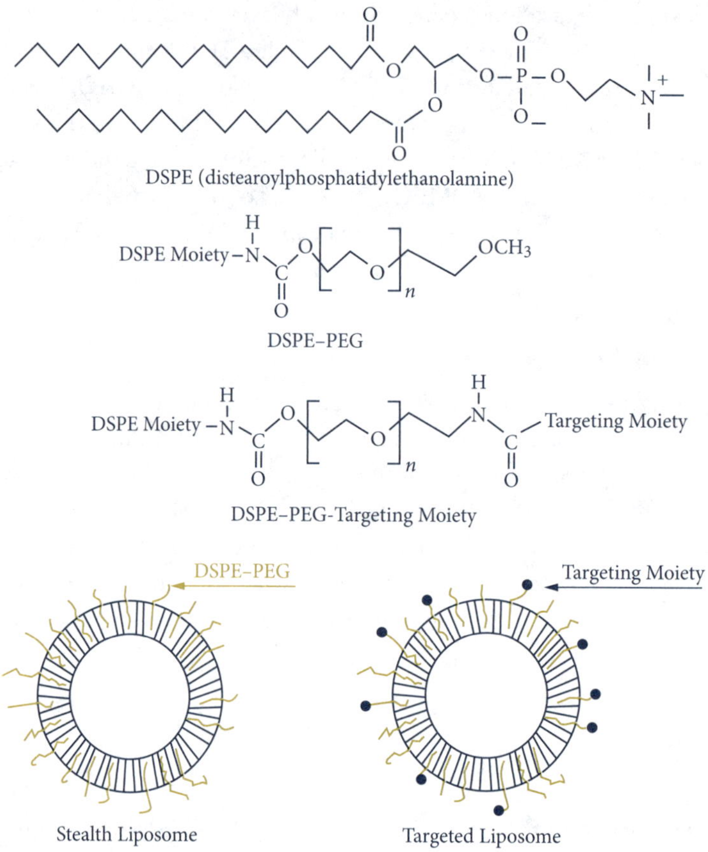

Figure 15-8 The PEG–DSPE conjugate for stealth and targeted liposome preparation.

the attractive van der Waals forces, thus stabilizing the vesicles by preventing them from aggregating.[111] X-ray analysis of the bilayers with grafted PEG 1900–DSPE further showed that the grafted polymer extends about 50 Å from the lipid surface and gives rise to strong intermembrane repulsive forces. As if a "cloud" is formed over the liposome surface, the steric hindrance effect of the PEG moieties reduces the interaction of liposomes with plasma proteins, making them stealth to the MPS and resulting in prolonged blood circulation and enhanced distribution in perfused tissues.[112] It should be mentioned that the surface structure characteristic plays an important role in the stealth effect. A more rigid polymer, such as dextran, grafted to liposomes in comparable quantities, e.g., would not lead to a similar reduction in liposome–protein interactions.[113]

Depending on the graft density and the length of the polymer, the PEG moieties at the liposome surface may exhibit varying degrees of conformational flexibility. There is a close relationship between circulation time of *PEGylated liposomes* and the amount and length of grafted PEG moiety. In most cases, longer-chain PEGs are associated with greater increase in blood circulating time. The blood levels of PEG liposomes made with PEG 2000 and PEG 5000, for example, are much higher than the ones containing PEG 750 and PEG 350.[114]

Clinical Use of Stealth Liposomes

Doxil/Caelyx is a stealth liposomal preparation approved for the treatment of Kaposi's sarcoma[115] and recurrent ovarian cancer.[116] It has also been studied for the treatment of other malignancies including multiple myeloma, breast cancer, and recurrent high-grade glioma and in combination therapy with agents such as paclitaxel, docetaxel, and vinorelbine.[117, 118] The lipid bilayer of Doxil consists of HSPC, CHOL, and mPEG2000–DSPE at a molar ratio of 55:40:5. Liposomes with a mean diameter of 85 nm are able to incorporate doxorubicin at a concentration of 2 mg/mL. The plasma elimination of Doxil follows a biexponential curve, with half-lives of 1.5 and 45 h (median values); in comparison, plasma half-lives are 0.2 h for free drug and 2–3 h for the non-PEGylated Myocet. Nearly 100% of the drug detected in the plasma after Doxil injection was in liposome-encapsulated form; plasma clearance was slow (0.1 L/h) and the distribution volume small (4 L). As can be expected from the pharmacokinetic data, drug-associated cardiotoxicity, myelosuppression, alopecia, and nausea were much lower than those of an equivalent-effective dose of conventional doxorubicin.

SPI-077 (Alza Corporation, Mountain View, CA) is a stealth liposome preparation composed of fully hydrogenated HSPC, CHOL, and DSPE–PEG and cisplatin (in the aqueous core). The apparent half-life of this preparation is 60–100 h. Phase I and II clinical trials for head and neck and lung cancers[119] showed a promising low-toxicity profile but a therapeutic efficacy that is hampered by low cisplatin release.[120] The lack of drug release from SPI-077 was also confirmed in experimental animal studies.[121] These results indicate a potential drawback of the stealth liposomes for not being able to release the drug content adequately, for the same reasons that made them stealth.

In fact, while stealth liposomes are able to lodge in the interstitial spaces among tumor cells, they are cumulated in the extracellular fluid surrounding the tumor cells without entering them. The anticancer drug must be released from the liposomes into the tumor extracellular fluid and then diffuses into the cells.[122] As a result, the ability of liposomes to release the drug into the tumor extracellular fluid, which depends on the fluidity of the liposome, is of equal importance to their targeting ability, which depends on the stability of the preparation. While the targeting action of stealth liposomes is well illustrated with elevated drug concentration at tumor sites, little is known about the kinetics of drug release at the interstitial spaces, or whether the measured concentration is from the released free drug or the drug inside the liposomes.[121] In addition, the released drug must be able to penetrate the solid tumors and to overcome cell-mediated drug resistance. For these reasons, the concept of a "removable" PEG surface conjugation, aimed to facilitate liposome capture by tumor cells following accumulation of PEG liposome at the target site, has been exploited as a potential improvement of stealth liposomes for targeted drug delivery. It has been shown that the conjugation of PEG to PE with a dithiobenzylurethane linkage can release PEG via mild thiolysis.[123]

PEG Alternatives

Hydrophilic polymers, other than PEG, having highly flexible chains and biocompatibility may also be useful to formulate long-circulating liposomes. As alternatives to PEG, a number of polymers including poly(acrylamide), poly[*N*-(2-hydroxypropyl) methacrylamide], and L-amino-acid-based lipid conjugates have been found to extend blood circulation time and diminish liver capture of the liposomes, in efficacies similar to that of PEG. The L-amino-acid-based polymers, e.g., showed prolonged circulation time and reduced uptake by the MPS, to the same extent as DSPE–PEG 2000.[124] These polymers appear to be attractive alternatives for designing long-circulating liposomes, because they are biodegradable and readily usable for conjugation with targeting moiety or pH-sensitive triggering mechanisms.

Targeted Liposomes

A targeting moiety may be attached to the surface of stealth liposomes to aid in targeting efficiency and the internalization of liposomes by targeted cells. Liposomes with grafted monoclonal antibody (mAb) or fragments are known as *immunoliposomes*. These liposomes are more advantageous over molecular targeting approaches in that the liposomes can deliver much greater amount of drug, and the multiple presences of targeting moieties also provide increased ligand avidity and cell uptake. Immunoliposomes also provide a bystander effect, as the drug molecules can diffuse into adjoining tumor cells.

The preparation of targeted liposomes involves the use of a PEG (3400)–DSPE conjugate containing a maleimide group at the end of the PEG chain. After liposome formation, reduced thiol groups of Fab or single-chain scF5 fragments (scFv) are joined to the maleimide group of the PEG-liposomes via a stable thioether linkage. Alternatively, drug-loaded PEG liposome, such as Doxil, can be modified by postinsertion of a mAb–DSPE–PEG conjugate into the premade liposomes.[125] A formulation of a PEGylated doxorubicin liposome system conjugated with the F(ab′)2 fragment of the human mAb GAH (MCC-465) has been investigated in clinical trials for the treatment of metastatic colorectal cancer.[126] GAH is a human antibody obtained by the hybridoma technique. The epitope recognized by GAH is not well characterized, but human gastric, colorectal, and mammary cancer cells are highly GAH-positive, whereas the normal counterparts are GAH-negative. Preclinical studies showed that MCC-465 did not have significant antitumor activity against GAH-negative Caco-2 xenografts. However, MCC-465 exhibited significantly superior antitumor effects against GAH-positive WiDr-Tc and SW837 xenografts compared with liposomes without GAH. Immunostaining of GAH revealed that 94% of surgical specimens of colorectal cancer were GAH-positive.

Another targeted antigen by immunoliposomes is the p185 HER2/neu glycoprotein (HER2), using the anti-HER2 mAb trastuzumab or fragments. The immunoliposomes were made using the anti-HER2 scFv fragment conjugated to PEG–DSPE via postinsertion into premade doxorubicin PEG liposomes.[127] Trastuzumab (Herceptin, Genentech Inc., CA) was the first humanized mAb approved by FDA as monotherapy for metastatic breast cancer, and has been used alone or in combination with other chemotherapeutic agents for the treatment of breast cancer. Antibody-based therapeutics have emerged as important components of therapies for an increasing number of human malignancies. It is likely that more immunoliposomes will be in clinical trials in the near future. Other ligands that have been used for targeting stealth liposomes to overexpressed receptors in cancer cells include folic acid, which has been used for liposome-specific targeting of Doxil, cisplatin, daunorubicin, and other agents,[128] and transferrin, which is a popular ligand for liposome preparation in the delivery of anticancer drugs, proteins, and genes to malignant cells.[129]

Cationic Liposomes

A gene delivery system must bypass cell membrane and facilitate endosomal escape to allow the targeting material to reach the intracellular site. Among various synthetic carriers used in gene therapy, cationic liposomes are the most suitable transfecting vectors. These lipid systems allow condensation of DNA plasmid into a highly organized structure, protect DNA against degradation in storage and systemic circulation, and deliver the gene intracellularly without DNA degradation. The transfection efficiency is achieved using a lipid structure that consists of a positively charged head group that interacts with negatively charged DNA, a linker group that regulates the biodegradability of the lipid, and a hydrophobic chain that anchors the cationic lipid into the bilayer. The commonly used cationic lipids include *N*-[1-(dioleoyloxy)propyl]-*N,N,N*-trimethylammonium salt (DOTMA) and dioleoylphosphatidylethanolamine (DOPE) in a 1 : 1 ratio (Lipofectin, Invitrogen Corp., Carlsbad, CA); 2,3-dioleoyloxy-*N*-[2-(sperminecarboxamido)ethyl]-*N,N*-dimethyl-1-propanammonium trifluoroacetate (DOSPA, LipofectAMINE); *N*-[1-(2,3-dioleoyloxy)]-*N,N,N*-trimethylammonium propane methylsulfate (DOTAP); and dioctadecylamino-glycyl-spermine (DOGS, or Transfectam).

Cationic liposomes are large and toxic at repeated administrations. They induce a complement system that results in their rapid removal from the circulation. As a result, PEGylation of cationic liposomes has been employed to overcome these problems. In liposomes composed of a cationic lipid (DOTAP or DOGS), a neutral lipid (DOPE), and PEG–PE, the surface modification using a relatively large amount of PEG (5.7 mol%) has been shown to improve the delivery of an oligodeoxyribonucleotide (ODN) without losing structural activity or stability of the resulting complexes. The PEGylated formulation was found to be MPS-avoiding and retain a high level of the originally loaded ODN in the complex after plasma incubation.

PEGylated cationic liposomes, however, have low tranfection efficiency due to the absence of net positive charge on the vesicle surface. This has led to the development of cationic PEG–lipid (CPL) conjugates with one or more positively charged moieties for postinsertion into premade stabilized plasmid–lipid vesicles. An interesting study involves the insertion of a CPL known as CPL_4 (a dansylated lipid–PEG conjugate with cationic groups linked to the PEG terminal group) into liposomes containing the surface PEG–CerC20 (ceramide) moieties.[130] When PEG 3400 was used, the inserted cationic groups extended beyond the PEG–CerC20 "cloud," which resulted in both improved cell uptake and dramatically enhanced transfection potency, but was rapidly cleared from circulation. The use of a shorter PEG linker (PEG 1000), on the other hand, resulted in a shielding of the positive charges by the PEG–CerC20 cloud, and the liposomes regained their stealth property. It is suggested that the PEG–CerC20 moieties, which facilitate long circulation, can be designed slowly to dissociate at the targeted site, thus exposing the cationic CPL with a shorter PEG chain for enhanced transfection of the targeted cells.[131]

Other Applications

Liposomes have been used for diagnostic imaging to aid in the determination of targeting specificity and the treatment of diseases. As a carrier for contrast agents, liposomes can increase the signal difference between areas of interest and background and can localize the contrast moieties in the target tissues or organs. Diagnostic agents, such as ^{111}In, ^{99}Tc, Mn, and Gd, can be complexed with a soluble chelator for encapsulation into the aqueous core, or with chelating agents containing hydrophobic groups for incorporation into the lipid bilayer. Liposomes are suitable for most contrast procedures, including gamma-scintigraphy, magnetic resonance imaging (MRI), and computed tomography imaging (CTI). Long-circulating Gd liposomes have been used in blood pool imaging to prolong the presence of the contrast agent in the body, and liposomes containing unsaturated phospholipids have shown high accessibility of water and increased relaxivity, making them highly suitable for MRI. A review of nanocarrier-assisted imaging methods can be found in the studies of Bae et al.[132]

Polymeric Micelles in Anticancer Chemotherapy

Micelles are formed by amphiphiles that exhibit a hydrophilic head group and a hydrophobic tail moiety. At low concentrations in an aqueous medium, an amphiphile exists as monomers in solution. As the concentration increases, these molecules aggregate via self-assembly to form micelles. The concentration at which micelles begin to form is known as the critical micelle concentration (CMC). The formation of micelles is driven by dehydration of the hydrophobic tails, leading to a favorable state of entropy and allowing the hydrophobic moieties to associate via van der Waals forces, while the resulting hydrophilic shell is stabilized by hydrogen bonds with the surrounding water.

Polymeric Micelles

Block copolymers with hydrophilic and hydrophobic units can undergo self-assembly in aqueous solution in a manner similar to that of low-molecular-weight surfactants to form micelles known as *polymeric micelles*. Block copolymers are polymers composed of two or more homopolymer units linked by covalent bond. The union of the homopolymers may require an intermediate nonrepeating unit, known as a junction block. Copolymers with two or three distinct blocks are

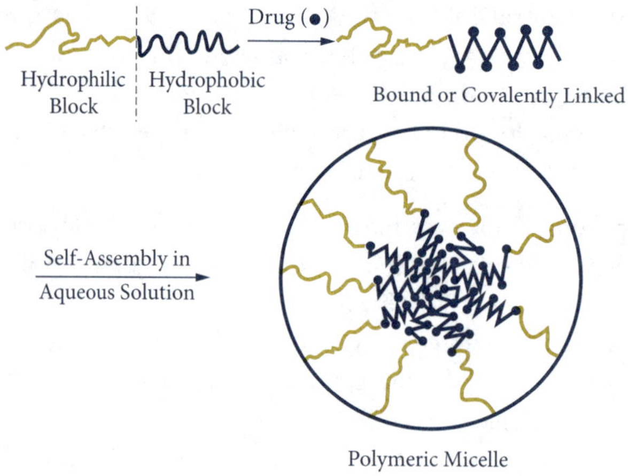

Figure 15-9 Formation of polymeric micelles by block copolymer.

called diblock and triblock copolymers, respectively. These blocks can be arranged in A-B diblock or A-B-A triblock types, or as grafted copolymers, in which the block A backbone is grafted with one or more block B side chains, or vice versa. A schematic illustration of the formation of polymeric micelles via self-assembly of block copolymers is shown in **Figure 15-9**. Because of the stability rendered by the hydrophobic core assembly and hydrophilic interaction with the surrounding, polymeric micelles have a much lower CMC (10^{-7} to 10^{-6} *M*) than the low-molecular-weight surfactants (10^{-4} to 10^{-3} *M*).[133] As a result, these micelles are stable at very low concentrations, making them relatively insensitive to dilution compared to surfactant micelles, as in circulation if they were to be injected into the bloodstream. The size of the polymeric micelles is 5–100 nm, which is well suited for percutaneous lymphatic delivery and easy extravasation from blood vessels to the tumor tissue.

Selection of Block Copolymers

Both the hydrophilic and the hydrophobic units are important in achieving a viable micelle targeting system. The hydrophilic shell should provide a steric effect to avoid MPS detection, so that the micelles can remain in circulation for a prolonged time. PEG, for reasons given previously, is the usual choice. The hydrophobic block should exhibit a high loading capacity and compatibility with the incorporated drug. Drug molecules may be incorporated physically through hydrophobic interactions or chemically through covalent linkage. Polymers that have been used as the hydrophobic block include polyesters such as poly(DL-lactic acid) (PDLLA) and poly(ε-caprolactone) (PCL); polyethers such as poly(propylene oxide) (PPO); polyamino acids such as poly(L-aspartate) (PAsp) and poly(glutamate) (PGlu); and poloxamers (triblock copolymers of PEG–PPO–PEG). The CMC of polymeric micelles depends on the type and molecular weight of the hydrophobic block; the more hydrophobic and the higher the molecular weight, the lower is the CMC.[134]

The polyamino acids are very versatile systems when used to form the hydrophobic core. In NK012, a formulation using PEG–PGlu, the drug 7-ethyl-10-hydroxy-campothecin (SN-38)—a campotothecin analog that acts as a DNA topoisomerase I inhibitor but cannot be administered IV due to its low water solubility and high toxicity—is covalently linked to PGlu by the condensation reaction between the carboxylic acid of polyglutamate and the phenol of SN-38. This condensation renders the PGlu block hydrophobic, resulting in micelle formation.[135] Polyaspartate (PAsp) and polyglutamate can also be modified to exhibit increased hydrophobicity for physical incorporation of hydrophobic drugs. Examples are the PEG–PAsp–paclitaxel (PTX) micelle system, in which one-half of the carboxylic groups of the polyaspartate block were esterified with 4-phenyl-1-butanol using 1,3-diisopropylcarbodiimide to increase its hydrophobicity, and Nanoplatin (NC-6004), which is a micellar system of PEG and poly(γ-benzyl L-glutamate)/cisplatin complex.[136]

Passive Targeting

The ability of polymeric micelles to deliver anticancer agents through the EPR effect has been well studied, and a number of these formulations are in various stages of clinical trials. Preclinical results have shown a general ability of the polymeric micelle systems to increase plasma AUC and C_{max} and drug distribution in tumor tissue, while reducing systemic drug toxicity, when compared to free drug at equal or higher doses in different animal models. It should be mentioned that the increased AUC and C_{max} reflect the stability of micelles in circulation, where the measured drug concentrations were usually not differentiated between free and encapsulated forms. Clinical trials in various stages have shown encouraging results for their antitumor activity, as summarized in **Table 15-11** for various micelle formulations. Among these, Genexol PM (paclitaxel) has been approved for use in the treatment of breast cancer.

Triggered Drug Release

Drug release from micelles is governed by the rate of drug diffusion, partition coefficient, micelle stability, and biodegradation of the copolymers.[151] In addition, many block copolymers exhibit unique properties, including pH, temperature, ultrasound, and light sensitivities, that can be utilized to achieve a *triggered drug release* if the property is properly matched with physiological conditions. The most commonly studied phenomena are the pH- and temperature-triggered release mechanisms, which are described below.

pH-Sensitive Polymeric Micelles

Differences in pH between healthy and tumor tissue, as well as the acidic environment in endosomal and lysosomal compartments, can be exploited as an internal stimulus for triggered drug release. The normal extracellular and intracellular pH values are 7.4 and 7.2, respectively, In tumor tissue, however, lactate, carbon dioxide, and other metabolic acids produced by cancer cells via a high rate of aerobic and anaerobic glycolysis are released into the interstitial fluid but are not well excreted due to the impaired vasculature and lymphatic drainages. This results in an interstitial pH of 6.8.[152] In the endosomal and lysosomal compartments, the pH is even lower, around 5–6.

A pH-triggered release of drug can occur if the hydrophobic polymer of the micelles becomes protonated (positively charged) under the pH conditions of the tumor area. This occurs if the pH is below the pK_a of a base group, which would lead to destabilization of the micelle through charge repulsion and micelle dissociation. Polymers such as poly(L-histidine), polypyridines, and polysulfonamides have been shown to exhibit this property. Poly(L-histidine), by virtue of its imidazole rings, is endowed with a pH-dependent amphoteric property, with a pK_a around 6.5.[153] This polymer is largely neutral at normal physiological pH, but is positively charged at pH 6.5 and below. An example of a polyhistidine-containing micelle preparation is given by Lee et al.[154] They reported that the release of doxorubicin from micelles prepared using a triblock copolymer PLA–PEG–polyHis occurs at pH 6.8 and lower. The amount of drug released increases as the pH is lowered (to pH 6.0) over a 24-h period, and the drug release is correlated to the drug's cytotoxicity. In comparison, only minimal release and cytotoxicity was observed at pH 7.4. The pH-sensitive micelles were described to be "flowerlike," as they open when the pH drops. Another mechanism of pH-triggered release is based on the use of acid-labile bonds (pH-sensitive polymer–drug conjugates), such as a hydrazone linkage, positioned in the main chain, at the side chain, or at the

Table 15-11 Polymeric Micelles for the Delivery of Chemotherapeutic Agents†

Drug	Micelle	Treatment	In Vivo Results Compared to Free Drug	Clinical Studies
7-Ethyl-8-hydoxy-campothecin (SN-38, NK012)	Polymer: PEG–PGlu Drug loading: by conjugation Size: 20 nm	Breast cancer	(1) 200-fold increase in plasma AUC (IV, 30 mg/kg) over CPT-11(66.7 mg/kg, which hydrolyzes to SN-38 in circulation). (2) Lower clearance and higher tumor-plasma ratio over free SN-38 in HT-29 tumor-bearing mice.[135, 137, 138]	Phase I study: Maximum tolerated dose (MTD): 37 mg/m^2 equivalent dose to SN-38, every 3 weeks; Dose-limiting toxicity (DLT): neutropenia.[139]
Paclitaxel (NK105)	PEG–PAsp esterified with 4-phenyl-1-butanol Drug loading: by hydrophobic incorporation Size: 85 nm	Advanced stomach cancer	(1) Showed 50-fold increase in AUC, 3-fold higher in C_{max} in tumor of CDF1 mice. (2) Antitumor activity of NK105 (equivalent dose, 25 mg/kg) in HT-29 tumor-bearing mice was comparable to that of 100 mg/kg of PTX in solution. (3) Showed significant reduction of side effects caused by PTX solution.[139]	Phase I study: Caused less hypersensitivity reactions than PTX solution in patients suffering from pancreatic, bile duct, gastric, and colonic cancers; MTD: 150 mg/m^2, for 1 h every 3 weeks.[139, 140]
Doxorubicin (SP1049C)	Pluronic L61 & F127 (1:8 w/w ratio) Size: (22–27 nm)	Adenocarcinoma of esophagus, gastroesophageal junction, and stomach	(1) Showed greater efficacy than free drug against tumor cell lines.[141] (2) Showed superior antitumor activity and efficacy and increased AUC in tumor tissue in multiple animal models and in doxorubicin-resistant tumors.[142]	Phase I study: MTD (70 mg/m^2) is the same as free drug, but showed significantly higher antitumor activity and better safety profile; DLT: neutropenia.[143] Phase II study: SP1049C was effective as monotherapy in patients suffering from adenocarcinoma of the esophagus.[144]
Cisplatin (CDDP) (Nanoplatin) (NC-6004)	PEG–poly(γ-benzyl-L-glutamate/CDDP complex Size: 30 nm	Solid tumor; breast cancer; pancreatic cancer	(1) Showed no difference in antitumor activity compared to CDDP at equivalent dose in BALB/c mice bearing human MKN-4 cells. (2) Showed 65-fold increase in AUC and 8-fold increase in C_{max} in plasma and 2.5-fold increase of C_{max} in tumor, as compared to systemic CDDP in rats. (3) Showed significant reduction of nephrotoxicity and neurotoxicity and dose-limiting factors of CDDP.[145]	Phase I study: NC-6004 was well tolerated by patients suffering from colorectal carcinoma, upper gastrointestinal cancers, non-small-cell lung carcinoma, melanoma, and other tumor types.[146]

Paclitaxel (Genexol-PM)[‡] In combination with carboplatin	PEG–PDLLA Size: 20–50 nm	Non-small-cell lung cancer; ovarian cancer	(1) Showed 3-fold increase in the MTD and significantly increased antitumor efficacy compared to free PTX. (2) AUC of Genexol-PM was similar to PTX, but the concentration was 2–3 times higher in tissues, including liver, spleen, kidneys, lungs, heart, and tumor.[147]	Phase I studies: MTD: 390 mg/m^2 every 3 weeks or 120 mg/m^2 every week.[148] Phase II studies: Genexol-PM was effective and safe in patients suffering from metastatic breast cancer and advanced pancreatic cancer; hypersensitivity occurred in 19.5% of breast cancer patients.[149] Genexol-PM in combination with cisplatin showed increased antitumor activity compared to PTX in solution in patients with advanced non-small-cell lung carcinoma.[150]

[†]Extracted from the study of Oerlemans C, Bult W, Bos M, Storm G, Nijsen JFW, and Hennick WE. *Pharm Res.*, 27:2569–2589, 2010.

[‡]Approved for use in the treatment of breast cancer.

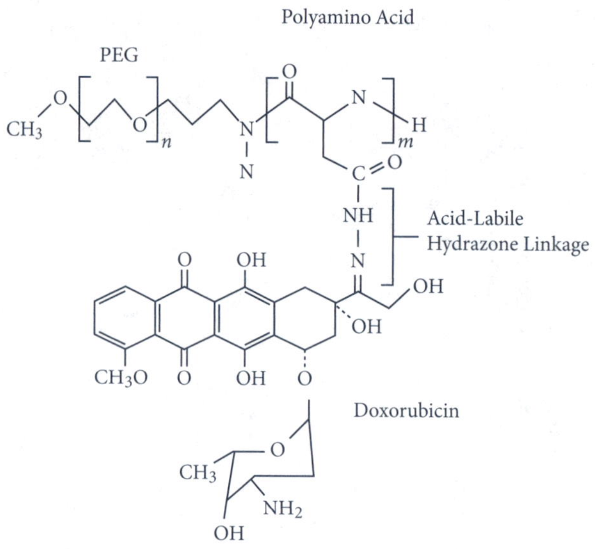

Figure 15-10 The amino acid–hydrazone–doxorubicin linkage for pH-triggered drug release.

terminal of the core-forming block.[155, 156] For example, Bae et al.[155] have prepared micelles based on PEG–poly(aspartate hydrazone doxorubicin), where the drug molecules were conjugated to the hydrophobic segments through acid-sensitive hydrazone linkers (see **Figure 15-10**). This preparation allows for a selective release of the drug at endosomal pH, which has been shown to suppress tumor growth in mice with enhanced therapeutic efficacy and decreased systemic toxicity compared to free doxorubicin.[157]

Thermosensitive Micelles

A thermosensitive polymer is one that exhibits a lower critical solution temperature (LCST) in solution, below which the polymer is soluble; but at temperatures above its LCST, the polymer is phase-separated due to loss of hydration and aggregation of polymer chains. In a block copolymer, either the hydrophilic or the hydrophobic unit can be a thermally sensitive segment; hence there are two types of thermal sensitive micelles: one with a thermosensitive outer shell and one with a thermosensitive inner core. For the former, when the external temperature is above LCST, the hydrophilic shell shrinks and results in a weakened micelle structure that triggers the release of drug and aggregation of dehydrated micelles.[158] In the latter, where the core block is thermosensitive, micelles are subjected to instability due to hydration at temperature below the LCST. Above the LCST, the micelles are gradually destabilized due to hydration of the hydrophobic block. The use of micelles with a thermosensitive shell for triggered drug release is quite clear. Micelles are passively targeted to the tumor tissue via the EPR effect; once in tumor tissue with elevated temperature, micelles having an LCST above 37°C will become dehydrated and aggregated to aid in their detainment and drug release at the targeted sites. Studies have also shown that cell uptake of dehydrated micelles occurs more readily than that of normal micelles.[159] Together, these phenomena trigger targeted drug release to the tumor tissue. For micelles with a thermosensitive core, controlled degradation of the hydrophobic block via a slow hydration process may be used to achieve controlled drug release of the tumor site (see section below).

A frequently studied polymer for the preparation of thermosensitive micelles is poly(*N*-isopropylacrylamide) (PNIPAAm), which shows a reversible and sharp phase transition at 32°C,[160] and it can be used as a hydrophilic or hydrophobic block in polymeric micelle formation. The LCST of a polymer can be increased or decreased by introducing a hydrophilic or hydrophobic comonomer through copolymerization. For the preparation of micelles with a thermosensitive shell, hydrophilic compounds such as acrylamide (AAm) and hydroxymethylacrylamide (HMAAm) have been used to produce an LCST above 37°C when copolymerized with PNIPAAm.[161] When a micelle preparation for docetaxel using (PNIPAAm-*co*-AAm)-*b*-poly(D,L-lactic acid)[†] was tested in vivo,[162] the results showed that the micelles indeed enhanced significantly the drug's antitumor efficacy in mice when the treatment was aided by hyperthermia compared to conventional docetaxel formulation.

Micelles with a thermosensitive core have been made using poly(*N*-(2-hydroxypropyl)-methacrylamide) (PHPMAm) and *N*-(2-hydroxyethyl)methacrylamide (HEMAm). These hydrophilic polymers can be rendered hydrophobic by esterification with oligolactates to yield copolymers with desired LCST between 10 and 65°C depending on the length of the lactate side group.[163] As lactate is biodegraded via hydrolysis, polymeric micelles containing lactate chains can dissolve gradually as a consequence. The lactate degradation can be utilized to control drug release, but fast degradation can also result in instability of the micelles and shorter circulation time. This has led to the development of micelles in which the core polymers are cross-linked to slow down the biodegradation, thus enhancing their stability in circulation. Indeed, Rijcken et al.[164] have developed a cross-linked thermosensitive micelle system based on the HEMAm block copolymer linked with various monodisperse oligolactates (HEMAm–Lac_n), where part of the hydroxyl end groups of the lactates was derivatized with methacrylic acid to allow cross-linking of the micellar core. These cross-linked micelles showed excellent physical stability, a superior circulation profile, and increased accumulation at tumor site, compared to non-cross-linked micelles. The hydrolyzable cross-linked micelles are considered to be attractive for controlled drug delivery. After in vivo injection, the micelles are expected to be stable during blood circulation; in tumor tissue, as the lactate side chains degrade by hydrolysis, encapsulated drug will be released from the swelling micelles.

Active Targeting

Polymer micelles with PEG shell have been modified with chemically linked folate for active targeting. In an in vitro study with human pharyngeal cancer cells, the cytotoxicity of folate-bound micelles loaded with doxorubicin was 8-fold higher than nontargeted micelles.[165] In mice after IV administration, the folate-derived micelles resulted in a therapy that was substantially better than that of free doxorubicin or micelles without folate conjugation.[166] Active targeting using folate can also be coupled with the pH-sensitive mechanism for triggered drug release. Micelles consisting of poly(L-histidine)-*b*-PEG-*b*-PLLA and doxorubicin were conjugated with folic acid for active targeting to overcome multidrug resistance.[167] It was shown that when the micelles were internalized by folate receptor–mediated endocytosis, the poly(L-histidine) block became protonated at endosomal pH, resulting in micelle destabilization, disruption of endosomal membrane, and release of the drug into the cytosol. By this targeting mechanism, drug interaction with the *P-glycoprotein* in cellular membrane, which is the transporter responsible for multidrug resistance, is minimized. Combination of folate with doxorubicin micelles where the drug was conjugated to the hydrophobic block through acid-sensitive hydrazone linkers has also been used for endosomal drug release via the pH-triggered mechanism.[168] A more elaborate system was developed by Sethuraman and Bae,[169] in which the transacting activator of transcription (TAT) peptide was conjugated to PLLA-*b*-PEG-*b*-PSD micelles. TAT is cationic and forms stable complex with the anionic PSD (poly(methacryloyl sulfadimethoxine)) at pH 7.4. At the tumor tissue pH (6.8), the sulfonamide groups are protonated and detached, thus exposing the TAT on the micelle surface to mediate the cellular uptake of the micelles.

[†] *b* is sometimes used to indicate the linkage of two homopolymers in the formation of a *block* copolymer.

Polymeric micelles that exhibit combined targeting and triggered-release functions are referred to as *multifunction micelles*. As shown by the examples given above, they exhibit greater antitumor effects than single-function micelles. Multifunction micelles also include those that combine targeting with imaging for the assessment of the targeting specificity and biodistribution of the micellar systems.[132] The targeting and multifunction micelles are very attractive drug delivery systems based on preclinical studies. The preparation of these systems, however, involves multiple-step procedures in which each single modification of the dosage form must be optimized, making it difficult to prepare as a parenteral product. To date, only passively targeted polymeric micelles have been investigated in clinical studies.

VI. Chapter Summary

As set forth by the chapter objectives, this chapter provides a discussion of drug delivery based on the major routes by which drugs can be delivered and the dosage forms that can be designed for such deliveries. It should be emphasized that not all drugs can be delivered by a single route, and all routes may offer certain benefits in terms of improved therapeutic efficacy, reduced toxicity, and patient acceptance. In general, drug delivery is carried out to achieve a local, systemic, or targeted drug effect. It is often advantageous and necessary to (1) use site-directed routes to deliver drugs for local effects (as in ocular drug delivery) and (2) explore noninvasive alternative routes (to oral and parenteral administration) for systemic drug delivery, to achieve quicker onset of action and reduced side effects. For the latter, the usefulness of the nasal and inhalation routes for systemic drug delivery is described. Drug development is driven by cost-benefit considerations, patient acceptance, and clinical necessities. For most drugs, conventional oral drug delivery is quite sufficient; innovations on sustained drug release have resulted in dosage forms that enhance patient acceptance and compliance. Pharmaceutical companies have well-established facilities and protocols for the development of these cost-effective dosage forms. For diseases such as cancer in which inherently cytotoxic agents are used, conventional dosage forms are problematic and their therapeutic effects depend largely on treatment schedules designed based on a patient's toxic tolerance. Hence, targeted drug delivery is a clinical necessity, and the science through which drug targeting can be achieved dominates the current research field. In some of the targeting approaches, as partially shown in this chapter, multiple chemical and physical steps are employed in achieving a desired molecular architecture of the drug or dosage form, which could present significant difficulties in terms of drug product development. Many of the targeting preparations that are in clinical trials or are approved drug products are simplified dosage forms. It is perhaps necessary that the targeting approach be simplified for easier product development, which remains a scientific challenge. One thing is certain: There will be no clinical benefit unless there is a product, and this calls for a cooperative effort in research and development by biomedical and pharmaceutical scientists.

VII. References

1. Rojanasakul Y, Wang LY, Bhat M, Glover DD, Malanga CJ, and Ma JKH. *Pharm Res.* 9:1029–1034, 1992.
2. Dijkman GA, Debruyne FM, Fernandez del Moral P, et al. *Eur Urol.* 27:43–46, 1995.
3. Chien WY, Su KSE, and Chang SF. *Nasal Systemic Drug Delivery.* New York, Marcel Dekker, Inc., 1989.
4. Illum L. *Eur J Pharm Sci.* 11:1–18, 2000.
5. Schipper NG, Verhoef JC, and Merkus FW. *Pharm Res.* 8:807–814, 1991.
6. Hehar SS, Mason JD, Stephen AB, et al. *Clin Otolaryngol.* 24:24–25, 1999.
7. Mathison S, Nagilla R, and Kompella UB. *J Drug Target.* 5:415–441, 1998.

8. Westin UE, Bostrom E, Grasjo J, Hammarlund-Udenaes M, and Bjork E. *Pharm Res.* 23:565–572, 2006.
9. Lee VHL. Enzymatic barriers to peptide and protein nose-brain pathway for psychotropic peptides: evidence absorption. *CRC Crit Rev Ther Drug Carrier Syst.* 5:69–97, 1988.
10. Illum L. In: Mathiowitz E, Chickering DE, and Lehr CM (eds). *Bioadhesive Formulations for Nasal Peptide Delivery: Fundamentals, Novel Approaches and Development.* New York, Marcel Dekker, 1999, pp 507–539.
11. Kublik H and Vidgren MT. *Adv Drug Deliv Rev.* 29:157–177, 1998.
12. Aurora J. Development of nasal delivery systems: A review. *Drug Deliv Technol.* 2(7):1–8, 2002.
13. McMartin C, Hutchinson LE, Hyde R, and Peters GE. *J Pharm Sci.* 76:535–540, 1987.
14. Inagaki M, Sakakura Y, Itoh H, Ukai K, and Miyoshi Y. *Rhinology.* 23:213–221, 1985.
15. Hussain A, Kimura R, Huang CH, and Kashihara T. *Int J Pharm.* 21:233–237, 1984; Hussain AA, Foster T, Hirai S, Kashihara T, Batenhorst R, and Jone M. *J Pharm Sci.* 69:1240–1243, 1980.
16. Jiang XG, Lu X, Cui JB, Qiu L, and Xi NZ. *Yao Xue Xue Bao.* 32:458–460, 1997.
17. Hirai S, Yashika T, Matsuzawa T, and Mima H. *Int J Pharm.* 7:317–325, 1981.
18. Huang CH, Kimura R, Nassar R, and Hussain A. *J Pharm Sci.* 74:608–611, 1985.
19. Yamamoto A, Morita T, Hashida M, and Sezaki H. *Int J Pharm.* 93:91–99, 1993.
20. Ohwaki T, Ishii M, Aoki S, Tatsuishi K, and Kaman M. *Chem Pharm Bull. (Tokyo)* 37:3359–3362, 1989.
21. Illum L, Fisher AN, Jabbal-Gill I, and Davis SS. *Int J Pharm.* 222:109–119, 2001.
22. Davis SS and Illum L. *Clin Pharmacokinet.* 42(13):1107–1128, 2003.
23. O'Hagan DT and Illum L. *Crit Rev Ther Drug Carrier Syst.* 7(1):35–97, 1990.
24. Schipper NG, Verhoef JC, Romeijn SG, and Merkus FW. *Calcif Tissue Int.* 56:280–282, 1995.
25. Merkus FW, Verhoef JC, Romeijn SG, and Schipper NG. *Pharm Res.* 8:588–592, 1991.
26. Farraj NF, Illum L, Davis SS, and Johansen BR. *J Control Release.* 13:253–261, 1990.
27. Gavini E, Rassu G, Sanna V, Cossu M, and Giunchedi P. *J Pharm Pharmacol.* 57:287–294, 2005.
28. Lopes T, Dias JS, Marcelino J, Varela J, Ribeiro S, and Dias J. *BJU Int.* 87:322–325, 2001.
29. Costantino HR, Illum L, Brandt G, Johnson PH, and Quay SC. *Int J Pharm.* 337:1–24, 2007.
30. Schoenwald RD. *Clin Pharmacokinet.* 18(4):255–269, 1990.
31. Allen LV Jr. *Int J Pharm Compd.* 2(3):184–188, 1998.
32. Thompson JE. Ophthalmic solutions. In: *A Practical Guide to Contemporary Pharmacy Practice.* Baltimore, MD, Williams & Wilkins, 1998, pp 27.1–27.16.
33. Allen LV Jr. Buffer solutions for ophthalmic preparations. *Int J Pharm Compd.* 2(3):190–191, 1998.
34. Ma WD, Xu H, Wang C, Nie SF, and Pan WS. *Int J Pharm.* 350:247–256, 2008.
35. Sruvudya B, Candoza RM, and Amin PD. *J Control Release.* 73:205–211, 2001.
36. Cohen S, Lobel J, Trevgoda A, and Peled Y. *J Control Release.* 44:201–208, 1997.
37. Lee SY, Chee SP, Balakrishnan V, Farzavandi S, and Tan DTH. *Br J Ophthalmol.* 87:1424–1426, 2003.
38. Tan DTH, Chee SP, Lim L, et al. *Ophthalmology.* 106:223–231, 1999.
39. Tan DTH, Chee SP, Lim L, et al. *Ophthalmology.* 108:2172–2181, 2001.
40. Weibel, ER. *Physiol Rev.* 53:419–495, 1973.
41. Enna SJ and Schanker LS. *Am J Physiol.* 223:1227–1231, 1972.
42. Baron J, Voigt JM, Whitter TB, et al. Identification of intratissue sites for xenobiotic activation. In Snyder R (ed): *Biological Reaction Intermediate III. Molecular and Cellular Mechanism of Action in Animal Models and Human Disease.* New York, Plenum Press, 1988; pp 119–144.
43. Sanderson MJ and Dirksen ER. *Am Rev Respir Dis.* 139:432–440, 1989.
44. Brain JD and Valberg PA. *Am Rev Respir Dis.* 120:1325–1373, 1979.
45. Kliment V. *Folia Morphol Praha.* 21:59–64, 1973.
46. Colthrope P, Farr SJ, Taylor G, Smith IJ, and Wyatt D. *Pharm Res.* 9:764–768, 1992.

47. Verdugo P, Johnson NT, and Tam PY. *J Appl Physiol.* 48:868–871, 1980.
48. Nadel JA. *Chest.* 80(suppl):849–851, 1981.
49. Duchateau GSMJE, Zuidema J, Hermens WAJJ, and Merkes FWHM. *Int J Pharm.* 31:275–276, 1986.
50. Van de Donk HJM, Muller-Phantema IP, Zuidema J, and Merkus FWHM. *Rhinology.* 18:119–133, 1980.
51. Byron PR. *Dv Drug Deliv Rev.* 5:107–132, 1990.
52. Schanker LS and Hemberger JA. *Biochem Pharmacol.* 32:2599–2601, 1983.
53. Wang LY, Ma JKH, Pan WF, et al. *Pharm Res.* 11:513–517, 1994.
54. Wang LY, Toledo-Velasques D, Schwegler-Berry D, Ma JKH, and Rojanasakul Y. *Pharm Res.* 10:1662–1667, 1993.
55. Morita T, Yamamoto A, Takakura Y, Hashida M, and Sezaki H. *Pharm Res.* 11:909–913, 1994.
56. Ma JKH, Bhat M, and Rojanasakul Y. Drug metabolism and enzyme kinetics in the lung, In: Hickey AJ (ed). *Inhalation Aerosols, Lung Biology in Health and Disease.* New York, Marcel Dekker, 1996, Vol 94, pp 155–195.
57. Clark JG, Wicks SR, and Farr SJ. *Int J Pharm.* 93:221–231, 1993.
58. Adjei AL, Qiu Y, and Gupta PK. Bioavailability and pharmacokinetics of inhaled drugs. In: Hickey AJ (ed). *Inhalation Aerosols, Lung Biology in Health and Disease.* New York, Marcel Dekker, 1996, Vol 94, pp 197–231.
59. Byron PR, Miller NC, Blondino FE, Visich JE, and Ward GH. Some aspects of alternative propellant solvency, in: Byron PR, Dalby RN, and Farr SJ (eds). *Proceedings of Respiratory Drug Delivery IV*, 1994, pp 231–241.
60. Short R. *InPharma.* 943:3, 1994.
61. Dalby RN, Tiano SL, and Hickey AJ. Medical devices for the delivery of therapeutic aerosols to the lungs. In: Hickey AJ, (ed). *Inhalation Aerosols, Lung Biology in Health and Disease,* New York, Marcel Dekker, 1996, vol. 94, pp 441–473.
62. Taburet AM and Schmit B. *Clin Pharmacokinet.* 92:95–106, 1994.
63. Okumura K, Twajkawa S, Yoshida T, Seki T, and Komada F. *Int J Pharm.* 88:63–73, 1992.
64. Zainudin BMZ, Biddiscombe M, Tolfree SEJ, Short M, and Spiro SG. *Thorax.* 45:469–473, 1990.
65. Pascal S, Diot P, and Lemarie E. *Rev Mal Respir.* 9:145–153, 1992.
66. Stoutenbeek CP, Van-Saene HK, Miranda DR, Zandstra DF, and Langrehr D. *Intensive Care Med.* 12:419–423, 1986.
67. Fei YJ, Kanai Y, Nussberger S, et al. *Nature.* 368:563–566, 1994.
68. Viahov IR, Santhapuram HK, Kleindl PJ, Howard SJ, Stanford KM, and Leamon CP. *Bioorg Med Chem Lett.* 16:5093–5096, 2006.
69. Reddy JA, Dorton R, Westrick E, et al. *Cancer Res.* 67:4434–4442, 2007.
70. Dosio F, Milla P, and Cattel L. *Curr Opin Investig Drugs.* 11:1424–1433, 2010.
71. Francis RJ, Sharma SK, Springer C, et al. *Br J Cancer.* 87:600–607, 2002.
72. Kan O, Kingsman S, and Naylor S. *Expert Opin Biol Ther.* 2:857–868, 2002.
73. Roy P and Waxman DJ. *Toxicol in Vitro.* 20:176–186, 2006.
74. Boekhout AH, Bijnen JH, and Shellens JH. *Oncologist.* 16:800–810, 2011.
75. Yang T, Choi MK, Cui FD, et al. *J Control Release.* 120:169–177, 2007.
76. Parveen S and Sahoo S. *J Drug Target.* 17:533, 542, 2008.
77. Dhar S, Gu FX, Langer R, Farokhzad OC, and Lippard SJ. *Proc Natl Acad Sci USA.* 105:17356–17361, 2008.
78. Farokhzad OC, Heng J, Teply BA, et al. *Proc Natl Acad Sci USA.* 103:6315–6320, 2006.
79. Yang W, Cheng Y, Xu T, Wang X, and Wen L. *Eur J Med Chem.* 44:862–868, 2009.
80. Patel Y, Sadhukha T, Ma L, and Panyam J. *J Control Release.* 136:21–29, 2009.
81. Yoo H and Park T. *J Control Release.* 96:273–283, 2004.

82. Liu Y, Li K, Pan J, Liu B, and Feng SS. *Biomaterials*. 31:330–338, 2010.
83. Danhier F, Vroman B, Lecouturier N, et al. *J Control Release*. 140:166–173, 2009.
84. Luzzi LA and Gerraughty RJ. *J Pharm Sci*. 56:634–638, 1967a; Luzzi LA and Gerraughty RJ. *J Pharm Sci*. 56:1174–1177, 1967b.
85. Luzzi LA, Zoglio MA, and Maulding HV. *J Pharm Sci*. 59:338–341, 1970; Madan PL, Luzzi LA, and Price JC. *J Pharm Sci*. 63:280–284, 1974.
86. Luzzi LA. Microencapsulation (review), *J Pharm Sci*. 61:1588–1593, 1972.
87. Leelarasamee N, Howard SA, Malanga CJ, et al. *J Microencapsulation*. 3:171–179, 1986.
88. Buhleier E, Wehner W, and Vogtle F. *Synthesis*. 2:155–158, 1978.
89. Mohammad N and Antony D. *Curr Opin Pharmacol*. 6:522–527, 2006.
90. Gillies ER and Fréchet JMJ. *Drug Discovery Today*. 10:35–43, 2005.
91. Basu MK and Lala S. *Curr Mol Med*. 4:681–689, 2004.
92. Patel HM. *Crit Rev Ther Drug Carrier Syst*. 9:39–90, 1992.
93. Chonn A, Semple SC, and Cullis PR. *J Biol Chem*. 270:25845–25849, 1995.
94. Devine DV, Wong K, Serrano K, et al. *Biochim Biophys Acta*. 1191:43–51, 1994.
95. Oja CDM, Semple SC, Chonn A, et al. *Biochim Biophys Acta*. 1281:31–37, 1996.
96. Harashima H, Sakata K, Funato K, et al. *Pharm Res*. 11:402–406, 1994.
97. Marjan J, Xie Z, and Devine D. *Biochim Biophys Acta*. 1192:35–44, 1994.
98. Bradley AJ, Devine DV, Ansell SM, et al. *Arch Biochem Biophys*. 357:185–194, 1998.
99. Damen J. *Biochim Biophys Acta*. 665:538–545, 2005.
100. Senior J. *FEBS Lett*. 145:109–114, 1982.
101. Veerareddy PR and Vobalaboina V. *Drugs Today*. 40:133–145, 2004.
102. Allen TM and Martin FJ. *Semin Oncol*. 31(suppl 13):5–15, 2004.
103. Jaeckle KA, Phuphanich S, Bent MJ, et al. *Br J Cancer*. 84:157–163, 2001.
104. Verschraegen CF, Kumagai S, Davidson R, et al. *J Cancer Res Clin Oncol*. 129:549–555, 2003.
105. Zhang JA, Anyarambhatla G, Ma L, et al. *Eur J Pharm Biopharm*. 59:177–187, 2005.
106. Liu D, Mori A, and Huang L. *Biochim Biophys Acta*. 1104:95–101, 1992.
107. Oku N and Namba Y. *Methods Enzymol*. 391:145–162, 2005.
108. Caliceti P and Veronese FM. *Adv Drug Del Rev*. 55:1261–1277, 2003.
109. Mahmood I and Green MD. *Clin Pharmacokinet*. 44:331–347, 2005.
110. Allen C, Dos SN, Gallagher R, et al. *Biosc Rep*. 22:225–250, 2002.
111. Needham D, McIntosh TJ, and Lasic DD. *Biochim Biophys Acta*. 1108:40–48, 1992.
112. Blume G. *Biochim Biophys Acta*. 1146:157–168, 1993.
113. Torchilin VP, Omelyanenko VG, Papisov MI, et al. *Biochim Biophys Acta*. 1195:11–20, 1994.
114. Allen TM, Hansen CB, and Guo LSS. *Biochim Biophys Acta*. 1150:9–16, 1993.
115. Krown SE, Northfelt DW, Osoba D, et al. *Semin Oncol*. 31(suppl 13):36–52, 2004.
116. Rose PG. *Oncologist*. 10:205–214, 2005.
117. Vorobiof DA and Rapoport BL. *Breast*. 13:219–226, 2004.
118. Katsaros D, Oletti MV, Rigault de la Longrais A, et al. *Ann Oncol*. 16:300–306, 2005.
119. Kim ES, Lu C, Khuri FR, et al. *Lung Cancer*. 34:427–432, 2001.
120. Harrington KJ, Lewanski CR, Northcote AD, et al. *Ann Oncol*. 12:493–496, 2001.
121. Zamboni WC, Gervais AC, Egorin MJ, et al. *Cancer Chemother Pharmacol*. 53:329–336, 2004.
122. Harrington KJ, Rowlinson-Busza G, Syrigos KN, et al. *Br J Cancer*. 83:684–688, 2000.
123. Zalipsky S, Qazen M, Walker JA, et al. *Bioconjug Chem*. 10:703–707, 1999.
124. Metselaar JM, Bruin P, de Boer LW, et al. *Bioconjug Chem*. 14:1156–1164, 2003.
125. Lukyanov AN, Elbayoumi TA, Chakilam AR, et al. *J Control Release*. 100:135–144, 2004.
126. Matsumura Y, Gotoh M, Muro K, et al. *Ann Oncol*. 15:517–525, 2004.
127. Nellis DF, Ekstrom DL, Kirpotin DB, et al. *Biotechnol Prog*. 21:205–220, 2005.
128. Stephenson SM, Low PS, and Lee RJ. *Methods Enzymol*. 387:33–50, 2004.

129. Ishida O, Maruyama K, Tanahashi H, et al. *Pharm Res.* 18:1042–1048, 2001.
130. Palmer LR, Chen T, Lam AM, et al. *Biochim Biophys Acta.* 1611:204–216, 2003.
131. Chen T, Palmer LR, Fenske DB, et al. *J Liposome Res.* 14:155–173, 2004.
132. Bae KH, Chung HJ, and Park TG. *Mol Cells.* 31:295–302, 2011.
133. Torchilin VP. *Pharm Res.* 24:1–16, 2007.
134. Torchilin VP. *J Control Release.* 73:137–172, 2001.
135. Koizumi F, Kitagawa M, Negishi T, et al. *Cancer Res.* 66:10048–10056, 2006.
136. Matsumura Y. *Adv Drug Deliv Rev.* 60:899–914, 2008.
137. Saito Y, Yasunaga M, Kuroda J, Koga Y, and Matsumura Y. *Cancer Sci.* 99:1258–1264, 2008.
138. Nakajima TE, Yasunaga M, Kano Y, et al. *Int J Cancer.* 122:2148–2153, 2008.
139. Matsumura Y and Kataoka K. *Cancer Sci.* 100:572–579, 2009.
140. Hamaguchi T, Kato K, Yasui H, et al. *Br J Cancer.* 97:170–176, 2007.
141. Venne A, Li S, Mandeville R, Kabanov A, and Alakhov V. *Cancer Res.* 56:3626–3629, 1996.
142. Alakhov V, Klinski E, Li SM, et al. *Colloids Surf B—Biointerfaces.* 16:113–134, 1999.
143. Danson S, Ferry D, Alakhov V, et al. *Br J Cancer.* 90:2085–2091, 2004.
144. Armstrong A, Brewer J, Newman C, et al. *J Clin Oncol.* 24(June 20 suppl; abstr. 4080), 2006.
145. Uchino H, Matsumura Y, Negishi T, et al. *Br J Cancer.* 93:678–687, 2005.
146. Wilson RH, Plummer R, Adam J, et al. *J Clin Oncol.* 26(May 20 suppl; abstr 2573), 2008.
147. Kim SC, Kim DW, Shim YH, et al. *J Control Release.* 72:191–202, 2001.
148. Kim TY, Kim DW, Chung JY, et al. *Clin Cancer Res.* 10:3708–3716, 2004.
149. Lee KS, Chung HC, Im SA, et al. *Breast Cancer Res Treat.* 108:241–250, 2008.
150. Kim DW, Kim SY, Kim HK, et al. *Ann Oncol.* 18:2009–2014, 2007.
151. Teng Y, Morrison ME, Munk P, Webber SE, and Prochazka K. *Macromolecules.* 31:3578–3587, 1998.
152. Engin K, Leeper DB, Cater JR, Thistlethwaite AJ, Tupchong L, and McFarlane JD. *Int J Hyperthermia.* 11:211–216, 1995.
153. Lee ES, Gao Z, and Bae YH. *J Control Release.* 132:164–170, 2008.
154. Lee ES, Oh KT, Kim D, Youn YS, and Bae YH. *J Control Release.* 123:19–26, 2007.
155. Gillies ER and Frechet JMJ. *Pure Appl Chem.* 76:1295–1307, 2004.
156. Filippov S, Hruby M, Konak C, Mackova H, Spirkova M, and Stepanek P. *Langmuir.* 24:9295–9301, 2008.
157. Bae Y, Nishiyama N, Fukushima S, Koyama H, Yasuhiro M, and Kataoka K. *Bioconjug Chem.* 16:122–130, 2005.
158. Cammas S, Suzuki K, Sone C, Sakurai Y, Kataoka K, and Okano T. *J Control Release.* 48:157–164, 1997.
159. Takeda N, Nakamura E, Yokoyama M, and Okano T. *J Control Release.* 95:342–355, 2004.
160. Pelton R. *Adv Colloid Interface Sci.* 85:1–33, 2000.
161. Chung JE, Yokoyama M, Yamato M, Aoyagi T, Sakurai Y, and Okano T. *J Control Release.* 62:115–127, 1999.
162. Liu B, Yang M, Li R, et al. *Eur J Pharm Biopharm.* 69:527–534, 2008.
163. Soga O, Nostrum CF, and Hennink WE. *Biomacromolecules.* 5:818–821, 2004.
164. Rijcken CJ, Snel CJ, Schiffelers RM, Nostrum CF, and Hennink WE. *Biomaterials.* 28:5581–5593, 2007.
165. Bae Y, Jang WD, Nishiyama N, Fukushima S, and Kataoka K. *Mol Biosyst.* 1:242–250, 2005.
166. Bae Y, Nishiyama N, and Kataoka K. *Bioconjug Chem.* 18:1131–1139, 2007.
167. Kim D, Gao ZG, Lee ES, and Bae YH. *Mol Pharm.* 6:1353–1362, 2009.
168. Wu XL, Kim JH, Koo H, et al. *Bioconjug Chem.* 21:208–213, 2010.
169. Sethuraman VA and Bae YH. *J Control Release.* 118:216–224, 2007.
170. Li R and Low P. *J Biol Chem.* 269:3198–3204, 1994.

VIII. Homework Problems

1. Name (*a*) the route of drug administration (other than injection) that provides the fastest onset of drug action and (*b*) the most and least permeable epithelia.
2. Describe the various mechanisms through which a permeability enhancer facilitates drug transport across an epithelium.
3. Is benzalkonium chloride a permeability enhancer? By what action?
4. Are there active transport (cell-mediated) mechanisms for transdermal drug delivery?
5. Describe the resistant factors for protein and peptide absorption through the nasal mucosa and drug delivery strategies to overcome these obstacles.
6. Which one is more likely to be absorbed through the cornea, (*a*) a hydrophilic or hydrophobic drug? and (*b*) a weak acid or a weak base?
7. Describe the pathways through which an ocularly applied drug may be lost to systemic circulation.
8. Calculate the amounts of NaH_2PO_4 (mol wt 120), Na_2HPO_4 (mol wt 142), and NaCl needed to make 100 mL of an isotonic buffer at pH 6.8 (use information given in Table 15-6).
9. Using the above buffer solution, show how you would prepare 60 mL of a 1% neomycin sulfate isotonic solution.
10. Why is boric acid used as a buffer agent in ophthalmic preparations but not in systemic parenteral solutions?
11. Describe the mechanisms of how the following systems may be used for in situ gel preparations for ophthalmic use: (*a*) Carbopol 940, (*b*) Pluronic F-127; (*c*) Gelrite, and (*d*) hydroxypropylcellulose.
12. Describe the advantages of the pulmonary route for systemic drug delivery over oral or parenteral drug administration.
13. Discuss the role of mucociliary clearance on drug absorption through inhalation drug delivery.
14. Select the right answer: An aqueous solution is best aerosolized via (*a*) MDI, (*b*) DPI, or (*c*) nebulizer.
15. In aerosol drug delivery using MDI, DPI, and nebulizer, less than 20% of the dose is absorbed through the lungs in all three cases. Where did the drug go in each type of delivery?
16. What are the effects of propellant, surfactant, and moisture content on sprayed particle size and lung deposition of drug delivered using an MDI?
17. What are P-142 and P-227?
18. *a*. What is the weight of nitrogen in an 8 fl oz aerosol container filled with 6 fl oz of viscous ointment? The container is pressurized to 90 psig, and the temperature is 25°C.

    Conversion factors: 1 fl oz = 29.57 mL
    Pressure (psia) = pressure (psig) + 14.7
    Pressure (atm) = pressure (psia)/14.7

    b. If 3 fl oz of the aerosol is dispensed from the above aerosol, what is the resulting pressure in the container?
    Hint: Following the discharge of 3 fl oz of ointment content, the gas volume occupies 5 fl oz. Letting V_1 and P_1 be, respectively, the initial volume and pressure values for nitrogen and V_2 and P_2 be the nitrogen volume and pressure in the container after emission, at constant pressure
    $V_1/V_2 = P_2/P_1$

    c. What is the pressure remaining in the container when all the product content has been dispensed? (*Hint*: The gas now occupies 8 fl oz.)

d. What is the vapor pressure† of a propellant blend of *P*-11 and *P*-12 in a 70 g to 30 g ratio?

	Vapor Pressure (psia)	Molecular Weight
P-11	13.4	137.38
P-12	84.9	120.93

19. What may be the major drawbacks of using the pulmonary route for systemic drug delivery?
20. Briefly describe the concepts of (*a*) a prodrug approach in drug targeting and (*b*) the bystander effect.
21. Select the correct answer: For active targeting, if the cytotoxicity of a prodrug for anticancer therapy is activated by a specific enzyme, this enzyme can be (*a*) indigenous to the tumor cells; (*b*) delivered to the tumor cells first, using a targeting moiety; (*c*) induced in tumor cells first via gene transfection before prodrug delivery; or (*d*) all of the above. What are these processes called?
22. Describe three different targeting moieties (e.g., for growth, nutrition, and angiogenesis) and their actions for tumor cell targeting.
23. PEG has been used as a component in all types of nanocarriers. Discuss briefly the positive and negative roles of PEG in drug targeting.
24. Describe some formulation factors that promote passive targeting via the enhanced permeation and retention effect.
25. It has been shown that liposomes made of phosphatidylcholine (PC) with saturated fatty acyl chains (such as distearoylphosphatidylcholine) are more stable in the blood than liposomes containing PC with unsaturated fatty acyl chains (such as dioleoylphosphatidylcholine). What would be your explanation?
26. The pharmacokinetic data for DaunoXome and daunorubicin solution therapies are as follows:

	Volume Distribution, L	Plasma Clearance, mL/min	Distribution Half-life, h	Elimination, Half-life, h
DaunoXome	6.4	17 ml/min	—	4.4
Daunorubicin solution	1006	236 ml/min	0.77	55.4

How would you interpret the above results with regard to the liposome targeting effect?

27. What are the common agents used to prepare PEGylated stealth liposomes and stealth liposomes with a targeting moiety?
28. How are polymeric micelles different from the liposome vesicles in structure, stability, and drug release?
29. Polyamino acids are hydrophilic polymers but can be used as hydrophobic blocks when linked to PEG or other hydrophilic units for the preparation of polymeric micelles. Describe the methods by which the polyamino acids are rendered hydrophobic.
30. What is the advantage of using polyhistidine as the hydrophobic block for tumor cell targeting and drug release at the targeted site?

---

†A mixture of liquefied gas propellants is a solution. According to Raoult's law, the partial vapor pressure of a component is equal to the vapor pressure of the pure substance times its mole fraction. The total vapor pressure of an ideal solution is the sum of the partial pressures of the components (Dalton's law). Hence, for a propellant blend containing propellants a and b,

$$P_{total} = p_a + p_b$$

where $p_a = X_a p_a^{o}$ and $p_b = X_b p_b^{o}$.

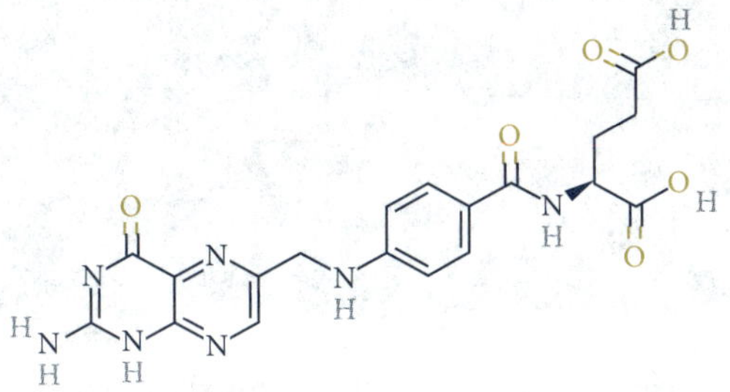

Figure 15-11 Folic acid.

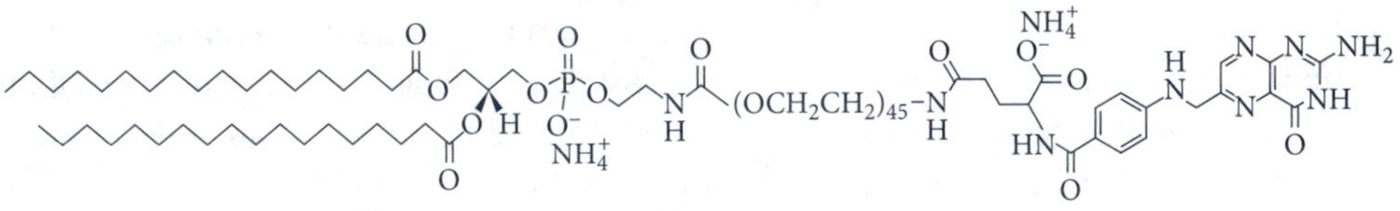

Figure 15-12 The DSPE–PEG (2000)–folate conjugate.[170]

31. What is LCST?

32. Poly(*N*-isopropylacrylamide) (PNIPAAm) is a hydrophilic thermosensitive polymer with an LCST of 32°C. Predict the change in hydrophobicity and LCST when this polymer is conjugated with (*a*) acrylamide (AAm); (*b*) methylacriamide (MAAm); (*c*) hydroxymethylacrylamide (HMAAm); and (*d*) oligolactates. How can the conjugated copolymers be used in micelle preparations?

33. Describe a literature method through which folate (see structure in **Figures 15-11** and **15-12**) is linked to PEG for active targeting using liposomes, polymeric micelles, or the nanocarriers.

Parenteral Drug Delivery Systems

CHAPTER 16

Hing Char, Jun Shao, and Joseph K. H. Ma

The Greek origin of the word parenteral consists of two parts: para meaning "outside" and enteron meaning "intestine." Parenteral literally means outside the intestine, and by convention, it refers to injections. Injections are usually delivered through a syringe and a needle, which causes pain and other undesired complications and inconvenience. And there are higher-quality standards for injections than for other noninvasive routes. One may ask, then, why some of the drugs should be given through injection but not through other more patient-friendly routes such as oral or inhalation. One obvious situation can be that the patient is unconscious. But most of the injections are delivered to conscious patients. So the question still remains. In this chapter, we answer this question, look into the special quality requirements of injections, and discuss how to prepare acceptable injection formulations.

CHAPTER OUTLINE

OBJECTIVES

1. Understand the need for parenteral drug delivery, the different routes of injections, and the dosage forms and devices suitable for such injections.
2. Understand the principles of designing various injectables.
3. Describe the specific requirements for injectables.
4. Understand the function and proper selection of excipients for parenteral solution preparation.
5. Know the general manufacturing process and quality control tests for injectables.
6. Understand the types and use of different sterilization methods.

I. Parenteral Drug Delivery

Drug Delivery by Injection

Need for Injections

There are many situations that call for the drug to be given by injection. First, in emergency situations, quick action of the drug is a must, which can be accomplished by injecting the drug directly into the blood circulation (intravenous injection). Although sublingual and inhalation delivery also can achieve fast action, not many drugs can be formulated or absorbed through these routes. Injections of drug solutions into muscles or subcutaneous tissues are usually absorbed quickly, reaching peak action within 30 min to 1 h. Second, by injection the drugs are usually completely absorbed and available for actions in the blood circulation, so that the bioavailabilities of injections are usually 100%. In practice, bioavailability refers to both the extent to which and the rate at which the drug is absorbed and becomes available at the action site. Because it is usually very difficult or impossible to measure the drug at the action site, the appearance of drug in the systemic blood circulation is used as the endpoint for the measurement of bioavailability. Many drugs, such as proteins and peptides, are not absorbed well through routes other than injections. When administered orally through the gastrointestinal tract, for example, these drugs can be extensively metabolized by enzymes in the intestinal lumen prior to absorption, by enzymes existing on the intestinal wall during absorption, or by liver enzymes after the peptides and proteins enter into the systemic blood circulation. Third, for unconscious patients, injections are probably the most convenient method to give medication. In addition, the parenteral injection route is needed for the delivery of specialized dosage forms for drug targeting purposes.

There are, of course, some disadvantages associated with injections. It is an invasive method that may cause pain and fear and may result in possible complications. The administration is inconvenient and requires professional skills. Not many parenteral products can be administered by the patients themselves. In addition, once the drug is administered, it is difficult to retrieve.

Injection Routes

Depending on where the needle goes, parenteral products can be administered through common routes such as intravenous (IV), subcutaneous (SC), intramuscular (IM), and intradermal (ID) injections. Less frequently used routes include intraarterial, intrathecal, intradural, and intracardiac injections.

Intravenous Injections

The drug is administered directly into a vein and enters systemic circulation. There is no absorption process, and the drug is ready to be distributed into various tissues once injected. A large volume up to several liters can be delivered through infusion over a certain time period. Infusion is a continuous slow delivery with a rate of 50–150 mL/h. Through IV injection, an accurate amount of drug can be delivered within a desired time period. This is particularly useful in cases where the accuracy of the dose must be monitored, such as in anesthesia and chemotherapy. In addition, IV injection of cytotoxic drugs, such as those used in chemotherapy, is necessary because these drugs can cause severe local tissue damage when administered through other routes, due to the high drug concentration at the delivery site. However, the IV administered drug concentration is quickly diluted following injection. That is why most of the chemotherapeutic agents are given by IV infusion. The possible dosage forms for IV injection include aqueous solutions, oil-in-water (O/W) emulsions, and aqueous colloidal dispersions such as liposomes and nanoparticles.

Oil-based preparations (solutions, W/O emulsions, suspensions, colloidal dispersions) cannot be given through IV injection because they are not miscible with the blood and will occlude the pulmonary microcirculation.

A few complications can occur with intravenous therapy. These include phlebitis, thrombosis, infiltration, and air emboli. Phlebitis is a local inflammatory reaction. Some symptoms include redness, warmth, and swelling at the administration site. To minimize phlebitis, the site can be changed or a smaller needle can be used. Thrombosis is the formation of a blood clot. It can result from extremes in solution pH, the inherent irritating properties of the drug administered, needle or catheter trauma, and particulate matter. Infiltration occurs when the dose leaks into the surrounding tissue. It is usually caused by improper placement or dislodgement of the catheter. Some symptoms include swelling, pain, itching, burning, or discoloration. If infiltration occurs, the IV infusion should be discontinued and started at another injection site. Injection of air into the blood circulation can cause serious problems and even death, depending on the amount and delivery rate. There is a controversy about the limit of the amount of air that can be injected. It should be a good practice to purge all the bubbles from the IV line to avoid injecting any air into the blood.

Subcutaneous Injections

The drug is injected into the loose connective tissues just below the dermis, and it is allowed to be absorbed into the blood circulation. Usually a small amount of drug from an injected solution is completely absorbed regardless of its polarity and molecular weight, and the peak concentration can be reached within 30 min to about 2 h following administration. However, if the molecular weight is larger than 15 kDa, the drug will be absorbed mainly through the lymphatic system which is a slow process. There are many pain receptors in the subcutaneous tissue; hence ideally only nonirritating drugs should be administered by this route. The typical sites of SC injection are the outer area of the upper arms, front area of the legs, and abdomen (just above and below the waist excluding the area next to the navel). The injection volume is 1–1.5 mL. Hyaluronidase (Hylenex) may be administered subcutaneously to increase the injectable volume to 5–10 mL by temporarily breaking down the hyaluronic acid in the subcutaneous tissue. Subcutaneous injection is the preferred route for self-administration by the user. Usually, 25- to 30-gauge needles ⅜ to ⅝ in long are suitable. Some newer drugs for diabetes such as Byetta are delivered using 30- or 31-gauge, ⅓-in ultrafine needles. The possible dosage forms for SC injection include solutions, suspensions, emulsions, and colloids.

Intramuscular Injections

The drug is injected into a muscle, usually the gluteal (buttocks), vastus lateralis (lateral thigh), or deltoid (upper arm) muscles. The injection volume is usually 1–3 mL. Intramuscular tissue is richly supplied with blood vessels so the absorption of the drug is relatively faster and usually more complete than the SC injection. Again, when the molecular weight of the drug is too large (> 15 kDa), the absorption occurs mainly through the lymphatic system, a slow process. There are few pain receptors in the muscles mentioned above, which gives a better tolerance to injected viscous and irritating drugs. Incorrect injection may lead to local muscle damage. For IM injection, a 21- or 23-gauge needle 1 to 1½ in long is usually used. The possible dosage forms include solutions, suspensions, emulsions, and colloids.

Intradermal Injections

The drug is injected into the dermal layer of the skin. This route of administration is usually used for diagnostic purposes (e.g., allergy, tuberculin test), with injection volumes typically less than 0.1 mL. The injection is normally made using a 23- to 26-gauge needle ⅜ in long. Absorption of the drug through ID injection is slow and limited. The possible dosage forms are the same as those for SC injections.

Dosage Form Types and Devices

Parenteral products can be classified as *small-volume parenterals* (SVPs) and *large-volume parenterals* (LVPs). SVPs are usually solutions, suspensions, or emulsions with unit package volume no more than 100 mL. They are formulated as injectables for IM, SC, or ID administration or as additives to IV solutions, if compatible. SVPs can be designed for multiple-dose purpose, in which case the volume should not be more than 30 mL and a preservative should be added. LVPs are usually electrolyte solutions, lipid emulsions, solutions for parenteral nutrition; or irrigating solutions with unit package volume of several hundred milliliters to 1 L. Due to the large volume to be administered, LVPs should not contain preservatives to avoid the potential adverse reaction caused by the preservatives.

Injectable Dosage Forms

The official parenteral products as defined by USP include solutions, emulsions, suspensions, and drug powders that are used by reconstituting the products in suitable solvent vehicles. The necessity of making a reconstituted product usually indicates that the drug or the formulation lacks long-term stability in the vehicle of use. There are five types of parenteral products, which can be seen from the examples given:

1. *Drug injection*. The product is in a solution form and ready for use.

   Example: Ciprofloxacin Injection, USP, contains 1% ciprofloxacin, lactic acid as a solubilizing agent, and hydrochloric acid for pH adjustment.

2. *Drug for injection*. The product is in a dried powder form to be reconstituted as an injectable solution.

   Example: Targocid for injection, which contains 200 mg per vial of lyophilized teicoplanin, is used as an injectable antibiotic when reconstituted with 3 mL of sterile water for injection.

3. *Drug injectable emulsion*. The product is an emulsion and ready for use.

   Example: Diprivan (propofol) injectable emulsion contains propofol in an O/W emulsion with soybean oil, glycerol, egg lecithin, and disodium edetate. The drug has only limited solubility in water.

4. *Drug injectable suspension*. The product is a suspension and ready for use.

   Example: Penicillin G procaine injectable suspension contains penicillin G procaine in a stabilized aqueous suspension with sodium citrate buffer, 0.5% lecithin, 0.5% carboxymethylcellulose, 0.5% povidone, 0.1% methylparaben, and 0.01% propylparaben.

5. *Drug for injectable suspension*. The product is in a dried powder form. Upon reconstitution, it forms a suspension or colloidal dispersion suitable for injection.

   Example: Abraxane for injectable suspension. In this product, the drug paclitaxel is prepared as albumin-bound and lyophilized powder (mean size ~ 130 nm), which is to be reconstituted with 0.9% sodium chloride injection, USP, prior to intravenous infusion.

Special Parenteral Products

There are some special parenteral products such as *implants* and in situ gels. Implants are the delivery devices implanted mostly under the skin for sustained-release purposes. They are often designed for drug release over a period of several months to 1–2 years and are particularly useful for long-term treatment of some diseases. For example, Viadur is an osmotic pump design for continuous delivery of leuprolide, a testosterone suppression agent, over 1 year for the palliative treatment of advanced prostate cancer.[1] The implant is a cylindrical titanium alloy reservoir (diameter 4 mm, length 45 mm) capped on one end by a rate-controlling membrane and at the other end by a diffusion moderator (see **Figure 16-1** for illustration). The rate-controlling membrane is a semipermeable membrane that allows water to diffuse into the system due to the osmotic gradient between the tissue fluid and the osmotic engine containing mainly NaCl. The advantage of implant systems is the prolonged release of drug for a long period up to 1–2 years. The disadvantages include two required surgeries (implanting and removing the device) and possible local inflammatory responses and low patient compliance.

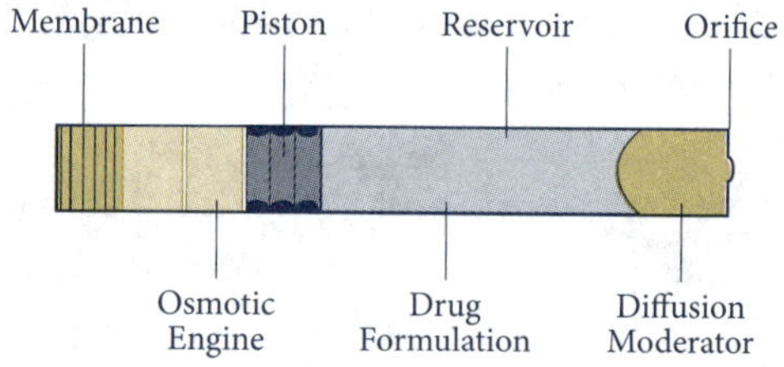

Figure 16-1 Cross-sectional diagram of the Duros implant.
Modified from: Wright JC, Tao Leonard S, Stevenson CL, Beck JC, Chen G, Jao RM, Johnson PA, Leonard J, Skowronski RJ. An in vivo/in vitro comparison with a leuprolide osmotic implant for the treatment of prostate cancer. *Journal of Controlled Release*, 2001; 75: 1–10.

In situ gels are polymeric systems that can be administered as liquid, but undergo a phase transition to semisolid upon exposure to physiological environments. It is recalled that the gelation of a system can be triggered by temperature change such as the poloxamers, by pH such as the Carbopols, and by the presence of salts such as the alginates. The use of polymers based on their sol-gel transition characteristics at body temperature after SC or IM injection provides a novel parenteral delivery strategy. The formation of gel allows for high drug loading and can provide a mechanism for prolonged release. The gel can be further modified to control the drug release rate by using copolymers, ionic strength, heat, and photosensitive agents. The disadvantage is that the release of the drug can be affected by the morphology formed in vivo. Some polymers such as the biodegradable low-molecular-weight PLGA (polyglycolic acid)–PEG (polyethlene glycol)–PLGA system[2] and Pluronic F-127[3] have been tested for use as in situ gels.

Injection Devices

Many chronic diseases such as diabetes, multiple sclerosis, and rheumatoid arthritis require self-medication by patients using injectable products. To be of convenience to patients and for improved compliance, easy-to-use injection devices such as prefilled syringes, pen injectors, and autoinjectors have been marketed. Note that except for parenteral products marketed for safe self-medication, parenteral injections are performed only by healthcare professionals.

Prefilled Syringe

Prefilled syringes are loaded with the final drug product and are ready for injection. They are a popular option for the packaging and delivery of injectable solution products, and they offer a more convenient alternative to vials for the preparation and administration of drugs. For products packaged in vials, the user needs to perform many steps to prepare and administer the drug, such as withdrawing the solution from the vial, removing air bubbles from the syringe, and changing needles. These preparation steps can be challenging for the elderly and patients with diseases such as rheumatoid arthritis. In addition, prefilled syringes are precise in dosing because the dose is already measured in the syringe, whereas a withdrawing error of dosage from the vial often occurs in self-medication. Prefilled syringes are usually for single use only. Some examples of prefilled syringes include Lovenox (enoxaparin sodium) and Pegasys (PEGylated interferon α-2a).

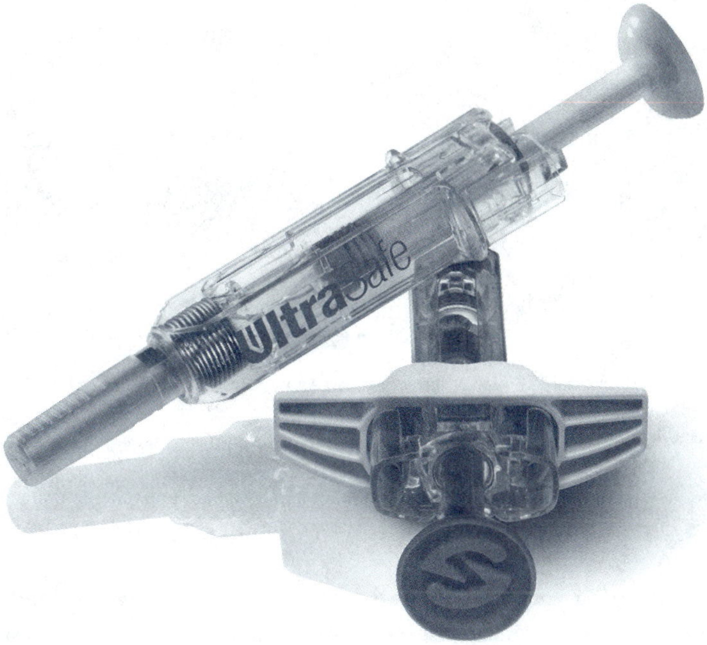

Figure 16-2 UltraSafe Needle Guards are activated manually and designed to attach easily to most prefilled glass syringes.
Courtesy of: SafetySyringes, Inc.

Device with Needle Protection System (Safe Needle Devices)

The Needlestick Safety and Prevention Act requires healthcare employers to improve protection against accidental needlesticks and other sharps injuries that expose healthcare workers to potentially deadly blood-borne pathogens. As a result of this law, new devices have entered the market (see **Figure 16-2** for an example) to enhance the safety of healthcare providers responsible for dispensing and administering parenteral products. The Lovenox prefilled syringes, e.g., also contain a safety system that shields the needle after injection. After the injection and removal of the needle from the injection site, the user activates the safety system by pushing the plunger rod. The protective sleeve will automatically cover the needle. The user can then easily dispose of the syringe in a sharps container.

Pen Injector

Pen injectors have been in use in the diabetes management and human growth deficiency market since the 1980s. These devices have become popular for use in infertility, osteoporosis, and hepatitis diseases, due to their small size, ease of use, and convenience compared to vials. Pen injectors use a cartridge as the primary drug container. For proper use of the pen injector, the user attaches a needle to the tip of the device, inserts the needle into the skin, and pushes the button to inject the drug. An example of a pen injector is the Byetta (exenatide), which delivers 60 doses, twice daily, for 30 days. It has a prefilled glass cartridge assembled into the device (see **Figure 16-3**). Some pen injectors have a "dial-a-dose" feature where the user can vary the dose.

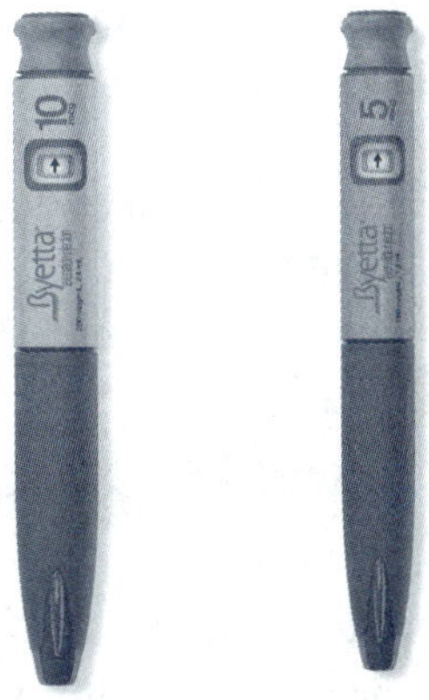

(*A*) (*B*)

Figure 16-3 Pen injector: Byetta pen.
Courtesy of: Amylin Pharmaceuticals, Inc. and Lilly USA, LLC.

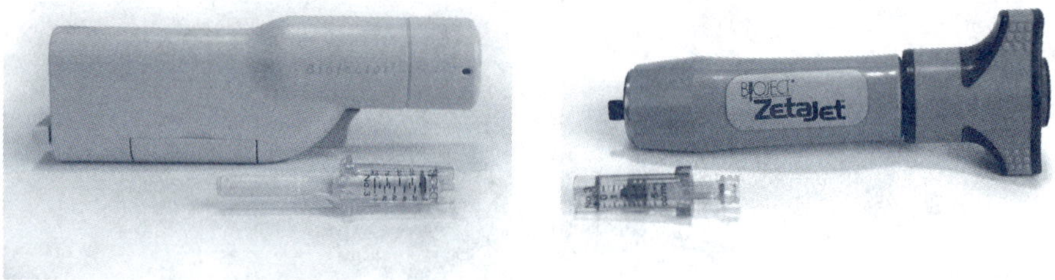

(*A*) (*B*)

Figure 16-4 Needle-free injectors: (*A*) Biojector intradermal injector (powered by compressed CO_2); (*B*) Zetajet (spring-powered).
Courtesy of: Bioject Medical Tecnologies Inc.

Autoinjector

Autoinjectors are spring-based or compressed-gas devices designed to deliver a single dose from a prefilled syringe or cartridge. They can be disposable or reusable. Disposable autoinjectors have been used historically for emergency conditions, such as the use of EpiPen in the treatment of life-threatening allergic reactions, but are now used in diseases such as rheumatoid arthritis and anemia. Disposable autoinjectors are for single use. The reusable autoinjectors contain a prefilled syringe or cartridge with the desired needle attached. An example is the Autoject 2 (Owen Mumford). Autoinjectors have a safety lock that prevents the administration of the drug unless the device is pressed against the skin. This prevents accidental firing (injection) of the device. The needle is completely hidden within the autoinjector. When pressed against the injection site and a trigger button is pressed, the syringe needle is automatically inserted into the skin and the drug is delivered.

Needle-Free Injector

Many patients have a fear of needles. Elimination of the needle from the injection process can thus improve the patient's acceptance of and compliance with a parenteral drug therapy. Two examples of needle-free injectors are shown in **Figure 16-4**. The reusable Biojector 2000 device can deliver intramuscular or subcutaneous injections up to 1 mL in volume. The needle-free technology utilizes a high-pressure gas such as carbon dioxide or a spring to drive the drug solution at high speed through a tiny orifice in the device held against the skin. The ultrafine stream of solution then penetrates the skin to provide an intradermal or intramuscular drug delivery. The Zetajet system is a compact, spring-powered, durable device, and it is intended to deliver vaccines and injectable medications either subcutaneously or intramuscularly for both professional use and home use for patients who self-inject. The spring-powered system is more suited for multiple uses such as in mass immunization programs.

II. Design and Use of Parenteral Dosage Forms

The decision on the method of drug administration is often the result of a set of therapeutic requirements. The design of a parenteral dosage form is to meet such requirements by providing a system that is safe for administration and efficacious in its use. There are several key factors associated with the formulation of a parenteral dosage form, namely, drug solubility, stability, route of administration, drug release pattern, and in vivo distribution characteristics.

General Considerations

Solubility Considerations

Water-based preparations are always preferred because they are less irritating and safer to use than nonaqueous preparations for parenteral administration. If the drug is soluble and stable in aqueous solution, then a simple aqueous solution should be the choice. If a drug is water-insoluble, cosolvents such as ethanol, propylene glycol, and polyethylene glycol 400 (PEG 400), or hydroxypropyl-β-cyclodextrin (which enhances solubility by forming inclusion complexes with the drug), can be used to dissolve the drug in the aqueous system. Fixed oils such as sesame oil can also be used to formulate poorly soluble drugs for IM administration. If the drug is not stable in solution forms, a lyophilized dosage form can be developed to increase its shelf life. The lyophilized powder is reconstituted with a diluent before administration.

Biopharmaceutical Considerations

The therapeutic requirements of a drug can be the onset time, duration of action, peak of action, therapeutic windows (between the minimum effective concentration and minimum toxic concentration), and local or systemic treatment. Among all the injection routes, IV injection has the shortest onset time followed by IM and then SC injections. The drug will reach the target tissue within seconds after IV injection to exert actions. The onset times for IM or SC injectable solutions are usually within 30 min but can be as short as 5 min. The peak concentration in blood after IV injection is at the beginning, whereas for IM or SC injection it can be in the range of 0.5 h to many hours after administration, depending on the formulation. Note that the peak of drug action, which depends on the mechanisms of its pharmacological and toxicological effect, does not necessarily correlate with the peak of plasma concentration.

Therapeutic Considerations

For drugs with narrow therapeutic windows, IV infusion may be the choice accurately to control the drug concentration in blood. Other routes usually result in a fluctuating blood concentration profile except those well-formulated sustained-release products (such as the osmotic pump). For chronic treatment, prolonged-release dosage forms may be the choice. To achieve this goal, the drug can be formulated into depot formulations such as suspensions, nano/micro particulate systems, in situ gel, or implants. When designing prolonged-release dosage forms, one should keep in mind that a long-term stabilized drug concentration is not necessarily desirable for some diseases that can be better treated with a pulse-type drug release. Diabetes is one such disease, where the natural insulin release from the pancreatic cells depends on the blood glucose level. A continuous high level of insulin may cause hypoglycemia and other problems.

Dosage Form Design and Use

Suspensions

Usually, drug in solution is absorbed faster than drug in a suspension. The latter, however, can be useful for formulation of sustained-release dosage forms, as the drug in suspension must undergo a dissolution process, which can result in the drug acting for a longer duration than that delivered by solutions. For example, insulin injection can be formulated to exhibit rapid, intermediate-, and long-acting effects. Regular insulin injection is in the form of solution, which is quickly absorbed after injection to produce a rapid drug action and is therefore used in emergency situations such as ketoacidosis. Different types of crystalline insulin have been developed to make suspension injections in order to prolong the duration of action. Isophane insulin suspension (NPH insulin), for example, consists of crystals made of insulin, zinc, and protamine, which have a rod shape with an average length of about 30 μm. After injection, the crystals are slowly dissolved, so that the absorption of insulin is slow with an onset time of 1–1.5 h, but the duration of drug action is much longer (close to 24 h) than that of insulin in solution. NPH is considered to be intermediate-acting. A crystal form consisting of only zinc and insulin has also been developed as extended insulin zinc suspension (ultralente). This crystal dissolves even more slowly than NPH, with an onset time of about 4–8 h and duration of action of about 36 h or more. Ultralente is known as the long-acting insulin preparation.

For insulin preparation, two other products should be mentioned, namely, Humalog Mix50/50 and Humalog Mix75/25. They are premixed insulins containing insulin lispro protamine suspension, an intermediate-acting preparation, and insulin lispro injection (Humalog), a rapid-acting solution preparation, at the ratio of 50 : 50 and 75 : 25, respectively. Chemically, insulin lispro is a human insulin analog, created when the amino acids at positions B28 (Pro) and B29 (Lys) on the human insulin B chain are reversed. Both the premixed preparations exhibit a short onset time, time for peak concentration at 30–90 min after dosing, and prolonged duration of action. Humalog Mix50/50 can achieve a peak insulin concentration which is twice that of Humalog Mix75/25, but the latter exhibits greater action than the former at late phase, due to the presence of a higher content of the longer-acting component. **Table 16-1** shows the effect of various insulin preparations after injection. The glucose infusion rate to maintain a normal plasma glucose level is a measurement of the insulin activity in vivo. It can be seen from the table that Humalog, the solution preparation, resulted in the greatest peak action but with the shortest duration, and the pure suspension preparation resulted in the lowest peak action but with the greatest late-phase action, whereas the two mixtures exerted intermediate actions. Compared to each other, the mixture with more solution (Mix50/50) exhibited a higher peak action whereas the mixture with more suspension (Mix75/25) exhibited a higher late-phase effect. These examples show that the peak and the duration of drug action can be optimized based on the solubility of the drug and the formulation type.

Oil solutions for IM injection also provide longer actions than solutions after injection. The drug absorption from such preparations can take the following routes: the drug first partitions into the interstitial fluid and then is absorbed; the oil (together with the drug) is absorbed

Table 16-1 Comparison of Humalog Insulins for Diabetes[†]

Brand (Composition)	Onset (h)	Peak (h)	Duration (h)	Percent of Total Activity in First 4 Hours[‡]
Insulin lispro protamine suspension	1 to 1.5	1.3 to 18.3 (mean 5.8)	Up to 24	22% (6.3–40%)
Humalog Mix 75/25 (75% lispro protamine and 25% lispro injection)	0.25 to 0.5	1 to 6.5 (mean: 2.6)	Up to 24	35% (21–56%)
Humalog Mix 50/50 (50% lispro protamine and 50% lispro injection)	0.25 to 0.5	0.8 to 4.8 (mean: 2.3)	22 or more	45% (27–69%)
Humalog (Insulin lispro injection)	0.25 to 0.5	0.8 to 4.3 (mean: 2.4)	3 to 6.5	70% (49–89%)

[†]Data are taken from a report (PV 5551 AMP) of Eli Lilly Company, Indianapolis, IN.[4]
[‡]Derived from glucose clamp studies in nondiabetic subjects.
Data from: Report by Eli Lilly and Company. HUMALOG® MIX75/25™ 2009. http://pi.lillg.com/us/humalog7525-pi.pdf, accessed on 7/12/2011.

through convective transport into the lymphatic system; the oil (together with the drug) is emulsified into O/W emulsion and absorbed into the blood circulation. The lymph moves at a slow rate and finally enters the blood circulation at the left and right subclavian veins at the rate of about 100–150 mL/h.

Microspheres

Lupron Depot is a microsphere depot formulation for leuprolide acetate, made with gelatin and DL-lactic and glycolic acids copolymer, that can deliver the drug over a period of one to several months depending on the dose. The drug is embedded in the matrix of the polymers, and it diffuses out slowly through the aqueous channels. The drug release rate is mainly controlled by the length the drug molecule has to travel to reach the surface of the microsphere, the porosity of the matrix, and the erosion/degradation rate of the matrix. Microspheres, with or without drug incorporation, may be used in chemoembolization treatment of hepatic cancers. In this method, the delivery of chemotherapeutic agents into the tumor-feeding artery is followed by blockage of the artery using biodegradable microspheres or other preparations such as gelatin cube.[5] The embolization is intended to reduce the blood supply to the tumor and to prolong the residence time of the drug in the tumor tissue. This treatment has been found to be effective in delaying tumor progression but not in increasing the survival rate,[6, 7] indicating that there is still a need to improve the technology from the perspectives of dosage forms, delivery techniques, drugs, and embolization agents.[8]

Localized Drug Delivery by Injection

For localized diseases or in the case where whole-body distribution of drug is unwanted, such as in the case of chemotherapy, local injections, if possible, can provide great advantages. Misonidazole, a radiosensitizing agent, has been injected directly into tumor tissue to enhance the radiotherapeutic efficacy and reduce the systemic exposure to the drug.[9] Injection of ethanol into liver cancer lesion, or percutaneous ethanol injection therapy (PEIT), under the guidance of ultrasound, CT scan, or laparoscopic ultrasonography, has been widely practiced in the treatment of liver tumors, especially of hepatocellular carcinoma, with a remarkable anticancer effect and considerably high long-term survival rates.[10] Direct injection of ethanol into tumor mass has also been found effective and safe in treating renal tumors of nonsurgical patients.[11] Localized injection has been found useful in other diseases as well. Anesthetic agents are usually given locally for dental procedures. Local corticosteroid injection has been suggested as second-line treatment for patients with disk-related sciatica, as well as for selected patients with chronic low back pain.[12]

III. Special Requirements of Parenteral Products

In addition to the formulation and therapeutic considerations, a parenteral dosage form should meet the following special requirements: It should be sterile, free of pyrogen, isotonic, free of particulate matter for solution preparations, and stable.

Sterility

Parenteral dosage forms are unique pharmaceutical dosage forms because of their requirement to be sterile, meaning the absence of microorganisms. Sterility is absolute; the product is either sterile or not sterile—it cannot be partially sterile. Sterility can be achieved through various methods discussed later in this chapter.

Free of Pyrogen

Pyrogens are fever-causing organic compounds from bacteria and other microorganisms. Among which, lipopolysaccharides (LPS), or endotoxins, from gram-negative bacteria are most noted to cause dosage contaminations. The administration of pyrogen-contaminated parenterals can result in a febrile reaction; hence, they are unacceptable as a finished parenteral product. Pyrogens are thermally stable and cannot be destroyed by regular sterilization methods such as autoclave. The commonly used method to remove pyrogens is via oxidative chemical reaction. Potassium permanganate, a strong oxidative agent, can be used to oxidize the pyrogens into volatile or non-volatile precipitates. Barium hydroxide is also added during the reaction to facilitate the formation of precipitates. To remove pyrogens, water is first distilled several times and then treated with potassium permanganate and barium hydroxide. After the reaction, the treated water is further distilled to remove all chemicals.

Pyrogen removal can also be achieved by *reverse osmosis* (RO), a membrane filtration method that removes large molecules and ions from solutions by applying pressure to the solution when it is on one side of a selective membrane. In this method, the soluble substances to be removed are retained on the pressurized side of a membrane, which excludes the passage of large molecules or ions but allows the solvent (water) to pass freely. The RO processes, when arranged in series, are very useful for the manufacturing of pyrogen-free Water for Injection.

Isotonicity

An isotonic solution is a solution that has the same osmotic pressure as that of the blood with respect to the membrane of the cells of interest. It is preferable to administer isotonic solutions to minimize injection site irritation or pain. Administration of a hypotonic solution can lead to the swelling of cells and may result in cell bursting due to water being transported into the cells by osmosis. Hypertonic solutions can lead to shrinking of cells due to loss of water through osmosis (crenation). Intravenous injections should be isotonic. Intravenous injection of hypotonic preparations can cause hemolysis. However, a small volume of hypertonic preparation can be given by IV injection because it is quickly diluted by the blood. Some examples of isotonic solution are 0.9% sodium chloride solution (normal saline) and 5% dextrose solution. A solution of 270–300 mosmol/L can be considered as iso-osmotic to blood. It should be pointed out that iso-osmotic (meaning the same osmotic pressure) is not necessarily isotonic. If one or more solutes are freely permeable through the cell membrane, then the iso-osmotic preparation is not isotonic toward that particular cell membrane. For example, borate can freely pass through red blood cell membrane and behaves as water toward red blood cell membrane from the perspective of osmosis.

Free of Particulate Matter

Parenteral solutions should be free from particulate matter. Some examples of particulate matter include lint, fibers, glass, rubber, and undissolved chemicals. These may be introduced to solution by contamination during the compounding and manufacturing process and/or by interactions between the product and the glass container or stopper. Particulate matter can be removed by filtration.

Stability

Parenteral products should be physically and chemically stable for the duration of their shelf life. In addition, the products must maintain the microbiological stability (sterility) for the shelf life. The container closure integrity is an important aspect of the manufacturing process because the container and closure are used to keep the product in and to keep potential microorganisms and other contaminants out. The manufacturer needs to validate its container closure system to ensure that the product is sterile for the stated shelf life. The most common stability problems associated with solution injectables are hydrolysis and oxidation. Hydrolysis can be prevented or slowed down by control of the formulation factors such as pH. Oxidation can be prevented by adding antioxidants and chelators to prevent heavy metals from catalyzing the oxidation reaction or by replacing the air in the headspace of the container with inert gas such as N_2.

IV. Excipients for Parenteral Preparations

Parenteral preparations may contain excipients such as buffering agents, chelating agents, solubilizers, stabilizers, protectants, substances to adjust tonicity, or antimicrobial agents (**Table 16-2**). No coloring agents should be added to injections. The addition of excipients to the formulation should be kept to a minimum. When excipients are used, they should not affect the stability, safety, or efficacy of the product. The excipients selected should meet compendial standards (for example, USP, EP, JP). The quality of excipients used in the formulation should be taken into consideration. For example, polysorbate 80 may contain a trace amount of peroxide, which may have an impact on the stability of the drug.[13, 14]

To search for excipients used in approved drug products, consult the FDA web site (http://www.accessdata.fda.gov/scripts/cder/iig/index.cfm). This site publishes an inactive ingredients database for approved drug products. The excipients are listed in alphabetical order. Also provided is the route of administration and the strength used in most cases. The database is updated quarterly.

Solvents and Vehicles

Water

Water is the main solvent/vehicle for most of the injections, simply because the body fluid is an aqueous solution, which indicates that water is safe and nonirritating. Note that water is not inert; there is no lack of interactions between water and the drug or between water and the biological system, but our understanding of in vivo drug action is entirely based on water being the medium. Water used for the preparation of injectables must be pyrogen-free, but not necessarily sterile in cases where the final products are subjected to the sterilization process. But even in cases where sterility is not required, the water used should have minimum bacterial contamination. There are several preparations of water for parenteral use. Water for Injection, *USP*, is the most often used water for manufacturing parenterals, which is pyrogen-free, contains total solids $\leq 10\,\mu g/mL$, and

Table 16-2 Pharmaceutical Excipients for Injectable Formulations

Excipient Group	Purpose	Examples
Buffering agents	Maintain pH	Acetate, citrate, phosphate
Tonicity agents	Adjust tonicity	Sodium chloride, mannitol
Surfactants	Act as solubilizer, stabilizer, protection from adsorption or aggregation	Polysorbate 20, polysorbate 80, poloxamer 188
Protectants and bulking agents	Act as cryoprotectant/lyoprotectant	Trehalose, sucrose, mannitol
Antioxidants	Prevent oxidation	Methionine, ascorbic acid, sulfites, bisulfites
Chelators	Act as stabilizer, prevent oxidation	EDTA
Preservatives	Act as antimicrobial agent	Benzyl alcohol, phenol, methylparaben, propylparaben

has no added substances. It is manufactured by distillation or the reverse osmosis process after the pyrogens have been removed through oxidation. It is not necessary for it to be sterile. The final products made with Water for Injection, USP, have to be sterilized.

Once water for injection, USP, is sterilized, it is called Sterile Water for Injection, *USP*, which is usually packed in a single-dose package equal to or less than 1 L. Sterile Water for Injection, USP, is pyrogen-free and sterile, and it can be used to reconstitute some of the dry powder injectables such as ampicillin for injection for clinical use, where the ingredients of the dry powder formulation will render the reconstituted solution isotonic. Because it contains no solute, Sterile Water for Injection, USP, has no tonicity. Some of the dry powder injectables require the vehicle to have a certain tonicity, in which case Sterile Water for Injection, USP, should not be used. It is important to keep in mind that 1-L package of Sterile Water for Injection, USP, should not be used for IV infusion.

When one or more preservatives are added to sterile water for injection, USP, it is called Bacteriostatic Water for Injection, *USP*. It is intended for the reconstitution of dry injectables for multiple-dose applications. The presence of the preservative(s) can kill the bacteria from possible contamination during repeated use. Due to the toxicity of the preservatives, Bacteriostatic Water for Injection, USP, is packed in containers equal to or less than 30 mL to avoid a large amount of the preservative(s) being administered. Usually, if more than 5 mL per dose is required, Sterile Water for Injection, USP, instead of Bacteriostatic Water for Injection, USP, should be used.

Isotonic Vehicles

When isotonic solvents/vehicles are required for reconstitution of injectables, 0.9% sodium chloride injection, USP, bacteriostatic 0.9% sodium chloride injection, USP, 5% dextrose injection, USP, and lactated Ringer's injection, USP, can be used. All solutions mentioned above are isotonic, sterile, and pryrogen-free, and they contain no preservatives except for bacteriostatic 0.9% sodium chloride injection, USP. Attention should be paid to the potential toxicity of the preservative (benzyl alcohol) when bacteriostatic 0.9% sodium chloride injection, USP, is used. The 0.9% sodium chloride injection, USP, contains 9 g/L NaCl with a calculated osmolarity of 308 mosmol/L. The 0.45% sodium chloride injection, USP (containing 4.5 g/L of NaCl), is also available, which has one-half of the tonicity of the blood. The 5% dextrose injection, USP, contains 5.0 g/L of dextrose (hydrated) with a calculated osmolarity of 252 mosmol/L. It is slightly hypotonic, but still safe for IV injection. Lactated Ringer's injection, USP, contains 6 g/L of NaCl, 3.1 g/L of sodium lactate anhydrous, 0.3 g/L of KCl, and 0.2 g/L of $CaCl_2$, with a calculated osmolarity of 273 mosmol/L.

Hydroalcoholic Vehicles

In addition to aqueous solutions, some nonaqueous solvents are available for injection preparations when the drug is not stable or not soluble in water. The nonaqueous solvent to be used should be safe, nonirritating, and nonsensitizing. It should have no adverse effect on drug actions, should be physically and chemically stable, and should lack pharmacological activities. In practice, none of the available solvents can meet all the requirements. The choice of solvent should be based on the balance of the advantages and disadvantages. The commonly used nonaqueous solvents are low-molecular-weight polyethylene glycols (PEGs), propylene glycol, glycerin, and ethanol. They are miscible with water and are usually used together with water as the cosolvent(s) to increase the solubility. Fixed vegetable oils such as cottonseed oil, sesame oil, and corn oil are also used for injection preparations that are not injected directly into the blood circulation. Oil-based injectables are administered by the IM route. Note that mineral oil and paraffin oil should not be used for injection preparations, although they are commonly used in pharmaceutical preparations intended for delivery of drug through topical, transdermal, and oral routes.

Buffering Agents and Other Excipients

Buffer Solutions

A buffer is used to maintain the pH for the stability and/or solubility of the formulation. It is best to choose a buffer system having a pK_a approximately equal to the required pH, in order to have a maximum buffering capacity. See **Table 16-3** for available buffers. As a general rule, the buffering range of a given buffer is ±1 pH unit of the pK_a of the buffering agent.[15, 16] The target pH for physiological acceptability is 7.4; however, in practice a wider pH range is considered acceptable. From a tissue irritancy point of view, a pH range of 3–10 is considered acceptable for the IV route due to rapid dilution effect of the blood. For IM and SC injections, pH ranges of 3–10 and 3–6, respectively, are considered acceptable.[17] The buffer concentration is usually 10–100 m*M*. The choice of the buffering agents should be taken into consideration for lyophilization. For example, certain buffers such as acetate are volatile. If used in lyophilized products, they may be removed from the formulation during drying. This will result in a formulation with little or no buffering capacity. Crystallization of the buffering agents can cause a change in pH, which may affect the stability of the drug. For example, dibasic sodium phosphate is prone to crystallization during lyophilization, and will cause a decrease in pH (e.g., from 7 to 4).[18, 19]

Preservatives

Preservatives are used to prevent or inhibit the growth of microorganisms. Antimicrobial agent is added to the formulation when the product is to be used multiple times (e.g., multidose vial) except for antibiotic preparations or otherwise instructed in the USP product monograph. Benzyl alcohol (1–2%) and the parabens (methylparaben 0.18% combined with propylparaben 0.02%) are commonly used in injectables. Benzyl alcohol should be avoided when the product is used

Table 16-3 Pharmaceutical Buffers for Parenteral Preparation

Buffering System	pK_a	Effective pH Range
Gluconic	3.86	2.6–4.6
Lactic	3.86	2.8–4.8
Ascorbic	4.17	3.2–5.2
Benzoic	4.20	3.2–5.2
Citric	3.13 4.76 6.40	2.1–6.2
Succinic	4.19 5.63	3.2–6.6
Acetic	4.76	3.8–5.8
Carbonic	6.36 10.33	5.4–7.4
Phosphoric	2.12 7.21 12.67	6.2–8.2
Tris (hydroxymethyl) aminomethane (TRIS)	8.07	7.1–9.1
Glycine	2.35 9.78	8.8–10.8

for children under the age of 2 years because its degradation product is benzyaldehyde, which is toxic to the central nervous system. No preservative should be used in injectables for infants or in large-volume parenteral preparations.

Antioxidants

Antioxidants are sometimes needed to prevent the drug from being oxidized. Commonly used antioxidants include sulfites, bisulfites, and metabisulfites, to be used in high-, intermediate-, and low-pH solutions, respectively. These agents can decompose quickly in the presence of air. Therefore, the air in the container should be replaced with inert gas while these compounds are used as antioxidants. They can also react with ortho- or para-hydroxybenzyl derivatives, and are incompatible with drugs such as chloramphenicol and phenylmercuric acetate. Ascorbic acid is another commonly used antioxidant. It lowers the pH because of its acidity. The aqueous solution of 5% ascorbic acid would have a pH around 2–3. It is relatively stable in powder form but not in solution form, especially in alkaline solution.

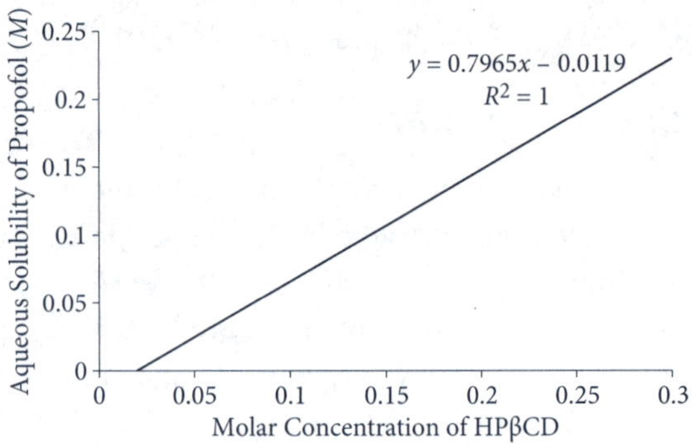

Figure 16-5. Effect of 2-hydroxylpropyl-β-cyclodextrin (HP-β-CD) on the aqueous solubility of propofol. Reprinted from: *International Journal of Pharmaceutics*, Vol 139/Issue 1–2, Giuseppe Trapani, Angela Lopedota, Massimo Franco, Andrea Latrofa, Gaetano Liso. Effect of 2-hydroxypropyl-*β*-cyclodextrin on the aqueous solubility of the anaesthetic agent propofol (2,6-diisopropylphenol), Pages No. 215–218. Copyright 1996, with permission from Elsevier.

Solubilizers

Many drugs have limited aqueous solubility and thus require the addition of cosolvents, such as those low-molecular-weight alcohols mentioned above or solubilizers to achieve certain concentrations. Commonly used solubilizers include various surfactants such as polysorbates (Tween 20 and 80), poloxamer 188, and lecithin. These agents, however, can cause significant toxic effects when used in parenteral solutions. For this reason, a group of compounds known as *cyclodextrins* has been extensively studied as solubilizing agents for parenteral preparations based on their ability to form inclusion complexes with hydrophobic drugs. Cyclodextrins are cyclic oligosaccharides derived from starch that have the shape of truncated cones. There are three basic types of cyclodextrins: α-, β-, and γ-cyclodextrins denoting rings of 6, 7, and 8 glucose units, respectively. The larger the cyclic structure, the bigger the central hydrophobic cavity for hosting a drug molecule. Both α- and γ-cyclodextrins have been used for parenteral preparations, whereas the β-cyclodextrin was found not suitable for parenteral use due to its renal toxicity, even though it is the most commonly used cyclodextrin for oral dosage forms. However, derivatives of β-cyclodextrin such as 2-hydroxylpropyl-β-cyclodextrin (HP-β-CD) have been proved safe for parenteral use. An example is Sporanox (itraconazole) injection, which contains 400 mg/mL of HP-β-CD in the formulation. The ability of 2-hydroxylpropyl-β-cyclodextrin to act as a solubilizing agent is illustrated in **Figure 16-5**, where, as can be seen, the molar aqueous solubility of propofol (2,6-diisopropylphenol), a water-insoluble anesthetic agent with a partition coefficient (log P) of 3.4, is linearly related to the increase in molar concentration of the cyclodextrin.[20]

Containers and Enclosure Systems

Various container systems are used for parenteral products: vials, ampoules, cartridges, and prefilled syringes. The most common packaging for parenteral products is the glass vial. With the exception of the ampoules, the other three container systems require the use of elastomeric components such as stoppers, plungers, or rubber disks for closures. USP has listed four different classifications for glass containers: type I, borosilicate glass; type II, treated soda lime glass; type III, soda lime glass; and NP, general-purpose soda lime glass. Type I, II, and III glasses are suitable for parenteral products, with type I glass being the preferred glass container. It is the least reactive with the formulation contents. NP is a general-purpose glass and is used for nonparenteral applications. Closures are made of natural, neoprene, or butyl rubber. Butyl rubber is commonly used due to its good oxygen/moisture barrier property. Note that natural rubber may contain latex, which can cause allergic responses in people with latex sensitivity. All container closure systems should ensure the stability of the products and provide the products with adequate protection from factors such as loss of solvent, exposure to reactive gases (e.g., oxygen), and microbial contamination.

V. Manufacturing and Quality Controls

Preparation of Parenteral Products

Parenteral solutions are prepared in a clean environment as defined by *current good manufacturing practice* (cGMP) guidelines, which requires an inspected and approved facility for parenteral product manufacturing. For heat-stable products, the following procedures are generally followed. The parenteral solution is compounded in a clean environment according to cGMP. The drug and excipients are dissolved in water for injection, or in another suitable vehicle previously discussed. The solution is adjusted with an acidifying or alkalizing agent to the desired pH. Water for injection is added to a final volume in the batch solution. The solution is filtered through one or two sterilizing-grade 0.2-μm membrane filters into a sterilized receiving vessel. After filtration, the solution is filled into sterilized vials, closed with sterilized stoppers, and sealed. It is terminally sterilized by autoclaving.

For heat-liable products, the manufacturing follows the aseptic process. In an aseptic process, the product is sterile filtered, aseptically filled into vials, and sealed. Before aseptic assembly into a final product, the individual parts of the final product are sterilized. For example, the glass vials are sterilized by dry heat, the rubber stoppers are sterilized by moist heat (autoclave), and the product solutions are sterile filtered.

Quality Controls

Sterility and Pyrogen Testing

The finished product needs to be sterile and free of pyrogen. Sterility testing is usually performed using the *membrane filtration* method. In this method, the product solution is filtered through an 0.45-μm filter. The concept behind this method is that the microorganisms will be collected onto the surface of an 0.45-μm filter. The filter is washed by filtering through a sterile fluid to remove substances that may have a bacteriostatic effect. The filter membrane is then divided and placed into test media, such as fluid thioglycollate medium (FTM) and soybean-casein digest medium (SCDM), and incubated. If the media become turbid during the 14-day incubation period, it is a positive test (readers are referred to the current USP Chapter 71 for details of the Sterility Test). Pyrogen can be tested by two methods (USP Chapter 85). In the first method, healthy rabbits are injected with the product through the ear vein, and the body temperature is monitored. The elevation of the body temperature indicates the contamination of pyrogen in the product. In the second method, the *Limulus Amebocyte Lysate* (LAL) *test* is used. LAL is an extract from the blood cells (amoebocytes) of the horseshoe crab, Limulus polyphemus. LAL reacts with the *bacterial endotoxins* and lipopolysaccharides, which are the main components of *pyrogen*. This test is more sensitive for detecting endotoxins than the rabbit test. However, some parenteral products such as oxacillin sodium, meperidine HCl, and vancomycin HCl can interfere with the LAL results, and they should be tested using the rabbit pyrogen method.

Analytical and Particulate Testing

In addition to the sterility and pyrogen tests, physiochemical and analytical determination of the quality and content of the finished products should be carried out. These tests include pH, viscosity, osmolality, solution color, content assay, impurity assay, and stability test. Finally, particulate matter should be examined, which can be done by naked eye or suitable instruments. The end user such as the nurse or the patient should check for any particles in the product before administration. The product should be discarded in case of the presence of particles.

Potential Problems

Parenteral solutions can interact with the surface of glass vials and extract elements such as silica, boron, barium, sodium, potassium, aluminum, and calcium. Some leachables from glass such as barium, calcium, and aluminum can react with the formulation (drug and/or buffers) and result in formation of particulate matter.[20, 21] The interaction of glass with citrate and phosphate buffers has been reported in the literature. Glass is not totally resistant to the action of citrates and phosphates, especially under autoclaving conditions. This can lead to pH drift and formation of insoluble salts, resulting in particulate matter (e.g., boron oxide or aluminum oxide). For this reason, the use of citrate and phosphate buffers in terminally sterilized parenteral products should be avoided.[21, 22]

Methods of Sterilization

Sterilization of pharmaceutical preparations is required for parenteral preparations. Depending on the content materials used, a product may be sterilized by steam, dry heat, filtration, or ionized radiation (e.g., gamma radiation).

Steam Sterilization

This method is called *autoclaving*. It employs water under pressure and elevated temperature. It is performed in an autoclave, a closed chamber. The pressurized system leads to higher boiling point of water, which causes microorganism death through coagulation of proteins in bacterial cells at high temperature. Usually, the sterilization requires 15 min at 121°C. For a large package, it may require a longer time period. The primary applications of the autoclave are for sterilization of equipment, processing tubing, filters, rubber stoppers, and final product if the product is heat-stable. It is not suitable for sterilization of dry substances because of the presence of steam.

Dry Heat Sterilization

This method is less efficient and requires longer exposure time and higher temperature (for example, 180°C for 45 min) than steam sterilization. It is performed in an oven. The mechanism of microorganism destruction is primarily the result of an oxidation process at high temperature. The dry heat method is used for sterilizing items such as glass containers, vials, stainless steel items, oils, and dry powders, and for removing pyrogens (depyrogenation), which cannot be removed by sterile filtration or autoclaving. The minimum time and temperature for depyrogenation is 30 min at 250°C. Pyrogens are water-soluble, can easily pass through 0.22-μm filters, and are also stable at the autoclaving temperature. In general, it is difficult to remove pyrogens from products once they are present. Therefore it is important to first remove the pyrogens from the individual ingredients, especially water, and then prevent *pyrogen contamination* during the manufacturing processes.

Sterilization by Filtration

Filtration is a common method of sterilization for drug product solutions. The microorganisms and visible particulate matter are removed by filtration using a sterile filter of 0.22-mm pore size. Most of the bacteria are 0.5–5.0 mm in length. Among the smallest bacteria are members of the genus Mycoplasma, which measure at about 0.2–0.3 μm. This method is used to sterilize product solutions that are not heat-stable such as protein and peptide products. The commonly used filters in manufacturing sterile dosage forms include PVDF (polyvinylidene fluoride), nylon, cellulose esters, and PES (polyethersulfone). By filtration, both the live and dead microorganisms can be removed. However, the sterility of the filtered solution is not guaranteed since the membrane filters used might be flawed or defective. It is important that integrity testing be performed before and after filtration to ensure that the filter has no defects such as leaks or perforations that might have occurred during the filtration.

Most 25- to 33-mm syringe disk filters used in pharmacy compounding can filter a volume up to 100 mL. For filtering a larger volume (> 100 mL) of solution, a cartridge filter with greater surface areas may be required. Filtering of a viscous solution will require more time. Some filter membranes such as cellulose acetate may adsorb the drug to lower the concentration of the preparation. However, it is convenient and quick and is used in clinical pharmacies for the preparation of sterile products in a laminar flow hood.

Ionized Radiation Sterilization

This method uses ionized radiation (e.g., gamma rays) to destroy microorganisms. It is used for drug products that cannot withstand high temperature or solids that cannot be filtered through the 0.22-mm membrane.

VI. Chapter Summary

Parenteral dosage forms provide unique advantages for drug delivery, especially for emergency cases and drugs that cannot be well absorbed through other delivery routes. The bioavailability of drug by injections is usually 100%. Modern drug delivery concepts such as using microsphere, nanoparticle, and in situ gel preparations must consider how such dosage forms will be administered. It is likely that targeted delivery will be more feasible through injections than through other routes, suggesting that such preparations must adhere to the parenteral drug delivery principles. Parenteral preparations are sterile and are free of pyrogen and visual particulate matter in solutions, which requires a strict and high-standard manufacturing process and aseptic technique during administration.

VII. References

1. Wright JC, Tao Leonard S, Stevenson CL, et al. An in vivo/in vitro comparison with a leuprolide osmotic implant for the treatment of prostate cancer. *J Control Release*. 75:1–10, 2001.
2. Choi S, Baudys M, and Kim SW. Control of blood glucose by novel GLP-1 delivery using biodegradable triblock copolymer of PLGA-PEG-PLGA in type 2 diabetic rats. *Pharm Res*. 21:827–831, 2004.

3. Barichello JM, Morishita M, Takayama K, and Nagai T. Absorption of insulin from Pluronic F-127 gels following subcutaneous administration in rats. *Int J Pharm.* 184:189–198, 1999.
4. Eli Lilly and Company. Humalog Mix75/25. 2009. http://pi.lilly.com/us/humalog7525-pi.pdf, accessed on 7/12/2011.
5. Uraki J, Yamakado K, Nakatsuka A, and Takeda K. Transcatheter hepatic arterial chemoembolization for hepatocellular carcinoma invading the portal veins: Therapeutic effects and prognostic factors. *Eur J Radiol.* 51:12–18, 2004.
6. Bruix J, Llovet JM, Castells A, et al. Transarterial embolization versus symptomatic treatment in patients with advanced hepatocellular carcinoma: results of a randomized, controlled trial in a single institution, *Hepatology.* 27:1578–1583, 1998.
7. Bruix J, Sala M, and Llovet JM. Chemoembolization for hepatocellular carcinoma. *Gastroenterology.* 127:S179–S188, 2004.
8. Gadaleta CD and Ranieri G. Trans-arterial chemoembolization as a therapy for liver tumours: New clinical developments and suggestions for combination with angiogenesis inhibitors. *Crit Rev Oncol Hematol.* 80:40–53, 2011.
9. Hong SS, Abe Y, Kaneta K, and Matsuzawa T. Combined treatment of radiation and local injections of misonidazole. *Int J Radiat Oncol Biol Phys.* 10:2369–2373, 1984.
10. Shiina S, Teratani T, Obi S, Hamamura K, Koike Y, and Omata M. Percutaneous ethanol injection therapy for liver tumors. *Eur J Ultrasound.* 13:95–106, 2001.
11. Fotiadis NI, Sabharwal T, Morales JP, Hodgson DJ, O'Brien TS, and Adam A. Combined percutaneous radiofrequency ablation and ethanol injection of renal tumours: Midterm results. *Eur Urol.* 52:777–784, 2007.
12. Valat JP and Rozenberg S. Local corticosteroid injections for low back pain and sciatica. *Joint Bone Spine.* 75:403–407, 2008.
13. Akers MJ. Excipient-drug interactions in parenteral formulations. *J Pharm Sci.* 91:2283–2297, 2002.
14. Nema S, Washkuhn, RJ, and Brendel, RJ. Excipients and their use in injectable products. *PDA J Pharm Sci Technol.* 51:166–171, 1997.
15. Flynn GL. Buffers: pH control within pharmaceutical systems. *J Parenteral Drug Assoc.* 34:139–162, 1980.
16. Wang YJ and Kowal RR. Review of excipients and pH's for parenteral products used in the United States. *J Parenteral Drug Assoc.* 34:452–462, 1980.
17. Strickley RG. Parenteral formulations of small molecules therapeutics marketed in the United States (1999)—Part I. *PDA J Pharm Sci Technol.* 53:324–349, 1999.
18. Carpenter JF, Pikal MJ, Chang BS, and Randolph TW. Rational design of stable lyophilized protein formulations: Some practical advice. *Pharm Res.* 14:969–975, 1997.
19. Pikal-Cleland KA, Cleland JL, Anchordoquy TJ, and Carpenter, JF. Effect of glycine on pH changes and protein stability during freezing-thawing in phosphate buffer systems. *J Pharm Sci.* 91:1969–1979, 2002.
20. Trapani G, Lopedota A, Franco M, Latrofa A, and Liso G. Effect of 2-hydroxypropyl-β-cyclodextrin on the aqueous solubility of the anaesthetic agent propofol (2,6-diisopropylphenol). *Int J Pharm.* 139:215–218, 1996.
21. Borchert SJ, Abe A, Aldrich DS, Fox LE, and Freeman JE. Particulate matter in parenteral products: A review. *J Parenteral Sci Technol.* 40:212–241, 1986.
22. Borchert SJ, Ryan MM, Davison RL, and Speed W. Accelerated extractable studies of borosilicate glass containers. *J Parenteral Sci Technol.* 43:67–79, 1989.

Recommended Readings

Akers MJ: *Sterile Drug Products: Formulation, Packaging, Manufacturing and Quality.* New York, Informa Healthcare, 2010.

Gupta PK and Brazeau GA (eds): *Injectable Drug Development: Techniques to Reduce Pain and Irritation.* Englewood, CO, Interpharm Press, 1999.

Shrewsbury R: Sterile compound formulations: Routes of administration, in: *Applied Pharmaceutics in Contemporary Compounding,* Englewood, CO, Morton Publishing Company, 2008, 2nd ed, chapter 24.

Strickley RG: Solubilizing excipients in oral and injectable formulations. *Pharm Res.* 21:201–230, 2004.

VIII. Homework Problems

1. What are the ranges of (*a*) injection volume, (*b*) the acceptable pH, and (*c*) the estimated time to reach peak absorption for SVP solutions when given by IV, IM, and SC injections?
2. Name the five special requirements for a parenteral product.
3. Which of the following are complications of intravenous administration?
   a. Phlebitis
   b. Thrombosis
   c. Air emboli
   d. Precipitation
   e. Infiltration
4. Must preservatives be added to all parenteral products?
5. What are the intended uses of Kollidon 17 PF (polyvinylpyrrolidone), benzyl alcohol, and propylene glycol in the following injectable solution? Show how you would prepare the solution.

Diclofenac Injectable Solution (25 mg/mL)		
Ingredients	**Quantity, per mL**	**Batch size, 1000 mL**
Diclofenac sodium	25 mg	25 g
Kollidon 17 PF	17 mg	17 g
Benzyl alcohol	40 mg	40 g
Propylene glycol	160 mg	160 g
Water for injection	q.s. to 1 mL	q.s. to 1000 mL

6. Describe the purpose of each excipient in the formulation.

Ingredients	**Quantity, per mL**
Epoetin alfa	20,000 units
Albumin (human)	2.5 mg
Sodium citrate	1.3 mg
Citric acid	0.11 mg
Sodium chloride	8.2 mg
Benzyl alcohol	10 mg
Water for injection q.s.	1 mL

7. Which of the following statements are true?
   a. Water for injection is sterile.
   b. Water for injection is pyrogen-free.
   c. Water for injection is free of particulate matter.
   d. Bacteriostatic water for injection contains a preservative.
8. You have formulated an injectable solution for SC administration with an osmolality reading of 220 mosmol/L. Is this formulation a hypotonic, isotonic, or hypertonic solution? How can you make this solution isotonic?
9. According to USP, what are the five types of injectable products?
10. Can an oil solution be administered parenterally? How is drug absorbed from such a dosage form?
11. Describe the usage of filtration and autoclaving in the preparation of parenteral products.
12. What are pyrogens of pharmaceutical significance? How can you make pyrogen-free water?
13. What are the two commonly used methods to test pyrogen in injections? Discuss the advantages and disadvantages of both.
14. Give an example of a solubilizer for parenteral preparations and its action on increasing the solubility of the drug.
15. What is the acceptable solid content in Water for Injection, USP? What may be the acceptable particle size in a parenteral solution?
16. What are the quality control tests for parenteral products?

CHAPTER 17

Delivery of Biotechnology Products

Sudjit Luanpitpong and Yon Rojanasakul

Recent advances in molecular biotechnology have provided greater understanding of disease pathogenesis at the cellular and molecular levels. This opens up the possibility of defining molecular dysfunctions and drug targets for several major disorders, leading to the discovery of a large number of drugs with macromolecular properties. Macromolecular drugs including recombinant proteins and nucleic acids hold great promise as novel therapeutics mainly on the basis of their site-specific activity and reduced side effects. However, successful development of these agents still remains a challenge. This chapter reviews key aspects and factors essential for the development of this new class of drugs, which are different from those of conventional drugs with small-molecule properties. As macromolecular drugs are poorly absorbed and rapidly metabolized in the body, enormous challenges for drug delivery are encountered. This chapter focuses on key barriers to macromolecular drug delivery and approaches to overcome these barriers. Also discussed in this chapter are the special interests for insulin delivery and targeted delivery for cancer therapy.

CHAPTER OUTLINE

OBJECTIVES

1. Describe the major factors contributing to the instability of protein and peptide drugs.
2. Describe the strategies for oral protein and peptide drug delivery and their alternate routes of administration.
3. Characterize the various classes of nucleic acid therapeutics and their mechanisms of action.
4. Describe the physiological barriers for efficient macromolecular delivery.
5. Understand the concept of drug delivery systems for nucleic acid therapeutics.

I. Protein and Peptide Drug Delivery

Protein is a class of organic macromolecules that perform a wide range of cellular functions. Proteins have a defined sequence of amino acid, defined by the sequence of a gene and a three-dimensional structure. Amino acids are joined in a form of polymer by the peptide bonds between the carboxyl and amino groups of adjacent amino acid residues (**Figure 17-1**). *Peptide* is a short linear chain of amino acid residues also with a defined sequence.

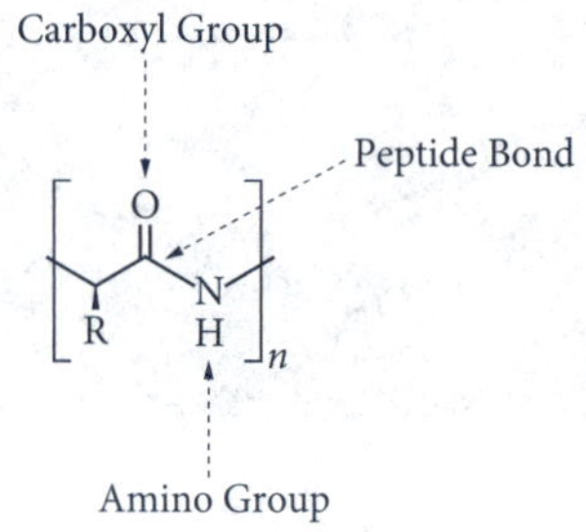

Figure 17-1 Chemical structure of the protein repeating unit in a peptide.

Structure of Proteins

Protein structures have four increasing orders of complexity: primary, secondary, and tertiary structure and quaternary form (**Figure 17-2**). The *primary structure* refers to the order in which the individual amino acids are arranged and bound together by peptide bonds. *Secondary structure* occurs when the sequence of amino acids is linked by hydrogen bonds between the backbone amides and carboxyl groups as a coiled α-helix or a β-pleated sheet. *Tertiary structure* refers to the three-dimensional arrangement of a single protein molecule when certain α-helix and β-sheets are folded into a compact globule. *Quaternary form* is the assembly of several ternary forms of protein molecules or polypeptide chains.

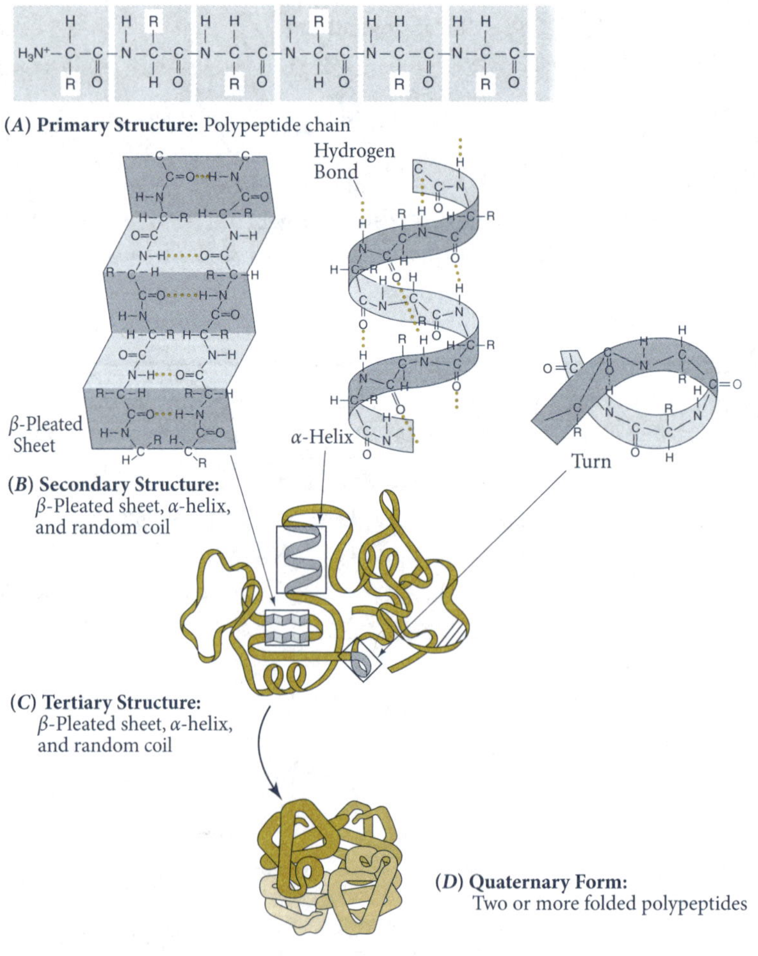

Figure 17-2 Diagrammatic representation of protein structure.

Stability of Proteins and Peptides

A major problem associated with the use of proteins and peptides is their instability during storage and manufacturing. Instability of proteins can be classified into two distinct classes: physical instability and chemical instability. *Physical instability* mainly results from changes in the higher-order structure of proteins (secondary protein structure and above). *Chemical instability* is the modification of the protein molecule via bond formation or cleavage, resulting in the formation of a new chemical structure. Peptides, however, degrade only by chemical processes.[1, 2]

Physical Instability

Physical instability is characterized by structural changes due to the polymeric nature of proteins and their ability to assemble some form of superstructure. Thus, physical instability is less of a problem in the case of small-molecule drugs. Proteins can undergo a variety of physical instability processes, some of which are listed below.

Denaturation

Denaturation is the disruption of secondary and tertiary structures of a protein leading to unfolding of its structure. Denaturation can be reversible or irreversible, where the original structure cannot be recovered. In general, globular proteins fold in such a way that the exposure of hydrophobic groups is lessened. Thus, denatured proteins are generally insoluble in an aqueous solution. Apart from the decrease in solubility, denaturation may also result in loss of biological activity, changes in molecular shape, and susceptibility to enzymatic reactions. Factors affecting the denaturation of proteins are temperature, pH, and presence of organic solvents such as alcohol and acetone.

Aggregation

Protein molecules may self-associate in an aqueous medium to form oligomers. Factors affecting protein aggregation are pH, solvent composition, ionic strength, and solvent dielectric properties. In addition, denaturants induce protein aggregation through the formation of unfolded intermediates. Aggregation is also important in determining drug action. For example, the zinc hexamer of insulin confers its long-acting properties. Conversely, some proteins such as growth hormone and interferon-γ are inactive when aggregated.

Surface Adsorption and Precipitation

Precipitation, the macroscopic equivalent of aggregation, usually occurs with protein denaturation, which facilitates the precipitation process. Insulin is known to adsorb onto the surface of containers, either glass or plastic, thus reducing the amount of insulin being delivered. At air/water interfaces, insulin could undergo further denaturation, causing precipitation and physical blockage of the delivery ports.

The physical stability of proteins could be improved through pharmaceutical formulations. For example, to prevent protein adsorption, additives such as serum albumin and some surfactants (e.g., poloxamers and polysorbate) are commonly used to prevent the binding of proteins to containers. As mentioned above, protein denaturation can occur at the air/water interface; therefore minimization of air exposure helps prevent protein denaturation. Protein denaturation can also be minimized by the addition of cosolvents such as polyethylene glycol and glycerol. Optimization of pH is also critical to avoid stability problems arising from charge neutralization and to ensure adequate aqueous solubility.

Chemical Instability

Deamidation

Deamidation is the reaction when the side-chain group of glutamine (Gln) or asparagine (Asn) is hydrolyzed to form a free carboxylic acid. Deamidation can alter biological activity and protein function. Proteins undergoing deamidation include human growth hormone, insulin, adrenocorticotropic hormone (ACTH), prolactin, and lysozyme.

Oxidation

Oxidation is one of the major causes of protein degradation. Factors affecting protein oxidation are pH, temperature, trace metals (catalysts), and buffers. Proteins containing histidine (His), methionine (Met), cysteine (Cys), tryptophan (Trp), and tyrosine (Tyr) residues are susceptible to oxidation. Methionine is highly sensitive to oxidation, and histidine is susceptible to oxidation in the presence of metals. Oxidation of the thiol group of cysteine represents the typical oxidative reaction as it readily reacts with oxygen to yield sulfenic acid (RSOH). Oxidation of proteins often results in a complete or partial loss of biological activity; thus minimizing protein oxidation is essential to the therapeutic use of proteins.

Racemization

Racemization is a process of conversion of L-amino acid to D, L mixtures. All amino acid residues except glycine (Gly) are subject to base-catalyzed racemization.

Proteolysis

Proteolysis leads to the cleavage of peptide bonds, often resulting in loss of biological activity. Aspartic acid (Asp) is the most labile residue to proteolysis as its carboxyl group is considered to be an intramolecular catalyst.

β-Elimination

Inactivation of proteins at high temperature is often due to the destruction of disulfide bonds from the cysteine residue as a result of β-elimination. Side chains containing serine (Ser), threonine (Thr), phenylalanine (Phe), and lysine (Lys) are prone to β-elimination under alkaline conditions.

Disulfide Formation

The interchange of disulfide bonds can lead to incorrect pairings, changes in three-dimensional structure, and rapid loss of biological activity.

Routes of Protein and Peptide Delivery

Due to some unique properties and restrictions, proteins and peptides are usually not therapeutically active when given orally. Development of successful delivery systems for proteins and peptides depends on the understanding of their physicochemical and biological properties. Some general considerations for the development of effective delivery systems are as follows[3]:

- *Molecular weight:* The larger the molecular weight or size, the lower the permeation rate of the molecule across biological membranes.
- *Immunogenicity:* Alterations of protein structure and composition might trigger allergic and immunologic responses.

Table 17-1 Factors Affecting Oral Delivery of Protein and Peptide Drugs

Structure	Physicochemical Factors	Physiological Factors
Molecular weight and size	Solubility	pH
Shape and conformation	Partition coefficient	Digestive enzymes
Electrostatic charge	Aggregation	Mucosal barrier
	Stability	Intestinal permeability
		Transport mechanisms
		Metabolism—gut and hepatic
		Dietary factors

- *Conformational stability:* Changes in protein conformation likely affect their biological activity.
- *Half-life:* Rapid degradation of proteins by proteolytic enzymes and rapid clearance by liver and kidney might occur.
- *Mechanism of drug action:* Precise mechanism of action and drug target are critical.
- *Others:* There are significant individual variables in pharmacokinetics and pharmacodynamics.

Oral Delivery

In general, an oral administration is preferred over other methods of administration because of its ease of delivery and patient compliance, i.e., compared to injection. However, oral bioavailability of protein drugs is extremely low, typically less than 1%. Two main reasons for this poor bioavailability are (1) instability of proteins and peptides in the gastrointestinal (GI) tract due to enzymatic digestion and (2) poor permeability of the intestinal epithelial membrane to large molecules.[4]

An orally administered protein must be able to resist both chemical and enzymatic degradation in the GI tract and to penetrate the mucosal membrane to be effective therapeutically. Once absorbed, the drug molecule should be able to avoid hepatic first-pass metabolism and clearance by gut mucosa and liver. Factors influencing protein drug delivery are listed in **Table 17-1**.

Several approaches have been used to overcome the GI tract barriers of protein and peptide drugs in order to improve their oral bioavailability. These approaches include the following:

Enzyme Inhibition

Coadministration of protease inhibitors is one possible approach to improve enzyme stability and thus intestinal absorption of protein drugs. Coadministration of insulin with bacitracin, sodium glycocholate, camostat mesilate, FK-448, and other protease inhibitors has been shown to increase insulin absorption.[5,6] However, long-term effects of protease inhibitors need to be evaluated as they may cause undesirable side effects.

Permeation Enhancers

Bile salts and fatty acids are the most common penetration enhancers for increasing the permeability of intestinal epithelium, likely via the transcellular route. Penetration enhancers that destabilize or weaken the intestinal epithelium tight junctions facilitating the paracellular transport of proteins are also available, based on detergent-like molecules and micelles such as pluronic acid.[7] In addition, zonula occluden toxin has been demonstrated effectively to open the tight junctions in a reversible manner and improve the permeation of insulin.[8] However, these penetration enhancers could impair or damage the GI barrier and increase the risk of local inflammation and infection.

Delivery Systems

Entrapment of protein and peptide drugs in delivery systems such as liposomes and micro- and nanoparticles is one of the most common strategies for oral protein delivery. These delivery systems offer the many advantages including these[9]:

1. They protect the drugs from enzymatic degradation and reduce their systemic clearance.
2. They enhance drug solubility.
3. They provide controlled drug release and minimize undesirable side effects.
4. They improve biodistribution of the drugs.
5. They lower the immunogenicity of the drugs.
6. They reduce acute toxicity due to the initial burst of the drugs.
7. They target the drugs to their site of action.

PEGylation

PEGylation is a process of attachment of polyethylene glycol (PEG) to a molecule that has been shown to improve the enzymatic stability of various proteins such as tumor necrosis factor, epidermal growth factor, and interferon. Such improvement is the result of increased molecular mass and lowered renal clearance, steric hindrance to proteolytic enzymes, and phagocytosis avoidance.[10]

Structure Modification

Terminal modification of proteins and peptides, commonly N-acetylation and C-amidation, in many cases can increase enzymatic stability. However, it might lead to the loss of biological activity as well. Another modification strategy is the replacement of labile amino acids in the polypeptide chain with those that are resistant to enzymatic degradation.[11]

Development of Oral Dosage Forms

Based on the discussion given above, a number of strategies have been used to improve the stability and oral absorption of proteins and peptides through the use of micro- and nanoparticulate systems.

Lipid-Based Drug Delivery Systems

Liposomes are spherical vesicles made of phospholipid bilayers that can entrap drug molecules between the bilayers. Cationic liposomes are most widely used due to the electrostatic interaction between the negatively charged molecules and the positively charged lipids, yielding a stable complex. Typically, the complex carries a net positive charge and is attracted to the negatively charged plasma membrane (and to other negatively charged molecules such as serum proteins). Common problems associated with the use of cationic liposomes are cytotoxicity and nonspecific binding. Liposomes have increasingly been used as a delivery system for protein-based cancer therapy. Proteins such as Bak, which can induce cancer cell death by causing cytochrome c release and caspase activation, have been shown to be effective when delivered as liposomal preparations.[12] However, in vivo efficacy of the system needs further evaluations as in vitro efficacy does not warrant in vivo performance. Other lipid-based systems for protein delivery include *solid–lipid nanoparticles* and *microemulsions*. An oral formulation of calcitonin and human growth hormone in a microemulsion system has been developed and tested in humans for commercialization under the name Macromol.[6]

Table 17-2 Biodegradable Polymers Used in Protein and Peptide Drug Delivery

Natural Polymers	Synthetic Polymers
Albumin	Maleic anhydride–alkyl vinyl ether copolymers
Alginate	Pluronic polyols
Cellulose derivatives	Poly(acrylic acid)
Collage	Poly(amino acids)
Fibrin	Poly(anhydrides)
Gelatin	Poly(depsipeptide)
Hyaluronic acid	Poly(esters): poly(lactic acid) (PLA), poly(lactic-*co*-glycolic acid) (PLGA), poly(β-hydroxybutyrate), poly(caprolactone), poly(dioxanone)
Polysaccharides	Poly(ethylene glycol)
	Poly(hydroxypropyl)methacrylamide
	Poly[(organo)phosphazene]
	Poly(ortho esters)
	Poly(vinyl alcohol)

Biodegradable Polymeric Delivery Systems

Several types of biodegradable polymer can be used for the preparation of protein and peptide delivery systems, as listed in **Table 17-2.**[13] Biodegradable polymers have the advantage over nonbiodegradable polymers of eliminating the need for postdelivery removal of the polymer. The mode of polymer degradation, depending on the material type and design, can be classified as bulk erosion, surface erosion, hydration and solubilization, and cleavage of specific linkages designed into the polymer–protein conjugates. *Microparticles* and *nanoparticles* are the most desirable types of delivery system. Poly(lactic acid) and poly(glycolic acid) homo- and copolymers are currently the most commonly used. The copolymers, poly(lactic-*co*-glycolic acid) (PLGA) of varying molecular weight, are biodegradable and biocompatible and also show potential properties for controlled-release applications. Peptide-containing PLGA microparticles previously have been reported to prevent the allergic sensitivity to the whole peptide and to have an initial burst release of the peptide followed by a slow and sustained release.[14] Another promising approach is the coating of protein and peptide with a polymer cross-linked with an azoaromatic group, which is resistant to acidic and enzymatic degradation in the stomach and small intestine.[13] Once entering the colon, these polymers are reduced by indigenous microflora and release the drug for absorption (**Figure 17-3**). Oral administration of vasopressin and insulin in a gelatin capsule coated with azopolymer produces biological responses in animal studies.

Alternative Routes of Administration

Parenteral Route

Although oral administration is the preferred method of protein drug administration, almost all commercial products are in parenteral dosage forms, as it provides greater bioavailability and therapeutic efficacy. Because many proteins undergo hydrolysis or form aggregates in an aqueous

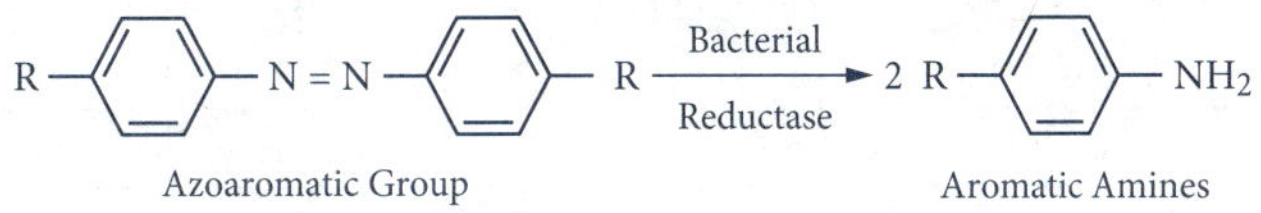

Figure 17-3 Reduction of the azo bonds to amines by reductases from bacteria residing in the colon.

Table 17-3 Alternative Routes of Administration for Protein and Peptide Drugs

Route	Advantages	Disadvantages
Nasal	Easily accessible Fast uptake Lower proteolytic activity than GI tract Avoidance of first-pass metabolism	Lack of reproducibility, particularly under pathological conditions Low bioavailability for large protein and peptide molecules Inappropriate for highly potent drugs
Pulmonary	Relatively easy to access Fast uptake Large absorptive surface area Highly permeable blood barrier Lower proteolytic activity than GI tract Avoidance of first-pass metabolism	Lack of reproducibility, particularly under pathological conditions Presence of macrophages with high affinity for drug delivery carriers
Rectal	Relatively easy to access Partial avoidance of first-pass metabolism Suitable for drugs that irritate GI mucosa Allows large-dose administration	Low bioavailability for drugs with large molecular size
Buccal	Easily accessible Avoidance of first-pass metabolism	Ineffective for large protein and peptide molecules even in the presence of penetration enhancers
Transdermal	Easily accessible Large available surface area Low proteolytic activity Avoidance of first-pass metabolism	Low bioavailability because of the strong barrier property of the skin and the high degree of lipophilicity of the stratum corneum

solution, they are often formulated as lyophilized powders. Lyophilization is a method of drying proteins without destroying their three-dimensional structure. Briefly, the protein solution is frozen and then warmed under a vacuum so that the ice sublimes.[2]

Nonparenteral Route

Because proteins and peptides generally exhibit a very short biological half-life, repeated administration through the parenteral (invasive) route is undesirable, especially for long-term treatment. Consequently, several alternative routes of administration have been explored and utilized. The advantages and disadvantages of these routes are summarized in **Table 17-3**.[1,4]

Therapeutic Proteins and Peptides

Recombinant DNA technology has made possible the large-scale production of protein drugs. Thus far, the U.S. Food and Drug Administration has approved nearly 100 protein drugs, and many are in clinical trials. Some of the commonly used protein drugs are listed in **Table 17-4**.

Table 17-4 Some Therapeutic Proteins and Peptides, Their Trade Names, and Their Indications

Protein/Peptide	Trade Name (Manufacturer)	Indications
α_1-Antitrypsin	Aralast (Baxter)	Cystic fibrosis therapy
Albumin	Plasbumin (Talecris)	Plasma volume expander
Calcitonin	Miacalcin (Novartis)	Calcium regulation, osteoporosis
DNase	Pulmozyme (Genentech)	Cystic fibrosis therapy

Protein/Peptide	Trade Name (Manufacturer)	Indications
Erythropoietin α	Epogen (Amgen)	Anemia
Factor VIII	Alphanate (Grifols), KoGENate (Bayer)	Hemophilia
Glucagon	GlucaGen (Nova Nordisk)	Diabetes therapy
Growth hormone	Portropin (Genentech), Humatope (Lilly)	Growth acceleration
Hirudin	Refludan (Bayer)	Management of thromboembolic disease
Insulin	Humulin (Lilly), Velosulin (Nova Nordisk)	Diabetes therapy
Interferon α-2a	Referon A (Hoffman LaRoche)	Leukemia
Interferon α-2b	Intron A (Schering-Plough)	Leukemia, hepatitis therapy
Interferon β-1	Betaseron (Berlex)	Multiple sclerosis
Interleukin-2	Proleukin (Chiron)	Melanoma, carcinoma
Leuprolide acetate	Lupron (Abbott)	Prostatic carcinoma
Octreotide	Sandostatin (Novartis)	Growth inhibition
Oxytocin	Pitocin, Syntocinon	Labor induction (uterine contraction)
Parathyroid hormone	Forteo (Lilly)	Calcium regulation
Tissue plasminogen activator (t-PA)	Activase (Genentech)	Management of acute myocardial infarction (fibrinolytic agent)
Vascular endothelial growth factor antibody	Avastin (Genentech)	Various forms of cancer (antiangiogenesis)
Vasopressin	Pitressin (Parke Davis)	Diuresis

II. Nucleic Acid Therapeutics

Nucleic acid sequence plays a critical role in the expression of a gene, which is encoded for the synthesis of RNA and subsequent protein. Briefly, a specific gene is transcribed from DNA to form a messenger RNA (mRNA) that has a complementary base sequence. Translation of mRNA by transfer RNA (tRNA) at the ribosome then carries out the protein synthesis. Modulating gene expression or protein synthesis at the transcriptional or posttranscriptional level has gained interest as a novel therapeutic strategy for several major diseases including cardiovascular diseases, inflammation, and cancer. Nucleic acid therapeutics can be classified into various types based on the target site and mechanism of action, as summarized in **Figure 17-4**.

Therapeutic Classes

Deoxyribonucleic Acid

Substitution of a defective or missing gene with a functional one is the straightforward goal of *gene therapy*. Accordingly, gene or DNA delivery is becoming the main focus of gene therapy. Therapeutic DNAs must cross extracellular and intracellular barriers to reach their target site in the nucleus, where transcription would take place.

Transcription Factor Decoy

Short, double-strand (ds) DNA decoy molecules have been used to disrupt gene expression at the level of transcription.[15] These decoy oligonucleotides containing a *cis*-transcription recognition sequence competitively bind to transcription factors, resulting in the decreased activation of gene promoter and reduced gene transcription. One drawback of the DNA decoy is the potential

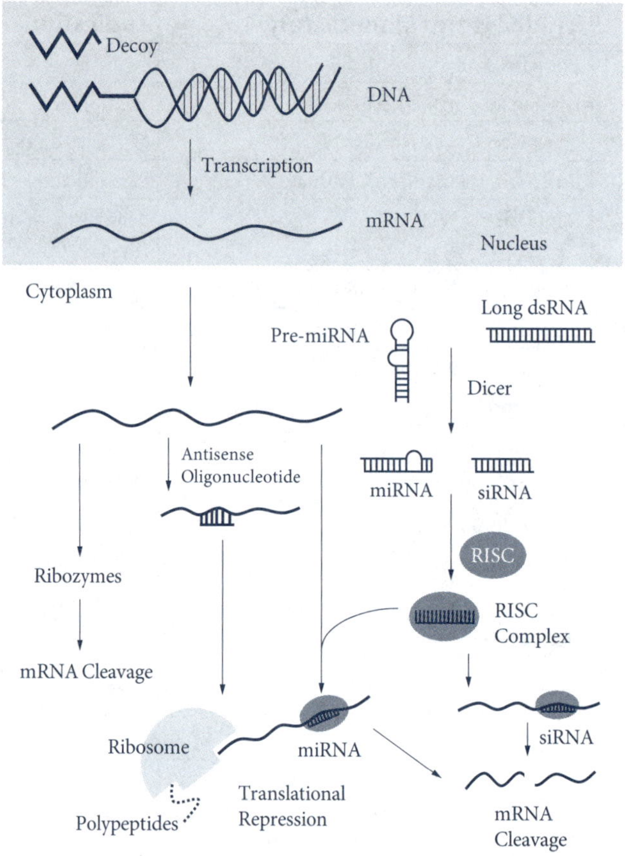

Figure 17-4 Diagrammatic representation of different nucleic acid therapeutics.

unwanted side effects from multiple signaling pathways and biological functions that might be regulated under a single transcription factor.[9]

RNA Interference

RNA interference (RNAi) or posttranscriptional gene silencing is a naturally occurring defense mechanism in eukaryotic organisms. RNAi is activated by long double-strand (ds) RNAs (approximately 500–1000 nucleotides), which are processed into 21–25 nucleotides called *short interfering RNA* (siRNA) by the enzyme Dicer (RNase III nuclease).[16] Then siRNA is incorporated into a multicomponent nuclease complex called RISC (RNA-induced silencing complex) present in the cytosol, forming a guide sequence that targets the RISC to a desired mRNA and promotes its destruction (Figure 17-4). For therapeutic purposes, synthetic siRNAs can be introduced directly to the cells or via an in vivo generation of siRNAs and *short hairpin RNAs* (shRNAs) from a plasmid DNA construct. In addition, *microRNAs* (miRNAs), naturally occurring endogenous short, double-strand noncoding RNA molecules, have been discovered.[17] Recent studies suggest that more than 1000 miRNAs are encoded in the human genome, which target about 60% of all genes. The miRNAs bind to a complementary sequence of target mRNA transcripts, resulting in translational repression and/or mRNA degradation (Figure 17-4).

Antisense and Antigene Oligonucleotides

An *antisense oligonucleotide* is an oligonucleotide that has a reverse-complementary sequence to the target mRNA. It hybridizes to the mRNA via Watson–Crick base-pairing, forming an mRNA–antisense duplex. The duplex blocks translation of a completed message and recruits the activation

Table 17-5 Comparison of Anti-mRNA Strategies

	Antisense Oligonucleotides	siRNA/miRNA	Ribozymes/DNAzymes
Structure	Short (~15–25 nt) Single-strand	Short (~21–25 nt) Double-strand	Three-dimensional catalytic motif
Mechanism of action	Hybridization to target mRNA	Incorporated into RISC, guiding nuclease to target mRNA	Catalyze cleavage of RNAs by chemical reactions

of endogenous nucleases such as RNase-H, which leads to the destruction of the mRNA strand.[18] An antigene oligonucleotide is an oligonucleotide that binds to double-strand DNA to form a DNA–antigene triplex, thus inhibiting transcription. For a specific binding to its target, both antisense and antigene oligonucleotides require a minimum length of about 10 nucleotides; however, the most common length is 15–25 nucleotides.

Ribozymes and DNAzymes

Ribozymes (RNA enzymes) and DNAzymes (DNA enzymes) are oligonucleotides with catalytic activity. These catalytic oligonucleotides bind to target mRNA in an antisense fashion and cleave or edit RNA molecules through chemical reactions such as hydrolysis and transesterification reactions. Several classes of ribozyme motifs have been identified, including hammerhead, hairpin, group I and II intron, ribonuclease P, and hepatitis delta virus ribozymes. Hammerhead and hairpin ribozymes have been extensively studied owing to their small size and rapid kinetics. Theoretically, ribozymes might have an advantage over RNase-H-dependent antisense oligonucleotides; however, this has not been shown consistently in vivo.[16] For DNAzymes, after binding to the RNA substrate, it would cleave sequences that contain purine–pyrimidine junctions. DNAzymes have some theoretical advantages over RNAzymes as DNA is more stable than RNA and as DNAzymes are easier to synthesize.

Comparison of the various anti-mRNA strategies is summarized in **Table 17-5**.

Physiological Barriers

As polyanionic macromolecules, all nucleic acid therapeutics face a series of barriers, both intracellular and extracellular, before reaching their target site (**Figure 17-5**). These barriers must be overcome for effective delivery of the therapeutic molecules.

Extracellular Barriers

For systemic delivery, drug molecules must navigate the circulatory system of the body while avoiding rapid clearance by endogenous nucleases, renal filtration, uptake by phagocytes, and aggregation with serum proteins. As nucleic acids are easily degraded by nucleases, they must be protected, i.e., by condensation or encapsulation with appropriate agents.

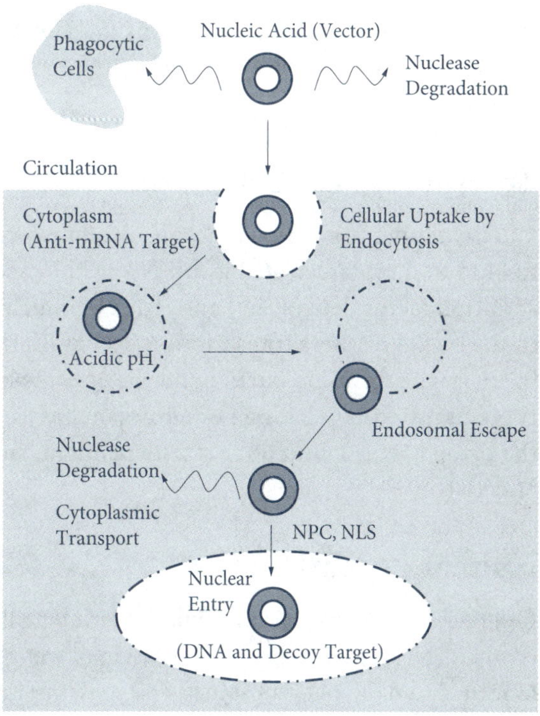

Figure 17-5 Physiological barriers for the delivery of nucleic acid therapeutics.

Phagocytic cells serve as a significant immunological barrier in the reticuloendothelial system (RES), not only in the bloodstream but also in the extracellular matrix of tissues. Phagocytes such as macrophages and monocytes effectively engulf and remove foreign materials, including drug carriers and macromolecules. Furthermore, to reach their target, drug molecules must overcome the vasculature barrier through extravasation, avoiding the lymphatic drainage and penetrating the interstitium. In general, molecules larger than 5 nm in diameter do not readily cross the capillary endothelium, and thus they remain in the circulation until they are cleared from the body or enter some tissues. Liver, spleen, and some tumors allow passage of molecules up to 200 nm in diameter; accordingly they might be considered as potential organ targets for systemic delivery of macromolecules.

Another barrier to the effective delivery of drugs is the lack of target cell selectivity. The requirement for cellular selectivity may vary, depending on the cell target. Great efforts have been made to achieve targeted drug delivery through the use of monoclonal antibodies and various membrane-bound receptors.

Local delivery to the target site of action offers certain advantages including higher bioavailability owing to greater target accessibility and reduced side effects. Potential organ targets for topical delivery are eye, skin, and mucous tissues and for direct delivery are lung, brain, spinal cord, and isolated tumor.[16]

Intracellular Barriers

Internalization and Endosomal Escape

Drug molecules must enter target cells in order to exert their therapeutic effects. This process normally occurs through endocytosis, in which drug molecules are engulfed in the endocytic vesicles with acidic pH (~ 5.5) and en route to lysosomes filled with digestive enzymes. Several strategies have been used to facilitate the endosomal escape of nucleic acids. For example, the cationic polymer polyethyleneimine (PEI) acts as a *proton sponge* to facilitate endosomal disruption. The large buffering capacity of the nonprotonated amino groups of PEI (pH 5–7) causes a large influx of hydrogen ions by endosomal ATPase. As protons enter the endosome along with the concurrent influx of chloride ions to maintain electroneutrality, water diffuses via osmosis, leading to osmotic swelling, endosomal burst, and subsequent release of its content into the cytosol.[19]

Transport in the Cytoplasm

Once escaping from the endosome, drug molecules must dissociate from their delivery system to bind to their target, that is, mRNA in the case of antisense or siRNAs. For DNAs, transcription factor decoys, and antigene oligonucleotides, the drug molecules must gain access to the nucleus, where transcription occurs. In the cytoplasm, drug molecules face two major barriers: the diffusion barrier and the enzyme barrier. The cytoplasm is rich with structural proteins, microtubules, and other organelles as well as nucleases. As diffusion of DNAs in the cytoplasm is found to be size-dependent, smaller and more condensed DNAs are more effective.

Nuclear Localization

Cell nucleus is enclosed with a nuclear envelope that displays tightly regulated pores. *Nuclear pore complex* (NPC) allows the transportation of water-soluble molecules across the nuclear envelope, including RNAs, ribosomes, and proteins; however, small molecules less than 9 nm in size can diffuse through the pores in its closed state. In the open state, the complex allows passage of molecules with size less than 26 nm.[20] Larger molecules can be recognized by a specific signal sequence called the *nuclear localization signal* (NLS), generally a short conserved cationic peptide, and can be translocated into the nucleus with the help of a carrier protein called importin. Several studies have shown that attachment of NLS to DNA enhances the nuclear entry and transcriptional activity of DNA.

Drug Delivery Systems

Viral Vectors

Viral vectors are powerful tools for delivering genetic material, either DNA or RNAi, into the cells. Naturally, viruses have evolved specialized mechanisms to enclose their nucleic acids in a coat that has multiple functions, including protecting the nucleic acids from enzymatic degradation, mediating viral entry into the host cell, and releasing their nucleic acid content into the infected host. Viral vectors are generally applicable for a wide range of cell types, including dividing and nondividing cells. Commonly used viral vectors for gene delivery are retrovirus, Moloney murine leukemia virus (MMLV) subgroup, adenovirus, adeno-associated virus (AAV), herpes simplex virus (HSV), and vaccinia virus (poxvirus), as summarized in **Table 17-6.**[20, 21]

Nonviral Vectors

Lipid-Based Delivery

Lipoplexes—cationic liposome–nucleic acid complexes—are complexes spontaneously formed between nucleic acids and cationic lipids, such as the monocationic lipids DOTAP (*N*-[1-(2,3-dioleoyloxy)]-*N*,*N*,*N*-trimethylammonium propane methylsulfate) and DMRIE

Table 17-6 Comparison of Viral Vectors

	Size Φ, nm	Loading Capacity	Advantages	Limitations
MMLV	~ 100	< 8 kb†	Long-lasting (stable) gene expression	Small packing capacity Infects only rapidly dividing cells
Adenovirus	70–100	< 8 kb	Infects various cell types independent of cell cycle	Immunogenic, not suitable for long-term gene expression Rapid clearance of vectors Small packing capacity
AAV	~ 20	< 4 kb	Infects various cell types independent of cell cycle Low toxicity and immunogenicity Stable expression	Very limited packing capacity
HSV	N/A	< 40 kb	Large loading capacity Infects various cells with preference for neurons independent of cell cycle	Transient expression Potentially pathogenic
Vaccinia	N/A	< 25 kb	Infects various cell types independent of cell cycle Relatively safe High efficiency	Highly immunogenic; however, this makes them attractive for cancer immunotherapy

†Kilobases.

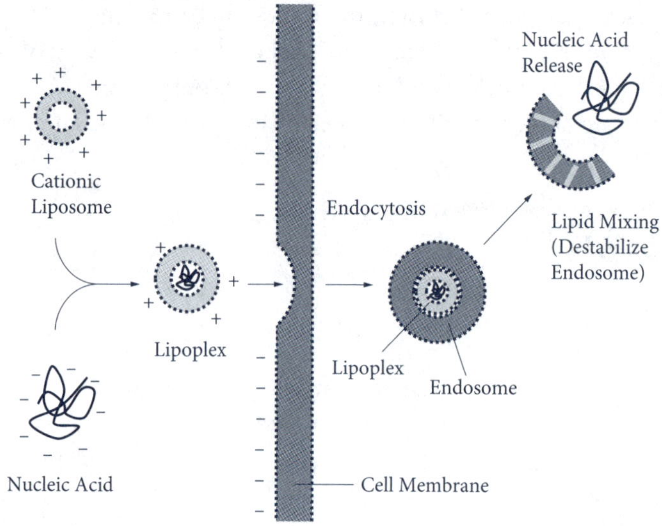

Figure 17-6 Lipoplex-mediated nucleic acid delivery.

(*N*-[1-(2,3,-dimyristyloxypropyl)]-*N*,*N*-dimethyl-(2-hydroxyethyl)ammonium bromide) or the polycationic lipid DOSPA (2,3-dioleoyloxy-*N*-[2(sperminecarboxamido)-ethyl]-*N*,*N*-dimethyl-1-propanaminiumtrifluoro acetate), as a result of opposing electrostatic charges. By virtue of their net positive charge, lipoplexes have a high affinity toward plasma membranes, facilitating their entry into the cells by endocytosis.[17] To escape from the endosome after endocytosis, cationic lipids are often used in combination with the so-called *helper lipids* such as DOPE (1,2-dioleoyl-*sn*-glycero-3-phosphoethanolamine) or cholesterol. These helper lipids undergo a conformational change that destabilizes the endosomal membrane (**Figure 17-6**). Examples of commercially available lipoplex-forming agents are Transfectin and Cytofectin.

In vivo studies have shown that liposomes and lipoplexes have a rapid RES clearance. Modification of liposomes with polyethylene glycol (PEG) has been reported to reduce opsonization and phagocytosis of the liposomes by phagocytic cells of the RES, resulting in a prolonged systemic circulation of the liposomes.[22]

Polymer-Based Delivery

Similar to the cationic lipids, cationic polymers can form complexes with nucleic acids, condensing the molecules into a more compact structure and masking their negative charge. *Polyplexes*—cationic polymer–nucleic acid complexes—are prepared from cationic polymers such as PEI, which additionally provide the proton sponge effect, facilitating the complex's escape from the endosome. Some delivery systems combine polymers with liposomes forming *lipopolyplexes*. Polymers such as protamine, histone, and adenoviral-derived μ-peptide carry positive charges that help condense the DNA to form a tightly packed particle for transfection.[23] One example of such a combination consists of DOTAP (1,2-dioleoyl-trimethylammonium propane; cholesterol liposomes), protamine sulfate, and plasmid DNA encoding for IL-2 and p53 for cancer treatment.[24]

Polymeric micelles are colloidal dispersions prepared from amphiphilic copolymers, consisting of hydrophilic and hydrophobic monomer units. Polyplex micelles forming through an electrostatic interaction between nucleic acids and PEG-based block copolymers have recently gained much attention due to their nanometric-scale size and excellent biocompatibility, e.g., the use of PEG-poly(methacrylic acid) (PMA) block copolymer for the construction of nanoparticles encapsulating siRNA, which is designed to assist endosomal escape via the conformational change of PMA at endosomal pH.[25]

Dendrimers are highly branched, roughly spherical, large molecules that are attractive as a nucleic acid delivery system. They are synthesized by defined polymerization reactions. Depending on the initial monomer and the building block monomers used, several categories of dendrimers have been synthesized with various functional groups. Thus far, most studies on dendrimeric delivery of nucleic acids have utilized polyamidoamine (PAMAM) starburst dendrimers, which possess a hydrocarbon core and cationic surface amino groups that facilitate nucleic acid binding.[26] Dendrimer–oligonucleotide complexes both exhibit a 75% reduction in enzymatic degradation of the phosphodiester oligonucleotide in serum and provide protection from lysosomal degradation.

Peptide-Based Delivery

Cell-penetrating peptides (CPPs), also known as *protein transduction domains* (PTDs), are small motifs in proteins of approximately 10–16 amino acids in length. These peptides promote the delivery of macromolecules as well as carrier systems across cell membranes via a receptor-, energy-, and transporter-independent mechanism.[27] This property theoretically allows the delivery of macromolecules in nearly all cell types without relying on endocytosis and its associated delivery problems, e.g., endosomal entrapment. CPPs typically contain alternate domains of hydrophobic and charged residues. As cellular uptake of CPP-conjugated cargos depends on the electrostatic attraction between positively charged cargo particles and negatively charged phospholipids, cell specificity is lacking. Thus far, several CPP motifs have been identified, including the HIV-1 Tat protein, *Drosophila melanogaster* homeotic transcription factor ANTP (penetratin), and herpes simplex virus type 1 (HSV-1) VP-22 transcription factor. In addition, chimeric CPPs such as MPG or transportan have been proposed in which domains isolated from different proteins are joined together.

Hundreds of publications have reported the potential of CPPs, notably Tat 48-60 CPPs, to promote the cellular uptake of oligonucleotides and peptides. One example is the delivery of the 16-amino-acid BH4 peptide, which is shared by several antiapoptotic proteins in the Bcl-2 family. Tat-BH4 constructs were found to be effective in preventing the apoptosis of endothelial cells.[28] Additionally, these CPPs were reported to form polyplexes with DNA. Such peptide–DNA polyplexes efficiently enter the cells through endocytosis or by direct membrane transduction. CPPs also allow cellular internalization of nonpermeant macromolecules such as proteins, as demonstrated by the successful delivery of fused construct between the Tat CPP and β-galactosidase both in vitro and in vivo.[29, 30]

Protein-Based Delivery

Proticles are nanoparticles prepared by self-assembly of complexes between protamine free bases and human serum albumin.[31] The net positive charge of the complex leads to the attraction of nucleic acids such as oligonucleotides and siRNA, forming ternary nanoparticles. Ternary proticles are reported to be stable in solutions of up to physiological ionic strength for several hours. Cellular uptake of oligonucleotides increases approximately 12-fold by proticle delivery in comparison to free oligonucleotides. In addition, the biodegradability of proticle components produces no or minimum cytotoxicity.

Receptor-Mediated Delivery

Receptor-mediated delivery could be used for effective targeting of nucleic acids to subsets of cells or specific organs. Generally, targeting strategies are divided into two classes: ligand–nucleic acid conjugates and ligand-targeted nanoparticles. For tumor targeting, the differences in molecular machinery between tumor cells and benign cells as a consequence of cell transformation have often been exploited for tumor delivery. Examples of the tumor targeting moieties are folate receptor (FR) for ovarian, colorectal, and breast cancer; transferrin for pancreatic cancer; anti-HER2 antibody for breast cancer; anti-CD19 for malignant B cells; anti-GD2 for neuroblastoma and melanoma; and prostate-specific membrane antigen (PMSA)-specific aptamer for prostate cancer and tumor vascular endothelium.[18, 26, 32]

Physical Methods

External physical energy and/or force has been used as an alternative method to overcome the physiological barriers for nucleic acid delivery. Basically, these methods induce a reversible change in cell membrane integrity that allows passage of nucleic acids across the permeabilized membrane. Based on the type of physical energy or force applied and how they are used, physical methods are categorized into microinjection, projectile injection (e.g., gene gun and jet injection), electroporation, hydrodynamic injection, laser irradiation, and ultrasound–, magnetic field–, and electric pulse–mediated delivery.[33]

III. Insulin Delivery

With the increasing incidence of diabetes mellitus (DM), insulin has become one of the most commonly used biotechnology products. Conventional insulin treatment is a replacement therapy, in which exogenous insulin is injected into the systemic circulation to restore insulin deficiency. However, the burden of daily injections, pain, inconvenience, and potential health hazards remain a major problem for insulin therapy. Consequently, novel insulin formulations and analogs as well as noninvasive routes of administration have been explored and developed.

Insulin Injection

Currently, almost all insulin products in the United States are biotechnology-derived human insulin produced by recombinant DNA technology. Insulin products are classified based on their onset and duration of action, as summarized in **Table 17-7**.[34]

Insulin Formulations

Human insulin molecules have a natural tendency to self-associate and form dimers. In the presence of *zinc*, three dimers join together to form a hexamer. To bind to its receptors, the hexamer must dissociate to monomeric insulin. Accordingly, zinc has been used in various commercial formulations to stabilize the insulin molecules for a longer shelf life or to prolong the action of insulin.

NPH insulin (neutral protamine Hagedom, or isophane, insulin) is a suspension of crystalline zinc insulin combined with a positively charged polypeptide, protamine. NPH insulin could be mixed with soluble insulin to complement its action.

Lente insulin (crystalline zinc acetate insulin) is a suspension of insulin with zinc but contains no polypeptides. The drawback of Lente insulin is the incompatibility when mixing it with other short-acting insulin, due to the excess of zinc. Currently, Lente insulin is no longer available in the U.S. market.

Table 17-7 Types of Insulin Preparations and Suggested Action Profile

Types	Onset of Action, h	Peak of Action, h	Duration of Action, h
Rapid-acting			
Analog: Lispro	0.25–0.5	0.5–1	3–5
Analog: Aspart	0.3–0.6	0.5–1	3–5
Short-acting			
Regular or soluble	0.5–1	2–4	6–8
Intermediate-acting			
NPH	1–2	6–12	18–24
Lente	1–3	6–12	18–26
Long-acting			
Ultralente	4–6	10–16	24–28
Analog: Glargine	4–6	None	> 24

Insulin Analogs

The insulin molecule consists of an A chain with 21 amino acids and a B chain with 30 amino acids. Structural modifications of the insulin molecule to control its stability and action are listed below.

In *insulin lispro*, the amino acids lysine and proline are reversed in the C-terminal end of the B chain of the insulin molecule (Lys (B28), Pro (B29) human insulin). The inversion leads to a substantial reduction in self-association of the molecule. In addition, insulin lispro dissociates more rapidly from its hexamer zinc complexes and is better absorbed into the circulation after subcutaneous injection.

In *insulin aspart*, amino acid proline at position B28 is replaced by the negatively charged aspartic acid, resulting in increased charge repulsion and less self-association.

In *insulin glargine*, amino acid asparagine in the A chain at position A21 is replaced by glycine, and two arginines are added to the B chain at positions B31 and B32 of the insulin molecule. Such modifications make the molecule more soluble in an acidic pH. Insulin glargine is generally prepared as a solution at pH 4.0. After subcutaneous injection, the acidic solution is neutralized, leading to the formation of *microprecipitates* that slowly release insulin glargine into the circulation.

Oral Insulin

Oral insulin offers great potential advantages over injectable insulin, including improved patient compliance and fewer side effects. Through oral administration, it is likely to achieve a high hepatic concentration of insulin without overinsulinizing the periphery, which is common with the injection and causes undesirable side effects such as weight gain and hypoglycemia.[35]

The main challenges for oral insulin are to overcome the enzymatic and permeation barriers of the GI tract. Several approaches have been developed to overcome these problems, including the use of (1) penetration enhancers such as bile salts, surfactant *N*-lauryl-β-D-maltopyranoside, salicylates, metal chelator sodium edetate, and zonula occludens toxin; (2) enzyme inhibitors such as Bowman–Birk inhibitor (BBI), sodium glycolate, camostat mesilate, bacitracin, and ovomucoids; (3) mucoadhesive polymers to extend the residence time and to intensify the mucosal contact of insulin in the GI tract; (4) particulate carrier systems such as liposomes, microemulsions, polymeric micelles, and polymeric nano- and microparticles that protect insulin from enzymatic degradation and facilitate its absorption through gut-associated lymphoid tissues (GALT) like the Peyer's patches; and (5) colon-targeted delivery systems.[36] The recent oral insulin products that undergo clinical trials are Eligen (tablet with permeation enhancer, Emisphere Technology), Macrulin (Macrosol W/O microemulsion, Cortecs International/Provalis PLC), IN-105 (PEGylated insulin with permeation enhancer, Biocon), and HDV-I (liposomal insulin tablet, Diasome Pharmaceuticals).

Buccal Insulin

The advantages of buccal mucosa as a drug delivery route include ease of access, relatively low proteolytic activity, and high vascularization. However, both partially keratinized and multilayered structures and the continuous flow of saliva limit drug absorption. Although promising in vitro, the in vivo results with various penetration enhancers, protease inhibitors, and bioadhesive polymers have not shown efficacy. A more promising technology has been developed by Generex Biotechnology using the combination of Oral-lyn (mixed micellar solution), absorption enhancers, and a propeller called RapidMist, which generates small particles from an aqueous spray to the oral cavity.[37] This system provides a more rapid onset but shorter duration of action of insulin as compared to regular injectable insulin.

Inhaled Insulin

The lungs provide a very large (~ 100–150 m^2) and highly vascularized absorptive surface area for drug delivery. In addition, the alveolar epithelium lining of the lung is very thin, thereby permitting rapid drug absorption. First-pass metabolism is also avoided with lung delivery. However, there are other barriers, which include (1) the presence of pulmonary mucus, which is the direct surface layer in which insulin comes into contact with prior to absorption; (2) degradation by proteases; and (3) clearance by alveolar macrophages that secrete short-lived peroxidases and cellular mediators to degrade the inhaled molecule. The transepithelial transport of insulin is incompletely understood, but likely through the junctional paracellular route,[36] although endocytosis of insulin is well known. So far, four inhaled insulin products have progressed through phase III clinical trials: Exubera (dry powder inhalation, Nektar therapeutics/Pfizer/Sanofi-Aventis), AERx iDMS (liquid aerosol, Aradigm Corp/Novo Nordisk), HIIP (AIR technology, Alekermes/Eli Lily), and Technosphere (encapsulated microsphere, PDC/MannKind Corp). The Exubera system was given U.S. FDA approval in 2006.[38] However, its use was initially inhibited by its cost, and it was withdrawn from the market in 2008. Also, several cases of lung cancer attributed to its use have been reported.

Nasal Insulin

Nasal insulin delivery has been widely investigated as an alternative route to injection and inhalation. The rationales for nasal administration are that (1) the nose has a reasonably large absorption area (~ 150 cm^2) because of the presence of microvilli on the epithelial surface; (2) the subepithelial layer is highly vascularized, and the venous blood from the nose passes directly to the systemic circulation, thus avoiding first-pass metabolism; (3) it provides a rapid onset of drug action; and (4) it is easily accessible. Despite these advantages, there are some limitations, including the presence of mucociliary clearance, mucus layer, and proteolytic enzymes, which limit drug absorption. Therefore, pharmaceutical additives such as absorption enhancers, enzyme inhibitors, and mucoadhesive polymers have been used.[36] Examples of nasal insulin formulations are Nasulin (nasal spray with physiological absorption enhancer, Bentley Pharmaceutical), QDose (dry powder insulin, Ventura/Microdose Technology), and ChiSys (chitosan-based system, West Pharmaceutical Services).

Transdermal Insulin

There are several transdermal insulin delivery systems being developed, including PassPort (transdermal patch using microporation technique to create micropores on the skin surface, Altea Therapeutics), U-Strip (transdermal patch using ultrasound to induce pore dilation, Encapsulation System), and Macroflux (transdermal patch using microprojections to promote microcapillary drug absorption, Alza Corp). A promising insulin formulation that has progressed to clinical trial is Transfersulin (IDEA AG), which encapsulates insulin into transferosome, an ultradeformable vesicle that could penetrate pores much smaller than its size.

IV. Augmentation of EPR Effect for Tumor Targeting

The enhanced permeability and retention (EPR) effect is the physiology-based mechanism of tumor targeting based on the principle that under certain inflammatory and hypoxic conditions, such as those observed in tumors, the endothelial lining of blood vessels becomes leaky or more permeable than normal, which is sometimes called *leakage vasculature.*[39] Thus, certain particles ranging from 10 to 500 nm in size can leave the vascular bed and accumulate in the tumor interstitial space, while the compromised lack of lymphatic drainage in tumor tissues allows them to remain there. This accumulation is spontaneous and also known as *passive targeting.* However, unlike macromolecules, small-molecule drugs are not retained in the tumor because of their ability to diffuse back to the circulation (**Figure 17-7**).

Generally, the EPR-based tumor targeting requires the macromolecular drugs or carriers to be long circulating to ensure sufficient accumulation of the drugs or carriers in the target. The molecules have to avoid opsonization and removal by the RES. The most common strategy is to modify the surface of the molecules by PEGylation or by conjugation of the drug molecules with polymers such as poly(styrene-*co* maleic acid anhydride) (SMA). Receptor-mediated targeting (active targeting) is also used in combination with the EPR effect to enhance drug accumulation in the areas with limited blood supply. Two different strategies have been used to augment the EPR effect: (1) slow infusion of angiotensin II artificially to elevate blood pressure and (2) administration of nitroglycerin or other nitric oxide ($NO^{\cdot}$) donors to increase vascular extravasation.[40]

The use of nitroglycerin is unique because in hypoxic tumor tissues nitroglycerin can be converted to nitrite, which is further reduced to $NO^{\cdot}$ (**Figure 17-8**). This effect is similar to that observed in the cardiac tissues with angina pectoris, exhibiting hypoxic and acidic conditions. The release of nitrite from nitroglycerin and further conversion of nitrite to $NO^{\cdot}$ promote vascular blood flow, elevate pO_2, and consequently enhance the EPR effect.

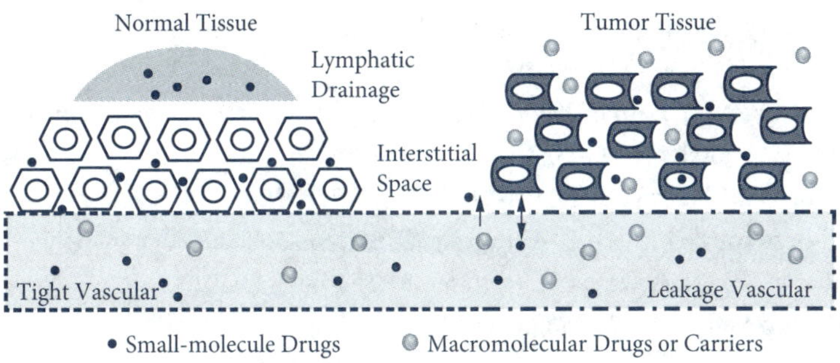

Figure 17-7 Diagrammatic representation of normal versus tumor vasculature.

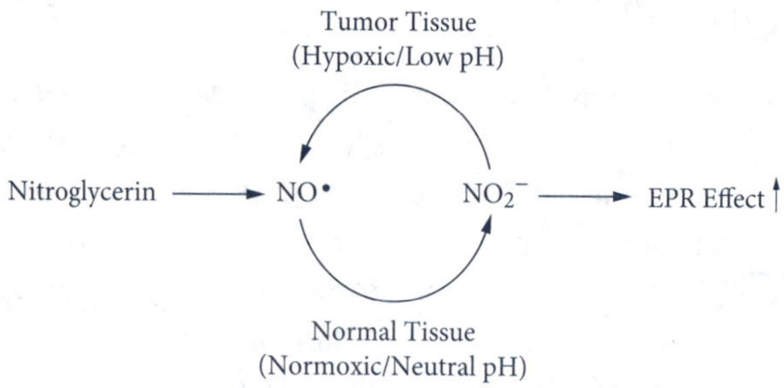

Figure 17-8 Mechanism of NO˙ generation from nitroglycerin.

V. Chapter Summary

Macromolecular drugs such as proteins and nucleic acids have emerged as a new class of therapeutic agents due to their unique biological and pharmacological properties. However, unlike with conventional drugs, the use of these macromolecules is faced with several obstacles in their delivery, including enzymatic instability, phagocytic clearance, and poor absorption. Several approaches have been used to aid the delivery of macromolecular drugs. These include biological approaches, such as the use of receptor-mediated endocytosis and viral vectors for nucleic acid and protein delivery; physical approaches, such as the use of liposomes and nanocarriers as well as electrical and ultrasonic techniques; chemical approaches, such as conjugation and side-chain modifications; and genetic approaches, such as site-directed mutagenesis. Although much progress has been made in the delivery of macromolecular drugs, several challenges remain. The success of macromolecular drugs will depend on understanding the physiological barriers to their delivery and advances in nanotechnology and molecular pharmaceutics.

VI. References

1. Reddy IK. in: *Pharmaceutical Biotechnology*. Lancaster, PA, Technomic Publishing, 1997, 2nd ed, pp 137–157.
2. Florence AT and Attwood D, in: *Physical Pharmacy*. London, Pharmaceutical Press, 2008, pp 137–148.
3. Reddy IK, in: *Pharmaceutical Biotechnology*. Lancaster, PA, Technomic Publishing, 1997, 2nd ed, pp 159–182.
4. Crommelin DJA, in: *Pharmaceutical Biotechnology*. Amsterdam, Harwood Academic Publishers, 1997, pp 71–99.
5. Yamamoto A, Taniguchi T, Rikyuu K, et al. *Pharm Res*. 11:1496–1500, 1994.
6. Lee HJ. *Arch. Pharm Res*. 25:572–584, 2002.
7. Soltero R and Ekwuribe N. *Innovat Pharm Technol*. 1:106–110, 2001.
8. Muller G. *Pharmacol*. 86:92–116, 2010.
9. Azad N and Rojanasakul Y, in: *Biopharmaceutical Drug Design and Development*. Totowa, NJ, Humana Press Inc., 2008, pp 293–323.
10. Simone Fishburn C. *J Pharm Sci*. DOI 10.1002/jps.21278, 2007.
11. Werle M and Bernkop-Schnurch B. *Amino Acids*. 30:351–367, 2006.
12. Tan ML, Choong PFM, and Dass CR. *Peptides*. 31:184–193, 2010.
13. Gombotz WR and Pettit DK. *Bioconjugate Chem*. 6:332–351, 1995.
14. Agudo MT and Lambert PH. *Immunobiology*. 184:113–125, 1992.
15. Sharma HW, Perez JR, Higgins-Sochaski K, Hsiao R, and Narayanan R. *Anticancer Res*. 16:61–69, 1996.

16. Whitehead KA, Langer R, and Anderson DG. *Natl Rev Drug Discov*. 8:129–138, 2009.
17. Reischl D and Zimmer A. *Nanomedicine: NMB*. 5:8–20, 2009.
18. Yu B, Zhao X, Lee J, and Lee RJ. *AAPS J*. 2:195–203, 2009.
19. Belsuise-Valladier P and Behr JB. *Cytotechnol*. 35:197–201, 2001.
20. Guan J, Pan X, Lee LJ, and Lee RJ, in: *Biopharmaceutical Drug Design and Development*. Totowa, NJ, Humana Press Inc., 2008, pp 141–173.
21. Boeckle S and Wagner E. *AAPS J*. 8:E731–E742, 2006.
22. Allen TM and Hansen C. *Biochim Biophys Acta*. 1068:133–141, 1991.
23. Bertrand JR, Pottier M, Vekris A, Opolon P, Maksimenko A, and Malvy C. *Biochem Biophys Res Commun*. 296:1000–1004, 2002.
24. Whitmore M, Li S, and Huang L. *Gene Therapy*. 6:1867–1875, 1999.
25. Kataoka K, Itaka K, Nishiyama N, Yamasaki Y, Oishi M, and Nagasaki Y. *Nucleic Acids Res Suppl*. 19:17–18, 2005.
26. Hughes MD, Hussain M, Nawaz Q, Sayyed P, and Akhtar S. *DDT*. 6:303–315, 2001.
27. Said Hassane F, Saleh AF, Abes R, Gait MJ, and Lebleu B. *Cell Mol Life Sci*. 67:715–726, 2010.
28. Ono M, Sawa Y, Ryugo M, et al. *Eur J Cardiothorac Surg*. 27:117–121, 2005.
29. Fawell S, Seery J, Daikh Y, et al. *Proc Natl Acad Sci USA*. 91:664–668, 1994.
30. Schwarze SR, Ho A, Vocero-Akbani A, and Dowdy SF. *Science*. 285:1569–1572, 1999.
31. Mayer G, Vogel V, Weyermann J, et al. *J Control Release*. 106:181–187, 2005.
32. Belting M and Wittrup A. *Mol Biotechnol*. 43:89–94, 2009.
33. Villemejane J and Mir LM. *Brit J Pharmacol*. 157:207–219, 2009.
34. Gossain VV. *Int J Diab Countries*. 23:26–36, 2003.
35. Iyer H, Khedkar A, and Verma M. *Diabetes Obes Metab*. 12:179–182, 2010.
36. Khafagy ES, Morishita M, Onuki Y, and Takayama K. *Adv Drug Deliv Rev*. 59:1521–1546, 2007.
37. Henkin RI. *Nutrition*. 26:33–39, 2010.
38. Lassmann-Vague V and Raccah D. *Diabeties Metab*. 32:513–522, 2006.
39. Torchilin V. *Adv Drug Deliv Rev*. doi:10.1016/j.addr.2010.03.011, 2010.
40. Maeda H. *Bioconjugate Chem*. 21:797–802, 2010.

VII. Homework Problems

1. What are the major challenges for oral delivery of peptide and protein drugs? Describe the approaches to overcome the problems.
2. Describe the principle of biodegradable polymers that target protein and peptide drugs to the colon.
3. What are the differences among the various anti-mRNA strategies including antisense oligonucleotides, siRNAs, and ribozymes?
4. What is the "proton sponge" effect?
5. A pharmaceutical company has explored an siRNA drug. What physiological barriers should be considered for the development of an effective delivery system?
6. If one considers viral vectors for immunotherapy against cancer, what would be the most attractive one and why?
7. Explain how helper lipids in the lipoplexes help the release of nucleic acids from the endosome.
8. Explain why insulin glargine is a long-acting insulin analog.
9. What tumor property leads to an EPR effect?

CHAPTER 18

Application of Nanoscience in Pharmaceutics

Anand Iyer, Neelam Azad, Yon Rojanasakul, and Joseph K. H. Ma

Nanotechnology may be defined as the design, characterization, production, and application of structures, devices, and systems, by controlled manipulation of size and shape to the nanometer scale, that exhibit at least one novel or superior characteristic compared to conventional system.[1, 2] The idea of using a nanosystem that exhibits an atomic, molecular, or supramolecular structure for medical treatment is not new, however, with the preeminent Nobel laureate Richard Feynman proposing, in the 1960s, the use of tiny nanorobots that may provide accurate, cost-effective, and reliable solutions to diagnosis and treatment of human diseases.[3, 4] Over the past decade, nanotechnology has driven the applications of nanomaterial across a broad domain, from areas as common as cosmetics, stain-resistant clothing, sporting goods, etc., to more specialized ones including communications, electronics, optics, chemistry, energy, and medicine. In this chapter, the applications of manomaterials for in vitro diagnostics, in vivo imaging, and drug delivery, along with the fate of the nanoparticles and their toxicities in the living systems are described.

CHAPTER OUTLINE

OBJECTIVES

1. Introduce the concept of nanotechnology.
2. Discuss the use of nanotechnology in medicine.
3. Briefly describe the medical application of nanotechnology.
4. Delve into the nanobiotechnological aspects of drug delivery.
5. Describe various drug delivery systems.
6. Discuss the therapeutic implications of nanodelivery systems in various disease states.
7. Briefly describe the toxicity associated with nanoparticle exposure.

I. Introduction

In the strictest sense, nanotechnology deals with structures with sizes between 1 and 100 nm in length in at least one dimension. However, nanotechnology encompasses structures that may be up to several hundred nanometers in size. Overall, nanotechnology deals with the following parameters: physical properties arising from the nanosize, chemical properties arising from the arrangement of matter in the atomic scale at predefined positions, and the emergence of complex functional systems with novel properties as a result of the physicochemical characteristics of these nanomaterials.[5]

Nanoparticles have several properties that are particularly attractive for biomedical applications. High strength, durability, and solubility as well as a large surface/mass ratio provide for an excellent potential to bind and carry biomolecular agents such as drugs and proteins. Nanoparticles hold the promise for an endless array of applications in medicine, including drug delivery, development of novel therapeutics, and biomedical imaging. The development of nanoparticles for biomedical applications including the use of nanomaterials as carriers to deliver therapeutic agents is currently undergoing tremendous expansion. Not only are engineered nanoparticles utilized as carriers of drug, but also the drug itself is being formulated at the nanoscale, thus enabling the drug to function as a carrier by itself.[6] High carrier capacity, feasibility of incorporation of both lipophilic and lipophobic drugs, and stability across various administrative routes are some of the favorable properties of the nanodelivery systems. The eventual aim in nanomedicine is to be able to develop nanoparticle-based delivery systems that improve drug incorporation and release, offer enhanced stability and biocompatibility of the drug, and improve the biodistribution, targeting, and therapeutic activity of the drug.[6] In terms of drug delivery, nanotechnology offers advantages such as (1) targeted delivery of drugs in a cell- and tissue-specific manner, (2) delivery of macromolecules to intracellular sites of action, (3) improved delivery of water-insoluble drugs, (4) delivery of drugs across biological membrane barriers, (5) visualization of drug delivery, and (6) real-time monitoring of efficacy of the drug.[7, 8]

The application of nanotechnology to medicine is diverse and depends on the physicochemical properties of the nanomaterial. We begin the discussion of medical use of nanoparticles by first examining the various types of nanomaterials.

Classification of Medical Nanomaterials

The term *nanoparticle* refers to a broad inclusion of particles with distinct chemical compositions, sizes, shapes, charges, and physicochemical properties. Nanomaterials may be classified, depending on their base materials, as carbon-based, metal-based, biological, polymeric, ceramic, and composite materials. Based on the particle shape, these materials are also referred to as nanofibers, nanowires, nanorods, nanoscrolls, nanotubes, or nanospheres. Chemically, nanomaterials may simply be referred to as organic and inorganic. A summary of the different types of nanoparticles is given in **Table 18-1**.

Carbon-Based Nanomaterials

Carbon-based nanoparticles take the form of hollow spheres, ellipsoids, or tubes. Spherical or ellipsoidal carbon nanoparticles are referred to as *fullerenes*, whereas cylindrical nanoparticles are referred to as *nanotubes*. Carbon nanotubes, either single-walled or multi-walled, have large surface areas, unique surface properties, and a needle-like shape; they have the potential to deliver large amounts of therapeutic agents to the targeted disease sites. Single-walled carbon nanotubes (SWCNT) are the fibrous analogues of spherical fullerene, which are currently being investigated

Table 18-1 Nanoparticle Classification, Properties, and Applications

Classification	Properties	Application
Carbon-base nanomaterial		
Carbon nanotube SWCNT MWCNT	Cylindrical and fibrous	Electronics; energy storage; delivery of DNA, siRNA, and protein; imaging
Fullerenes	Ellipsoidal or spherical hollow carbon compounds	As superconductors, lubricants, catalysts, and carriers for drug delivery
Metal-base nanomaterial		
Quantum dots (QDs)	Close-packed semiconductor devices; fluorescent	Contrast agent for MRI and positron emission tomography (PET)
Gold nanoparticles (GNP)	Binds strongly to peptides, antibodies, pathogens, and oligonucleotides	Imaging and diagnostic
Nanosilver	Containing up to 15,000 Ag; antibacterial	Antibacterial for wounds and burns; disinfectant sprays
Metal oxides (iron oxide)		Imaging and diagnostic
Biological nanomaterial		
Proteins, nucleic acid, and carbohydrates	Nanostructured; fluorescence-labeled; biodegradable	Cancer imaging and treatment
Polymeric nanoparticles		
Self-assembled (liposomes, polymeric micelles), Non-self-assembled (dendrimers, nanospheres)	High drug-loading; stealth; biodegradable; surface modification for drug targeting	Drug targeting, imaging, and diagnostic
Nanoceramics (oxide and non-oxide ceramic materials)		
Calcium phosphate ceramics (Hydroxyapatite)	Greater mechanical strength than normal material; biocompatible	Bioactive coating of bioinert materials such as titanium and its alloys, metallic prosthetics, and implants
Nanocomposites		
	Combination of a nanomaterial with other nanoparticles or with larger, bulk materials	Packaging; construction; automotive; electronics; medicine
Nanoclays		Used as materials of enhanced mechanical, thermal, sound barrier, and flame-retardant properties
Nanocrystalline calcium phosphates		Artificial bone composites
Magnetic hollow silica nanocomposites (MHSNC)	Nanoparticles of spherical or needle-like calcium carbonate surface-coated with Fe_3O_4 and silica	Drug delivery and imaging
Microcatheters	Nanotube-filled polymer composites	Used as medical devices

as imaging agents for the identification and localization of tumors. Functionalized single-walled carbon nanotubes have been used as carriers for specific delivery of anticancer drugs, proteins, DNA, and siRNA to diseased tissues, and to enhance drug bioavailability by improving drug solubility or decreasing clearance.[9] Fullerenes are compounds containing from 60 to hundreds of carbon atoms. The common fullerene C_{60} is a spherical molecule consisting of 60 carbon atoms. These nanoparticles are under investigation for their potential uses as superconductors, lubricants, catalysts, and drug-delivery systems.[10]

Metal-Based Nanomaterials

Also known as *nanometals*, metal-based nanoparticles include *quantum dots* (QDs), nanogold, nanosilver, and metal oxides. Anisotropic metal-based nanoparticles have been used as targeting contrast agents due to their strong surface *plasmon resonance* that results from free electron oscillation, which gives a sharp and intense absorption band in the visible range. For molecular imaging, the contrast agents must contain disease-specific biomarkers for targeting and provide good image contrast between labeled and unlabeled tissues. QDs are small, closely packed semiconductor devices that fluoresce at various wavelengths according to their size. This makes them highly suitable as contrast agents for magnetic resonance imaging (MRI) or positron emission tomography (PET).[11] Both gold nanoparticles (GNP) and QDs are good contrast materials because of their unique physicochemical properties, which are quite different from their bulk counterparts. These nanomaterials also possess the ability to bind to proteins, peptides, antibodies, and oligonucleotides that can be used for targeting specificity. Silver nanoparticles, with sizes generally smaller than 100 nm, represent another prominent nanoproduct. These particles exhibit potent antibacterial activity due to the high number of surface atoms and are marketed for treatment of wounds and burns, as contraceptives, and as water disinfectants and room sprays.[12]

Biological Nanomaterials

Nanomaterials of biological origin include proteins, nucleic acids, and carbohydrates. The use of DNA as a structured nanomaterial has opened a new avenue toward the rational design of DNA nanostructures with different polymeric topologies.[13] A number of nanoparticles of various chemistries and architectures for cancer imaging and treatment have also been reported.[14] One example is the use of peroxalate ester nanoparticles with an encapsulated fluorescent dye for detecting cancer.[15] This technique is based on the rationale that the generation of hydrogen peroxide in human cells is precancerous; the dye becomes fluorescent when it is in contact with hydrogen peroxide, which can then be detected using imaging equipment. This system is biodegradable and biocompatible, and its hydrolytic degradation products are considered to be nontoxic or of low toxicity to the human body.

Polymeric Nanoparticles

Nanostructured polymers are self-assembled structures, such as liposomes and micelles, or non-self-assembled structures, such as dendrimers and nanospheres. Many synthetic and natural polymers, e.g., poly(lactic-*co*-glycolic acid) (PLGA), have been tested as drug carriers for cancer treatment. PLGA nanoparticles are biodegradable, biocompatible, and safe for human use; they can be PEGylated to exhibit long circulation times and be prepared with efficient drug loading. These advantages are common to most polymeric nanoparticles.

Nanoceramics

Nanoceramics are composed of oxide and non-oxide ceramic materials, silicates, or hard metals. Nanoceramics possess superior mechanical properties compared to conventional ceramics. Nanoceramic products used in industry and research include titanium, silica, alumina, tungsten carbide, zinc oxide, silicon nitride, ferric oxide, and silicon carbide, among others. Calcium phosphate nanoceramics have gained attention in the biomedical field due to their superior biological and biomechanical properties. Hydroxyapatite ($Ca_{10}(PO_4)_6(OH)_2$) is used, at present, for bioinert coatings of metallic prosthetics and implants containing titanium and its alloys.[16]

Nanocomposites

Nanocomposites are the combination of nanoparticles of one type with another, or the composite of nanoparticles with the larger-size bulk material. They are widely used in materials of packaging, building and construction, electronics, auto parts, and medicine. An example of a medical nanocomposite is the use of nanocrystalline calcium phosphates to manufacture artificial bone composites.[17] Magnetic hollow silica nanocomposites (MHSNC) have also been prepared for drug delivery studies. These particles contain surfaces coated with Fe_3O_4 and silica on nanosized spherical and needle-like nanoparticles of calcium carbonate.

As can be seen from Table 18-1, nanomaterials are widely used in medical practice. The major applications are in drug discovery, molecular diagnostics, molecular imaging, implants, active implants, tissue engineering, genomics, and proteomics. Nanoparticles that are frequently studied for biomedical applications include titanium dioxide, nanogold, nanosilver, nanotubes, fullerenes, QDs, polymeric nanoparticles, nanocrystals, and metal colloidal particles.

II. *In Vitro* Diagnostics

Nanotechnology has played an important role in refining and enabling *in vitro* techniques for disease diagnostics. *In vitro* diagnostics, which ranges from assaying blood for pathogens before a transfusion to monitoring drug levels in patients to diagnosis and treatment of most diseases, is an integral part of health care. Various nanoplatforms have been developed to allow for real-time evaluation of disease markers by noninvasive techniques. Applications of nanotechnology in diagnostics fall under the general categories of nanoarrays and biochips. The methods and their applications are described below.

Nanoarrays

Methods that provide collections of miniaturized test sites arranged on solid substrates so that many tests can be performed at the same time were first developed as microarrays (biochips or DNA chips). The microarrays are composed of an orderly arrangement of proteins or thousands of DNA or RNA fragments on glass, silicon, or nylon substrates. This technique was evolved from Southern blotting technology, in which a fragmented DNA is attached to the substrate and then probed with a known gene or DNA fragment, using fluorescent tags to allow visual detection. The microarrays are fabricated using a variety of techniques including photolithography, which enables the deposition of material in desired patterns that could be used to attach biosensors. Nanotechnology operates at the atomic, molecular, or macromolecular range. The key to this technique is high-voltage electron beam (E-beam) lithography. The electrons produce a chemical change in which a beam of electrons is scanned across a surface covered with a thin film, called a resist, which allows the surface to be patterned and the deposit of metals such as gold for the binding of biomaterial. This results in nanoarrays, with molecules placed at defined locations on a surface with nanometer spatial resolution. Nanoarray spots can include biological samples such as protein, DNA, RNA, and whole viruses, as well as nonbiological samples such as solutions, colloids, and particle suspensions. In the miniaturization of bioaffinity tests for proteins, nucleic acids, and receptor-ligand bindings, these arrays utilize approximately 1/10,000 of the surface area occupied by a conventional microarray, and over 1500 nanoarray spots may be placed in the area required for a single microarray spot. For example, NanoArray (BioForce Nanosciences, Ames, Iowa) prints biological and nonbiological sensors onto silicon chips with ultra-micro spot sizes ranging from 1 to 20 μm and in the nanometer range up to 250 nm.

Nanoarrays offer a number of advantages over conventional microarrays. They are sensitive and precise in attaching biomolecular material and specific molecular segments such as single-strand DNA.[18, 19] Nanotechnology also allows the investigation of individual cells and molecules because of the nanosized measuring device. This is potentially useful to differentiate healthy cells from diseased cells at a single-cell resolution level. The primary benefit of such sensitivity is that (1) it helps in the detection of small differences between cell types or weak effects of drugs that might not be detectable using methods with lesser resolution, and (2) it affords a suitable alternative to general biochemical methods that evaluate cell mixtures, which typically lack insight into the definitive basic structure due to the presence of multiple components.[5] Nanoarrays offer label-free detection of the targeted species, such as via measurement of atomic vibrational frequency, thus retaining their biological activity for subsequent analysis.

Significant advances have been made, with the aid of bioinformatics and improved semiconductor manufacturing, in the expression analysis of single cells.[20, 21] Biochip analysis, such as expression chips for bacterial infections in the mouth, has become a part of routine diagnostic examinations in the clinic. These techniques are currently being applied toward profiling the expression of proteins at a single-cell level. Antibody arrays, first reported in 2002, have several clinical applications including discovery of disease markers for diagnosis and drug response, and tracking of disease progression. These principles have been applied to the evaluation of tumor subtypes and cancer progression.[5, 22–24]

Micro-Electromechanical Systems

Microfluidic and microcantilever devices are micro-electromechanical (MEM) systems developed using nanotechnology for *in vitro* diagnostics. Microfluidics is the science of manipulating and controlling fluids and particles (proteins, DNA, cells, viruses, etc.) at micrometer and submicrometer dimensions based on the particle's electrokinetic properties including size, density, charge, light scattering, and antigenic properties. A microfluidic device consists of channels that can control the flow of fluid measured in micro-, nano-, or even pico-liter quantities. Such a device is fabricated using photolithographic and etching techniques. One of the most promising applications of microfluidic devices is in point-of-care diagnosis. Separation of targeted cells from complex tissue samples is the most important preparation stage. Normal laboratory techniques for cell sorting can require complex technologies and special equipment such as centrifugation, fluorescence-activated cell sorting, electrophoresis, and chromatography. Whether it is incorporated into the total analysis or stands alone, the microfluidic technique offers time and cost savings, small sample analysis, high sensitivity, and rapid results. Materials such as poly(dimethylsiloxane), which has excellent biocompatibility with minimal endotoxin contamination and immune response, have made microfluidic chips easy to produce and use.[25–27] Such systems have been used for capturing cancer cells, monitoring allergic responses, and measuring prostate-specific antigen levels.[27, 28]

It is perhaps fruitful to examine the various size ranges (see **Table 18-2**) in order to gain a perspective of the microfluidic (and nanofluidic) channels. As can be seen, the microfluidic channels with nano- and pico-liter flow correspond to cell volumes, which allow for quite efficient cell sorting based on cell sizes as compared to conventional fluidic devices that have microfluidic channels greater than 1 mm.

Microcantilevers are measurement units for targeted biomarkers such as a proteins, DNA, receptor ligands, cells, or viruses. The tip of the microcantilever is coated via E-beam lithography with a thin film (e.g., gold) that binds to a biosensor or receptor, and the fixed end contains an ion implant to sense weight-induced vibrational changes. The device also includes a piezoelectric actuator at the base to provide controlled oscillation. When a targeted biomarker binds to the tip of the microcantilever, the weight of the biomarker will induce a change in vibrational frequency,

Table 18-2 Particle Size, Fluidic Channels, and Biological Entities

Size Range (m)	Volume Range (L)	Biological Entity
10^{-10} to 10^{-9} (1 Å to 1 nm)		Atoms and molecules
Nanofluidic Range		
10^{-9} to 10^{-8} (1 to 10 nm)		DNA
10^{-9} to 10^{-7} (1 to 100 nm)	10^{-21} to 10^{-18} (1 aL)†	Viruses
10^{-7} to 10^{-6} (0.1 to 1 μm)	10^{-18} to 10^{-15} (1 fL)	Viruses
Microfluidic Range		
10^{-6} to 10^{-5} (1 to 10 μm)	10^{-15} to 10^{-12} (1 pL)	Bacteria
10^{-5} to 10^{-4} (10 to 100 μm)	10^{-12} to 10^{-9} (1 nL)	Cells
10^{-4} to 10^{-3} (0.1 to 1 mm)	10^{-9} to 10^{-6} (1 μL)	Hair

†1 aL (attoliter) = 10^{-18} L; 1 fL (femtoliter) = 10^{-15} L; 1 pL (picoliter) = 10^{-12} L.

which is then accurately measured by the device. Nanocantilevers have been designed for the measurement of biomarker proteins, DNA, and oligonucleotides at clinically significant levels without fluorescent labels.[5, 29]

Both microfluidic and microcantilever techniques, as well as nanowires, are surface-patterning tools that can be incorporated in nanoarrays and other biochips. Nanowires are usually placed in microfluidic channels for the binding of various analytes. The mechanism of detection is through an electronically determined shift in conductance across the filaments, when the receptor is occupied by the targeted biomarker.[29–32]

III. *In Vivo* Imaging

Imaging constitutes one of the main areas of application for nanoparticle systems and is particularly applicable in cancer treatment. Such a technique may be used for locating cancer tumors that are too small to be detected by other means. When combined with drug targeting using a multifunctional delivery system, imaging can be used to assess the targeting specificity and the biodistribution of the delivery system. In surgical procedures, imaging techniques can be used by the physician to better find and remove all traces of cancerous growth.

Luminescent Systems

Several nanosystems are currently under investigation for their capability in providing *in vivo* imaging. Quantum dots (QDs), which are fluorescent colloidal semiconductor nanocrystals, serve as excellent contrast agents, providing greater resolution than existing fluorescent dyes.

In a semiconductor crystal lattice of sufficiently small size, the surface electrons are confined in all three spatial dimensions. The electron crowding leads to split energy levels when electrons are excited by an external energy (or wavelength), which would not occur without the electron confinement. This energy difference is referred to as bandgap, which measures the energy required for electron to flow in a semiconductor. Since the electrons are confined in all three dimensions, excited electrons will return to their ground state by emitting the acquired energy as fluorescence. The bandgap increases as the nanostructure size decreases. When the particle size is smaller than a critical radius (known as the Exciton Bohr radius), typically less than 10 nm, quantum confinement dominates the electronic and optical properties. Hence quantum dots will fluoresce at different wavelengths based on particle size, with smaller particles emitting fluorescence at shorter wavelengths (greater energies) than larger particles.

Quantum dots have been used for targeting and imaging of prostate cancer cells.[33] The use of QDs *in vivo*, however, is limited to studies in experimental animals. Concerns about the toxicity of the cadmium-containing material that QDs are made from are a major reason for restricting their use in human subjects. The luminescent approach has also been achieved using engineered spongy (porous) silicon nanoparticles of which the intrinsic near-infrared photoluminescence enables the monitoring and degradation of the particles *in vivo*. The porous nature of the silicon particles allows drug molecules and targeting moieties to be enclosed into the system. They are also biodegradable (into silicic acid), thus making the system relatively nontoxic.

Magnetic Resonance Imaging

In addition to fluorescent imaging, magnetic resonance imaging (MRI) and computed tomography play an important role in identifying diseased tissue and require sensitive contrast agents to achieve high signal/noise ratios. As opposed to traditional contrast agents such as gadolinium, newer nanosize contrast agents seem to possess far better imaging and diagnostic capabilities.[3,5] For example, *iron oxide* (Fe_2O_3 and Fe_3O_4) *nanoparticles* are superparamagnetic, meaning they exhibit much stronger magnetic susceptibility than do paramagnets due to the nanoparticle size, and thus can be magnetized easily by an external magnetic field and used as contrast agents for MRI. Iron oxide nanoparticles are coated with tumor-targeting antibodies or peptides suitable for tumor cell targeting. These particles are drained through lymph nodes, allowing them to be used in the evaluation of immune responses in patients with lung, prostate, breast, or cervix cancers, which would not be achievable using traditional methods.[34,35] Similar superparamagnetic particles conjugated with human epidermal growth factor receptor 2- and luteinizing hormone-releasing hormone antibodies have been used for MRI imaging of breast cancer cells.[36]

IV. Nanoparticle-Based Drug Delivery

Targeted drug delivery in the context of nanomedicine consists of two components: one is the active pharmaceutical ingredient,[37,38] and the other is the nanocarrier, although the formulation could be the drug itself, if possible.[39] The detailed strategies and methods in drug delivery and targeting using nanoparticle (NP) systems have been discussed previously. As a brief summary, one recalls that a targeting system is used to deliver a drug to the specific site and to minimize the drug's systemic toxicity. There are several requirements that need to be met for such a drug delivery system, including the capabilities to (1) navigate the bloodstream, (2) evade biological barriers, (3) target the appropriate site, and (4) trigger the appropriate response.[40] In general, the selection of a drug carrier should be made based on a number of factors including drug loading, drug release, solubility, targeting approach, stability of the formulation, and the biocompatibility and disposition of the carrier in the biological system. Biocompatible and biodegradation properties of an NP system are obviously desirable. Successful targeting also depends on having a better understanding of the fate of the particles in the body, which is summarized in the next section.

Disposition of Nanoparticles

Absorption

Nanoparticles (NPs) have been studied in oral and transdermal preparations for potential enhancement of product stability and/or drug absorption. Concerted efforts have been given to the development of oral vaccines using the NP system.[41,42] A number of studies have shown that the GI uptake of particles is size dependent, with NPs absorbed much more readily than microparticles.[42–44] For example, using polystyrene latex particles in the range of 50 nm to 3 µm, Jani et al. (1990) showed that in rats, the ingested particles with sizes of 50 and 100 nm were absorbed by 36% and 24%, respectively. In comparison, particles with sizes above 1 μm were trapped in the Peyer's Patches of the small intestine, which did not translocate to the circulation system.[43] The ingested NPs can enter the body by a process called *persorption*, which denotes a paracellular uptake of NPs from the GI tract into the lymphatic and blood circulation. Electron microscopic studies of ingested colloidal gold nanoparticles (4 to 58 nm) in mice indeed showed a size-dependent particle uptake in the small intestine by persorption, with smaller particles being more extensively absorbed than larger particles. The mechanism of absorption involves the penetration of NPs through holes created by single, degrading enterocytes in the process of being extruded from a villus.[42] The surface charge of the NPs also dictates their GI uptake, with positively charged NPs showing more effective absorption than neutral or negatively charged particles.[45]

In the study of transdermal absorption of nanoparticles, there is no consensus about whether nanoparticles can penetrate the skin barrier. Studies reported virtually no penetration of titanium dioxide through intact skin in a mini pig model.[46] Other studies, however, found that small amounts of zinc (soluble compound) from ZnO NPs, which is used in sunscreen products, are absorbed through human skin.[47] However, it is not known whether it is absorbed as nanoparticles, soluble Zn, or both. Despite some inconsistencies in the literature, studies continue to show that skin penetration by NPs may depend on several factors including the movement of skin, follicular openings, and the particle type and charge. For example, the penetration of fluorescent beads (500 to 1000 nm) through the epidermis occurred only after the application of a flexing motion,[48] as was the case with the penetration of skin by peptide-attached fullerene C_{60} nanospheres.[49] The surface charge of NPs is an important factor in its transdermal absorption in that negatively charged latex particles (50 and 500 nm) were found to penetrate the epidermis, but positively charged or neutral particles did not.[50] In addition, QDs with sizes of 4.6 nm (spherical) and 12 nm by 6 nm (ellipsoidal) were shown to penetrate intact skin.[51] These studies show that the skin is permeable to small and/or anionic nanoparticles, and that penetration may be enhanced by mechanical flexion.

Metabolism

There is no evidence that metal-based NPs are destroyed in the body after they reach the systemic circulation. However, these NPs may be involved in enzyme-mediated reactions. For example, the protein cap of a functionalized QD can be cut by proteases. The metallic core of QDs (and other metal oxides) may be bound by cysteine-rich metallothioneins and excreted. Enzymes such as metalloproteinases also bind metal to regulate cellular metal homeostasis. Of the carbon-based NPs, single-walled carbon nanotubes (SWCNT) have been shown to react with hypochlorite and reactive radical intermediates of the neutrophilic enzyme myeloperoxidase, in media containing neutrophils.[52] The extent to which carbon nanotubes are biodegraded may reflect the severity of the NP-induced inflammatory responses *in vivo*. In biodegradable systems, degradation of polymers, such as PLGA, is catalyzed by nonspecific esterases. Lipid NPs, on the other hand, are known to fuse with cell membranes and undergo lipid exchange.

In Circulation

After reaching the systemic circulation, NPs may interact with plasma proteins, coagulation factors, platelets, and red and white blood cells. The binding to plasma components may have a substantial effect on the metabolism, distribution, and excretion of nanoparticles.[41] Such binding may neutralize or inhibit the adverse effects of the NPs, facilitate phagocytosis following opsonization, or lead to particle excretion. A serum component, apolipoprotein-A1, has been shown to bind to silica and possibly other particles. Nanoparticles, such as gold and TiO_2, can enter human erythrocytes.[53] As these cells are not phagocytes, it is suggested that, instead of phagocytosis or endocytosis, the NPs may cross the cell membrane by processes such as diffusion, trans-membrane channels, adhesive interactions, or yet undefined mechanisms.[41] One other important observation is that NPs with diameters less than 200 nm may gain access to the central nervous system through the blood–brain barrier.[54]

Distribution and Elimination

After inhalation delivery of an aerosol consisting of Tc-labeled carbon NPs (<100 nm) to healthy subjects, radioactivity was detected in the blood at 1 minute, it reached a maximum between 10 and 20 minutes, and the radioactivity distribution in various organs followed.[55] This suggests that carbon NPs are quickly translocated into systemic circulation, and the distribution of NPs into tissues is through the circulation system. The major sites of NP accumulation are lung, liver, spleen, heart, kidney, and brain. The uptake of fluorescein isothiocyanate-labeled polystyrene particles (50 nm) in liver following IV injection was found exclusively in hepatocytes in the first hour via phagocytosis.[56] Biliary excretion of these nanoparticles was responsible for their elimination, which accounts for about 4% of the dose after 24 hours. The lung appears to be the first site of accumulation for IV-administered NPs through the lung filtration process. Zinc oxide NPs, after IV administration into mice for example, exhibited a primary retention in lung (43.6% of dose per gram of wet lung) in the first hour, followed by translocation to the intestinal tract for feces excretion at a later stage.[57] In nasal delivery, the major sites of NP distribution are liver, kidney, and olfactory bulb.[58]

The distribution of polymeric NPs may vary with their rate of biodegradation. A short-term study showed that in mice, the distribution of NPs made of PLGA at 7 days post-oral administration was 40% in the liver, 26% in the kidneys, and 13% in the brain.[59] The particles remained detectable in the brain, heart, kidneys, liver, lungs, and spleen well past the 7-day mark. For lipid NPs delivered endotracheally to the lungs, translocation of particles to the stomach, liver, auxiliary lymph nodes, and inguinal lymph nodes was observed 1 hour after delivery. Para-aortic lymph nodes were the site with the highest accumulation, with the lymphatic drainage being the main route for translocation of endotracheal-delivered lipid particles.[60]

The plasma elimination half-life for intratracheally instilled[59] Fe_2O_3 NPs in rats is 22.8 days.[61] For silica NPs (50, 100, or 200 nm), although the IV-administered dose (to mice) was partially cleared via urine and bile, a significant portion was found in macrophages in the spleen and liver and remained there for 4 weeks after a single injection.[62] The intravenously injected QD NPs in mice were detectable after 133 days in the lymph nodes and bone marrow.[63] All of these studies indicate that nondegradable NPs have a long and extended stay in the biological system. In a study of the particle size effect on tissue accumulation of NPs, Sarlo et al. (2009) showed that latex fluorospheres of 20 nm, 100 nm, or 1000 nm, administered by IV or repeated pharyngeal aspiration, can be detected in tissue up to 90–120 days after the final dose.[64] In thymus, the largest extra-pulmonary depot for the particles, 25% of the 20 nm particles were recovered after 4 months. In comparison, only 6% and 1–3% of the dose were recovered for particles of 100 and 1000 nm, respectively. These results show that particle distribution may be size dependent, and there is a late phase distribution of small nanoparticles even though a large amount of the NPs could be excreted rapidly. It is likely that not all NPs will be eliminated, and this would result in an accumulation in the body under repeated use.

The above discussion may be summarized to provide some perspectives on the use of nanoparticles for drug delivery. First, the extended resident time and distribution of NPs in the biological system is a serious toxicological concern. Thus, biodegradable NPs, such as those of the polymeric types, are preferred for drug delivery purposes. Second, the interaction of NPs with plasma constituents may play a role in drug delivery in several ways. Removal of opsonized NPs by phagocytes will lower the stability of NPs in circulation and their drug targeting capability. Interaction of NPs with plasma substances may aid in their elimination through the renal system, which may be of value for nondegradable particles, or allow them to remain in the vasculature for drug delivery purposes. Third, several studies have shown distribution of NPs in brain tissue following different routes of administration, indicating that nanoparticles penetrate the blood–brain barrier.[42, 59, 65] This may be used to provide targeted delivery of drugs, despite concerns over their potential toxicity, to the central nervous system.

Delivery Systems

The following is a brief discussion of several classes of the NP delivery systems.

Liposomes

Liposomes are spherical phospholipid vesicles (composed of amphiphilic phospholipids and cholesterol), and they have a self-associated bilayer with an aqueous interior (similar to that seen with biological membranes). Properties such as permeability, charge density, and steric hindrance of the phospholipid constituents dictate overall physicochemical properties of the liposome itself.[2] Varying between 50 and 100 nm, liposomal vesicles may be classified as uni- or multilamellar depending upon the size and number of layers of the constituent phospholipids.

Liposomes demonstrate excellent circulation, penetration, and diffusion properties, and owing to their amphiphilicity, liposomes have the ability to incorporate both hydrophilic drugs, by trapping them within their aqueous interior, and lipophilic drugs, by incorporating them into the phospholipid membrane. Liposomes may be loaded with drug through several processes, including (1) solvent exchange mechanisms involving organic solvents, (2) use of drugs with high lipophilicity, (3) formation of liposome in a solution saturated with the drug, or (4) formation of a drug–liposome complex using a pH gradient.[66] Based upon the pH of the drug being encapsulated, liposomes may be further classified into anionic, neutral, and cationic forms. Anionic and neutral liposomes have poor encapsulation efficiencies[67]; cationic liposomes, on the other hand, are the most widely used and preferred form for drug delivery. Not only is a more stable complex achieved with a negatively charged drug and a positively charged liposomal carrier, but also cationic liposomes carry a net positive charge, which facilitates their interactions with the negatively charged plasma membrane and promotes internalization of the complex via endocytosis.[68] However, cationic liposomes do show nonspecific binding to other tissue compartments including blood plasma and endothelial blood vessels, leading to decreased biological activity of the drug. Nevertheless, liposomal delivery systems are relatively inert and demonstrate low toxicity and limited antigen stimulation, making them favorable systems for drug delivery.

The liposomal membrane is amenable to modification by addition of ligands and polymeric moieties, which may increase both the targeting selectivity and the activity of the encapsulated drug. Liposomes home in to their intended site of action by extravasating into the interstitial space from the bloodstream, and they can target specific tissue by both passive and active strategies. However, owing to their relatively large size, liposomes are rapidly cleared by the phagocytic macrophages, leading to a decrease in half-life. This may be successfully countered by the incorporation of poly(ethylene) glycol moieties to the liposome structure (known as PEGylation), which not only leads to increased stability of the system in circulation, but also enhances the selectivity of the drug. A good example is the PEGylated Doxil (liposomal preparation of doxorubicin for treatment of leukemia), where PEGylation leads to antitumor effects in both drug-resistant and non-drug-resistant cells.[69] The success of Doxil has stimulated intense research into the development of liposomal formulations for several forms of cancer.

Lipid Nanoparticles

Lipospheres are solid lipid nanoparticles at body temperature (37.8°C) with a diameter of up to 1000 nm, and they can be synthesized using a combination of a wide range of lipids, including mono-, di-, and triglycerides and fatty acids. Lipospheres are produced by replacing the liquid lipid (oil) of an oil-in-water emulsion by a solid lipid, which may be produced using several commercially viable methods.[70] Lipospheres are biodegradable and biocompatible, and they exhibit low toxicity in humans.[71] Several factors affect drug loading onto lipospheres, including (1) lipophilicity of the drug, (2) physicochemical properties of the lipid, (3) type of lipid used to make the nanosphere, and (4) crystalline characteristics of the lipid at 37.8°C.[70] Lipospheres have been investigated for the delivery of various anticancer drugs, including doxorubicin, cholesteryl butyrate, mitoxantrone, and paclitaxel.[71, 72]

The term *nanocapsule* refers to any NP system having a shell and space that allow drug to be encapsulated. Colloidal vesicular nanocapsules can be made to contain a unique polymer membrane with desired drug release characteristics. For example, oil-based nanocapsules may be prepared by interfacial polymerization of alkylcyanoacrylate, and the oily nature and ultrafine particle size of poly(acryl cyanoacrylate) shell allow for sustained drug release.[73] There are several advantages to using nanocapsules as drug delivery systems. Nanocapsules have a high loading capacity–polymer content ratio and may be utilized for both lipophilic and hydrophilic drugs.[74] Nanocapsules are also very amenable to modifications in size, shape, and structure. For example, pH-sensitive nanocapsules with varying release characteristics may be synthesized so as to swell or shrink in response to changes in pH. Also, encapsulation of the drug prevents unwanted allergic reactions and protects the drug from degradation during both storage and administration.[75] Nanocapsules also provide for increased bioavailability of drug, higher levels of safety and efficacy, and improved patient compliance. They are, however, susceptible to phagocytic clearance in circulation, which limits their use in IV drug delivery. The surface properties of the nanocapsules largely dictate the drug release rate. Methods that can be used for precise manipulation of surface properties and particle size are some of the subjects of current research.

Micelles

Micelles formed by simple amphiphilic molecules (surfactants) are nanosize, colloidal dispersions with a hydrophobic core and a hydrophilic shell, and they are used to increase the solubility and bioavailability of poorly soluble drugs.[3, 76] Their individual size is less than 50 nm in diameter, which, together with their thermodynamically stable hydrophilic shell, provides a significant advantage over liposomes in terms of evading the mononuclear phagocytic system (MPS).[77] This allows the micelles to circulate in the vascular system over extended time. In micelle formation, the lipophilic fragments of the amphiphilic molecules are combined to form a hydrophobic core, whereas the hydrophilic fragments are arranged and stabilized by the aqueous environment to form the outer shell. Incorporation of a hydrophobic drug into the micelle core in fact stabilizes the micelle system. Hydrophilic molecules may associate with the micelles at the surface, while drugs with intermediate polarity may be incorporated along areas where both hydrophilic and hydrophobic interactions exist. Micelles may be modified in a manner similar to liposomes. For example, pH-sensitive drug-binding linkers may be added to the micelle for controlled release of drugs.[78] They may also be modified to contain targeting ligands to achieve tissue specificity.

The term *polymeric micelles* refers to micelles formed by a block copolymer that contains a hydrophilic homopolymer block and a hydrophobic homopolymer block. The critical micelle concentration for polymeric micelles is significantly lower than that of the common micelles formed by simple surfactants. Polymeric micelles are thus more versatile in their application in drug delivery, especially in passive and active targeting of tumor tissue.

Gold Nanoparticles

Gold nanoparticles (GNP) may be formulated into nanospheres, nanoshells, nanorods, or nanocages. They contain a surface made up of gold atoms that may be functionalized with a monolayer of several types of moieties including thiol groups, peptides, glyconanoparticles, and phosphonioalkyl selenoates.[79] Gold nanoparticles are synthesized via reduction of gold tertrachloride by sodium borohydride in the presence of thiols, and may be further functionalized using other moieties.[80] Gold nanoparticles are relatively nontoxic in a number of human cell lines and are favored for their stability, targeting ability, and evasion of host defenses.[80, 81] Application of gold nanoparticles as drug delivery carrier is under intense investigation (e.g., gold nanoparticles bound to the anticancer agent paclitaxel), and current uses are restricted mainly to gene therapy and imaging.[82, 83]

Carbon Nanotubes

Carbon nanotubes are formed by a coaxial sheet of graphite less than 100 nm in length, arranged in the form of a cylinder.[7] Carbon nanotubes may be designed either as a single- (one graphite sheet) or multiwall nanotubes. Fullerenes, similar to carbon nanotubes in their molecular framework, are synthesized either by vaporization of graphite or by combustion of simple hydrocarbons.[84] Carbon nanotubes demonstrate excellent electrical properties, and their semiconductor nature makes them ideal candidates for biosensing. Further, they can be rendered hydrophilic and functionalized, making them potentially useful as drug carriers and tissue-repair scaffolds.[85]

Nanocrystals

Nanocrystals are crystalline aggregates of hydrophobic drug molecules, coated with a thin hydrophilic layer that aids in the distribution and bioavailability of the enclosed drug, ultimately leading to increased efficiency of overall drug delivery.[86] The use of an appropriate coating layer is critical to achieving high dose levels and increased bioavailability of nanocrystals. An important drawback, however, is the need for crystallization of the active compound (which might not always be feasible) and limited stability of the nanocrystal itself. One of the first nanoparticle-based drugs to be approved was the immunosuppressant sirolimus formulated using a NanoCrystal technology (by Elan Pharmaceuticals).[2] Since then, nanocrystal-based formulations for paclitaxil and doxorubicin have been tested in clinical trials.[87, 88]

Quantum dots, which are aggregates of colloidal fluorescent semiconductor nanocrystals ranging in size from 2 to 10 nm, are a specialized form of nanocrystals widely used in biological imaging and as labels for bioassays.[89, 90] They are composed of a central semiconductor core surrounded by a thin coating of surfactant. The central core may be composed of a combination of cadmium, indium, lead, and gallium compounds, coated over with a thin layer of zinc sulfide.[84, 91] In some cases, the core may be PEGylated so as to increase the biocompatibility and stability in biological systems.[92] Quantum dots have been extensively tested for *in vivo* imaging of cancers in experimental animals. They absorb white light and reemit it within nanoseconds with different bulk band gap energies corresponding to fluorescent light between 400 and 1350 nm. Quantum dots support various applications such as multicolored imaging,[93, 94] cell labeling and tracking,[95] gene expression,[96] fluorescence resonance energy transfer, and *in vivo* imaging.[97, 98]

Polymeric Nanoparticles

Nanoparticles made of mostly biodegradable organic polymers take the form of nanospheres, nanocapsules, liposomes, or polymeric micelles. The fabrication of these particles as well as their intended use as a drug delivery system depend on the physicochemical properties of the polymer(s) used. For example, nanospheres and nanocapsules can be readily made using chitosan, a cationic polysaccharide consisting of repeating glucosamine and *N*-acetyl-glucosamine units, with a pK_a of 6.5. Chitosan, at acidic pH, interacts with polyanionic polymers, proteins, and cell membrane. As a result, this polymer exhibits mucoadhesive properties, increases cellular permeability, and can be used to improve the bioavailability of orally delivered proteins. Chitosan may be used to coat lipid particles or mix with other polymers such as carbomers, Pluronics, and sodium alginate to form pH-, thermal-, and ion-sensitive nanocapsules for controlled drug delivery. It can also be used to incorporate proteins, such as insulin, or DNA to form nanoparticles for oral protein or gene delivery.[99] An example of a thermosenstive nanocapsule preparation is the combination of chitosan with Pluronic F127. The nanocapsules are expanded at 4°C (~240 nm), which allows for the incorporation of a drug, but become small at 37°C (~37 nm) for slow drug release.[100] Polymer-based nanocarriers are easily amenable to functional modifications for evading MPS and/or drug targeting purposes.

Dendrimers, which are spherical-shape polymers generated using a series of convergent or divergent polymerization reactions, contain repeated branches of polymer chains around a central core.[101] Dendrimers may either act as reservoirs, encapsulating drug molecules inside their core, or present multiple ligands per dendrimer due to the high number of functional groups. The potential applications of dendrimers in drug delivery include drug targeting and formulations for non-steroidal anti-inflammatory drugs, antimicrobials, antivirals, and prodrugs.

Application Areas

In this section, the applicability of the aforementioned nanotechnology-based delivery systems and imaging probes in the treatment of a number of disease states is described.

Cancer Treatment

One of the major application areas for nanoparticle delivery systems is in the treatment of cancer. Several agents developed over the years have greatly improved the imaging, diagnosis, and treatment of cancer.

Polymeric Systems

Liposomal delivery systems were among the first to experience success in the targeting of cancer. Doxil, a liposomal formulation of the anthracycline drug doxorubicin, has already been approved for the treatment of cancer in AIDS-related Kaposi's sarcoma and multiple myeloma, and it is currently undergoing clinical trials for breast cancer. Other cancer drugs that are currently being developed using liposomal nanodelivery systems include daunorubicin (DaunoXome), vincristine (Onco-TCS) (SPI-77), and lurtotecan (OSI-211).[102] A micellar preparation of paclitaxil has also been developed that allows for significant dose escalation of paclitaxel, and patients previously unresponsive to traditional paclitaxel demonstrated strong antitumor responses.[5] In another study, micellar preparations of the topoisomerase inhibitor mitoxantrone, when injected into mice with breast cancer and lymph node metastasis, showed a threefold reduction in lymph node size compared to control animals, which were given free mitoxantrone alone.[70]

The primary purpose of cancer drug delivery is to improve drug efficacy while reducing the drug's systemic toxicity. In this light, some polymeric preparations for paclitaxel and cisplatin have shown an ability to induce apoptotic death of the cancer cells, but, more importantly, they have elicited minimal toxic responses from patients who would otherwise demonstrate symptomatic effects of drug toxicity when administered the noncarrier form of paclitaxel and cisplatin.[103, 104] The U.S. FDA has already approved Abraxane (paclitaxel conjugated to albumin nanoparticles), which shows longer circulation half-life, greater efficacy against metastatic breast cancer, and reduced toxic side effects compared to free paclitaxel.[105]

Gene Delivery

In addition to drugs, nanoparticles may act as gene carriers to target cancer.[106] For example, nanoliposomes modified with the transcriptional activator TAT quickly and efficiently translocated to human breast adenocarcinomas.[107] Albumin nanoparticles containing several antisense oligonucleotides could also effectively target tumors from various tissues.[108] Another system used is the poly(ethylamine)–poly(ethylene glycol) nanospheres functionalized with the Arg-Gly-Asp (RGD) peptide motif, which could specifically target tumor vasculature overexpressing integrins, and successfully deliver siRNA that countered the expression of vascular endothelial growth factor receptor-2.[109]

Experimental Systems

Gold nanoparticles functionalized with paclitaxel (for breast cancer) and 6-mercaptopurine (for leukemia) have been shown to exhibit greater antitumor effects against cancer compared to free drug.[110, 111] The rationale of using GNP for anticancer drug delivery lies in the possibility that some combined therapy may be achieved based on the surface properties of the gold nanoparticles. These relatively nontoxic particles bind easily to antibodies that recognize the cancer cells; they can be used for cancer cell detection via the surface plasmon resonance effect, and they can also destroy tumor cells via noninvasive radiowave thermal ablation. Of the other NP types, fullerenes loaded with Taxol have been tested for delivering drug to skin melanomas,[112] and quantum dot-tagged doxorubicin was shown to provide both targeting and delivering specificity to prostate cancer cells as evidenced by simultaneous imaging.[98] In addition, XPclad NPs have been engineered to carry both hydrophilic and hydrophobic drugs. XPclad carriers loaded with cisplatin resulted in significant prostate tumor regression in mice without seriously affecting normal cells.[113] As mentioned earlier, dendrimers have the potential to be an effective delivery system for a wide array of small-molecule drugs. In tumor cell targeting, dendrimeric preparations of doxorubicin,[114] etoposide,[115] and paclitaxel[116] are being investigated, and a methotrexate-containing dendrimer preparation has been shown to target human tumors via overexpressed folic acid receptor and reduce tumor cell growth.[117]

Gene and Vaccine Delivery

The successful delivery of exogenous DNA to the cell is an important approach to regulate cellular function, and it has been one of the important goals of gene therapy. The delivery of genetic material may be achieved by using engineered viral delivery systems that allow for packaging of the DNA and delivering it by using the inherent abilities of the virus to infect a cell and deliver its genetic package. However, issues such as risk of reversion of virus to its native form, initiation of an immune response leading to de novo carcinogenesis, and failure to achieve large-scale production of the viruses have prompted the development of nonviral delivery systems.[118] Several nonviral nanoformulations that allow for efficient DNA delivery without the cytotoxicity, immunogenic reactions, and cost associated with viral systems have been developed and tested.[119, 120] Owing to their malleability in terms of structure manipulation and high stability of the DNA enclosed, cationic lipids and polymers are some of the most popular delivery systems being investigated for gene delivery.[121–123] Various nanocarriers such as 2-diethylaminoether-dextran, poly(ethylenimine), and other artificial lipids have been used for DNA delivery, both *in vitro* and *in vivo*. Further, coupling of the DNA polyplexes with molecules such as transferrin, folate, antibodies, nuclear localization sequence tags, or calcium phosphate has been found to enhance the transfection efficiency of these delivery systems.[124–126]

Nanoparticle systems have also been developed, particularly as adjuvants, to enhance the delivery of vaccines for various diseases. This is mainly due to the fact that currently used aluminum-based adjuvants trigger allergic reactions in some populations, and increased levels of IgE and T-helper type 2 responses in others, without the induction of cell-mediated immunity.[127] Novel nanoparticle adjuvant systems such as poly(methyl methacrylate) and poly(lactic-*co*-glycolic acid) coupled to staphylococcal enterotoxin B toxoid demonstrated a strong cellular immune response compared to aluminum salts, suggesting that they could be used as suitable alternatives to the current aluminum-based adjuvants.[128, 129]

Cardiovascular Therapy

Cardiac disease represents one of the major causes of mortality and disability in the United States. Although several drugs are available for treating heart disease and other associated comorbid conditions, most drugs do not provide the appropriate level of drug in the target arteries for sufficient periods of time. Several microscale instruments have been developed to open blocked arteries, but they are extremely bulky and prone to infection. Hence, nanotechnology-based tools are being developed to overcome these significant impedances to therapy, including nanosensors that can monitor biological signals such as the release of proteins or antibodies in response to cardiac inflammation.[130]

One of the primary causes of heart disease is the formation of atherosclerotic plaques. Nanoparticles, designed to circulate in the bloodstream to allow them to adhere to specific regions of the vasculature,[131] can be used to treat this problem. An important consideration for such a delivery system is the targeting ability of the nanoparticles to the atherosclerotic lesions. To date, a number of systems have been shown to provide targeting specificity for imaging of atherosclerotic lesions. For example, cysteine-arginine-glutamate-lysine-alanine (CREKA) functionalized micellular preparations of heparin have been shown effectively to target atherosclerotic plaques,[132] and the use of magnetofluorescent nanoparticles targeted to vascular adhesion molecule-1 has provided enhanced MRI contrast and fluorescent imaging contrast capabilities.[133] Similar success was also achieved using a paramagnetic liquid perfluorocarbon nanoparticle preparation, which incorporates a vitronectin antagonist that targets integrins.[134, 135] Hydrophobically modified chitosan nanoparticles and magnetofluorescent nanoparticles coupled to dextran have also been shown to accumulate preferentially at atherosclerotic lesions.[136, 137]

Nanoparticle-based delivery systems can also be used to combat other cardiac problems including myocardial infarction, arrhythmias, and retenosis, with appropriate targeting ligands and drugs.[138] Abciximab, a chimeric monoclonal antibody, has sensors that bind and inhibit the fibrinogen receptors through steric hindrance, leading to decreased inflammation. Tenecteplase, produced using recombinant DNA technology, is a tissue plasminogen activator that dissolves blood clots formed in blood vessels of the heart. Although therapies to combat restenosis have largely been ineffective, localized drug therapies using nanopreparations with sustained-release capabilities are currently being investigated.[130]

Neurological Diseases

The central nervous system is a tissue unlike most in the body in the sense that it is protected by a unique membrane known as the blood–brain barrier. The unique morphology of the capillary system in the barrier with its abundant tight junctions prevents the entry of almost all foreign bodies including therapeutic agents into the central nervous system.[139–142] Substances may therefore gain access to the central nervous system only by lipid-mediated free diffusion or through receptor-mediated endocytosis. Nanotechnology provides an effective alternative that may help bypass this barrier, thereby allowing for the treatment of diseases using drugs that might not otherwise have any therapeutic effects.

Glioblastoma multiforme is one of the most lethal neoplasms with a mean survival period of 1 year, and it is characterized by upregulation of low-density lipoprotein (LDL) receptors, which makes them susceptible to LDL.[143, 144] However, the isolation and reconstitution of natural LDL from plasma have proved extremely difficult, and alternative versions are desirable. To this end, synthetic LDL nanoparticles carrying paclitaxel have been shown effectively to inhibit glioblastoma multiforme tumor cell growth.[145]

Another important health concern with respect to the nervous system is the incidence of stroke, caused due to the rupture of atherosclerotic plaques in the neuronal vasculature. Fibrin is one of the critical components of atherosclerotic plaques, and it is a primary target for therapeutics against stroke. Magnetic nanoparticles conjugated to an antibody fragment of fibrin via avidin–biotin linkages have been successfully used to target fibrin in atherosclerotic plaques.[146, 147] Further, paclitaxel-loaded nanoparticles also inhibited vascular smooth-cell proliferation, an important approach to inhibiting strokes. Nanoparticle formulations of fumagillin, an antiangiogenic agent, also resulted in a reduction of growing plaques.[84]

Neurodegenerative diseases such as Alzheimer's and Parkinson's are extremely degenerative and debilitating, and this represents one of the growing areas of research toward identifying therapeutic interventions. Alzheimer's disease, the most common form of dementia in populations over 65 years of age, is caused by the accumulation of β-amyloid plaques. Therapeutic agents such as acetylcholinesterase inhibitors, antioxidants, c-secretase inhibitors, and vaccines against β-amyloid protein are being investigated to treat this disease.[148, 149] Neurodegenerative diseases are also associated with oxidative stress induced by elevated levels of iron, copper, and zinc. To this end, polymeric nanoparticles are currently being investigated to carry metal chelators such as desferrioxamine, which is normally toxic and is incapable of traversing the blood–brain barrier due to its high hydrophilicity.[150]

V. Toxicological Assessment of Nanomaterials

The rapid progress in the field of nanotechnology and the exponential growth in the applicability of nanomaterials in biomedical fields such as imaging, drug delivery, diagnostics, cancer therapy, and gene delivery have led to an associated increase in the propensity for potentially toxic health effects from the use of nanomaterials. Studies to investigate these effects and their underlying mechanisms have not been sufficiently conducted. This is the primary pitfall of nanobiotechnology as with other emerging technologies that hold immense potential, where the focus is still on expanding the applicability of these tools to tap into the many benefits that nanotechnology offers.

Nanoproperty and Toxicity

Size and Shape-Dependent Effects

It is now well documented that factors such as size, shape, surface chemistry, synthesis methodology, degree of agglomeration, and chemical entity and composition all play a critical role in determining the overall toxicological profile of both organic and inorganic nanoparticles.[151] Nanoparticle-induced toxicity arising from the small size and high surface area/volume ratio of nanoparticles, increased persistence of these nanostructures in various tissues in the body, and particle agglomeration also preclude the applicability of current standards of safety to these materials that are altered at the nanometer level.[6] All carbon-, metal-, and metal oxide-based nanoparticles are potentially genotoxic, as evidenced by DNA damage measurements. Particles less than 100 nm in size have a very high likelihood of aggregating, which (depending upon the diameter of the vasculature) may potentially occlude blood flow, thus triggering a change of the coagulation pathways.[84] Further, changes in circulation times and clearance from the body, e.g., in the case of radiotherapeutic nanoparticles, may lead to severe side effects. Some nanoparticles are fibrous, such as the carbon nanotubes, which are allotropes of carbon with a cylindrical nanostructure. The SWCNT are tube structures with a diameter of close to 1 nm and are composed of a one-atom-thick layer of graphite, and MWCNT are tube structures with diameters of tens of nanometers and composed of two or more layers of graphite atoms. These particles induce pulmonary fibrosis but have somewhat different mechanisms. In the case of SWCNT, the single-wall structure allows the particles to penetrate the lung epithelium and directly stimulate fibroblasts proliferation for the fibrotic process. This is different from the action of other fibrotic agents, which induce fibrosis by causing a persistent inflammation in the lung.[152] MWCNT with relatively longer lengths (1–5 μm) have been found to induce mesothelioma. This structure allows the particles to migrate to the subpleural tissue, penetrate the visceral pleura, and enter the intrapleural space.[153] Particles of barium sulfate, used in gastroendoscopy, are quite often found in liver tissue; this also suggests a possible breach of the interstitial barrier by NPs.[154]

Safety Issues

The concern of nanoparticle toxicity applies not only to the patient population, but also to individuals who are exposed to the nanomaterials during the manufacturing and disposal processes. Nanoparticles can be easily aerosolized or incorporated into the groundwater when disposed, and specialized filtration and protection techniques might be required sufficiently to manage the disposal of nanoparticle-based systems.[155] Therefore, there is a need for more work to be done to assess the toxicological effects of nanomaterials that will be used in the fields of medicine and health care. The known toxicity of a number of NP systems with potential applications in drug delivery is summarized in the next section.

Toxicity of Nanomaterials

Acute and Chronic Toxicity

A number of nondegradable nanoparticle systems have been studied for potential application as drug delivery systems. The toxicity profiles of these systems, as reported in the literature, are summarized in **Table 18-3**.

Table 18-3 Toxicological Profiles of Some Medical Nanomaterials

Nanomaterial	Acute and Chronic Toxicity	Genotoxicity/Carcinogenesis
Mesoporous Silica		
In vivo (IV injection) silica NP, 70 nm	Liver injury detected by serum aminotransferase and inflammatory cytokines; hepatic fibrosis	
Silica NP, 300 and 1000 nm	No effect at 100 mg/kg body weight	
Gold Nanoparticles (GNP)		
In vitro	GNP-induced apoptosis or necrosis in different cell types; cationic, but not anionic, functionalized GNP showed moderate toxicity.	Genotoxicity: Comet assay of bronchoalveolar lavage cells from mice via 54 μg/mouse instillation
In vivo (IV injection)	PEGylated GNP accumulated in the liver and spleen for up to 7 days and induced acute inflammation and apoptosis in liver with numerous NP-containing cytoplasmic vesicles and lysosomes within liver Kupffer cells and spleen macrophages.	
In vivo (oral administration)	All animals survived at 28 days posttreatment with no significant changes in clinical signs, hematological parameters, body and organ weights, or histopathology; LD50: > 2000 mg/kg body weight.	
Colloidal Nanosilver		
In vitro	Decreased cell viability of murine peritoneal macrophages at 1 to 25 ppm after 24-hour cell culture	
In vivo (intratracheal instillation)	Pulmonary inflammation	

(*Continues*)

Table 18-3 (*Continued*)

Nanomaterial	Acute and Chronic Toxicity	Genotoxicity/Carcinogenesis
Fullerenes		
Polyalkylsulfonated fullerene C_{60}	No toxicity was observed for fullerene C_{60}. No toxicity was observed after oral administration, but rats died within 30 hours after intraperitoneal injection; LD50 = 600 mg/kg body weight; rats injected with this NP intraperitoneally or intravenously exhibited distinct lysosome-overload nephrosis and phagolysosomal nephropathy.	Genotoxicity: transgenic mouse mutation system, at 10 μg/ml, gpt delta transgenic mouse primary embryo fibroblasts; Comet assay, 24 hours, doses between 0 and 200 μg/ml or long-term subculture (576 hours) at 100 μg/mL, FE1 mouse lung epithelial cells; Comet assay, at 2.2 μg/L in human lymphocytes
Carbon Nanotubes		
In vitro	Both SWCNT and MWCNT induce cytotoxicity, oxidative stress, apoptosis, and necrosis.	Genotoxicity: Comet assay at 0 to 40 μg/cm² in human lung epithelial cells (A549); transformation of bronchial epithelial cells after long-term, low-dose exposure.
In vivo (intrapulmonary delivery)	Aspiration of SWCNT or MWCNT results in transient inflammation and lung injury, persistent granulomas, and rapid and progressive interstitial fibrosis in mice; both SWCNT and MWCNT promote allergic responses in mice and increase lung susceptibility to pulmonary infection.	Intraperitoneal or intrascrotal injection of MWCNT produces mesothelioma in rodents.
In vivo (IV injection)	Survival rates and clinical and lab parameters revealed no evidence of toxicity in mice over 4 months after IV injection of SWCNT, but data suggested further confirmation using larger groups of animals was necessary.	
Titanium Dioxide		
In vivo (intrapulmonary delivery)	Pulmonary inflammation	Genotoxicity: among others, sister chromatid exchange, and micronucleus test at 0.5 and 1 μg/mL; Comet assay at 40, 60, 80, and 100 μg/cm² in human bronchial epithelial BEAS 2B cells; cell transformation assay, long-term exposure, and cultured fibroblast cells; DNA adduct formation at 5 and 10 μg/cm² and human lung fibroblasts; gene mutation at 10 μg/ml and gpt delta transgenic mouse primary embryo fibroblasts. Carcinogen in rodents; possible carcinogen in humans.

Silicon Dioxide (Silica)

Multifunctional silicon dioxide (SiO_2) nanoparticle systems are used for drug delivery and as food additives under current regulations. Mesoporous SiO_2 is a synthetic form of SiO_2 derived from nanotechnology; its porous nature allows for high drug loading onto the particles. The common types of mesoporous nanoparticles include Mobile Crystalline Material (MCM-41) and Santa Barbara Amorphous type material (SBA-15). Crystalline SiO_2 can be carcinogenic and is known to cause inflammation, lung injury, and fibrosis.[156] Studies have shown that SiO_2 NPs with a diameter of 70 nm (SP70) induced liver injury at 30 mg/kg body weight when given by IV injection, while larger particles (300 or 1000 nm) had no effect even at 100 mg/kg body weight.[158] The silica-induced toxicity includes dose-dependent increases in serum markers of liver injury, serum aminotransferase, and inflammatory cytokines. Repeated administration of SP70 twice a week for 4 weeks at 10 mg/kg body weight produced hepatic fibrosis. In contrast to these findings, mesoporous SiO_2 NPs have been considered to exhibit low toxicity and are used as carriers for targeted drug delivery to the heart.[157]

Gold Nanoparticles

Gold nanoparticles (GNP) have been shown to induce apoptosis or necrosis in different cell types.[159, 160] Cationic functionalized GNP also exert moderate toxicity compared to anionic functionalized GNP. In vivo studies in mice showed that PEG-coated GNP (13 nm) induced acute inflammation and apoptosis in the liver.[161] These particles were accumulated in the liver and spleen for up to 7 days. Transmission electron microscopy revealed numerous cytoplasmic vesicles and lysosomes within liver Kupffer cells and spleen macrophages, where the PEGylated GNP resided. Studies by Chen et al. (2009) showed that, in mice, naked GNP ranging from 8 to 100 nm injected intraperitoneally at a dose of 8 mg/kg body weight did not cause any adverse effects; however, GNP ranging from 8 to 37 nm induced severe sickness, fatigue, change of fur color, loss of appetite, and weight loss.[162] In another study in mice using different doses (40, 200, or 400 μg/kg body weight per day) of 12.5 nm GNP and intraperitoneal administration every day for 8 days, there was a dose-dependent tissue accumulation of GNP, but no evidence of toxicity was observed based on measurements of survival, behavior, body weight, organ morphology, blood biochemistry, and tissue histology.[65] In rats receiving GNP orally for 28 days, all animals survived the duration of the study with no significant changes in clinical signs, body weight, food consumption, hematological parameters, organ weight, or histopathology. The LD50 value of GNP in rats was greater than 2000 mg/kg body weight.[163]

Silver Nanoparticles

As a new generation of antimicrobials, nanosilver has been progressively used in products of nanomedicine. *In vitro* studies showed that the commercial colloidal nanosilver causes significant decrease in cell viability of murine peritoneal macrophages at concentrations of 1 to 25 ppm in 24-hour cell culture.[164] This acute cytotoxicity has urged *in vivo* studies to delineate the potential toxicity of silver nanoparticles. Intratracheally delivered silver NPs were found to induce pulmonary inflammatory response.[165]

Fullerenes

Nanoparticles of pristine fullerene C_{60} have no acute or chronic toxicity or genotoxicity in mice, rats, or guinea pigs.[166–168] However, some fullerene C_{60} derivatives are highly toxic.[168] Polyalkylsulfonated fullerene C_{60} is a highly hydrophilic fullerene derivative. When given orally to rats, no animal death or toxicity was observed. But when given by intraperitoneal injection, rats died within 30 hours, with an LD50 of about 600 mg/kg body weight. The animals exhibited distinct lysosome-overload nephrosis and phagolysosomal nephropathy, characterized by a tinctorial difference between the outer cortex and the inner cortex and the medulla.[169]

Carbon Nanotubes

Carbon nanotubes, including SWCNT and MWCNT, recently emerged as delivery vehicles for potential use in cancer treatment and gene therapy.[170] These carriers are generally delivered IV. Interactions of these particles with human cells and tissues are not well known, but both SWCNT and MWCNT were shown to induce cytotoxicity, oxidative stress, apoptosis, and necrosis *in vitro*.[171, 172] Aspiration of MWCNT results in transient inflammation and lung injury, a rapid and persistent granulomatous response, and rapid and progressive interstitial fibrosis in a mouse model.[173, 174] Similarly, aspiration or inhalation of SWCNT in mice causes transient inflammation, granulomas at deposition sites, and progressive interstitial fibrosis due to the rapid migration of smaller SWCNT structures into the alveolar septa.[175, 176] Both SWCNT and MWCNT induce an allergic response in mice, and the aspiration of SWCNT prior to pulmonary exposure to bacteria significantly increased the susceptibility of mice to pulmonary infection.[177] A study of IV-injected SWCNT in mice revealed no evidence of toxicity over 4 months, but the data suggested that further studies with larger groups of animals were necessary.[178]

Quantum Dots

A few studies exist that specifically address the toxic effects of quantum dots. They have been shown to be toxic *in vitro*,[179–181] with toxicity driven by the surface modifications of the quantum dot and potential leakage of metallic components for the nanoparticle core.

Genotoxicity

Toxicological test systems or end points used in *genotoxicity* studies include the Comet assay, micronucleus test, Ames test, mammalian (including human, rat, and mouse) cell gene mutation, sister chromatid exchange, chromosomal alterations, and cell transformation. The genotoxicity of TiO_2, fullerene $C_{60,}$ and silver nanoparticles have been well studied, whereas those of other nanoparticles are in need of further characterization. The micronucleus test is recognized as one of the most reliable assays for identifying genotoxic carcinogens. Both silver NPs and fullerene C_{60} tested negative with this method.[182] The Comet assay, also called single-cell gel electrophoresis, is a sensitive and rapid technique for quantifying and analyzing DNA damage in individual cells. Most Comet assay results were positive when used to evaluate the genotoxicity of nanoparticles, implying that nanoparticles possess the potential to induce DNA damage. The Ames test is a biological assay to evaluate the mutagenic potential of chemical compounds. Interestingly, all Ames test results in tested nanoparticles were negative; it is possible that Ames tests are not suitable for systems containing water-insoluble nanoparticles. As shown in Table 18-3, titanium dioxide, derivatized fullerenes, and carbon nanotubes exhibit genotoxicity.

Carcinogenicity

Studies of the carcinogenicity of nanoparticles have just begun. Due to a lack of epidemiological data, it has not been established whether exposure to engineered nanoparticles produces cancer in humans. TiO_2 nanoparticles are manufactured worldwide in large quantities for use in a wide range of personal-care products and nanomedicine. Carcinogenicity studies in rodents indicate that TiO_2 NPs produced lung tumors when given by inhalation[183, 184] or by intratracheal instillation[185] in rats. In these studies, several dosing strategies were used, and the incidence of lung tumors was characterized as adenomas/carcinomas and squamous cell epitheliomas/carcinomas. Based on these studies, the International Agency for Research on Cancer (IARC) concluded that TiO_2 NPs are carcinogenic in experimental animals,[186, 187] and, because of the lack of human epidemiological data, TiO_2 NPs are classified by WHO/IARC as a Group 2B compound (possibly carcinogenic to humans).

Pulmonary delivery of SWCNT in studies up to 6 months long did not result in tumor induction. However, cellular atopia, characterized by hypertrophic bronchoalveolar epithelial cells and multinucleated alveolar macrophages, has been reported.[188, 189] In addition, inhaled SWCNT resulted in significant mutations in the k-ras gene in mice, which has been associated with lung cancer.[175] MWCNT (3500 ppm iron content; diameter: 100 nm; length: 1–5 μm) have been reported to induce mesothelioma in p53 (+/–) mice at 25 weeks after intraperitoneal injection of a 3 mg/mouse dose.[190] The incidence of mesothelioma in the peritoneal cavity (87.5%) in the MWCNT group was significantly elevated compared to the control. Induction of mesothelioma by MWCNT (3500 ppm iron content; diameter 70–100 nm; length 1–4 μm) by a single intrascrotal injection of 20 mg/animal was also reported in rats at week 104.[191] The length of the MWCNT is of importance in mesothelioma induction. In a study in which rats were given MWCNT with an 11.3 nm mean diameter and a length of 0.7 μm by a single intraperitoneal injection at a dose of 20 mg/rat and observed for 104 weeks, the incidence of mesothelioma in the MWCNT groups was not statistically different from the vehicle-only control group.[192] The above discussion shows that there is insufficient data to evaluate the carcinogenicity of SWCNT, but that intraperitoneal or intrascrotal injections of MWCNT produce mesothelioma in rodents.

As a last note on toxicity, the concern for possible adverse health effects of the nanoparticle systems is perhaps the most important factor for the development of a viable drug delivery system. It is also the most difficult problem to overcome, despite the versatility of nanotechnology in pharmaceutical applications.

VI. Chapter Summary

The use of nanotechnology in pharmaceutical development offers some very exciting possibilities. Some techniques are at various stages of development, some are being actively used today, and others are only imagined. This chapter describes the three major uses of nanomaterials in pharmaceutical development: imaging, diagnostics, and drug delivery. Imaging and diagnosis are of equal, if not greater, importance compared to drug treatment because these techniques can provide precise diagnosis on the disease states and call for their early and effective treatment. They are important in preventing diseases from occurring or progressing, and thus they are important in limiting the use of harsh drug treatment regimens that is often associated with diseases such as cancer.

The conclusions that can be drawn from current developments are fourfold: (1) the strategies in drug delivery, imaging, and diagnostics using nanomaterials usually yield delivery systems that are significantly better, and in some cases 10 to 100 times better, than conventional methods; (2) the toxic risk of nanoparticles depends on their type; some are toxic and thus call for long-term toxicity studies; (3) nanoparticles derived from biodegradable polymers, which are the mainstay in pharmaceutical development, are suitable and versatile for drug delivery and targeting purposes; and (4) one must consider and reduce the complexity of the system in the context of pharmaceutical product development.

The idea of using manufactured *nanorobots* to make repairs at the cellular level, which is the ultimate goal of nanomedicine, is under investigation in long-range research. Nanotechnology has the potential to revolutionize the way we detect and treat diseases. There will likely be significant progress in these areas with the discovery of new physicochemical properties in the near future. With this notion, one may also anticipate the growth of physical pharmacy to provide a closer analysis of the physicochemical phenomena associated with nanomaterials.

VII. References

1. Bawa R. Patents and nanomedicine. *Nanomedicine* (*Lond*). 2:351–374, 2007.
2. Bawarski WE, Chidlowsky E, Bharali DJ, and Mousa SA. Emerging nanopharmaceuticals. *Nanomedicine*. 4:273–282, 2008.
3. Sandhiya S, Dkhar SA, and Surendiran A. Emerging trends of nanomedicine—an overview. *Fundam Clin Pharmacol*. 23:263–269, 2009.
4. Suri SS, Fenniri H, and Singh B. Nanotechnology-based drug delivery systems. *J Occup Med Toxicol*. 2:16, 2007.
5. Riehemann K, Schneider SW, Luger TA, et al. Nanomedicine—challenges and perspectives. *Angew Chem Int Ed Engl*. 48:872–897, 2009.
6. De Jong WH and Borm PJ. Drug delivery and nanoparticles: Applications and hazards. *Int J Nanomedicine*. 3:133–149, 2008.

7. Yih TC and Al-Fandi M. Engineered nanoparticles as precise drug delivery systems. *J Cell Biochem.* 97:1184–1190, 2006.
8. Farokhzad OC and Langer R. Impact of nanotechnology on drug delivery. *ACS Nano.* 3:16–20, 2009.
9. Liang F and Chen B. A review on biomedical applications of single-walled carbon nanotubes. *Curr Med Chem.* 17:10–24, 2010.
10. Yudoh K, Karasawa R, Masuko K, and Kato T. Water-soluble fullerene (C60) inhibits the osteoclast differentiation and bone destruction in arthritis. *Int J Nanomed.* 4:233–239, 2009.
11. Bottrill M, Kwok L, and Long NJ. Lanthanides in magnetic resonance imaging. *Chem Soc Rev.* 35:557–571, 2006.
12. Chen HQ, Luo FB, Liu Y, et al. Application of functional CdS nanoparticles in determination of silver ion by resonance light-scattering technique. *Spectrochim Acta A Mol Biomol Spectrosc.* 71:1701–1703, 2009.
13. Campolongo MJ, Tan SJ, Xu J, and Luo D. DNA nanomedicine: Engineering DNA as a polymer for therapeutic and diagnostic applications. *Adv Drug Deliv Rev.* 62:606–616, 2010.
14. Wang M and Thanou M. Targeting nanoparticles to cancer. *Pharmacol Res.* 62:90–99, 2010.
15. Sajja HK, East MP, Mao H, et al. Development of multifunctional nanoparticles for targeted drug delivery and noninvasive imaging of therapeutic effect. *Curr Drug Discov Technol.* 6:43–51, 2009.
16. Kalita SJ, Bhardwaja A, and Bhatta HA. Nanocrystalline calcium phosphate ceramics in biomedical engineering. *Mater Sci Eng: C.* 27:441–449, 2007.
17. Schwarz F, Sahm N, Bieling K, and Becker J. Surgical regenerative treatment of peri-implantitis lesions using a nanocrystalline hydroxyapatite or a natural bone mineral in combination with a collagen membrane: A four-year clinical follow-up report. *J Clin Periodontol.* 36:807–814, 2009.
18. Bruckbauer A, Zhou D, Ying L, et al. Multicomponent submicron features of biomolecules created by voltage controlled deposition from a nanopipet. *J Am Chem Soc.* 125:9834–9839, 2003.
19. Nijdam AJ, Ming-Cheng Cheng M, Geho DH, et al. Physicochemically modified silicon as a substrate for protein microarrays. *Biomaterials.* 28:550–558, 2007.
20. Kikuchi A and Okano T. Nanostructured designs of biomedical materials: Applications of cell sheet engineering to functional regenerative tissues and organs. *J Control Release.* 101:69–84, 2005.
21. Usui-Aoki K, Shimada K, and Koga H. A novel antibody microarray format using non-covalent antibody immobilization with chemiluminescent detection. *Mol Biosyst.* 3:36–42, 2007.
22. Kato K, Toda M, and Iwata H. Antibody arrays for quantitative immunophenotyping. *Biomaterials.* 28:1289–1297, 2007.
23. Haab BB. Antibody arrays in cancer research. *Mol Cell Proteomics.* 4:377–383, 2005.
24. Watanabe M, Guo W, Zou S, et al. Antibody array analysis of peripheral and blood cytokine levels in rats after masseter inflammation. *Neurosci Lett.* 382:128–133, 2005.
25. Vickers JA, Caulum MM, and Henry CS. Generation of hydrophilic poly(dimethylsiloxane) for high-performance microchip electrophoresis. *Anal Chem.* 78:7446–7452, 2006.
26. Takayama S, Ostuni E, LeDuc P, et al. Subcellular positioning of small molecules. *Nature.* 411:1016, 2001.
27. Du Z, Colls N, Cheng KH, et al. Microfluidic-based diagnostics for cervical cancer cells. *Biosens Bioelectron.* 21:1991–1995, 2006.
28. Majumdar A. Bioassays based on molecular nanomechanics. *Dis Markers.* 18:167–174, 2002.
29. Wu G, Datar RH, Hansen KM, et al. Bioassay of prostate-specific antigen (PSA) using microcantilevers. *Nat Biotechnol.* 19:856–860, 2001.
30. Cui Y, Wei Q, Park H, and Lieber CM. Nanowire nanosensors for highly sensitive and selective detection of biological and chemical species. *Science.* 293:1289–1292, 2001.
31. Woolley AT, Cheung CL, Hafner JH, and Lieber CM. Structural biology with carbon nanotube AFM probes. *Chem Biol.* 7:R193–204, 2000.

32. Koehne JE, Chen H, Cassell AM, et al. Miniaturized multiplex label-free electronic chip for rapid nucleic acid analysis based on carbon nanotube nanoelectrode arrays. *Clin Chem.* 50:1886–1893, 2004.
33. Gao X, Cui Y, Levenson RM,, et al. In vivo cancer targeting and imaging with semiconductor quantum dots. *Nat Biotechnol.* 22:969–976, 2004.
34. Harisinghani MG, Barentsz J, Hahn PF, et al. Noninvasive detection of clinically occult lymph-node metastases in prostate cancer. *N Engl J Med.* 348:2491–2499, 2003.
35. Torchilin VP. Targeted pharmaceutical nanocarriers for cancer therapy and imaging. *AAPS J.* 9:E128–147, 2007.
36. Leuschner C, Kumar CS, Hansel W, et al. LHRH-conjugated magnetic iron oxide nanoparticles for detection of breast cancer metastases. *Breast Cancer Res Treat.* 99:163–176, 2006.
37. Duncan R. The dawning era of polymer therapeutics. *Nat Rev Drug Discov.* 2:347–360, 2003.
38. Ferrari M. Cancer nanotechnology: Opportunities and challenges. *Nat Rev Cancer.* 5:161–171, 2005.
39. Kipp JE. The role of solid nanoparticle technology in the parenteral delivery of poorly water-soluble drugs. *Int J Pharm.* 284:109–122, 2004.
40. Ferrari M. Nanogeometry: Beyond drug delivery. *Nat Nanotechnol.* 3:131–132, 2008.
41. Hagens WI, Oomen AG, de Jong WH, et al. What do we (need to) know about the kinetic properties of nanoparticles in the body? *Reg Toxicol Pharmacol.* 49:217–229, 2007.
42. Hillyer JF and Albrecht RM. Gastrointestinal persorption and tissue distribution of differently sized colloidal gold nanoparticles. *J Pharm Sci.* 90:1927–1936, 2001.
43. Jani P, Halbert GW, Langridge J, and Florence AT. Nanoparticle uptake by the rat gastrointestinal mucosa: Quantitation and particle size dependency. *J Pharm Pharmacol.* 42:821–826, 1990.
44. Desai MP, Labhasetwar V, Amidon GL, and Levy RJ. Gastrointestinal uptake of biodegradable microparticles: Effect of particle size. *Pharm Res.* 13:1838–1845, 1996.
45. Janes KA, Fresneau MP, Marazuela A, et al. Chitosan nanoparticles as delivery systems for doxorubicin. *J Control Release.* 73:255–267, 2001.
46. Sadrieh N, Wokovich AM, Gopee NV, et al. Lack of significant dermal penetration of titanium dioxide from sunscreen formulations containing nano- and submicron-size TiO2 particles. *Toxicol Sci.* 115:156–166, 2010.
47. Gulson B, McCall M, Korsch M, et al. Small amounts of zinc from zinc oxide particles in sunscreens applied outdoors are absorbed through human skin. *Toxicol Sci.* 118:140–149, 2010.
48. Tinkle SS, Antonini JM, Rich BA, et al. Skin as a route of exposure and sensitization in chronic beryllium disease. *Environ Health Persp.* 111:1202–1208, 2003.
49. Rouse JG, Yang J, Ryman-Rasmussen JP, et al. Effects of mechanical flexion on the penetration of fullerene amino acid-derivatized peptide nanoparticles through skin. *Nano Lett.* 7:155–160, 2007.
50. Kohli AK and Alpar HO. Potential use of nanoparticles for transcutaneous vaccine delivery: Effect of particle size and charge. *Int J Pharm.* 275:13–17, 2004.
51. Ryman-Rasmussen JP, Riviere JE, and Monteiro-Riviere NA. Penetration of intact skin by quantum dots with diverse physicochemical properties. *Toxicol Sci.* 91:159–165, 2006.
52. Kagan VE, Konduru NV, et al. Carbon nanotubes degraded by neutrophil myeloperoxidase induce less pulmonary inflammation. *Nat Nanotechnol.* 5:354–359, 2010.
53. Rothen-Rutishauser BM, Schurch S, Haenni B, et al. Interaction of fine particles and nanoparticles with red blood cells visualized with advanced microscopic techniques. *Environ Sci Technol.* 40:4353–4359, 2006.
54. Tsuji JS, Maynard AD, Howard PC, et al. Research strategies for safety evaluation of nanomaterials, part IV: Risk assessment of nanoparticles. *Toxicol Sci.* 89:42–50, 2006.
55. Nemmar A, Hoet PH, Vanquickenborne B, et al. Passage of inhaled particles into the blood circulation in humans. *Circulation.* 105:411–414, 2002.

56. Ogawara K, Yoshida M, Furumoto K, et al. Uptake by hepatocytes and biliary excretion of intravenously administered polystyrene microspheres in rats. *J Drug Target*. 7:213–221, 1999.
57. Chen JK, Shih MH, Peir JJ, et al. The use of radioactive zinc oxide nanoparticles in determination of their tissue concentrations following intravenous administration in mice. *Analyst*. 135:1742–1746, 2010.
58. Liu Y, Gao YX, Zhang LL, et al. Potential health impact on mice after nasal instillation of nano-sized copper particles and their translocation in mice. *J Nanosci Nanotechnol*. 9:6335–6343, 2009.
59. Semete B, Booysen L, Lemmer Y, et al. In vivo evaluation of the biodistribution and safety of PLGA nanoparticles as drug delivery systems. *Nanomedicine*. 6:662–671, 2010.
60. Videira MA, Gano L, Santos C, Neves M, and Almeida AJ. Lymphatic uptake of lipid nanoparticles following endotracheal administration. *J Microencapsul*. 23:855–862, 2006.
61. Zhu MT, Feng WY, Wang Y, et al. Particokinetics and extrapulmonary translocation of intratracheally instilled ferric oxide nanoparticles in rats and the potential health risk assessment. *Toxicol Sci*. 107:342–351 2009.
62. Cho M, Cho WS, Choi M, et al. The impact of size on tissue distribution and elimination by single intravenous injection of silica nanoparticles. *Toxicol Lett*. 189:177–183, 2009.
63. Hardman R. A toxicologic review of quantum dots: Toxicity depends on physicochemical and environmental factors. *Environ Health Persp*. 114:165–172, 2006.
64. Sarlo K, Blackburn KL, Clark ED, et al. 2009. Tissue distribution of 20 nm, 100 nm and 1000 nm fluorescent polystyrene latex nanospheres following acute systemic or acute and repeat airway exposure in the rat. *Toxicology*. 263:117–126, 2009.
65. Lasagna-Reeves C, Gonzalez-Romero D, Barria MA, et al. Bioaccumulation and toxicity of gold nanoparticles after repeated administration in mice. *Biochem Biophys Res Commun*. 393:649–655, 2010.
66. Qiu L, Jing N, and Jin Y. Preparation and in vitro evaluation of liposomal chloroquine diphosphate loaded by a transmembrane pH-gradient method. *Int J Pharm*. 361:56–63, 2008.
67. Akhtar S, Hughes MD, Khan A, et al. The delivery of antisense therapeutics. *Adv Drug Deliv Rev*. 44:3–21, 2000.
68. Greish K, Fang J, Inutsuka T, Nagamitsu A, and Maeda H. 2003. Macromolecular therapeutics: Advantages and prospects with special emphasis on solid tumour targeting. *Clin Pharmacokinet*. 42:1089–1105, 2003.
69. Ogawara K, Un K, Tanaka K, et al. In vivo anti-tumor effect of PEG liposomal doxorubicin (DOX) in DOX-resistant tumor-bearing mice: Involvement of cytotoxic effect on vascular endothelial cells. *J Control Release*. 133:4–10, 2009.
70. Malam Y, Loizidou M, and Seifalian AM. Liposomes and nanoparticles: Nanosized vehicles for drug delivery in cancer. *Trends Pharmacol Sci*. 30:592–599, 2009.
71. Wong HL, Bendayan R, Rauth AM, et al. Chemotherapy with anticancer drugs encapsulated in solid lipid nanoparticles. *Adv Drug Deliv Rev*. 59:491–504, 2007.
72. Lu B, Xiong SB, Yang H, et al. Solid lipid nanoparticles of mitoxantrone for local injection against breast cancer and its lymph node metastases. *Eur J Pharm Sci*. 28:86–95, 2006.
73. Azad N and Rojanasakul Y. Nanobiotechnology in drug delivery. *Am J Drug Deliv*. 4:79–88, 2006.
74. Couvreur P, Barratt G, Fattal E, et al. Nanocapsule technology: A review. *Crit Rev Ther Drug Carrier Syst*. 19:99–134, 2002.
75. Mayer C. Nanocapsules as drug delivery systems. *Int J Artif Organs*. 28:1163–1171, 2005.
76. Moghimi SM, Hunter AC, and Murray JC. Long-circulating and target-specific nanoparticles: Theory to practice. *Pharmacol Rev*. 53:283–318, 2001.
77. Gaucher G, Dufresne MH, Sant VP, et al. Block copolymer micelles: Preparation, characterization and application in drug delivery. *J Control Release*. 109:169–188, 2005.

78. Bae Y, Jang WD, Nishiyama Fukushima NS, and Kataoka K. Multifunctional polymeric micelles with folate-mediated cancer cell targeting and pH-triggered drug releasing properties for active intracellular drug delivery. *Mol Biosyst*. 1:242–250, 2005.

79. Ju-Nam Y and Lead JR. Manufactured nanoparticles: An overview of their chemistry, interactions and potential environmental implications. *Sci Total Environ*. 400:396–414, 2008.

80. Ghosh P, Han G, De M, et al. Gold nanoparticles in delivery applications. *Adv Drug Deliv Rev*. 60:1307–1315, 2008.

81. Connor EE, Mwamuka J, Gole A, et al. Gold nanoparticles are taken up by human cells but do not cause acute cytotoxicity. *Small*. 1:325–327, 2005.

82. Lee SH, Bae KH, Kim SH, et al. Amine-functionalized gold nanoparticles as non-cytotoxic and efficient intracellular siRNA delivery carriers. *Int J Pharm*. 364:94–101, 2008.

83. Huang X, Jain PK, El-Sayed IH, and El-Sayed MA. Gold nanoparticles: Interesting optical properties and recent applications in cancer diagnostics and therapy. *Nanomedicine (Lond)*. 2:681–693, 2007.

84. Faraji AH and Wipf P. Nanoparticles in cellular drug delivery. *Bioorg Med Chem*. 17:2950–2962, 2009.

85. Polizu S, Savadogo O, Poulin P, and Yahia L. Applications of carbon nanotubes-based biomaterials in biomedical nanotechnology. *J Nanosci Nanotechnol*. 6:1883–1904, 2006.

86. Rosenthal SJ, Tomlinson I, Adkins EM, et al. Targeting cell surface receptors with ligand-conjugated nanocrystals. *J Am Chem Soc*. 124:4586–4594, 2002.

87. Damascelli B, Cantu G, Mattavelli F, et al. Intraarterial chemotherapy with polyoxyethylated castor oil free paclitaxel, incorporated in albumin nanoparticles (ABI-007): Phase II study of patients with squamous cell carcinoma of the head and neck and anal canal: Preliminary evidence of clinical activity. *Cancer*. 92:2592–2602, 2001.

88. Kattan J, Droz JP, Couvreur P, et al. Phase I clinical trial and pharmacokinetic evaluation of doxorubicin carried by polyisohexylcyanoacrylate nanoparticles. *Invest New Drugs*. 10:191–199, 1992.

89. Chan WC and Nie S. Quantum dot bioconjugates for ultrasensitive nonisotopic detection. *Science*. 281:2016–2018, 1998.

90. Dubertret B, Skourides P, Norris DJ, et al. In vivo imaging of quantum dots encapsulated in phospholipid micelles. *Science*. 298:1759–1762, 2002.

91. Manna L, Scher EC, Li LS, and Alivisatos AP. Epitaxial growth and photochemical annealing of graded CdS/ZnS shells on colloidal CdSe nanorods. *J Am Chem Soc*. 124:7136–7145, 2002.

92. Jamieson T, Bakhshi R, Petrova D, et al. Biological applications of quantum dots. *Biomaterials*. 28:4717–4732, 2007.

93. Kaji N, Tokeshi M, and Baba Y. Single-molecule measurements with a single quantum dot. *Chem Rec*. 7:295–304, 2007.

94. Kaji N, Tokeshi M, and Baba Y. Quantum dots for single bio-molecule imaging. *Anal Sci*. 23:21–24, 2007.

95. Muller-Borer BJ, Collins MC, Gunst PR, et al. Quantum dot labeling of mesenchymal stem cells. *J Nanobiotechnology*. 5:9, 2007.

96. Derfus AM, Chen AA, Min DH, et al. Targeted quantum dot conjugates for siRNA delivery. *Bioconjug Chem*. 18:1391–1396, 2007.

97. Alivisatos AP, Gu W, and Larabell C. Quantum dots as cellular probes. *Annu Rev Biomed Eng*. 7:55–76, 2005.

98. Bagalkot V, Zhang L, Levy-Nissenbaum E, et al. Quantum dot-aptamer conjugates for synchronous cancer imaging, therapy, and sensing of drug delivery based on bi-fluorescence resonance energy transfer. *Nano Lett*. 7:3065–3070, 2007.

99. Bowman K and Leong KW. Chitosan nanoparticles for oral drug and gene delivery. *Int J Nanomed*. 1:117–128, 2006.

100. Zhang W, Gilstrap K, Wu L, et al. Synthesis and characterization of thermally responsive Pluronic F127-chitosan nanoparticles for controlled release and intracellular delivery of small molecules. *ACS Nano.* 4:6747–6759, 2010.
101. Kojima C, Kono K, Maruyama K, and Takagishi T. Synthesis of polyamidoamine dendrimers having poly(ethylene glycol) grafts and their ability to encapsulate anticancer drugs. *Bioconjug Chem.* 11:910–917, 2002.
102. Peer D, Karp JM, Hong S, et al. Nanocarriers as an emerging platform for cancer therapy. *Nat Nanotechnol.* 2:751–760, 2007.
103. Danhier F, Lecouturier N, Vroman B, et al. Paclitaxel-loaded PEGylated PLGA-based nanoparticles: In vitro and in vivo evaluation. *J Control Release.* 133:11–17, 2009.
104. Gryparis EC, Hatziapostolou M, Papadimitriou E, and Avgoustakis K. Anticancer activity of cisplatin-loaded PLGA-mPEG nanoparticles on LNCaP prostate cancer cells. *Eur J Pharm Biopharm.* 67:1–8, 2007.
105. Hawkins MJ, Soon-Shiong P, and Desai N. Protein nanoparticles as drug carriers in clinical medicine. *Adv Drug Deliv Rev.* 60:876–885, 2008.
106. Hood JD, Bednarski M, Frausto R, et al. Tumor regression by targeted gene delivery to the neovasculature. *Science.* 296:2404–2407, 2002.
107. Torchilin VP. Tatp-mediated intracellular delivery of pharmaceutical nanocarriers. *Biochem Soc Trans.* 35:816–820, 2007.
108. Wartlick H, Michaelis K, Balthasar S, et al. Highly specific HER2-mediated cellular uptake of antibody-modified nanoparticles in tumour cells. *J Drug Target.* 12:461–471, 2004.
109. Schmieder AH, Winter PM, Caruthers SD, et al. Molecular MR imaging of melanoma angiogenesis with alphanubeta3-targeted paramagnetic nanoparticles. *Magn Reson Med.* 53:621–627, 2005.
110. Podsiadlo P, Sinani VA, Bahng JH, et al. Gold nanoparticles enhance the anti-leukemia action of a 6-mercaptopurine chemotherapeutic agent. *Langmuir.* 24:568–574, 2008.
111. Wei XL, Mo ZH, Li B, and Wei JM. Disruption of HepG2 cell adhesion by gold nanoparticle and Paclitaxel disclosed by in situ QCM measurement. *Colloids Surf B Biointerfaces.* 59:100–104, 2007.
112. Sitharaman B, Zakharian TY, Saraf A, et al. 2008. Water-soluble fullerene (C60) derivatives as nonviral gene-delivery vectors. *Mol Pharm.* 5:567–578, 2008.
113. Singh R and Lillard JW, Jr. Nanoparticle-based targeted drug delivery. *Exp Mol Pathol.* 86:215–223, 2009.
114. Bhadra D, Bhadra S, and Jain NK. Pegylated lysine based copolymeric dendritic micelles for solubilization and delivery of artemether. *J Pharm Pharm Sci.* 8:467–482, 2005.
115. Bhadra D, Bhadra S, and Jain NK. PEGylated peptide dendrimeric carriers for the delivery of antimalarial drug chloroquine phosphate. *Pharm Res.* 23:623–633, 2006.
116. Wang F, Bronich TK, Kabanov AV, et al. Synthesis and characterization of star poly(epsilon-caprolactone)-b-poly(ethylene glycol) and poly(L-lactide)-b-poly(ethylene glycol) copolymers: Evaluation as drug delivery carriers. *Bioconjug Chem.* 19:1423–1429, 2008.
117. Nakanishi T, Fukushima S, Okamoto K, et al. Development of the polymer micelle carrier system for doxorubicin. *J Control Release.* 74:295–302, 2001.
118. Gansbacher B. Report of a second serious adverse event in a clinical trial of gene therapy for X-linked severe combined immune deficiency (X-SCID). Position of the European Society of Gene Therapy (ESGT). *J Gene Med.* 5:261–262, 2003.
119. Lee M and Kim SW. Polyethylene glycol-conjugated copolymers for plasmid DNA delivery. *Pharm Res.* 22:1–10, 2005.
120. Pitard B, Oudrhiri N, Lambert O, et al. Sterically stabilized BGTC-based lipoplexes: Structural features and gene transfection into the mouse airways in vivo. *J Gene Med.* 3:478–487, 2001.
121. Duzgunes N, De Ilarduya CT, Simoes S, et al. Cationic liposomes for gene delivery: Novel cationic lipids and enhancement by proteins and peptides. *Curr Med Chem.* 10:1213–1220, 2003.

122. Pedroso de Lima MC, Neves S, Filipe A, et al. Cationic liposomes for gene delivery: From biophysics to biological applications. *Curr Med Chem.* 10:1221–1231, 2003.
123. Liu D, Ren T, and Gao X. Cationic transfection lipids. *Curr Med Chem.* 10:1307–1315, 2003.
124. Dauty E, Remy JS, Zuber G, and Behr JP. Intracellular delivery of nanometric DNA particles via the folate receptor. *Bioconjug Chem.* 13:831–839, 2002.
125. Qian ZM, Li H, Sun H, and Ho K. Targeted drug delivery via the transferrin receptor-mediated endocytosis pathway. *Pharmacol Rev.* 54:561–587, 2002.
126. Zanta MA, Belguise-Valladier P, and Behr JP. Gene delivery: A single nuclear localization signal peptide is sufficient to carry DNA to the cell nucleus. *Proc Natl Acad Sci USA.* 96:91–96, 1999.
127. Ambrosch FG, Wiedermann G, Jonas S, et al. Immunogenicity and protectivity of a new liposomal hepatitis A vaccine. *Vaccine.* 15:1209–1213, 1997.
128. Raghuvanshi RJ, Mistra A, Talwar GP, et al. Enhanced immune response with a combination of alum and biodegradable nanoparticles containing tetanus toxoid. *J Microencapsul.* 18:723–732, 2001.
129. Kreuter J, Mauler R, Gruschkau H, and Speiser PP. The use of new polymethylmethacrylate adjuvants for split influenza vaccines. *Exp Cell Biol.* 44:12–19, 1976.
130. Sahoo SK, Parveen S, and Panda JJ. The present and future of nanotechnology in human health care. *Nanomedicine.* 3:20–31, 2007.
131. Phillips MA, Gran ML, and Peppas NA. Targeted nanodelivery of drugs and diagnostics. *Nano Today.* 5:143–159, 2010.
132. Peters D, Kastantin M, Kotamraju VR, et al. Targeting atherosclerosis by using modular, multifunctional micelles. *Proc Natl Acad Sci USA.* 106:9815–9819, 2009.
133. Tsourkas A, Shinde-Patil VR, Kelly KA, et al. In vivo imaging of activated endothelium using an anti-VCAM-1 magnetooptical probe. *Bioconjug Chem.* 16:576–581, 2005.
134. Neubauer AM, Myerson J, Caruthers SD, et al. Gadolinium-modulated 19F signals from perfluorocarbon nanoparticles as a new strategy for molecular imaging. *Magn Reson Med.* 60:1066–1072, 2008.
135. Neubauer AM, Sim H, Winter PM, et al. Nanoparticle pharmacokinetic profiling in vivo using magnetic resonance imaging. *Magn Reson Med.* 60:1353–1361, 2008.
136. Park K, Hong HY, Moon HJ, et al. A new atherosclerotic lesion probe based on hydrophobically modified chitosan nanoparticles functionalized by the atherosclerotic plaque targeted peptides. *J Control Release.* 128:217–223, 2008.
137. Jaffer FA, Sosnovik DE, Nahrendorf M, and Weissleder R. Molecular imaging of myocardial infarction. *J Mol Cell Cardiol.* 41:921–933, 2006.
138. Kong DF and Goldschmidt-Clermont PJ. Tiny solutions for giant cardiac problems. *Trends Cardiovasc Med.* 15:207–211, 2005.
139. Brightman MW. Morphology of blood–brain interfaces. *Exp Eye Res.* 25 Suppl:1–25, 1977.
140. Pardridge WM. Brain drug targeting and gene technologies. *Jpn J Pharmacol.* 87:97–103, 2001.
141. Pardridge WM. Formulation of therapeutic synthetic polymers for drug and gene delivery. *Drug Discov Today.* 7:1120–1121, 2002.
142. Pardridge WM. Drug and gene targeting to the brain with molecular Trojan horses. *Nat Rev Drug Discov.* 1:131–139, 2002.
143. Maletinska L, Blakely EA, Bjornstad KA, et al. Human glioblastoma cell lines: Levels of low-density lipoprotein receptor and low-density lipoprotein receptor-related protein. *Cancer Res.* 60:2300–2303, 2000.
144. Pitas RE, Boyles JK, Lee SH,et al. Lipoproteins and their receptors in the central nervous system. Characterization of the lipoproteins in cerebrospinal fluid and identification of apolipoprotein B,E(LDL) receptors in the brain. *J Biol Chem.* 262:14352–14360, 1987.
145. Nikanjam M, Gibbs AR, Hunt CA, et al. Synthetic nano-LDL with paclitaxel oleate as a targeted drug delivery vehicle for glioblastoma multiforme. *J Control Release.* 124:163–171, 2007.

146. Lanza GM and Wickline SA. Targeted ultrasonic contrast agents for molecular imaging and therapy. *Prog Cardiovasc Dis.* 44:13–31, 2001.
147. Lanza GM, Wallace KD, Scott MJ, et al. A novel site-targeted ultrasonic contrast agent with broad biomedical application. *Circulation.* 94:3334–3340, 1996.
148. Prasad KN, Hovland AR, Cole WC, et al. Multiple antioxidants in the prevention and treatment of Alzheimer disease: Analysis of biologic rationale. *Clin Neuropharmacol.* 23:2–13, 2000.
149. Selkoe DJ. Alzheimer's disease: Genes, proteins, and therapy. *Physiol Rev.* 81:741–766, 2001.
150. Blake DR, Winyard P, Lunec J, et al. Cerebral and ocular toxicity induced by desferrioxamine. *Q J Med.* 56:345–355, 1985.
151. Lewinski N, Colvin V, and Drezek R. Cytotoxicity of nanoparticles. *Small.* 4:26–49, 2008.
152. Wang L, Mercer RR, Rojanasakul Y, et al. Direct fibrogenic effects of dispersed single-walled carbon nanotubes on human lung fibroblasts. *J Toxicol Environ Health A.* 73:410–422, 2010.
153. Poland CA, Duffin R, Kinloch I, et al. Carbon nanotubes introduced into the abdominal cavity of mice show asbestos-like pathogenicity in a pilot study. *Nat Nanotechnol.* 3:423–428, 2008.
154. Gatti A. Nerve growth factor (NGF) induces a rapid and sustained downregulation of the focal adhesion kinase (FAK). *Cell Mol Neurobiol.* 24:461–475, 2004.
155. Caruthers SD, Wickline SA, and Lanza GM. Nanotechnological applications in medicine. *Curr Opin Biotechnol.* 18:26–30, 2007.
156. Castranova V, Porter D, Millecchia L, et al. Effect of inhaled crystalline silica in a rat model: Time course of pulmonary reactions. *Mol Cell Biochem.* 234/235:177–184, 2002.
157. Galagudza MM, Korolev DV, Sonin DL, et al. Targeted drug delivery into reversibly injured myocardium with silica nanoparticles: Surface functionalization, natural biodistribution, and acute toxicity. *Int J Nanomedicine.* 5:231–237, 2010.
158. Nishimori H, Kondoh M, Isoda K, et al. Silica nanoparticles as hepatotoxicants. *Eur J Pharm Biopharm.* 72:496–501, 2009.
159. Goodman CM, McCusker CD, Yilmaz T, and Rotello VM. Toxicity of gold nanoparticles functionalized with cationic and anionic side chains. *Bioconjug Chem.* 15:897–900, 2004.
160. Alkilany AM, Nagaria PK, Hexel CR, et al. Cellular uptake and cytotoxicity of gold nanprods: Molecular origin of cytotoxicity and surface effect. *Small.* 5:707–708, 2009.
161. Cho WS, Cho M, Jeong J, et al. Acute toxicity and pharmacokinetics of 13 nm-sized PEG-coated gold nanoparticles. *Toxicol Appl Pharmacol.* 236:16–24, 2009.
162. Chen YS, Hung YC, Liau I, and Huang GS. Assessment of the in vivo toxicity of gold nanoparticles. *Nanoscale Res Lett.* 4:858–864, 2009.
163. Pokharkar V, Dhar S, Bhumkar D, et al. Acute and subacute toxicity studies of chitosan reduced gold nanoparticles: A novel carrier for therapeutic agents. *J Biomed Nanotechnol.* 5:233–239, 2009.
164. Shavandi Z, Ghazanfari T, and Moghaddam KN. In vitro toxicity of silver nanoparticles on murine peritoneal macrophages. *Immunopharmacol Immunotoxicol.* 33:135–140, 2011.
165. Roberts JR, Chapman RS, Young S, et al. Pulmonary toxicity following intratracheal instillation of dispersed silver nanoparticles in rats. *The Toxicologist.* 120:A 1759, 2011.
166. Levi N, Hantgan RR, Lively MO, et al. C60-fullerenes: Detection of intracellular photoluminescence and lack of cytotoxic effects. *J Nanobiotechnol.* 4:14, 2006.
167. Gharbi N, Pressac M, Hadchouel M, et al. [60]fullerene is a powerful antioxidant in vivo with no acute or subacute toxicity. *Nano Lett.* 5:2578–2585, 2005.
168. Kolosnjaj J, Szwarc H, and Moussa F. Toxicity studies of fullerenes and derivatives. *Adv Exp Med Biol.* 620:168–180, 2007.
169. Chen HH, Yu C, Ueng TH, et al. Acute and subacute toxicity study of water-soluble polyalkylsulfonated C60 in rats. *Toxicol Pathol.* 26:143–151, 1998.
170. Firme CP, III. and Bandaru PR. Toxicity issues in the application of carbon nanotubes to biological systems. *Nanomedicine.* 6:245–256, 2010.

171. Casey A, Herzog E, Lyng FM, et al. Single walled carbon nanotubes induce indirect cytotoxicity by medium depletion in A549 lung cells. *Toxicol Lett.* 179:78–84, 2008.
172. Ravichandran P, Periyakaruppan A, Sadanandan B, et al. Induction of apoptosis in rat lung epithelial cells by multiwalled carbon nanotubes. *J Biochem Mol Toxicol.* 23:333–344, 2009.
173. Ma-Hock L, Treumann S, Strauss V, et al. Inhalation toxicity of multiwall carbon nanotubes in rats exposed for 3 months. *Toxicol Sci.* 112:468–481, 2009.
174. Mercer RR, Hubbs AF, Scabilloni JF, et al. 2011. Pulmonary fibrotic response to aspiration of multi-walled carbon nanotubes. *Particle Fibre Toxicol.* 8:21, 2011.
175. Shvedova AA, Kisin E, Murray AR, et al. Inhalation vs. aspiration of single-walled carbon nanotubes in C57BL/6 mice: Inflammation, fibrosis, oxidative stress, and mutagenesis. *Am J Physiol: Lung Cell Mol Physiol.* 295:L552–L565, 2008.
176. Mercer RR, Scabilloni J, Wang L, et al. Alteration of deposition pattern and pulmonary response as a result of improved dispersion of aspirated single walled carbon nanotubes in a mouse model. *Am J Physiol: Lung Cell Mol Physiol.* 294:L87–L97, 2008.
177. Shvedova AA, Fabisiak JP, Kisin ER, et al. Sequential exposure to carbon nanotubes and bacteria enhances pulmonary inflammation and infectivity. *Am J Respir Cell Mol Biol.* 38:579–590, 2008.
178. Schipper ML, Nakayama-Ratchford N, Davis CR, et al. A pilot toxicology study of single-walled carbon nanotubes in a small sample of mice. *Nat Nanotechnol.* 3:216–221, 2008.
179. Hardman R. A toxicologic review of quantum dots: Toxicity depends on physicochemical and environmental factors. *Environ Health Perspect.* 114:165–172, 2006.
180. Lovric J, Bazzi HS, Cuie Y, et al. Differences in subcellular distribution and toxicity of green and red emitting CdTe quantum dots. *J Mol Med.* 83:377–385, 2005.
181. Lovric J, Cho SJ, Winnik FM, and Maysinger D. Unmodified cadmium telluride quantum dots induce reactive oxygen species formation leading to multiple organelle damage and cell death. *Chem Biol.* 12:1227–1234, 2005.
182. Zhao J, Shi X, Castranova V, and Ding M. Occupational toxicology of nickel and nickel compounds. *J Environ Pathol Toxicol Oncol.* 28:177–208, 2009.
183. Heinrich UFR, Rittinghausen S, Creutzenberg O, et al. Chronic inhalation exposure of Wistar rats and two different strains of mice to diesel engine exhaust, carbon black, and titanium dioxide. *Inhal Toxicol.* 7:533–556, 1995.
184. Rittinghausen S, Mohr U, and Dungworth DL. Pulmonary cystic keratinizing squamous cell lesions of rats after inhalation/instillation of different particles. *Exp Toxicol Pathol.* 49:433–446, 1997.
185. Pott F and Roller M. Carcinogenicity study with nineteen granular dusts in rats. *Eur J Oncol.* 10:249–282, 2005.
186. Roller M. Carcinogenicity of inhaled nanoparticles. *Inhal Toxicol.* 21 Suppl 1:144–157, 2009.
187. Tsuda H, Xu J, Sakai Y, et al. Toxicology of engineered nanomaterials—a review of carcinogenic potential. *Asian Pac J Cancer Prev.* 10:975–980, 2009.
188. Porter DW, Hubbs A, Mercer R, et al. Mouse pulmonary dose- and time course-response induced by exposure to multi-walled carbon nanotubes. *Toxicol.* 269:136–147, 2010.
189. Shvedova AA, Kisin ER, Mercer R, et al. Unusual inflammatory and fibrogenic pulmonary response to single walled carbon nanotubes in mice. *Am J Physiol: Lung Cell Mol Physiol.* 289:L698–L708, 2005.
190. Takagi A, Hirose A, Nishimura T, et al. Induction of mesothelioma in p53+/- mouse by intraperitoneal application of multi-wall carbon nanotube. *J Toxicol Sci.* 33:105–116, 2008.
191. Sakamoto Y, Nakae D, Fukumori N, et al. Induction of mesothelioma by a single intrascrotal administration of multi-wall carbon nanotube in intact male Fischer 344 rats. *J Toxicol Sci.* 34:65–76, 2009.
192. Muller J, Delos M, Panin N, et al. Absence of carcinogenic response to multiwall carbon nanotubes in a 2-year bioassay in the peritoneal cavity of the rat. *Toxicol Sci.* 110:442–448, 2009.

VIII. Homework Problems

For Questions 1–5, select the most appropriate answer choice.

1. Nanotechnology deals with structure sizes between ____________ in length in at least one dimension.
   A. 1–10 nm
   B. 10–100 nm
   C. 1–10 μm
   D. 100–1000 nm
2. As opposed to traditional contrast agents such as ____________, newer nanosize contrast agents seem to possess far better imaging and diagnostic capabilities.
   A. Cadmium
   B. Gadolinium
   C. Zinc
   D. Aluminum
3. Functionalization of the surface of drug carriers by conjugation of ____________ greatly reduces opsonization and subsequent clearance by the body.
   A. Polymethyl methacrylate
   B. Polylactic acid
   C. Polyethylene glycol
   D. Polyethylenimine
4. Quantum dots are specialized forms of ____________.
   A. Nanocrystals
   B. Liposomes
   C. Dendrimers
   D. Gold nanoparticles
5. Glioblastoma multiforme is characterized by the upregulation of ____________.
   A. Albumin
   B. Vascular endothelial growth factor
   C. High-density lipoprotein
   D. Low-density lipoprotein
6. Why are quantum dots fluorescent? How does the particle size affect the quantum dot fluorescence?
7. Besides quantum dots, name another luminescent nanosystem that can be used for *in vivo* imaging.
8. Porous silicon nanoparticles have been studied as a drug delivery system. Are the silicon particles biodegradable?
9. Microcantilever devices are used in nanoarray and other biosensor systems. By what mechanism do they provide a measurement of a biomarker for diagnostic purpose?
10. List at least five advantages of using nanotechnology-based approaches for drug delivery.
11. By what mechanism may an orally delivered nanoparticle system be absorbed?
12. Name one product each from the liposome, polymeric micelle, and polymer nanoparticle systems that have been approved for use in the treatment of cancer.
13. What is a liposphere?

14. List and describe at least three application areas in health care for which nanodelivery systems are of particular use.
15. Describe a targeting strategy that may be used for the treatment of atherosclerosis.
16. Does the nanoparticulate system have any value for drug delivery to the central nervous system?
17. What would be the major concerns of using silica nanoparticles or carbon nanotubes as a drug delivery carrier?
18. Write a short report on the potential use of gold nanoparticles in drug delivery and imaging and their potential *in vivo* toxicity.

GLOSSARY

Term	Symbol	Definition or Description
Absorption		*Absorption* is the process through which a drug moves from the site of administration into the extracellular compartment of the body. For orally delivered drugs, this process involves (1) the disintegration of, and the release of the drug from, the dosage form, (2) dissolution of drug in the GI fluid, and (3) permeation of drug across GI membranes into the systemic circulation.
Absorption bases		When a water-in-oil (W/O) emulsifier is added to an oleaginous ointment base, the mixture becomes an absorption (anhydrous) base capable of absorbing large amounts of water or hydroalcoholic solution. Hydrophilic petrolatum, e.g., which consists of cholesterol, stearyl alcohol, white wax, and white petrolatum, can absorb water up to 10% of its weight. Lanolin is a fatty, semisolid mass containing 25–30% water. The anhydrous lanolin is insoluble in water but absorbs water to form W/O emulsion. The water absorption property of these bases allows for inclusion of water-soluble drugs with rapid-release characteristics.
Acid–base conjugation		In a solution, a weak acid or base will interact with the solvent that acts as a base or acid. The system consists two conjugated acid–base pairs as shown $$\underset{\text{base}_1}{NH_3} + \underset{\text{acid}_2}{H_2O} \rightleftarrows \underset{\text{acid}_1}{NH_4^+} + \underset{\text{base}_2}{OH^-}$$ where ammonia is a weak base and water is a weak acid. The product ammonium ion is the conjugate acid of ammonia, and the hydroxide ion is the conjugate base of water.
Acidity constant	K_a	*Acidity constant* is the equilibrium constant for the dissociation of a proton (H^+) from a molecule or a protonated ion in an aqueous solution, where the proton associates with water to form the hydronium ion (H_3O^+).
Active targeting		A drug can be modified to become a part of a complex molecule or included in a polymeric structure that exhibits strong affinity toward certain cell types via antigen–antibody interactions and

Term	Symbol	Definition or Description
		receptor-mediated endocytosis. This targeting approach in drug delivery is referred to as *active targeting*.
Activity	a	Because of the electrostatic interactions of ionic species, the equilibrium for the dissociation of a neutral molecule into ions, for example, $AB \rightarrow A^+ + B^-$, cannot be expressed with accuracy using the concentrations of the ions. Instead, the *activities* of the ions, which are proportional to the concentrations, are used in an equilibrium expression. For an insoluble electrolyte AB, the equilibrium expression is thus $K = a_+a_-$ (see *Activity coefficient* for further definitions).
Activity coefficient	γ	The *activity coefficient* is the proportional constant of activity to concentration, that is, $a = \gamma C$. For the equilibrium $AB \rightarrow A^+ + B^-$ of an insoluble salt, $$K = a_+a_- = (\gamma_+C_+)(\gamma_-C_-) = \gamma_+\gamma_-[A][B]$$ The *mean* ionic activity (a_+) and *mean* ionic activity coefficient ($\gamma_\pm$) for a univalent electrolyte are defined as $$a_\pm = (a_\pm a_-)^{1/2} \qquad \gamma_\pm = (\gamma_+\gamma_-)^{1/2}$$ Thus, $$K = a_\pm^2 = \gamma_\pm^2[A][B]$$
Adsorption		*Adsorption* of gases or solutes, as from a suspension, is a basic property of small particles. The extent of adsorption depends on the surface area, which varies with varying particle shapes, surface irregularities, and porosity. Most adsorptions occur through surface interactions involving either condensation or chemical bonding. The latter is commonly known as chemisorption.
Adsorption isotherm		*Adsorption isotherm* is the display of a gas pressure P-dependent adsorption of a gas (in volume V), the absorbate, onto a given amount of particles (m), the absorbent, at constant temperature, as in a plot of V/m versus P.
Agglomeration		*Agglomeration* is the process through which larger masses or desired particle sizes are produced from small particles (powders or dust) during granulation. The mechanisms of agglomeration include the formation of sinter bridges between partially melted particles, chemical bonding between particles, liquid bridges between particles in a wet process, masses due to van der Waals, electrical, or mechanical attractive forces, aggregates through interlocking by irregularly shaped particles, and binder matrices with embedded particles.

Term	Symbol	Definition or Description
Andreasen pipette		The *Andreasen pipette* is a temperature-controlled apparatus for particle size measurement of suspended particles. It consists of a special graduated cylinder (500 mL) with a ground tapered neck for particle suspension and a special stopper with a pipette immersed at a depth h below the surface of the suspension. The pipette permits the withdrawal of samples of the suspension at depth h. For particle analysis, a powder sample is dispersed by vigorous agitation into a liquid with a suitable deflocculating agent in an initial concentration of C_0 (0.5–1%) and is allowed to settle beginning at time 0. At desired time intervals, samples of the suspension are taken from the depth h below the surface, evaporated to dryness, and weighed to yield the concentration C_t. Based on the sedimentation theory, at any time t, the particles from the withdrawn sample will have a terminal settling velocity equal to or less than h/t. Thus, the ratio C_t/C_0 yields the weight fraction of particles that exhibits such a velocity and a Stokes diameter of d_{St}, which is $\leq[(h/t)(18\eta)/g(\rho_2 - \rho_1)]^{1/2}$.
Angle of repose	α	When bulk powders are poured onto a horizontal surface, they will form a conical pile. The *angle of repose* is the angle formed between the slope of the material and the horizontal plane, which is a measure of the flowability of the blend in that the better the flow, the lower the angle of repose. As a manufacturing rule, values in the range of 20° and 40° give acceptable flowability.
Antioxidant		*Antioxidants* are additives in food and drug preparations to prevent degradation by oxidation. They are reducing agents that either undergo preferential oxidation or serve as free radical chain reaction inhibitors. A chain reaction inhibitor is a compound that can provide an electron and hydrogen (H·) in stopping the chain reaction.
Antisense oligonucleotides		*Antisense oligonucleotides* are the reverse-complementary sequences that target the sequences of mRNA of a particular gene and effectively inhibit its expression.
Antithixotropy and rheopexy		Both rheopexy and antithixotropy have been used to describe time-dependent increase in viscosity under constant shear rate. Shear thickening may result from particle aggregations. When flow causes a reversible, time-dependent increase in viscosity, which is indicated by a reversed hysteresis loop of the flow curve, the phenomenon is called *antithixotropy*. The term *rheopexy* refers to the phenomenon that the gel formation of a system may be facilitated by tapping or low shear compared to keeping the sample at rest. In some colloidal

Term	Symbol	Definition or Description
		dispersions, the viscosity increases with time at low shear rates after shearing at high shear rate. This behavior is termed rheopectic but not antithixotropic, because the reversibility was not defined.
Apparent partition coefficient	K'	In the distribution of a weak acid or weak base drug between an aqueous phase and an oil phase, the aqueous phase contains both the acid form and the conjugated base form, depending on the pH of the aqueous solution. Partition of drug from the aqueous phase to the oil phase involves only the neutral species, but at equilibrium, the concentration ratio of drug in the oil phase to that of the aqueous phase will be a constant under constant pH. This ratio (K') is called the *apparent partition coefficient*.
Apparent solubility		*Apparent solubility* is the measured solubility following a prolonged incubation period (up to 24 h) but without the determination of whether the solution has reached an equilibrium solubility via a time-course study.
Arrhenius theory		Arrhenius discovered a linear relationship between log k and $1/T$ *for a reaction having a rate constant k at temperature T* as follows: $$k = Ae^{-E_a/RT}$$ where A is a preexponential factor and E_a is the activation energy. The *Arrhenius theory* suggests that any and all reaction processes involve the formation of some high-energy species known as the *activated complex*, which can break down into the products. If the energy difference between the activated complex and the reactants is E_a, the ratio of the number of activated complexes to the number of reactant molecules, according to the Boltzmann distribution, is $e^{-E_a/RT}$, and the rate of a reaction is proportional to the number or concentration of the activated complex.
Autocatalysis		The catalysis of a chemical reaction by the product of the reaction when a sufficient amount is generated is termed *autocatalysis*. In such a reaction, the rate will accelerate with time and temperature.
Autoclaving		*Autoclaving* is a method of steam sterilization. It employs water under pressure and elevated temperature in a closed chamber. The pressurized system is used to elevate the boiling point of water, so that the steam can reach a high temperature that causes death of microorganisms through coagulation of proteins in bacterial cells. Usually, the sterilization requires 15 min at 121°C. For a large package, it may require a longer time. Autoclaving is used for sterilization of equipment, tubing, filters, rubber stoppers, and final products if they are heat-stable. It is not suitable for sterilization of dry substances because of the presence of steam.

Term	Symbol	Definition or Description
BET isotherm		The *Brunauer, Emmet, and Teller (BET) isotherm* describes a multilayer formation and an S-shaped adsorption curve, in which multiple gas layers are condensed above the first layer with each layer exhibiting the same heat of condensation. If the particle surface contains a finite number of sites for the gas molecules to occupy, then the saturation of gas (or in liquid state) at the particle surface will lead to the saturated vapor pressure of the liquefied gas as the absorbed amount reaches infinity. In this approach, the isotherm can be written as $$\frac{P}{V(P^o - P)} = \frac{1}{cV_m} + \frac{c-1}{V_m c}\frac{P}{P^o}$$ where P^o is the saturation vapor pressure of the liquefied gas, c is a constant expressing the difference between the heat of condensation and the heat of adsorption, and V and V_m are volumes at pressure P and P^o, respectively. A plot of $P/V(P^o - P)$ versus P/P^o yields a straight line with a slope of $(c - 1)/V_m c$ and an intercept of $1/V_m c$, from which both V_m and c can be determined. The BET theory has been the basis for surface area determinations.
Binder		*Binders* are excipients that blend the active and inactive ingredients together. They can be used in their dry or powdered form. Binders that are hydrophilic can be used in a wet granulation process. A typical binder concentration is 2–5% of the formulation. Examples of commonly used binders are povidone, hypromellose, and hydroxypropylcellulose.
Bingham plastic		A material is called a *Bingham plastic* if it behaves as a rigid body at low stress until a critical stress value (yield stress) is reached; then, under a continuing increase in stress, it flows as a fluid with a constant viscosity.
Bioadhesives		*Bioadhesives* are polymers that exhibit gel-forming properties on contact with aqueous fluid. These polymers include starch, chitosan, and Carbopols, which may be used to enhance drug permeability through the nasal epithelium with extended residence time.
Bioavailability		*Bioavailability* is defined as the rate and extent to which the active ingredient or active moiety is absorbed from a drug product and becomes available at the site of action.
Bioavailability indices	C_{max}, t_{max}, AUC	Bioavailability is usually evaluated based on *three indices*: the maximum drug concentration in plasma (C_{max}), the time needed to reach this maximum (t_{max}), and the area under the plasma concentration–time curve (AUC).

Term	Symbol	Definition or Description
Biocompatibility		*Biocompatibility* relates to the nature of the interaction of biomaterials with the human body, and how these interactions determine the clinical success of a medical device.
Biodegradable		*Biodegradable* describes materials that can be decomposed by living organisms. For drug delivery, a biodegradable system would be one that leaves no residual materials following the release of drugs and the degradation of materials.
Biodistribution		*Biodistribution* refers to tracking of compounds of interest that have been administered in either an experimental animal or a human subject for purposes of therapy or diagnostics.
Bioequivalence		*Bioequivalence* is defined as the absence of a significant difference in the rate and extent to which the active ingredient or active moiety from two pharmaceutical equivalents becomes available at the site of action when administered at the same molar dose under similar conditions. Thus, two drug products having the same active moiety and at the same molar dose are deemed *bioequivalent* if they exhibit similar enough bioavailability to ensure comparable in vivo performance.
Bioinformatics		*Bioinformatics* is the application of computer science and informatics to the field of medicine. It utilizes algorithms, databases and information systems, computation theory, software engineering, data mining and processing, circuit theory, and statistics to generate new knowledge in biology and medicine and to develop new models of computation.
Biomarker proteins		*Biomarker proteins* are small-molecule indicators of a biological state, measured and evaluated as indicators of normal or pathogenic biological processes or pharmacologic responses to a therapeutic intervention.
Biopharmaceutics Classification System	BCS	BCS denotes the classification of drug substances into class I: high solubility–high permeability; class II: low solubility–high permeability; class III: high solubility–low permeability; and class IV: low solubility–low permeability groups. It is adopted by the FDA, the European Medicines Agency, and the World Health Organization for setting bioavailability and bioequivalence standards for immediate-release oral drug product approval. The solubility classification of a drug is based on the highest dose strength in an immediate-release product. A drug substance is considered highly soluble if the highest strength is soluble in 250 mL or less of aqueous media throughout the pH

Term	Symbol	Definition or Description
		range of 1.2–6.8. Otherwise, the drug substance is considered poorly soluble. A drug substance is considered highly permeable if the extent of intestinal absorption is determined to be 90% or higher.
Biowaiver		*Biowaivers* of in vivo bioavailability and bioequivalence requirements for immediate-release bioequivalent drug products may be granted to a BCS class I drug if it dissolves very rapidly (defined as more than 85% dissolution in less than 30 min) in media with pH 1.2, 4.5, and 6.8. Hence, a biowaiver depends on three parameters: high solubility, high permeability, and rapid dissolution at specified pH conditions, all of which may be modified by the presence of excipients.
Blending		*Blending* is defined as the mixing of drug and excipients to get a uniform distribution of the components. It can be achieved using rotating-shell or fixed-shell blenders. To ensure adequate blending, as required by the FDA, appropriate test methods and in-process controls have to be established, and blend sampling from different locations of the blender must be carried out to determine the uniformity of the active ingredient.
Block copolymer		A *block copolymer* is a polymer composed of two or more *homopolymer* units linked by covalent bond. The union of the homopolymers may require an intermediate nonrepeating unit, known as a junction block. Copolymers with two or three distinct blocks are called diblock and triblock copolymers, respectively. These blocks can be arranged in A-B diblock or A-B-A triblock types, or as grafted copolymers, in which the block A backbone is grafted with one or more block B side chains, or vice versa.
Bloom strength		*Bloom strength* is defined as the force or *bloom* (in grams) required to depress by 4 mm the surface of a 6.67% gelatin gel that has been kept 17 h at 10°C, with a standard AOAC (Association of Official Agricultural Chemists) plunger.
Brønsted–Lowry acid–base theory		According to the *Brønsted–Lowry acid–base theory*, an acid is a molecule or ion that has a dissociable proton, whereas a base is a molecule or ion having the capacity to accept a proton. The acid–base equilibrium consists of two conjugated acid–base pairs (see *Acid–base conjugation*).
Bricks-and-mortar model		The structure of the stratum corneum is conceptually modeled as *bricks and mortar*. The corneocytes are considered to be a *brick* and the lipid matrixes between the cells are considered to be *mortar*. The bricks-and-mortar model helps one to understand the stratum corneum barrier and predicts skin permeation of drugs.

Term	Symbol	Definition or Description
Buffer capacity	β	*Buffer capacity* is defined as the amount of base needed to increase the pH of a solution by 1 pH unit. The value of β depends on the pH of the solution, the pK_a of the buffer system, and the concentration of the buffer agents.
Bulk density	ρ_{bulk}	*Bulk density* is the weight of the material divided by its bulk volume, measured as follows: A sample of about 50 mL of powder, which has been passed through a U.S. no. 20 sieve, is introduced into a 100-mL graduated cylinder. The cylinder, held 1 in above a hardwood surface, is dropped three times onto the surface at 2-s intervals. The bulk density is then obtained as the ratio of the sample weight in grams to the measured volume in cubic centimeters by the graduated cylinder.
Bulk modulus	K	*Bulk modulus* refers to strain response to compressive stress applied to a liquid; it is measured as the change in hydrostatic pressure divided by the resulting change in volume.
Carr index		The *Carr index* (CI), also known as the *compressibility index*, is the percentage of the void volume in the bulk volume of a powder sample. It is calculated based on the tapped density (ρ_t) and the bulk density (ρ_b) of the material by the following equation: $$\text{CI} = [(\rho_t - \rho_b)/\rho_t\,] \times 100$$ Typically, values of 15–25% indicate a compressible blend.
Cell-penetrating peptides	CCPs	*Cell-penetrating peptides* (CPPs), also known as protein transduction domains (PTDs), are small motifs in protein that facilitate cellular uptake of macromolecules as well as carrier systems across biological membranes. Several peptide motifs have been identified with the typical polycationic or amphiphilic structures.
Charge transfer complex		*Charge transfer* (*CT*) *complexes* are formed between molecules that act as electron pair donors and acceptors, respectively. This type of complexation occurs mainly by sharing *p* electrons that are known to be more polarizable than the sigma (single) bond electrons. Aromatic compounds, in which the π electrons are delocalized in the ring system through the resonance effect, are able to make charge-transfer interactions. An example of a CT complex in pharmacy is butesin picrate, a yellow, water-insoluble powder that consists of two molecules of butyl *p*-aminobenzoate with one molecule of picric acid, which is used as a local anesthetic owing to the antiseptic effect of picric acid and the antibacterial action of butesin.

Term	Symbol	Definition or Description
Chelate		Metal complexes can be made to contain a ligand that occupies two or more coordination positions on the central atom. For example, in Cu(ethylenediamine)$_2^{2+}$, each ethylenediamine forms two coordination bonds through the two amino groups. The coordination number is 4. The term *chelate* applies to such a structure, where ethylenediamine is said to be bidentate for having two coordinating groups per molecule. The common metal-removing agent EDTA, which binds to even Ca^{2+}, despite the metal's tendency of not participating in complexation, is a sexadentate (coordination number = 6) chelating agent.
Chemical potential	μ	The *chemical potential* of a solution component represents the free energy change of the system brought about by a small increment of the component under constant temperature and pressure. For an ideal solution of a binary system, e.g., the chemical potential of the solvent $\mu_1(l)$ can be written as $\mu_1(l) = \mu_1°(l) + RT \ln X_1$ where $\mu_1°(l)$ is the chemical potential of the pure solvent in the standard state and X_1 is the mole fraction of the solvent. One can write a parallel equation for the solute as well. In phase equilibrium, i.e., between liquid and vapor, one important thermodynamic conclusion is that the chemical potential of each component must be the same in every phase in which it is present. Consider a solution at its boiling point under 1 atm pressure. The chemical potential of the solvent in solution must be the same as that of the vapor $\mu_1(g)$, which, at 1 atm, also equals to the standard state chemical potential of the vapor $\mu_1°(g)$. Thus, $\mu_1°(g) - \mu_1°(l) = RT \ln X_1$ This equation shows that the free energy change for the solvent going from liquid to vapor is a function of the temperature and its mole fraction. From this equation, it can be shown that the boiling point of a solvent is elevated by the addition of a solute, and the elevation is proportional to the mole fraction of the solute ($X_2 = 1 - X_1$) with the proportional constant equal to $R(T_o)^2/\Delta H_{vap}$, where T_o is the boiling point of the pure solvent and ΔH_{vap} is the heat of vaporization.
Clausius–Clapeyron relationship		The vapor pressure of a liquid decreases with the addition of a small amount of a solute, but increases with an increase in temperature. The *Clausius–Clapeyron equation* shows that the increase in vapor pressure in $d(\ln P)$ per small increase in temperature (dT) equals $\Delta H_{vap}/RT^2$, which is a constant over the range of the small temperature change. The addition of a small amount of a solute (dX_2) causes a decrease in vapor pressure by $d(\ln P)$. Thus, to regain the lowered vapor pressure, the temperature must be increased by dT. This is another approach to explain the boiling point elevation of a solution over that of the pure solvent.

Term	Symbol	Definition or Description
Clearance		*Clearance* refers primarily to the renal excretion ability of a certain pharmaceutical compound or biomolecule. Clearance may follow zero-order kinetics, where a constant amount of drug is eliminated per unit time, or first-order kinetics where a constant fraction of the drug is eliminated per unit time.
Colligative properties		Solution properties that depend on only the mole fraction of the solution but not on any of the properties of the solute are known as *colligative properties*. There are four such properties: vapor pressure lowering, boiling point elevation, freezing point depression, and osmotic pressure.
Competitive inhibition		A compound that decreases the rate of an enzymatic reaction is called an inhibitor. If the inhibitor binds to the enzyme at the active site and competes with the substrate for the free enzyme, the rate of substrate metabolism will be lowered. This is known as *competitive inhibition*. The kinetic evidence of such a process is that the slope of the Lineweaver–Burk plot for the substrate reaction will be increased by the presence of the inhibitor, but the *y* axis intercept, which is the reciprocal value of the maximum velocity, will remain constant.
Complementary base		*Complementary base* is the nucleic acid base that is linked by a hydrogen bond on an opposite strand of DNA or RNA. Guanine is the complementary base of cytosine, and adenine is the complementary base of thymine in DNA and of uracil in RNA.
Complex modulus	G^*	*Complex modulus* is the overall resistance of a material to deformation, which includes the storage or elastic (recoverable deformation) modulus G' and the loss or viscous (nonrecoverable deformation) modulus G''. And G^* is expressed as $G^* = G' + iG''$.
Complex reactions		Chemical reactions that involve more than one step in their reaction schemes, and for each step the product formed is measurable, are called *complex reactions*. These reactions, such as the reversible, parallel, consecutive, autocatalytic, induced, and chain reactions, are not a concerted process and cannot be treated by the steady-state approximation.
Computed tomography	CT	*Computed tomography* is an X-ray–based radiologic medical imaging technique that utilizes tomography created by computer processing to generate a three-dimensional image from a series of two-dimensional images taken around a single axis.
Contrast agents		*Contrast agents* are substances used to enhance the contrast of structures such as blood vessels and the gastrointestinal tract within the body for the purposes of medical imaging.
Coordination number		The *coordination number* is the secondary valence of a metal ion. It indicates the number of bonds or ligands that can be formed in the metal complexation. For example, Cu^{2+} has a coordination number of 4 and thus forms $Cu(NH_3)_4^{2+}$ with ammonia.

Term	Symbol	Definition or Description
Creep test		A *creep test* determines the strain response of a viscoelastic material under a constant low stress (below the yield stress) over a short time. The creep (deformation and flow) is then allowed to recover by removing the applied stress. A material is repeatedly tested until the strain rate is decreased to an equilibrium state. The strain may be expressed as a percentage of strain or as strain per unit of stress known as the *compliance* (J). The extrapolated J value (J_o) from the equilibrium curve gives the theoretical limit of recovery; the slope of the equilibrium curve allows for the determination of the zero-shear viscosity (η_o) by the relation η_o = applied stress/slope.
Crenation		*Crenation* is a process of cell shrinkage in a hypertonic environment because of the osmotic movement of water from the cells to the hypertonic medium.
Crossover frequency		In a dynamic oscillatory frequency sweep, the *crossover frequency* refers to the frequency at which the storage (G') and loss (G'') moduli cross, which usually marks the transition of the material from being elastic to fluidic, or vice versa.
Cryoprotectant and lyoprotectant		A *cryoprotectant* is a substance used to protect biological samples or protein solutions from freezing damage. A *lyoprotectant* is a substance used to prevent aggregation and loss of activity of biological molecules prepared in a lyophilized (freeze-dried) product. For example, sucrose and trehalose have been shown to protect and preserve anti-IgE and anti-HER2 antibodies in lyophilized isotonic formulations, which are ready for use as injections after reconstitution.
Current good manufacturing practice	cGMP	cGMP is a set of FDA regulations designed to ensure that a product is safe for use and that it has the ingredients and strength it claims to have. The cGMP regulations for drugs, which set managerial rather than scientific standards, contain minimum requirements for the methods, facilities, and controls used in manufacturing, processing, and packaging of a drug product. The approval process for new and generic drug applications includes a review of the manufacturer's compliance with the cGMP. FDA inspectors determine whether the firm has the necessary facilities, equipment, and skill to manufacture the new drug for which it has applied for approval, based upon the inspection of the facilities, sample analyses, and the compliance history of the firm. This information is summarized in reports that include the firm's past records. The FDA can issue a warning letter or initiate other regulatory actions against noncompliance. Failure to comply can also lead to a decision by the FDA to not approve an application to market a drug.

Term	Symbol	Definition or Description
Cyclodextrins		Natural *cyclodextrins* (CDs), also known as the *Schardinger sugars*, are products of starch and cyclodextrin glycosyltransferases. The CDs are constituted by 6-, 7-, and 8-glucopyranoside units, designated, respectively as α-, β-, and γ-CDs, arranged as a toroid in which the larger and smaller openings are lined with secondary and primary hydroxyl groups, respectively. CDs are in general water-soluble, but the interior of the toroid is relatively hydrophobic compared to the aqueous environment and is able to host a hydrophobic drug, forming an inclusion complex. CDs can be used to enhance drug solubility as well as drug permeation by acting on opening the epithelial tight junction.
Dalton's law		The total pressure exerted by a mixture of gases is equal to the sum of the pressures that each component would exert if placed separately into the container. — *Dalton's law*, 1810.
Dendrimers		*Dendrimers*, also known as cascade molecules, are repeatedly branched polymers that have a spherical three-dimensional morphology. They are synthesized from a starting initiator, to which chemical moieties are added by a repeating series of reactions. As the process repeats, successive layers are added, and the expanded sphere assumes a structure that consists of (1) an initiator core, (2) interior layers (generations) composed of radically attached repeating units, and (3) terminal functionality groups attached to the outermost generation. The outer layer can be cationic (—NH_3^+), hydrophilic (—OH or PEGylated), anionic (—CO_2^-), or hydrophobic. An example of the dendrimer types is the poly(amidoamine) (PAMAM) dendrimers, which are synthesized by starting with ammonia or ethylenediamine as the initiator.
Diffusion		*Diffusion* is one of the physicochemical transport phenomena that include molecular, momentum, and thermal conductivity transports. In diffusion, one deals with molecular transport or the drift of molecules from one place to another.
Dilatancy		*Dilatancy* is a non-Newtonian behavior where the viscosity of a liquid increases with increasing shear rate. It is irreversible and occurs in concentrated suspensions of deflocculated particles and at sufficiently high shear rates.
Dipole–dipole interaction		A chemical bond formed through uneven sharing of the pair of electrons, because of the greater electronegativity of one atom compared to the other, will have a partial separation of positive and negative charges. A compound possessing such a bond is said to be a *permanent dipole* (a polar compound). The dipole molecules in pure state or in a mixed system may position themselves with neighboring molecules in such a way that the opposite charge centers point toward one another. This is known as the *dipole–dipole interaction* or *Keesom force*.

Term	Symbol	Definition or Description
Disintegrant		*Disintegrants* are excipients that are not water-soluble but have a high affinity for water. By wicking or swelling mechanisms, these compounds can reduce the cohesive forces holding a tablet together and induce the breakup of a tablet into smaller particles, thus increasing the surface area for drug dissolution.
Distribution law	K	In oil–water phase equilibrium for the distribution of a drug, the chemical potential, or partial free energy, of the drug in the aqueous phase must be the same as the chemical potential of the same species in the oil phase. The change in standard free energy going from the aqueous to the oil phase is proportional to the logarithmic value of the concentration ratio of the drug in the two phases. Because at equilibrium, the free energy change is zero, the concentrations ratio of the drug in the oil and aqueous phases must be a constant, which is known as the partition coefficient (K). This is the *distribution law*. In order for the partition coefficient to be valid, the drug must exist in the same form in the two phases.
Drug and medicine		*Drug* refers to any chemical agent that is capable of interacting with living systems to produce a biological effect. A *medicine* is a pharmaceutical preparation of drug with the ultimate purpose of providing pharmaceutical care to patients.
Drug for injection		*Drug for injection* is a dried powder product to be reconstituted as an injectable solution using sterile water or an isotonic vehicle.
Drug targeting		*Drug targeting* refers to the delivery of drug to a specific site, which can be a macromolecule, an organ, a specific cell type, or a subcellular organelle. The overall goal of drug targeting is to achieve increased drug efficacy with reduced drug dose and systemic toxicity. In most targeting methods and approaches, the dosage form is usually delivered by parenteral injection, a relatively direct route to get the drug to the targeting tissue. Site-specific administration is sometimes possible, but such deliveries typically involve highly invasive procedures. Hence, a targeting dosage form must be suitable for injection without causing adverse effects and must be stable in systemic circulation. A prolonged circulation time often enhances the dosage form's targeting ability.
Dry powder inhalers	DPIs	The *dry powder inhalers* are devices used to deliver drug powder to the lungs via aerosolization by the patient's inspirational efforts. The basic features of a DPI include dose-metering mechanism, an aerosolization mechanism, a deaggregation mechanism, and an adapter to direct the aerosol into the patient's mouth. Drugs are milled to desirable sizes (< 5 μm) and formulated into large particles using lactose particles (60–80 μm) as carriers. During aerosolization, the deaggregation action

Term	Symbol	Definition or Description
		of the inhaler causes a stripping of drug particles from the lactose surface, allowing them to traverse through the respiratory tract, while the lactose particles are left behind in the mouthpiece of the device or in the mouth and throat of the patient. In unit-dose inhalers, the drug–lactose powder is filled into a hard gelatin capsule. These are two common DPI systems. The Spinhaler contains an impeller in the body of the inhaler. The capsule is pierced by the device when the system is ready to use, and the impeller rotates as the patient breathes through the device, projecting particles into the airstream. The Rotahaler has a mechanism for breaking the capsule into two pieces. The capsule body containing the dose falls into the device, while the cap is retained in the entry port. As the patient inhales, an erratic motion of the capsule containing the drug in the airstream causes the dislodged particles to be entrained through a grating system and inhaled.
Effective intestinal permeability	P_{eff}	Because of the expansion of surface area by villous structure in the intestine, the intestinal permeability is usually about 10^{-4} cm/s and is referred to as the *effective intestinal permeability*, as opposed to permeability measured by in vitro systems such as Caco-2 cell monolayer, which are in the range of 10^{-5} to 10^{-6} cm/s.
Efficacy		*Efficacy* is the ability of a pharmacologic drug or biomolecule to produce a desired effect, typically a beneficial change in response to a given intervention.
Electrical double layer		The charge of a particle in solution is made up of the actual charge of the particle and the ionic charges that are held sufficiently close to the particle that they will remain with the particle as it moves through the solution. This results in the existence of an *electrical* or *diffuse double layer* consisting of a tightly bound layer and the diffuse layer. When particles move, the plane of shear is within the double layer at the tightly bound layer surface.
Electrokinetic effects		*Electrokinetic effects* refer to the relative motion between a charged surface and an electrolyte solution. The surface is either a solid particle suspended in solution or a stationary wall of tube down which the solution flows. For stationary surface, electro-osmosis occurs under applied potential; there is also an induced effect known as the streaming potential. For suspended particles, electrophoresis occurs under applied potential; and there is an induced effect known as the sedimentation potential.
Electron affinity	A	*Electron affinity* is the energy (in electron volts) with which a neutral atom binds another electron. For fluorine at gaseous state, e.g., it is the energy given out in the reaction $$\mathrm{F}(g) + e^-(g) \rightarrow \mathrm{F}^-(g) \qquad A = 3.45\ \mathrm{eV}$$

Term	Symbol	Definition or Description
Electronegativity	x	*Electronegativity* is an index that attempts to represent the attracting tendency of an atom toward the pair of electrons that forms the bond between this atom and another atom. In the Mulliken expression, $x = (I + A)/5.6$, where I is the ionization potential, A is the electron affinity, and the factor 5.6 is an arbitrary scale. For example, $x_{Cl} = 3.0$ and $x_H = 2.5$.
Electroporation		*Electroporation* is a mechanical method employing externally applied high-voltage electrical pulses to induce transient formation of aqueous pores in the lipid bilayers.
Emulsifier		A well-dispersed homogeneous emulsion system consists of the oil and aqueous phases as well as a third phase known as the *emulsifier*, whose function is to maintain the stability of the oil–water interface. The emulsifier interacts with both the oil and water phases, serving as a solvation agent for the nondissolvable liquid particulate at the oil–water interface. Emulsifiers are usually surfactants.
Emulsion		*Emulsion* is a polydisperse system consisting of two or more liquids that are immiscible, e.g., water and oil.
Emulsion instability—aggregation, coalescence, and phase inversion		Emulsions are not physically stable. The instabilities include (1) *aggregation* of droplets, resulting in uneven distribution of the drug (known as *creaming*); (2) *coalescence*, resulting in larger droplets that cannot be redispersed into small droplets by gentle shaking; and (3) *phase inversion*, in which the original internal and external phases are reversed to external and internal phases, respectively, due to the use of a large volume of the original internal phase and/or misuse of the emulsifier(s).
Endosomes		*Endosomes* or endocytic vesicles are membrane-bound compartments of the endocytic membrane transport system. Once molecules are taken up by cells through an endocytosis process, they are engulfed in the endosomes and en route to lysosomes for degradation.
Enhanced permeability and retention	EPR	The *enhanced permeability and retention* (EPR) effect refers to the extravasation of nanoparticle drug carriers to, and their retention in, highly irregular tumor tissues. Increased angiogenesis occurs typically in solid tumors because of their high demand for nutrition and oxygen as the cells multiply and cluster. The blood vessels in tumors, however, are irregular, dilated, and leaky due to discontinuous lining of endothelial cells. The perivascular cells and the smooth-muscle layers are frequently absent or abnormal in the vascular wall. These defects result in extravasation of blood plasma components and, when present, nanoparticles. As the tumors progress, the lymphatic drainage in tumor tissues becomes increasingly impaired, which, along with slow venous return,

Term	Symbol	Definition or Description
		accounts for a high retention of nanocarriers in the tumor tissues. Hence, nanocarriers may be used for *passive targeting* of drug to the tumor tissue due to the high permeability of the vasculature and the lack of lymphatic drainage in tumor areas for particle clearance.
Epidermis		*Epidermis* is the outermost, nonvascular layer of the skin comprising mainly keratinocytes. Basal keratinocytes proliferate and give rise to differentiated cells, which, upon migration, generate several layers of epidermis that work in concert to provide strength and flexibility to the skin.
Fenton reaction		The *Fenton reaction* describes the generation of the hydroxyl radical by H_2O_2 in the presence of Fe(II) salts: $Fe^{2+} + H_2O_2 \rightarrow Fe^{3+} + {}^{\cdot}OH + OH^-$ There are multiple reactions associated with the Fenton reaction, such as: $Fe^{3+} + H_2O_2 \rightarrow Fe^{2+} + O_2^- + H^+$ ${}^{\cdot}OH + H_2O_2 \rightarrow H_2O + H^+ + O_2^-$ The Fenton-like reaction in the generation of $\cdot OH$ also occurs with copper(I) ions, in that $Cu^+ + H_2O_2 \rightarrow Cu^{2+} + {}^{\cdot}OH + OH^-$ The hydroxyl radical reacts with extremely high rate constants with almost every type of molecule found in living cells.
Fick's law of diffusion		*First law*: The rate of diffusion across a plane is proportional to (1) the concentration gradient dc/dx across a diffusion boundary layer and (2) the cross-sectional area A. If the diffusion rate is dW/dt, the number of grams of solute transferred across the boundary per second, then $dW/dt = -DA\ dc/dx$. If the amount of solute is measured in grams per second per unit area, that is, $dw = dW/A$, then $J = dw/dt = -D\ dc/dx$, where J is called the *flux*. *Second law*: The change in concentration per time in the diffusion distance (referred to as the boundary layer, x to $x + dx$) is directly proportional to changes in the concentration difference between x and $x + dx$. In other words, if the concentrations are C_1 and C_2 at x and $x + dx$, respectively, then $C_1 - C_2$ is the concentration gradient and dc/dt is proportional to $C_1 - C_2$.
Film pressure	π	The *film pressure* (π) refers to the surface tension lowering by the spread of a surfactant to form a monolayer film on a liquid surface. For example, when a surfactant is added to the water surface and is compressed against the floating barrier, the compressive force per unit area is known as the surface or film pressure, which corresponds to a lowering of the surface tension of water from γ^o to γ, that is, $\pi = \gamma^o - \gamma$.

Term	Symbol	Definition or Description
Floccules and flocculants		*Floccules* or flocs are loosely bound particle aggregates in a suspension formed by flocculation. This loose aggregation prevents the particles from forming tight aggregation that can eventually lead to cake formation. The floccules settle down quickly but with a high sedimentation volume, which allows for easy resuspension. Floccules are prepared with the aids of flocculating agents, or *flocculants*. Multivalent cations such as Al^{3+} and Ca^{2+} can effectively neutralize the negative charges on the surface of the particles, so that they can be used to reduce the repulsion force between particles and to promote particle association in the formation of floccules. Clays such as bentonite magma and polymers such as chitosan and gelatin can also be used as flocculating agents.
Flow curve		The *flow curve*, also known as the *rheogram* or *consistency curve*, of a liquid or deformable solid is the plot of the rate of shear (dv/dx) versus the shear stress (f/A). The velocity gradient is perpendicular to the direction of flow. A rheogram can also be expressed as a plot of shear stress versus the shear rate.
Free adhesion energy		The work required for the adhesion process, which involves the loss of surface area of the free solid and free liquid but a gain in the surface area of the interface, is the *free adhesion energy* (W_a), which is equivalent to $\gamma_S + \gamma_L - \gamma_{SL}$.
Freundlich isotherm		The adsorption of solute from solution onto an adsorbent may be limited to the formation of a monolayer, with any further addition of solute being strongly opposed by the power of solvation. An empirical isotherm based on this concept was introduced by Freundlich, called the *Freundlich isotherm*, in that if y is the weight of solute adsorbed per gram of adsorbent and c is the concentration of the solute in solution, then $y = kc^{1/n}$, where k and n are empirical constants. The equation is usually used in the logarithmic form: $\log y = \log k + (1/n) \log c$, which yields a straight line with the plot of $\log y$ versus $\log c$, from which k and n can be determined.
Gelatin for capsules		*Gelatin* used in manufacturing hard and soft capsules is obtained by partial hydrolysis of collagen derived from bovine or porcine skin and bones. Type A gelatin is derived from bovine or porcine skin by acid hydrolysis with a pI in the range of 4.8–5.2. Type B gelatin is derived from bovine or porcine bones by alkali hydrolysis, with pI in the range of 6.5–9.5. Gelatin derived from skin has plasticity, and gelatin derived from bones has firmness. Typically, capsules are manufactured by using both types of gelatin obtained from bovine spongiform encephalopathy (BSE)-free cattle. They have a bloom strength in the range of 150–280 g.

Term	Symbol	Definition or Description
General and specific acid–base catalysis		The term *general acid–base catalysis* refers to the catalytic action derived from the whole and part of the acid or base molecule, whereas in *specific acid–base catalysis*, the catalytic action is attributed specifically to H^+ or OH^- and is thus pH-dependent. Catalysis by the conjugated base of a weak acid may be obscured in an acidic solution, but is readily seen in neutral and alkaline pH.
Geometric diameter	d_g	For particle size distribution, the median value for a lognormal distribution is known as the *geometric diameter* d_g, which indicates that 50% of the particles will be either less than or greater than this size.
Geometric dilution		*Geometric dilution* is a process by which two powders of unequal quantity are mixed by trituration. The smaller-quantity powder, usually the active ingredient, is first triturated with an equal portion of the larger-quantity powder, which is then mixed and triturated with an equal portion of the larger-quantity powder. This process is continued until all of both powders have been mixed.
Gibbs' adsorption equation	Γ_2	The common form of the *Gibbs adsorption equation* is $$\Gamma_2 = -(C/RT)\, d\gamma/dC = [n_2^S - n_2(n_1^S/n_1)]/A$$ The quantity Γ_2 indicates the difference between the number of solute residing at the surface and that in the bulk solution of a comparable area. Here, n_2^S and n_1^S are the moles of solute and solvent, respectively, at the surface. The term $n_2(n_1^S/n_1)$ is the moles of solute in a bulk region that contains n_1^S solvent molecules. For this reason, Γ_2 is known as the algebraic *surface excess* of the solute at the interface over the number of moles that would be present in a bulk region containing the same number of moles of solvent. The importance of the Gibbs adsorption is that if a solute prefers to concentrate at the interface, Γ_2 will be positive and the surface tension will decrease with increasing solute concentration. Conversely, if Γ_2 is a negative excess, as in electrolyte solutions, then the surface concentration of electrolytes will be less than it is in solution, and $d\gamma/dC$ assumes a positive value. Thus, any compounds having a tendency to reside at the interface will reduce the surface tension of the liquid and are thus called surface-active. Small electrolytes are not surface-active and tend to move away from the surface.
Glidant		*Glidants* are excipients used to enhance the flow of the powder blends by reducing interparticulate friction. Commonly used glidants include colloidal silicon dioxide and many lubricants that exhibit similar activity.

Term	Symbol	Definition or Description
Hemolysis		*Hemolysis* is the swelling and burst of erythrocytes caused by the osmotic movement of water from a hypotonic medium to the intracellular space.
High-shear granulation		*High-shear granulation* is a process of combining a liquid and solid in granule preparation. Liquid undergoes shear when one area of the liquid has higher velocity than another area. The equipment consists of a low-speed rotating impeller that imparts higher velocity to the liquid at the tip of the impeller than at the center of the impeller, thus creating shear. The agglomeration in a high-shear process involves nucleation (formation of granules from combined liquid and solid particles) and coalescence (formation of larger granules by smaller granules). As more liquid is added, the agglomerates go quickly from having liquid bridges, liquid-filled pores, to complete enclosure by the liquid. This process results in the formation of round and dense particles, regardless of the morphology of the starting material.
Hixson–Crowell cube root law		The *Hixson–Crowell cube root law* describes particle dissolution based on a change in the radius of the particles as a function of time. The corresponding change in mass in the dissolution process can be expressed as $$(W_s/W_0)^{1/3} = 1 - DC_s t/\rho h r_0$$ where W_0 and W_s are the weights of the undissolved particles at 0 and time t, the diffusion coefficient is D, the solubility is C_s, the density is ρ, the diffusion boundary layer is h, and the initial radius of the particles is r_0.
Hooke's law		*Hooke's law* states that for relatively small deformation of an object, the displacement or size of the deformation is directly proportional to the deforming force or load. Under these conditions the object returns to its original shape and size upon removal of load.
Hydrophilic–lipophilic balance	HLB	The classification of surfactants based on their affinities to the aqueous and oil phases is known as the *hydrophilic–lipophilic balance* (HLB) system, originally conceived for non ionic surfactants. In this system, each surfactant is assigned a number, which represents the percentage weight of the hydrophilic (polyoxyethylene) group divided by 5, in order to limit the range from 0 to 20. Thus, for a 100% hydrophilic molecule, as in polyethylene glycol, the HLB value is 20. The HLB values for other surfactants have been determined by comparison of their physical chemical properties that reflect the molecular polarity of surfactants having known HLB values. These properties include aqueous solubility, interfacial tension, and dielectric constant. Surfactants exhibiting values greater than 20, such as sodium lauryl sulfate (HLB = 40), are deemed to have greater hydrophilic behavior than that of the polyoxyethylene groups alone.

Term	Symbol	Definition or Description
Hydrophobic bonding		Hydrophobic moieties of macromolecules and cellular membrane structures cannot be solvated by water. As a result, the water molecules in the nonpolar region may associate through hydrogen bonds to form quasi-crystalline structures and produce a higher degree of order than water molecules in the bulk phase. When two nonpolar moieties come close together, the region is shielded to a greater extent by interacting water molecules, through the collapse of the quasi-crystalline water structures of the isolated nonpolar moieties. The free energy change of this process is in favor for a close contact of the two nonpolar moieties, and their association is known as *hydrophobic bonding*. Hydrophobic interaction plays an important role in the biological system. The hydrophobicity of a compound is closely related to the drug's aqueous solubility and its partition into nonpolar phases; and it determines the rate and extent of drug absorption and tissue distribution. In the blood, drug is bound to plasma proteins, in which hydrophobic bonding is a primary interactive force. Drug interaction with the cell surface receptor is highly structure-specific, but the hydrophobic interaction is involved in stabilizing the drug–receptor complex.
Ideal solution		An *ideal solution* is a solution that obeys Raoult's law. Such a solution exhibits the characteristics of zero heat of mixing and a solution volume that is the sum of those of the components. In general, a liquid solution does not behave ideally as does a gaseous solution, but for a nonvolatile solute in dilute concentrations, the solution may be taken as an ideal solution.
Immersion free energy		*Immersion free energy* refers to the free energy change when a solid particle is immersed in liquid with complete wetting.
Immersed sword system		In coating pan design, the *immersed sword system* is a metal device consisting of concentric inlet and exhaust ducts attached to a perforated column immersed in the tablet bed. Through this device, dry air is introduced from the perforated column and flows upward through the tablet bed. Because the dry air is intimately mixed with the wetted tablets, a more efficient drying environment is provided. This device is one of several immersed systems developed for improved tablet coating and drying, which led to the development of fully or partially perforated side-vented pans that exhibit the advantages of rotation along a horizontal axis and superior drying efficiency needed for aqueous film coating.
Immunoliposomes		Liposomes (stealth or otherwise) with grafted monoclonal antibody (mAb) or fragments for active targeting are known as *immunoliposomes*.

Term	Symbol	Definition or Description
Inclusion complex		*Inclusion complexes* are formed primarily via physical entrapment, although chemical interactions may play a role. The formation of cyclodextrin inclusion complex, e.g., depends largely on the cavity size of the CD in relation to the molecular size of the guest molecule. The internal diameters of the α-, β-, and γ-CD cavities are about 5, 6, and 8 Å, respectively, with the cavity size of β-CDs corresponding to that of a benzene ring.
Inductive effect		The dissociation of a proton from organic acids can be enhanced by adjacent functional groups that have an electron-withdrawing property, indicating that structural modification can alter acid–base equilibrium. This is known as the *inductive effect*.
Interfacial film theory		The interactions of the emulsifier with the interfacial molecules (water or oil) reduce the internal pulling force by the like molecules, and therefore the interfacial tension. In forming stable emulsions, the emulsifier molecules will arrange in a special orientation. The *interfacial film theory* suggests that the emulsifier molecules form a film between the two phases, or wrap around the dispersed droplets, to reduce the interfacial tension.
Intrinsic solubility		Solubility is the concentration of a saturated solution in which the dissolved solute is in equilibrium with its solid phase (in excess) at constant temperature. For nonelectrolytes and organic weak acids and weak bases in their free (neutral) forms, the solubility is an equilibrium constant that describes an intrinsic property of the drug (which cannot be changed), and thus it is referred to as the *intrinsic* or *equilibrium solubility*.
Ionic strength	μ	*Ionic strength* is a measure of the nonideality imposed by all ions in the solution on ions from a given electrolyte. It is a solution property in that $\mu = ½(\Sigma C_i Z_i^2)$, where C_i is the concentration of the *i*th ion, Z_i is its charge, and the summation extends to all ions in the solution. The relationship between activity coefficient and ionic strength is given by the Debye–Hückel theory (see text for details).
Ionization energy	I	*Ionization potential* is the energy (in electron volts) required to remove an electron from a neutral atom. For example, $I_K = 4.34$, $I_H = 13.60$, and $I_F = 17.42$ eV.
Iontophoresis		*Iontophoresis*, also known as electromotive drug delivery, is a method using a small electric charge to drive solute molecules across the skin. This method is considered noninvasive.
Isoelectric point	pI	Compounds with both acid and base groups, such as the amino acids and proteins, can exist predominantly in the zwitterion form, in which the acid group is void of the proton (negatively charged) and the base group is protonated (positively charged),

Term	Symbol	Definition or Description
		at a pH known as the *isoelectric point* (pI). pI is the average of the two pK_a values of the acid and base groups. For proteins, pI is the pH at which the molecules have a net neutral charge. At pH above its pI, a protein becomes negatively charged, as in plasma albumin (pI = 4.9) at the physiological pH (7.4).
Isotonic solution		*Isotonic solutions* are pharmaceutical preparations that exhibit the same osmotic pressure as that of a physiological fluid to prevent osmosis-driven cell and tissue damage such as crenation or hemolysis.
Kelvin equation		The Kelvin equation relates the surface free energy change to the pressure-induced change in the size (radius) of a spherical bubble. The surface free energy change $RT \ln (P_2/P_1)$, from P_1 to P_2 can be expressed as $\Delta G = RT \ln(P_2/P_1) = V\Delta P$. According to the Laplace equation, the pressure change is inversely proportional to the radius, that is, $\Delta P = 2\gamma/r$, where γ is the surface tension. Thus, $RT \ln(P_2/P_1) = 2\gamma V/r$, which is known as the *Kelvin equation*.
Kinetic solubility		The solubility of a drug may be determined using a concentrated solution in a rich solvent such as DMSO. The DMSO sample is diluted with a solvent for which the solubility of the drug is to be determined; precipitation of drug occurs; and then the saturated concentration is measured as a function of incubation time. The measured aqueous solubility of drugs using the DMSO stock is higher than the equilibrium solubility at shorter incubation time (10 min), but approaches the equilibrium solubility at an incubation time of 20 h. This supersaturated concentration at shorter incubation time is referred to as the *kinetic solubility*. The supersaturation will eventually settle down via precipitation to reach the intrinsic or equilibrium solubility.
Lamellar structure		Skin lipids are elaborately organized into a *lamellar structure*, representing the skin barrier. Skin lamellar structure is composed of alternating layers of aqueous and lipid bilayers.
Langmuir isotherm		The *Langmuir isotherm* describes the formation of a gas monolayer over the surface of an adsorbent. This type of isotherm shows an initial steeply rising curve that indicates a strong binding of the gas to the surface and a gradually flattened out curve due to saturation. The theory suggested that the rate of evaporation is proportional to the fraction of the surface covered with gas (θ), whereas the rate of condensation is proportional to the amount of available gas (as indicated by pressure P) and the fraction of the surface not covered by the gas ($1 - \theta$). Thus, at equilibrium, when the rate of evaporation is the same as the rate of condensation, $k\theta = k'P(1 - \theta)$ (k and k' are the proportionality

Term	Symbol	Definition or Description
		constants). By letting $K = k/k'$, one obtains $\theta = P/(K + P)$. If the saturated volume of the gas adsorbed is V_m and the volume of adsorbed gas at any pressure P is V, then $V/V_m = \theta$ and $P/V = (K/V_m) + (P/V_m)$ A plot of P/V versus P will be linear with a slope of $1/V_m$ and an intercept of K/V_m, which permits the determination of K and V_m.
Laplace equation		For a soap bubble of radius r, the total surface free energy is $4\pi r^2\gamma$, where γ is the surface tension. If the radius were to decrease by dr, which must be brought about by a pressure change of ΔP on the bubble film, then the change in surface tension is $8\pi r\gamma\, dr$ and the work against this pressure change is $(\Delta P)4\pi r^2\, dr$. Thus, $(\Delta P)4\pi r^2\, dr = 8\pi r\gamma\, dr$, or $\Delta P = 2\gamma/r$. This relationship between ΔP and r is the *Laplace equation*, which indicates that the mechanical pressure across a curvature interface is related to the surface tension and the radius of the curvature interface.
Lewis acid–base theory		The *Lewis acid–base theory* defines the acid–base interaction as involving the donation of a pair of electrons from the base to the acid. There are three classes of Lewis acids that are of interest. The first class consists of compounds having *less than a full octet of electrons*, such as boric acid. The second class includes *hydrated metal ions* such as $Fe(H_2O)_x^{3+}$, which undergoes the following reaction: $Fe(H_2O)_x^{3+} + H_2O \rightleftarrows Fe(H_2O)_{x-1}^{2+} + H_3O^+$ The third class includes compounds that have *double bonds*, excluding those of the carbon–carbon linkage, such as the dissolved CO_2 in an aqueous solution that forms carbonic acid.
Ligand field theory		The *ligand field theory* describes metal complexation as arising from electrostatic or ion-dipole interactions between the metal ion and the ligands. This accounts for the octahedral configuration associated with a coordination number of 6 and the tetrahedral configuration assumed by most ligands with a coordination number of 4, because these symmetric layouts allow minimum repulsion among the ligands. Different ligands may impart a different ligand field strength that splits the d orbitals into low-energy and high-energy groups, where the d electrons will select the low-energy orbitals either alone or in electron pairs. This leads to the formation of two types of complexes of different electron configurations: spin-free and spin-paired. For an octahedral complex, the five d orbitals of a transition metal may be divided into two groups: the first three (d_{xy}, d_{xz}, d_{yz}) lie along the *diagonals* between the axes, and the other two (d_{y2}, d_{x2-z2})

Term	Symbol	Definition or Description
		lie directly on the axes. Electrons going into the *diagonals* will have lower energy than those going into the axial orbitals.
***Limulus* amebocyte lysate test**	LAL	The LAL assay is a quantitative test for bacterial endotoxins in parenteral products. The assay uses the *Limulus amebocyte lysate*, which has been characterized as an LAL reagent. There are two techniques for this test. The gel-clot technique is based on gel formation determined from dilutions of the test material directly compared with parallel dilutions of a reference endotoxin. The photometric techniques measure the turbidity or color development resulting from cleavage of an endogenous substrate or a synthetic peptide–chromogen complex, respectively. The quantities of endotoxin are expressed in USP Endotoxin Units (USP-EU). Five USP water products were given specific endotoxin limits: Water for Injection, Sterile Water for Injection, and Sterile Water for Irrigation have an allowable limit of 0.25 EU/mL; Sterile Water for Inhalation and Bacteriostatic Water for Injection have an endotoxin limit of 0.5 EU/mL.
Linear viscoelastic region	LVR	A material has a *linear viscoelastic region* (LVR) of G' at low stress values. As stress increases, a marked decrease in G' occurs at a critical stress value, which marks the breakdown of the viscoelastic structure. This phenomenon shows that if the deformation is small or applied sufficiently slowly, the molecular arrangements will not be changed from its equilibrium state. The critical stress value gives the length of the LVR; the longer the length, the greater the cohesive energy displayed by the internal structure of the viscoelastic body. Pharmaceutical formulations with longer LVR will be more resistant to breakdown by stress, such as those encountered during transportation and handling, than the ones with lesser LVR.
Lipophilicity and hydrophilicity		*Lipophilicity* refers to the ability of a chemical entity to dissolve in lipids such as fats and oils and nonpolar solvents such as hexane and toluene. *Hydrophilicity* refers to compounds that have a tendency to interact with or be dissolved in water and other polar substances.
Lipoplexes		*Lipoplexes*, also called cationic liposome–nucleic acid complexes, are spontaneously formed complexes between the negatively charged nucleic acids and cationic lipids as a result of opposing electrostatic charges. Lipoplexes often carry a net positive charge and can therefore interact electrostatically with negatively charged cell membranes.
Liposomes		*Liposomes* are thermodynamically stable vesicles consisting of lipid bilayers surrounding aqueous central cores. Conventional

Term	Symbol	Definition or Description
		liposomes are composed of phospholipids, often with cholesterol to stabilize the system. Novel liposomes contain additional components to phospholipids to improve the flexibility and skin penetration properties, namely as transfersomes and ethosomes.
log K_{ow}		The log K_{OW}, also known as log P, is the partition coefficient of a drug measured in the octanol–water system and expressed in the logarithmic scale. This parameter is used in mathematical models of quantitative structure–activity relationships (QSAR) to predict permeability, in vivo drug transport through aqueous and lipid compartments, drug binding, molecular structures, liquid chromatography, and the aqueous solubility of organic drugs.
Lognormal		Pharmaceutical powders often do not show normal particle size distribution. Statistical methods have shown, however, that many nonsymmetrical continuous distributions may be logarithm normal, or *lognormal*, in that the function log x assumes a normal distribution. The reverse is also true. In such a case, one can transform the unsymmetrical distribution of $f(x)$ into a normal distribution by substituting $\log x$ for x on a linear abscissa scale. The frequency for the distribution of $\log x$ is $$f(\log x) = \frac{1}{\sigma_{\log x}(2\pi)^{1/2}} \exp^{\{-[(\log x - \mu_{\log x})/\sigma_{\log x}]^2/2\}}$$
London force		The *London force* refers to induced dipole–induced dipole interaction, which originates from molecular internal vibrations. It is responsible for the liquefaction of nonpolar gases.
Lubricant		*Lubricants* are waxy substances used in tablet or capsule formulations. In a tablet formulation, lubricants reduce the friction between the die wall and tablet during ejection. They also reduce wear and tear on punches and dies and prevent sticking to the punch faces. In a capsule formulation, a lubricant prevents sticking to tamping pins and dosators. Because lubricants are hydrophobic, use in large quantities or mixing for prolonged periods can cause a slowing of drug dissolution from the dosage form. An overuse of lubricants can also result in softer tablets. Commonly used lubricants are magnesium stearate, stearic acid, and sodium stearyl fumarate, at 0.25–5%.
Lyophilic colloids		*Lyophilic colloids* are colloidal systems formed by solvent-loving single molecules. Hydrophilic macromolecules such as proteins, Carbopol, methylcellulose, gelatin, and acacia form lyophilic colloids in water. The dispersed single molecules are covered with a solvent sheath. If the concentration of the dispersed phase is sufficiently high, the system can become semisolid, known as a *gel* or, in the case of inorganic particles, *magma*.

Term	Symbol	Definition or Description
Lyophobic colloids		*Lyophobic colloids* are made with materials that have little, if any, affinity toward the dispersion medium. These systems include hydrophobic polymers such as ethylcellulose and inorganic particles such as silver, gold, and sulfur. Preparation of lyophobic colloids requires various considerations for the reduction of particle size to the colloidal range. For direct dispersion, the coarse particles are reduced to desired sizes by methods such as high-intensity ultrasonic generators, colloidal mills, and condensation and precipitation methods. Lyophilic materials can also be made lyophobic by chemical cross-linking that yields water-insoluble colloidal-size particles, or by polymerization, in which a suitable monomer is emulsified and polymerized within the colloidal droplet through the addition of a polymerization initiator.
Macromolecules		*Macromolecules* refer to large molecules made up of smaller organic subunits. There are four classes of biological macromolecules: nucleic acids, proteins, carbohydrates, and lipids.
Magnetic resonance imaging	MRI	*Magnetic resonance imaging* is a radiologic medical imaging technique that visualizes detailed internal structures by using the property of nuclear magnetic resonance to image the nuclei of atoms inside the body.
Membrane filtration		*Membrane filtration* is a common method for sterilization of drug solutions. Microorganisms and visible particulate matter are removed by filtration using a sterile filter of 0.22-μm pore size, as most bacteria are 0.5–5.0 μm in length. Among the smallest bacteria are members of the genus *Mycoplasma*, which measure at about 0.2–0.3 μm. The commonly used filters in manufacturing sterile dosage forms include polyvinylidene fluoride, nylon, cellulose esters, and polyethersulfone. The sterility of the filtered solution is not guaranteed because the membrane filters used might be flawed or defective. Most 25- to 33-mm syringe disk filters used in pharmacy compounding can filter a volume of up to 100 mL. For filtering a volume greater than 100 mL, a cartridge filter with greater surface areas may be required. The filtration method is convenient and is readily applicable in clinical pharmacies for the preparation of sterile products in a laminar flow hood.
Membrane-controlled (permeability)		The barrier of membrane permeability includes the membrane and unstirred water layers. On both sides of the membrane if a drug is highly water-soluble, diffusion across the unstirred water layer will be fast and the rate-limiting step will be its membrane permeability. In this case, $J = (D_m K_m / h_m) C_1$, and the permeability is *membrane-controlled.*

Term	Symbol	Definition or Description
Metered-dose inhalers	MDIs	*Metered-dose inhalers* are propellant-driven inhalers, capable of delivering accurate doses of aerosolized drugs to the lungs. The aerosol formulation consists of a product concentrate and the propellant. The product concentrate (solution or suspension) contains the active drug and additives, whereas the propellant aerosolizes the product concentrate to the desired form, size, and distribution. The essential components of an MDI are the container, metering valve, and actuator. The metering valve delivers a fixed volume of the aerosol after each actuation via a dual-valve mechanism. When the actuator is closed (at rest), a seal blocks the emission from the metering chamber to the atmosphere, but the chamber is open to the container and is filled with the aerosol content. When the actuator is depressed, the chamber is open to the atmosphere for the release of its content, but is sealed from the container. When the actuator is again closed, the chamber is reloaded for the next dose. Two types of metering valves exist: One is for inverted use to deliver suspensions and the other is for upright use (via a capillary dip tube) to delivery solution aerosols.
Michaelis–Menten constant	K_m	The general principle of enzyme kinetics involves the formation of an active enzyme–substrate complex and its subsequent rate limiting, breaking apart into enzyme and product. The *Michaelis–Menten constant* represents the dissociation constant for the enzyme–substrate complexation.
Microcantilevers		*Microcantilevers* are measuring units for targeted biomarkers such as a protein, DNA, receptor ligand, cell, or virus, in nanoarrays or other biosensing devices. The microcantilever detects and measures the binding of a biomarker by physical methods.
Microfluidics		*Microfluidics* is the science of manipulating and controlling fluids and particles (proteins, DNA, cells, viruses, etc.) at micrometer and submicrometer dimensions based on the particle's electrokinetic properties. A microfluidic device consists of channels that can control the flow of fluid measured in micro-, nano-, or even picoliter quantities, which allows for easy, rapid, and sensitive separation of targeted cells from complex tissue using small samples.
Micromeritics		*Micromeritics* is the science and technology of small particles with regard to particle size and distribution, surface area and activity, density, and flow properties.

Term	Symbol	Definition or Description
Milliequivalent	mEq	*Milliequivalent* is short for milligram-equivalent weight, which is a measure of the number of positive or negative charges produced by an electrolyte based on its milligram weight. The mEq is calculated using the equivalent weight of the electrolyte, defined as the molecular weight divided by the number of *positive or negative* charges (q) per molecule. For example, for calcium chloride (mol wt = 111), $q = 2$, the equivalent weight is 55.5. Thus, a quantity of 55.5 mg of calcium chloride produces 1 mEq of positive or negative charges, or numerically, 6.0225×10^{20} charges.
Molecular expressions		*Molecular expressions* are quantities expressed in the number of molecules (moles or millimoles), total number of molecules and ions in a solution (osmoles or millosmoles), and number of charges of a given electrolyte solution (gram-equivalent weight or mEq). 1 mol = 6.0225×10^{23} molecules. When these quantities are expressed relative to the volume of the solution or the weight of the solvent, they are known as molecular concentrations, which include molarity, osmolarity, molality, osmolality, normality, and mole fractions (see text for specific definitions).
Mucociliary clearance	MCC	The mucociliary apparatuses of the nasal epithelium and the tracheobronchial airways serve to entrap and eliminate particles from the regions via a combined activity of mucous secretion and the beating of cilia protruding from the luminal surface of the columnar cells. The complex but coordinated beating of the cilia moves the mucus layer toward the pharynx, thereby providing a *mucociliary clearance* mechanism for the nose and the lung. In the nasal cavity, the content of ciliated cells is relatively low in the anterior lower turbinate area, but increases toward the nasopharynx. In the lungs, the submucosal glands are found in the trachea and bronchi, and the ciliated cells extend as far down as the terminal bronchioles, indicating that the mucociliary apparatus protects the central region of the lungs.
Multifunction micelles		Polymeric micelles that exhibit combined targeting and triggered-release functions or targeting and imaging capabilities for the assessment of the micellar targeting specificity and their biodistribution are referred to as *multifunction micelles*. The term *multifunction* also applies to other nanocarrier systems.
Multilamellar vesicles		Multilamellar vesicles (MLV, 200–5000 nm), are liposomes which consist of two or more concentric lipid bilayers that are useful for entrapment of hydrophobic drugs.

Term	Symbol	Definition or Description
Nanoarrays		*Nanoarrays* are biosensing devices that provide collections of miniaturized test sites arranged on solid substrates with molecules placed at defined locations on a surface with nanometer spatial resolution. Nanoarrays are fabricated using photolithography and high-voltage electron beam (E-beam) lithography. The electrons produce a chemical change in the resist, which allows the surface to be patterned and the deposit of metals such as gold for binding of biomaterial. Nanoarray spots can include biological samples such as protein, DNA, RNA, and whole viruses as well as nonbiological samples such as solutions, colloids, and particle suspensions.
Nanocomposites		*Nanocomposites* are combined nanoparticles of one type with another, or the composite of nanoparticles with the larger-size bulk material. They are widely used in materials of packaging, building and construction, electronics, auto parts, and medicine. An example of a medical nanocomposite is the manufacturing of artificial bone composites from nanocrystalline calcium phosphates.
Nanoparticle systems		*Nanoparticle systems* contain particles in which at least one of the particle dimensions is 100 nm or less. In practice, the nanocarriers have a size range of 5–400 nm, which is within the colloidal size range. With the availability of various polymeric materials, some major forms of polymeric nanocarriers have been developed including nanospheres, liposomes, polymeric micelles, and dendrimers. Common to these polymeric systems is that they can be made using biodegradable material, thus causing little or no systemic toxicity. Among the nanocarriers, liposomes, polymeric micelles, and biodegradable nanoparticles have been extensively studied, and a number of such systems are under clinical investigation or approved for clinical use.
Nanotechnology		*Nanotechnology* refers to the design, characterization, production, and application of structures, devices, and systems by controlled manipulation of size and shape at the nanometer scale (atomic, molecular, and macromolecular scale) that yields a product with at least one novel or superior characteristic or property.
Nebulizer		The *nebulizer* system converts a liquid formulation to vapor using energy provided either by a high-velocity airstream (jet nebulizer) or by ultrasonication through the vibration of a piezoelectric crystal (ultrasonic nebulizer). These systems require a nebulizing device, a respiratory solution or suspension, auxiliary tubing, and mouthpieces or face masks. With a controlled airflow rate through the nebulizer, aerosolization of particles or droplets is achieved in 10 to 20 min. Unlike the

Term	Symbol	Definition or Description
		cumbersome equipment used in the past, modern nebulizers offer miniaturized hardware, the ability to generate small droplets for deep lung delivery, high-dose delivery capacity, and shorter treatment time.
Nernst potential		The electric potential of a charged particle at the particle surface in reference to the electrically neutral zone in the bulk medium is the *Nernst potential.*
New chemical (or molecular) entity		A candidate of an active pharmaceutical ingredient that has not been approved for its use prior to its current application is a *new chemical* (or *molecular*) *entity.*
Newton's law of viscosity		"The resistance which arises from the lack of slipperiness of the parts of the liquid, other things being equal, is proportional to the velocity with which the parts of the liquid are separated from one another."
Newtonian flow		The flow curve of a liquid is the plot of the rate of shear (dv/dx) versus the shear stress (f/A). Because viscosity is the ratio (f/A)/(dv/dx), the ideal behavior is indicated by a straight line through the origin, i.e., a constant viscosity with respect to shear stress versus rate of shear. This is known as the *Newtonian flow.*
Noninvasive		*Noninvasive* refers to the use of techniques that do not involve passage across a tissue barrier such as the skin.
Nonisothermal kinetics		*Nonisothermal kinetics* can be used to reduce the experimental effort in accelerated stability studies. This is achieved by a study design in which the temperature of the system is programmed to provide a series of isothermal kinetic stages at different temperatures. The kinetic parameters, i.e., the activation energy and rate constants, can thus be determined from a single set of kinetic data. Under consecutive equal-step temperature increases, the arithmetic mean of the rate constants for these isothermal stages may be taken as the ratio of the total degradation of the drug to the duration of the experiment. Thus, for a first-order kinetic process with n stages, $$\ln C - \ln C_o = (k_1 + k_2 + k_3 + \cdots + k_n)t/n$$ where C and C_o are the concentrations of the drug at time t and time 0, respectively. The values of $\ln C - \ln C_o$ and t/n are determined experimentally, from which the rate constants at different temperatures are determined with computer-assisted calculations.
Nuclear localization signal	NLS	Large molecules destined for transport into the nucleus contain cationic amino acid targeting sequences called the *nuclear localization signal* (NLS). Nucleoportins named importins recognize the NLS and facilitate the transport of molecules to the nucleus.

Term	Symbol	Definition or Description
Nuclear pore complex	NPC	The nucleus is enclosed within a nuclear envelope that displays tightly regulated pores. *Nuclear pore complex* (NPC), one of largest protein complexes in the cell, is responsible for the exchange of components, e.g., RNA, ribosomes, and proteins, between the nucleus and cytoplasm. The pores are constructed from a class of proteins called nucleoporins.
Nucleic acids		*Nucleic acids* are biological molecules essential for the expression of genes including DNA (deoxyribonucleic acid) and RNA (ribonucleic acid).
Octanol–water system		1-Octanol has a polar head and a hydrophobic alkyl chain, which resembles the lipids of biological membranes. A wider range of compounds are soluble in octanol compared to hydrocarbon solvents such as cyclohexane and isooctane. The solubility of water in octanol is 2.3 *M*, or 0.27 in mole fraction. This relatively high concentration of water allows the transfer of hydrated molecules from the aqueous to the organic phase without breaking of hydrogen bonds or solvation, and reduces the tendency of drug molecules from self-association. The solubility of octanol in water, on the other hand, is small and negligible, allowing easier solubility calculations and predictions. Hydrocarbon solvents are generally associated with molecular associations, which yield partition coefficients that do not correspond to the drug solubility. Given its tendency to allow the existence of drugs in one species in both phases, the octanol–water system is ideal for measuring the lipophilicity of drugs. For these reasons, the *octanol–water system* has served as the basis for various theoretical predictions of drug properties and their biological effects.
Ocular inserts		*Ocular inserts* are used for sustained-release purposes. Ocusert (Alza), e.g., is an oval pilocarpine-delivering device consisting of a titanium dioxide frame and a pilocarpine core sandwiched between two ethylene-vinyl acetate copolymer membranes. In use, the device is placed under the lower eyelid, where drug dissolves in lacrimal fluid and is released from the device at a controlled rate according to Fick's law. For sparingly soluble drugs, the concentration of dissolved drug in the device is maintained at solubility; hence, the release of drug follows zero-order kinetics, which is ideal for dosage planning. Soluble inserts are preparations that dissolve or erode within 1 h of application. These inserts are made of natural polymers. The sterile Lacrisert, e.g., is made of hydroxypropyl cellulose for the treatment of moderate to severe cases of dry eye.

Term	Symbol	Definition or Description
Ointments and creams		According to the FDA Center for Drug Evaluation and Research, an ointment is a semisolid preparation intended for external application to the skin or mucous membranes, whereas a cream is a semisolid dosage form containing one or more drug substances dissolved or dispersed in a suitable base. Ointment and cream may be differentiated by the bases used for the semisolid formulations. Traditionally, the definition of cream includes both oil-in-water and water-in-oil emulsions, which are regarded as more cosmetically acceptable than an ointment made using an oleaginous or anhydrous base.
Ophthalmic suspensions and ointments		*Ophthalmic suspensions* are aqueous formulations that contain finely divided particles (10 μm or less) for water-insoluble drugs. These products provide more extended corneal contact time than solutions do. The suspension has a solution concentration equal to the drug's solubility. As the drug is absorbed, particle dissolution will occur, and it is desirable that the particles have a rapid dissolution rate to maintain saturated concentration within the formulation's residence time in the eye. *Ophthalmic ointments* provide a longer contact time with the eye than suspensions do, but have slower onset of actions and rates of drug release. The ointment must be nonirritating, which requires that the ointment base be soft (of low yield stress) and the particle size small (micronized). Most ophthalmic ointment bases are a mixture of mineral oil and white petrolatum and have a melting point close to body temperature. Ophthalmic ointments have the drawbacks of blurred vision and oleaginous texture, which cannot be removed easily from the precorneal film. Therefore, they are used mostly at night as an adjunctive therapy to eyedrops. The ophthalmic suspensions and ointments are mainly used to deliver antimicrobial and/or anti-inflammatory agents.
Opsonins		*Opsonins* are molecules that target antigens for an immune response, and they include molecules that act as enhancers for phagocytosis (such as antibodies) or ones that activate the complement system.
Oriented-wedge theory		Surfactants containing strong *hydrophilic* head and *lipophilic* long chains can stabilize oil-in-water emulsions in which the nonpolar chains are inserted into the oil droplets while the polar heads are immersed in the surrounding aqueous phase, which is known as the *oriented-wedge theory*.
Ostwald power law		The *Ostwald power law* is used to gain quantitative perspectives of the flow curves of non-Newtonian systems. In this model,

Term	Symbol	Definition or Description
		the rate of shear ($\dot{g}$) is empirically taken to be proportional to the shear stress (τ) to the power of n, that is, $\dot{g} = K\tau^n$. This relationship is useful because of its simplicity, but it only approximately describes the behavior of a real non-Newtonian fluid.
Partition coefficient	K	See *Distribution law.*
Penetration enhancers		*Penetration enhancers* are substances that reversibly decrease the barrier function of the stratum corneum to promote skin penetration.
Permeability		In BCS, *permeability* is the rate and extent of mass transfer across human intestinal membrane. Drug permeability can be measured in human as well as nonhuman systems (e.g., in vitro epithelial cell culture methods) capable of predicting the extent of drug absorption in humans. The permeability of a drug substance in human subjects can be determined using mass balance, absolute bioavailability, or intestinal perfusion approaches.
Permeability-enhancing effects		For the delivery of protein and peptide drugs via site-directed routes such as intranasal or transdermal, *permeability-enhancing effects* achieved by either increasing tissue permeability or modifying drug-membrane charge selectivity are generally necessary. The major permeability-enhancing effects are (1) chemically modified tight junction opening (e.g., by chitosan and chelating agents), (2) disruption of membrane and tight junction (e.g., by solubilizing agents, bile salts, and surfactants), (3) bioadhesion (e.g., by gel-forming polymer solutions or microspheres), and (4) enzyme inhibition using various enzyme inhibitors.
Persorption		The term *persorption* refers to the ability of nanoparticles to penetrate the small intestine through holes created by single, degrading enterocytes in the process of being extruded from a villus. Positively charged nanoparticles show more effective absorption than neutral or negatively charged particles.
pH rate profile		The *pH rate profile* is a plot of log k_{obs} versus pH for the degradation of a drug at various pH. Linear changes in log k_{obs} with pH may be used to elucidate the specific acid and base catalyses.
Pharmaceutical dosage form		A *pharmaceutical dosage form* is a drug delivery system designed based on the route of administration and optimized drug absorption for the delivery of a measured amount of a medication. The dosage form can be solid or liquid preparations, suspensions, emulsions, and semisolids. Solid dosage forms can be designed for immediate (conventional), delayed (as in enteric coated tablets), or sustained (prolonged) drug release.

Term	Symbol	Definition or Description
Pharmaceutical excipients		*Pharmaceutical excipients* are substances other than the active ingredient included in a drug delivery system that provide any or a combination of the following functions: (1) to aid in the processing of the dosage form during its manufacture; (2) to protect or enhance the stability, bioavailability, or patient acceptability of the product; (3) to assist in product identification; and (4) to enhance any other attribute of the overall safety and effectiveness of the drug during storage or use.
Pharmaceutical powders		*Pharmaceutical powders* are compounded formulations for internal or external uses or for dosage form fabrications. They include bulk powders, oral powders, dusting powders, douche powders, insufflations, and inhalation powders.
Pharmaceutics		*Pharmaceutics* is an area of science that deals with the design, evaluation, development, and manufacturing of pharmaceutical dosage forms for the delivery of therapeutic agents.
Phase angle and tan delta	δ, $\tan\delta = G''/G'$	The *phase angle* is the phase separation between the applied stress and the responding strain in an oscillatory test, which measures the presence and extent of elasticity of a fluid. The tangent of the phase angle, commonly referred to as *tan delta*, is the ratio of the loss (viscous) modulus to the storage (elastic) modulus, that is, $\tan\delta = G''/G'$.
Phase-solubility method		Based on increased drug solubility in solutions containing cyclodextrin (CD), the *Higuchi–Connors phase-solubility* method determines drug–CD binding by measuring the intrinsic solubility (S_o) of the drug and its total solubility in the presence of CD (S_t). In this method, it is assumed that increased solubility is due to the formation of the 1 : 1 and 1 : 2 drug–CD complexes with binding constants of K_{11} and K_{12}, respectively. With this approach, it can be shown that $$(S_t - S_o)/S_o = K_{11}[\mathrm{CD}] + K_{11}K_{12}[\mathrm{CD}]^2$$
Photolithography		*Photolithography* is a microfabrication process that is used to remove selectively parts of a thin film or the bulk of a substrate. It utilizes light to transfer patterns onto a substrate, which is then engraved by treatment of various chemical entities.
pK_a		$pK_a = -\log K_a$
Plane of shear		The *plane of shear* defines the boundary between a charged surface and the solution. If an electric field is applied to charged particles in a suspension, they will move; or if a solution is made to flow down a tube, an electric field develops. Thus a plane of shear develops between the surface and the solution, which lies within the electrical double layer.

Term	Symbol	Definition or Description
Plasticity		*Plasticity* is the propensity of a material to undergo permanent deformation.
Poisson's theorem		*Poisson's theorem* states that the rate of change of electrostatic potential at a given point is proportional to the charge density at that point. This theorem leads to the equation $E = E_o e^{-\kappa x}$ where E is the potential at a solution plane having a distance x from the surface, E_o is the surface potential, and κ is known as the *Debye–Hückel constant*. This equation indicates that the electric potential decays exponentially with distance into the solution. When E drops to $1/e$ of E_o, the distance between the plane and the surface is $1/\kappa$. The significance of κ is that the reciprocal of κ is a distance that defines the boundary of the diffuse double layer. If one imagines a spherical surface on which the charge is $+ze$, then there will be a double layer of solution surrounding the particle where the outer edge will have a net excess charge (from the counter ions) of $-ze$ and be located at a distance of $1/\kappa$ from the particle surface.
Polymeric micelles		*Polymeric micelles* are self-assembled micelles of block copolymers. The micelle formation is driven by dehydration of the hydrophobic block, leading to a favorable state of entropy, allowing the hydrophobic moieties to associate via physical forces, while the resulting hydrophilic shell is stabilized by hydrogen bonds with the surrounding water. Because of the stability of the self-assembled structure, polymeric micelles have a much lower CMC (10^{-7} to 10^{-6} *M*) than micelles of common surfactants (10^{-4} to 10^{-3} *M*). As a result, they are stable at very low concentrations, making them relatively insensitive to dilution compared to surfactant micelles. The size range of the polymeric micelles is 5–100 nm, which is well suited for injection and easy extravasation from blood vessels to the tumor tissue.
Polyplexes		*Polyplexes* or cationic polymer–nucleic acid complexes are spontaneously formed complexes between anionic nucleic acids and cationic polymers as a result of opposing electrostatic charges. Similar to cationic lipids, cationic polymers can condense nucleic acids into smaller structures and mask the negative charges of molecules.
Porosimetry		*Porosimetry* is a technique used to determine the properties of porous particles such as the total pore volume, surface area, and true density. The technique involves the intrusion of nonwetting liquid (e.g., mercury) at high pressure into the powder through the use of a porosimeter. The total pore volume can be determined based on the external pressure needed to force the liquid into

Term	Symbol	Definition or Description
		the pores against the opposing force of the liquid surface tension. For density determinations, mercury or other liquid is often denied entry into the smallest spaces, thus underestimating the pore volume. As a result, the density thus measured may be smaller than the true density determined by using a helium densitometer.
Porosity	Φ	The *porosity* (Φ) of a powder sample is defined as the ratio of the void volume to the total volume. For example, the total porosity is indicated by $$\Phi_{total} = (V_{bulk} - V_{true})/V_{bulk} = 1 - V_{true}/V_{bulk} = 1 - \rho_{bulk}/\rho_{true}$$ where ρ is the density. Similarly, one can define the intraparticle and interparticle porosities as $$\Phi_{intraparticle} = 1 - \rho_{envelope}/\rho_{true}$$ $$\Phi_{interparticle} = 1 - \rho_{bulk}/\rho_{envelope}$$
Potts and Guy equation		The *Potts and Guy equation* has been used to predict the skin permeability (P_s) for drugs delivered from an aqueous vehicle using parameters such as the drug's molecular weight (MW) and octanol–water partition coefficient ($K_{O/W}$): $$\log P_s \cong -2.7 + 0.71 \log K_{O/W} - 0.0061\ \text{MW}$$ The transformed equation includes the effect of the drug's melting point (MP): $$\log P_s \cong -2.355 + 0.82 \log K_{O/W} - 0.00933\ \text{MW} - 0.00387\ \text{MP}$$
Powder flowability		*Powder flowability* refers to the ease with which a powder may flow through an orifice under gravitational forces. A powder may be free-flowing or cohesive due to attractive forces between particles. Factors that influence powder flow include particle size, shape, porosity, density, and surface texture. The powder flowability is indirectly indicated by a number of measurements such as the angle of repose, which measures the frictional forces in a loose powder, and the Hauser ratio, which is the ratio of the tapped to bulk densities.
Prodrugs		*Prodrugs* are inactive or the less active form of drugs. Once administered, the prodrugs are metabolized into active drugs (bioactivation), which exert pharmacological effects. Generally, prodrugs are designed to improve the bioavailability of active drugs or to provide drug targeting effects.
Protein binding	K, n	The term *protein binding* commonly refers to drug binding with plasma proteins, mainly human serum albumin (HSA), which serves to transport drugs, their metabolites, and endogenous molecules, such as the fatty acids, to various sites via circulation. The protein-bound drug is held in circulation; hence it is

Term	Symbol	Definition or Description
		inactive. However, the binding equilibrium is reversible; drug binding to HSA thus controls the free (active) concentration of the drug, provides a reservoir for a long duration of action, and ultimately affects the drug's absorption, metabolism, distribution, and excretion. Many drugs bind to HSA at the same site(s); the free concentration of a drug can be affected by coadministered drugs or by pathological conditions that modify the binding properties of the protein, resulting in clinically significant drug interactions. Drug protein binding is commonly expressed in percentage of bound drug. But in protein binding studies, the two important parameters are the binding constant (K), which indicates the strength of the binding, and the number of biding sites (n) in the protein for the bound drug.
Pseudoplasticity		Colloidal systems may become more fluid as they are stirred faster. This shear-thinning effect is called *pseudoplasticity.* A pseudoplastic solid, e.g., can undergo shear-thinning flow when the applied stress is above its yield stress value.
Pyrogen and bacterial endotoxin		Pyrogenic substances can be produced by some gram-positive bacteria, mycobacteria, fungi, and also viruses; pyrogens produced by gram-negative bacteria are the endotoxins. Although *microbial pyrogen* has become a general descriptive term for many different substances, the endotoxins are of greatest significance to the pharmaceutical industry due to possible contaminations. Bacterial endotoxins, found in the outer membrane of gram-negative bacteria, are members of a class of phospholipids called lipopolysaccharides (LPS). LPS are not exogenous products; instead, they are released from the bacteria after death and lysis of the cells. Examples of pyrogens producing gram-negative bacteria are *Escherichia coli*, *Proteus*, *Pseudomonas*, *Enterobacter*, and *Klebsiella*. There is also little recognition of the clinical significance of endotoxin, as the most emphasized pathogenic effect of gram-negative disease is the production of fever. But, of all the effects of endotoxin, fever is probably the least important biologically and clinically.
Pyrogen contamination		Water used as solvent or for washing processes and the raw materials are the main sources of endotoxins in parenteral products. When pyrogens were found in dosage forms traceable to the raw materials, the source was often the active drug substance, particularly when the drug is processed using water at some late stage of the synthetic process. If the drug substance is biologically produced, the incomplete removal of the microorganism during purification can result in the drug substance having high endotoxin levels. Examples include antibiotics produced by fermentation or genetically engineered

Term	Symbol	Definition or Description
		by-products of gram-negative bacteria. Water for Injection (WFI) may be a source of pyrogen. Circulating hot water systems (above 75°C) provide the environment least conducive to microbial growth and endotoxin formation, whereas ambient temperature presents potential problems. Many of the objectionable microorganisms grow well in cold WFI systems. This is particularly true of reverse osmosis systems.
Q_{10} approximation		For common degradation reactions, the rate constant increases 2- to 4-fold with a 10°C increase in temperature. This rate constant ratio is known as Q_{10}. The shelf life of a solution product will decrease by the same factor if the temperature is increased by 10°C. Thus, one can estimate the change in shelf life due to changes in storage condition by using a Q_{10} value of 2, 3, or 4, depending on the drug potency and its intended use, if the activation energy value for the reaction kinetics is not available.
Quantitative structure–activity relationships	QSAR	*Quantitative structure–activity relationships* (QSAR) are mathematical models used to predict structure-based in vitro and in vivo properties of drugs including drug permeability, in vivo transport of xenobiotics through aqueous and lipid compartments, drug binding, molecular structures and connectivity, liquid chromatography, and drug solubility. These methods are based on the log K_{OW} (log P) that measures a drug's lipophilicity. The partition coefficient of a drug is an additive and constitutive property, which can be calculated based on structural characteristics using published methods.
Random walk		Einstein treated diffusion as a process of spatial drift of molecules due to their kinetic motion. Because this drift is not a direct velocity, a molecule finds itself some distance x from its starting point after an elapse of time t in that x increases as a function of $t^{1/2}$, as a result of *random walk*.
Raoult's law		*Raoult's law* states that the partial vapor pressure of a component is equal to the vapor pressure of the pure component times its mole fraction. For a two-component system of A and B, $p_A = X_A P^o_A$ and $p_B = X_B P^o_B$
Rate of reaction		The *rate of reaction* is a function of the temperature and the product of the reactant concentrations involved in the reaction kinetics. Under isothermal conditions, the rate equation is the rate constant times the product of the reactant concentrations.
Reaction mechanism		The *reaction mechanism* consists of stepwise reactions, the formation of reactive intermediates whose concentration changes reach zero during the steady-state condition, and the rate-determining step that determines the overall reaction

Term	Symbol	Definition or Description
		kinetics. The reaction mechanism is verified by experimentally determined reaction rate and order with respect to each reactant.
Reaction order		*Reaction order* indicates the participation of reactant (concentration) in the reaction kinetics. It is an experimentally determined value. For a given reaction, the reaction order may be changed depending on the concentration of the reactants.
Reactive oxygen species	ROS	*Reactive oxygen species* include superoxide anion ($O_2^{\cdot -}$), hydrogen peroxide (H_2O_2), and hydroxyl radical ($^{\cdot}OH$).
Reinforced ionic bonding		Organic molecules can form complexes with other compounds through hydrogen bonding; ionic, ion–dipole, dipole–dipole, and hydrophobic interactions. These molecules can form ions through ionization of the acid or base groups at appropriate pH, and most compounds exhibit permanent dipole capable of forming weak bonds with ions (ion–dipole) or other dipoles (dipole–dipole). One of the key functions of the hydrogen bonding is to provide an increased stability of the molecular complexation. The combined binding force involving ion-pairing, hydrogen bonding, and hydrophobic interaction is known as the *reinforced ionic bond*, which occurs readily in many drug–receptor interactions.
Resonance effect		Aromatic and conjugated double-bond systems can stabilize a structure via delocalization of the electron pair into the conjugated system. For example, the dissociation of a proton from barbituric acid leads to the formation of an aromatic ring. This makes barbituric acid a much stronger acid than substituted barbiturates. Phenols are stronger acids than aliphatic alcohol for the same reason. An aromatic amine, on the other hand, is a weaker base than an aliphatic amine because the positive charge formed by accepting a proton cannot be delocalized into the aromatic system.
Reverse osmosis	RO	*Reverse osmosis* is a membrane filtration method that removes large molecules and ions from solutions by applying pressure to the solution when it is on one side of a selective membrane. The result is that the soluble substances to be removed are retained on the pressurized side of a membrane, which excludes the passage of large molecules or ions but allows the solvent (i.e., water) to pass freely. The RO processes, arranged in series, are used to manufacture pyrogen-free Water for Injection.
RNA interference	RNAi	*RNA interference* (RNAi) is the post-transcriptional gene-silencing process that regulates the activity of the associated gene. The process is a naturally occurring defense mechanism in eukaryotic organisms. So far, two types of small RNA—small interfering RNA (siRNA) and micro RNA (miRNA)—have been discovered as central to RNA interference.

Term	Symbol	Definition or Description
Roller compactor		In dry granulation, the agglomeration is carried out by compaction or densification, in which the powder mixture is compacted in large pieces and subsequently broken up and sized into granules. In a *roller compactor*, powders are fed via an auger into two counterrotating rollers and compressed under force. The result is a dense compaction in the shape of a ribbon or sheet, which can be milled to the desired granule size. The apparatuses can have a horizontal feed, a combination of horizontal and vertical feed, or an angular feeding option, and the gap of the compact rolls can be fixed or adjustable according to the amount of powder drawn.
Scatchard equation		The *Scatchard equation* (Equation (5-17)) is used in the determination of the binding constant and the number of primary binding sites in drug–protein binding studies. It is based on the assumption that the intrinsic binding constant for all sites is the same.
Sedimentation coefficient		In ultracentrifugation of a solution containing macromolecular compound, the centrifugal force is balanced by the frictional force ($= 6\pi r\eta dr/dt$) in that $$dr/(r'\omega^2)\,dt = S = m(1 - v\rho)/6\pi r\eta.$$ The term $dr/(r'\omega^2)\,dt$ is a characteristic value of a macromolecule, known as the *sedimentation coefficient* (S), defined as the velocity (dr/dt) with which a macromolecule moves per unit centrifugal field $r'\omega^2$. By combining S and the diffusion coefficient (D) of the macromolecule, its molecular weight (M) can be determined by the relation $M = RTS/D(1 - v\rho)$, where v is the volume of 1 g of the macromolecule and ρ is the density of the solvent.
Shear strain and shear stress		*Shear strain* is a unitless quantity indicating the deformation of an ideal elastic body in response to an applied stress. *Shear stress* is the shear force per unit area.
Skin appendages		*Skin appendages* are skin-associated structures that serve particular functions including sensation, contractility, lubrication, and heat loss. In humans, the common skin appendages are sweat ducts, hair follicles, and sebaceous glands. These appendages provide a continuous pathway directly across the stratum corneum.
Small- and large-volume parenterals	SVPs and LVPs	*SVPs* are solutions, suspensions, or emulsions with unit package volume no greater than 100 mL. They are formulated as injectables for IM, SC, or ID administration or as additives to IV solutions, if compatible. SVPs can be designed for multiple-dose purposes, in which case the volume should not be greater than 30 mL and a preservative should be added. *LVPs* are usually

Term	Symbol	Definition or Description
		electrolyte solutions, lipid emulsions, solutions for parenteral nutrition, or irrigating solutions with unit package volume of several hundred milliliters to 1 L. LVPs do not and should not contain preservatives.
Solubility parameter	δ	The *solubility parameter* (δ) is the square root of the cohesive energy density of a substance, that is, $\delta = [(\Delta H_v - RT)/V]^{1/2}$, where ΔH_v is the heat of vaporization and V is the molecular volume. This parameter represents the energy needed to remove a unit volume of molecules from its neighbors for a complete separation, and provides a numerical estimation of interactions between materials, in that compounds with similar values of solubility parameter will interact with one another, resulting in solvation and miscibility.
Solubility-controlled (permeability)		If the drug has only limited solubility in the medium, then the permeability will be *solubility-controlled*, in which the diffusion of the drug through the unstirred water layers (UWL) will be the limiting step, that is, $J = (D_w/2h_w)C_1$, where the measured flux will depend on the diffusion coefficient in the medium and the UWL thickness.
Solution		A (true) *solution* is a homogeneous one-phase system that consists of two or more components forming a molecular dispersion.
Specific surface area		*Specific surface area* is the surface area per unit volume (S_v) or per unit weight (S_w) of a powder material. These two expressions are related in that $S_v = \rho S_w$, where ρ is the density of the particle. With known particle size and distribution, the total or specific surface area of a powder sample, based on spherical diameter, can be calculated as follows: Volume of sphere = $\pi d^3/6$ Surface area = πd^2 For a particle group with a size d and N particles, w (weight of particle group) = $N(\pi d^3/6)\rho$ S (total surface area) = $N\pi d^2$ It follows that $S = 6w/\rho d$, or $S_w = 6/\rho d$ and $S_v = 6/d$.
Spreading and surface tension change		The surface free energy change resulting from the spread of a liquid droplet on another immiscible liquid, such as an oil droplet on water, is $\Delta W = \gamma_O A + \gamma_{WO} A - \gamma_W A = A(\gamma_O + \gamma_{WO} - \gamma_W)$ where γ_W and γ_O are the surface tensions of water and oil, respectively, γ_{WO} is the interfacial tension, and A is the spreading

Term	Symbol	Definition or Description
		surface area. If $\gamma_W - (\gamma_O + \gamma_{WO}) > 0$, the surface free energy change will be negative and the spreading will occur spontaneously. This difference in surface and interfacial tension between two states, that is, γ_W and $(\gamma_O + \gamma_{WO})$, is known as the spreading coefficient, which denotes the change of free energy per change of surface area at constant pressure and temperature.
Stability constant	β	The *stability constant* is the equilibrium constant determined for metal ion–ligand complexation. For multistep equilibrium, the stability constant for the overall stability of the complex is the product of the individual constants. For a complexation involving two steps with equilibrium constants K_1 and K_2, $\beta_{12} = K_1K_2$.
Stability of drug product		The *stability of drug product* is the extent to which a preparation retains the same properties that it had at the time of formulation. The USP/NF describes the *product stability* as to retain unchanged (1) physical properties, (2) chemical properties and composition, (3) microbiological sterility, and (4) therapeutic activities. This definition emphasizes that, in addition to chemical degradation of the active ingredient, changes in sterility and physical appearance have an impact on the drug therapeutic effect.
Steady-state approximation		Consider the reaction mechanism $$\mathrm{A + B} \underset{k_{-1}}{\overset{k_1}{\rightleftarrows}} \mathrm{X} \xrightarrow{k_2} \mathrm{C + D}$$ where X is the active intermediate. The net rate of formation of X involves the formation and destruction of X, that is, $$d\mathrm{X}/dt = k_1[\mathrm{A}][\mathrm{B}] - k_{-1}[\mathrm{X}] - k_2[\mathrm{X}]$$ The formation of X may be small under fast elimination to form the products; or if the formation of the products does not occur rapidly compared to the activation process, the rate of change of X will be small, and $d\mathrm{X}/dt$ can be set equal to zero. This method is known as the *steady-state approximation*.
Stealth or PEGylated liposomes		*Stealth liposomes* are long circulating liposomes created by incorporating the hydrophilic polyethylene glycol (PEG) chains onto the liposome surface. These flexible chains occupying the space immediately above the surface were shown to prevent the binding of plasma opsonins to the liposomes and thus allow them to avoid the action of the mononuclear phagocytic system (MPS). PEG is a biocompatible, hydrophilic polymer that has no significant immunogenic and antigenic activity. When

Term	Symbol	Definition or Description
		conjugated with therapeutic proteins and peptides, PEG has the capacity to increase drug solubility, stability, and bioavailability with increased half-life and decreased plasma clearance. This conjugation is commonly referred to as PEGylation. PEG can be incorporated onto the liposomal surface through physical adsorption, incorporation of a PEG–lipid conjugate during liposome formation, or after attachment to premade liposomes. The commonly used method is to anchor the polymer in the liposomal membrane via the PEG–DSPE (distearoylphosphatidylethanolamine) conjugate. The PEGylated liposome surface has been shown to produce a strong interbilayer repulsion that counters the attractive van der Waals forces, thus stabilizing the vesicles by preventing them from aggregation.
Stokes' diameter		*Stokes' diameter* is the diameter measured by the sedimentation method (see Andreasen pipette), which assumes that the particles are spherical.
Stokes' law		*Stokes' law* is a mathematical expression of the settling velocities of small particles in a fluid due to gravitation. The frictional force experienced by particles depends, in a complicated way, on the shape of the particle and the viscosity of the liquid. However, if the particle is spherical, a simple formula due to George G. Stokes (1851) applies: Frictional force = $6\pi r\eta\, dx/dt$, where the term $6\pi r\eta$ is known as the frictional coefficient.
Stratum corneum		The *stratum corneum*, or horny layer, refers to the outermost layer of epidermis, consisting mainly of inactive and dead keratinocytes called corneocytes. The stratum corneum is the major barrier of skin that serves to protect the underlying tissues from dehydration, infection, mechanical stress, and chemicals including drug penetration.
Supersaturation		*Supersaturation* refers to a solution that contains more dissolved solute than can be normally dissolved by the solvent under the given conditions of temperature and pressure. Supersaturation is thermodynamically unstable; thus it can increase the chance of precipitation or crystallization.
Surface excess		The tendency of a solute molecule to maintain a greater concentration at the surface than in the bulk solution (see Gibbs' adsorption equation) is called the *surface excess*.
Surface tension	γ	Unlike molecules below the surface that encounter forces from all sides, the surface molecules of a liquid are pulled by forces from molecules beneath the surface and less so by molecules in

Term	Symbol	Definition or Description
		the vapor phase above. As a result, there is a surface area change. The work per surface area (in dynes per centimeter) required to maintain this vapor–liquid interface is called the *surface tension*. The tension measured at the liquid–liquid or liquid–solid interfaces is called the *interfacial tension*. *Surface tension* has a unit of ergs per square centimeter or dynes per centimeter.
Surface-active agent (or surfactant)		According to Gibbs' adsorption theory, any solute that prefers to stay at the surface rather than in the bulk solution is a *surface-active agent*. Chemically, these compounds are amphiphilic, exhibiting both a hydrophobic and a hydrophilic moiety.
Tapped density	ρ_{tapped}	The *tapped density* is the ratio of weight to a tapped volume, which is measured using a tapped density tester by repeatedly tapping until a consistent tapped volume (less than 2% change) is achieved.
Terminal settling velocity		The size of a particle may be measured by the speed with which it moves through a liquid medium under the influence of gravity. A particle of mass m will displace a volume of m/ρ_2, or $\pi d^3/6$, of the medium, which corresponds to a mass of the medium of $(m/\rho_2)\rho_1$. Here, ρ_1 and ρ_2 are the densities of the medium and particle, respectively. The net force due to gravity is then $\pi d^3 g(\rho_2 - \rho_1)/6$. The particle will fall through the medium if $\rho_2 > \rho_1$, but as it accelerates, a viscous drag develops that is proportional to fv, where f is the friction coefficient and v is the velocity. A *terminal settling velocity* is reached when the force due to gravity and that of the viscous drag have become equal, i.e., when $v = \pi d^3 g(\rho_2 - \rho_1)/6f$ For a spherical particle, $f = 6\pi\eta r$ or $3\pi\eta d$, where r is the radius and d is the diameter of the particle. This leads to $v = d^2 g(\rho_2 - \rho_1)/18\eta$ Using the above equation, the diameter of a particle can be determined by measuring its terminal settling velocity.
Thermodynamic solubility		*Thermodynamic solubility* refers to solubility measured using a solid sample rather than a concentrated stock solution.
Thixotropy		*Thixotropy* refers to reversible and time-dependent viscosity change at a constant shear rate. A thixotropic liquid becomes more fluid with increasing time until an equilibrium viscosity is reached.

Term	Symbol	Definition or Description
Transcription factor decoy		*Transcription factor decoy* is a specific DNA sequence that binds competitively to a specific transcription factor and disrupts gene expression that is regulated by the transcription factor.
Transdermal delivery		*Transdermal delivery* is the movement of compounds across the skin into the systemic circulation. In the skin, compounds would pass through the layers of epidermis to reach the microcirculation of the dermis.
Transdermal patches		*Transdermal patches*, also called skin patches, are dosage forms designed to deliver therapeutic agents through the skin. Drugs are formulated in the patches, which are placed on the skin for an extended period.
Transition-state theory		In the *transition-state theory*, the activated complex is treated as a molecule despite its transitory existence. Consider the reaction $A + B \rightleftarrows (AB)^{\ddagger} \rightarrow \text{products}$ The equilibrium of the transition state can be written as $K^{\ddagger} = (AB)^{\ddagger}/[A][B]$ The thermodynamic expression for $K^{\ddagger}$ is $K^{\ddagger} = e^{+(\Delta S)\ddagger/R}\, e^{-(\Delta H)\ddagger/RT}$, and for the rate constant, $k_2 = (kT/h)\, e^{+(\Delta S)\ddagger/R}\, e^{-(\Delta H)\ddagger/RT}$ This equation shows that the exponential temperature dependence involves enthalpy rather than the activation energy, whereas the preexponential factor involves the entropy of activation. The latter represents the tendency through which the reactant molecules rearrange to form the activated complex, which depends largely on the molecular structure of the reactants as well as that of the complex. A positive entropy corresponds to a greater rate constant.
Triggered drug release		Drug release from the nanocarriers is governed by the rate of drug diffusion, the partition coefficient, the stability of the nanocarrier, and the biodegradation of the polymer. In addition, many polymers exhibit unique properties, including pH, temperature, ultrasound, and light sensitivities, which can be utilized to achieve a *triggered drug release* if the property is properly matched with physiological conditions. The most commonly studied phenomena are the pH- and temperature-triggered release mechanisms for tumor cell targeting due to the low-pH and high-temperature environment of the tumor tissue. Triggered drug release at the active site enhances the passive targeting of a nanoparticle system via the EPR effect.

Term	Symbol	Definition or Description
True density	ρ_{true}	*True density* is the ratio of the weight to the absolute volume of a powder material that excludes the volume of pores and interparticle spaces.
Ultrafiltration		*Ultrafiltration* is a rapid and physical method used to separate and determine the bound and free drug fractions in a drug–protein sample. The method uses the hydraulic pressure or centrifugation as the separation technique, based on the principle that protein-bound drug remains protein-bound during the separation procedure. Drug–protein binding can then be analyzed using the Scatchard equation based on the determined data.
Unilamellar and multilamellar vesicles		Liposomes are commonly classified, based on their size and lamellarity, into small *unilamellar vesicles* (SUV, 25–100 nm), *large unilamellar vesicles* (LUV, 100–400 nm), and *multilamellar vesicles* (MLV, 200–5000 nm). The unilamellar vesicles have a single lipid bilayer, suitable for the encapsulation of hydrophilic molecules in the aqueous core. MLVs consist of two or more concentric lipid bilayers that are useful for entrapment of hydrophobic drugs.
Unstirred water layer	UWL	An *unstirred water layer* exists at both sides of a membrane in an in vitro permeability study. On the donor side, the composition, pH, and layer thickness of the UWL are all determining factors on the permeability of water-insoluble drugs. The UWL at the receptor side of the membrane can prevent the drug from reaching the bulk of the receptor solution, thus resulting in high retention of drug in the membrane. In drug absorption in vivo, the absorbed drug will be quickly washed away by the blood.
Upper consolute temperature		For a partially miscible binary liquid system containing A and B in which the solubility of both A in B and B in A increases with increasing temperature, there is a critical temperature above which the two components become completely miscible. This temperature is known as the *critical solution temperature* or *upper consolute temperature.*
Viscoelasticity		*Viscoelasticity* refers to the phenomenon of a material that exhibits viscosity-dependent flow properties as a liquid as well as strain-recoverable elastic properties as a solid.
Viscosity	η	As a transport of momentum by a flowing liquid, *viscosity* is a measure of the friction that is present when adjacent layers of the fluid are moving at different speeds. The reciprocal of viscosity is called the *fluidity*. The quantity of viscosity, which is the ratio of the shearing stress to the velocity gradient (where the velocity of the fluid is a function of the distance away from the stress), is termed a coefficient rather than a constant, because it indeed changes with shear stress and time depending on the flowing material. This is the fundamental premise of rheology.

Term	Symbol	Definition or Description
Warfarin–azapropazone and tryptophan–benzodiazepine binding sites		Human serum albumin exhibits a single polypeptide chain of about 585 amino acids without prosthetic carbohydrate groups and a molecular weight of 67 kDa. The secondary structure of albumin is highly helical (α-helix content: 67%). The tertiary structure assumes a triangular shape, about 80 Å across the base and 30 Å in average thickness (molecular volume: about 88,000 $Å^3$). The globular protein shows three domains (I, II, and III); each is divided into subdomains A and B, with 6 and 4 α-helices, respectively. Two primary binding sites for anionic, hydrophobic drugs have been located in domains IIA and IIIA, which contain pockets formed by hydrophobic and positively charged residues. These two high-affinity binding sites have been named as (1) the *warfarin–azapropazone binding site* (site I), which is the highest-affinity binding site for warfarin and nonsteroidal anti-inflammatory drugs such as phenylbutazone, and (2) the *tryptophan–benzodiazepine binding site* (site II), where a number of profens (ibuprofen, fenoprofen, and ketoprofen) are known to interact. The warfarin binding site has been well characterized to contain Phe (211), Try (214), Leu (219), Leu (238), Arg (218), and His (242) residues that form a hydrophobic pocket and Arg (222), His (242), and a water molecule for electrostatic interactions. These preformed high-affinity sites account for the binding of most drugs at therapeutic concentrations.
Werner's theory		*Werner's theory* on metal complexation states that metal ions exhibit primary (ionizable) and secondary (non-ionizable) valences, where the latter indicate the coordination number. The secondary valences allow the metal ion to interact with anions or neutral molecules known as ligands, arranged spatially around the metal ion in a linear or bent chain, tetrahedral or square planar, or octahedral configuration that corresponds to the coordination number of 2, 4, or 6, respectively.
Wet granulation		Agglomeration in the presence of a liquid and a binder is termed *wet granulation*. A binder can be added in a dry powder form or as an aqueous solution. After the initial blending step, binder solution is added with agitation, followed by continued agitation or wet massing, wet sizing, and drying. After drying, a sizing step is often necessary to reduce the granule size before blending with a lubricant for compression or encapsulation. The agglomeration occurs in the presence of agitation, where liquid-coated particles aggregate by forming liquid bridges, which upon drying become solid bridges between binder particles.

Term	Symbol	Definition or Description
Wetting		*Wetting* is the process of adsorption of pure liquid by solid particles, resulting in the formation of a liquid film over the particle surface.
Yield stress		*Yield stress* is the minimum stress that must be applied to a solid or paste to initialize a significant flow and hence a significant drop in viscosity in the shear-thinning behavior.
Young's modulus	Y	The strain of a stretched filament having a cross-sectional area of A is the ratio of the stretched length to its original length. This is known as *Young's modulus*. If the length under tension is l_s and the length after the removal of stress is the original length l_o, then $Y = (f/A) / [(l_s - l_o)/l_o] = fl_o / A(l_s - l_o)$, where $(l_s - l_o)/l_o$ is the strain and f/A is the stress.
Zero-shear viscosity	η_o	*Zero-shear viscosity* is the limiting viscosity of low shear rate, which is the ultimate viscosity of a product at rest or undisturbed.
Zeta potential	ζ	The electric potential at the plane of shear within the electrical double layer of a charged surface in reference to a point in the bulk solution is the *zeta potential*. In practical terms, it is the potential difference between the dispersion medium and the layer of solution tightly bound to the dispersed particles.

INDEX

Note: Italicized page locators indicate figures; tables are noted with *t*.

E

F

H

I

X

Y

Z